INTRODUCTION TO HEALTH SERVICES

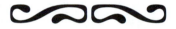

For N. Williams, the memory of D. Williams,
and J., C., J.C., and N. Torrens

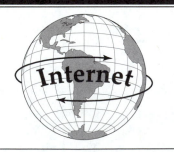

INTRODUCTION TO HEALTH SERVICES

FIFTH EDITION

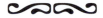

Edited by

Stephen J. Williams, Sc.D.
Professor of Public Health
Head, Division of Health Services Administration
Graduate School of Public Health
San Diego State University
San Diego, California

Paul R. Torrens, M.D., M.P.H.
Professor of Health Services
School of Public Health
University of California, Los Angeles
Los Angeles, California

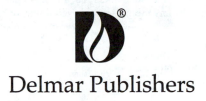

Delmar Publishers

an International Thomson Publishing company I(T)P®

Albany • Bonn • Boston • Cincinnati • Detroit • London • Madrid
Melbourne • Mexico City • New York • Pacific Grove • Paris • San Francisco
Singapore • Tokyo • Toronto • Washington

NOTICE TO THE READER

Delmar Staff

Publisher: William Brottmiller

Assistant Editor: Hilary A. Schrauf

COPYRIGHT © 1999

By Delmar Publishers

an International Thomson Publishing Company

The ITP logo is a trademark under license.

Printed in the United States of America

For more information, contact:

Delmar Publishers
3 Columbia Circle, Box 15015
Albany, New York 12212-5015

International Thomson Publishing—
  Europe
Berkshire House
168-173 High Holborn
London, WC1V 7AA
England

Thomas Nelson Australia
102 Dodds Street
South Melbourne 3205
Victoria, Australia

Nelson Canada
1120 Birchmount Road
Scarborough, Ontario
Canada, M1K 5G4

International Thomson Editores
Campos Eliseos 385, Piso 7
Col Polanco
11560 Mexico D F Mexico

International Thomson Publishing
  GmbH
Konigswinterer Strasse 418
53227 Bonn
Germany

International Thomson Publishing—
  Asia
60 Albert Street
#15-01 Albert Complex
Singapore 189969

International Thomson Publishing—
  Japan
Hirakawacho Kyowa Building, 3F
2-2-1 Hirakawacho
Chiyoda-ku, Tokyo 102
Japan

2 3 4 5 6 7 8 9 10 XXX 03 02 01 00 99 98

Library of Congress Cataloging-in-Publication Data

Introduction to health services/edited by Stephen J. Williams, Paul
  R. Torrens.—4th ed.
    p. cm.
    Includes Index.
    ISBN 0-8273-7852-1 (textbook)
    1. Medical care—United States.   2. Health services
administration—United States.   I. Williams, Stephen J. (Stephen
Joseph), 1948–   II. Torrens, Paul R. (Paul Roger), 1934–
    [DNLM: 1: Health Services—United States. W 84 AA1 I9]
RA395.A31495 1993
362.1'0973—dc20
DNLM/DLC
for Libarary of Congress   92–18592
                                        CIP

INTRODUCTION TO THE SERIES

This series in Health Services is now in its second decade of providing top quality teaching materials to the health administration/public health field. Each year has witnessed further strengthening of the market position of each of the principal books in the series, also reflecting the continued excellence of the products. Each author, book editor, and contributor to the series has helped build what is widely recognized as the top textbook and issues collection of books available in this field today.

But we have achieved only a beginning. Everyone involved in the series is committed to further expansion of the scope, technical excellence, and usefulness of the series. Our goal is to do more for you, the reader. We will add new books in important areas, seek out more excellent authors, and increase the physical attributes of the books to make them easier for you to use.

We thank everyone, the authors and users in particular, who have made this series so successful and so widely used. And we promise that this second decade will be dedicated to further expansion of the series, and to enhancement of the books it contains to provide still greater value to you, our constituency.

Stephen J. Williams
Series Editor

DELMAR SERIES IN HEALTH SERVICES ADMINISTRATION

Stephen J. Williams, Sc.D., Series Editor

Ambulatory Care Management, third edition
   Austin Ross, Stephen J. Williams, and Ernest J. Pavlock, Editors

The Continuum of Long-Term Care
   Connie J. Evashwick, Editor

Health Care Economics, fourth edition
   Paul J. Feldstein

Health Care Management: Organization Design and Behavior, third edition
   Stephen M. Shortell and Arnold D. Kaluzny, Editors

Health Politics and Policy, third edition
   Theodor J. Litman and Leonard S. Robins, Editors

Motivating Health Behavior
   John P. Elder, E. Scott Geller, Melbourne F. Hovell, and Joni A. Mayer, Editors

Really Governing: How Health System and Hospital Boards Can Make More of a Difference
   Dennis D. Pointer and Charles M. Ewell

Strategic Management of Human Resources in Health Services Organizations, second edition
   Myron D. Fottler, S. Robert Hernandez, and Charles L. Joiner, Editors

Financial Management in Health Care Organizations
   Robert A. McLean

Principles of Public Health Practice
   F. Douglas Scutchfield and C. William Keck, Editors

The Hospital Medical Staff
   Charles H. White

Essentials of Health Services
   Stephen J. Williams

Essentials of Health Care Management
   Stephen M. Shortell and Arnold D. Kaluzny, Editors

Essentials of Human Resources Management in Health Services Organizations
   Myron D. Fottler, S. Robert Hernandez, and Charles L. Joiner, Editors

Health Services Research Methods
   Leiyu Shi

Supplemental Reader:

Contemporary Issues in Health Services
   Stephen J. Williams, Editor

CONTENTS

FOREWORD

When the first edition of this book appeared in 1980, physicians had almost unfettered freedom to order whatever care they wanted for their patients, academic health centers were churning out specialists and living well off of post–World War II public largesse, and terms like *managed care* and *managed competition* were not essential to the vocabulary of a student well schooled in health services. As this fifth edition attests, such is no longer the case.

Some might say that those were the "good old days," but in fact the prevailing defects of that system propelled us to where we are today. The incentives for physicians in a fee-for-service system were to do more, rather than less, and in a system being fed by a constant stream of new costly technology, health care costs were out of control.

The runaway costs finally catalyzed action by both business and government. Employers, facing ballooning employee health expenses, were unwilling to continue to do business as usual and began using their considerable force in the marketplace. The Clinton administration attempted comprehensive national health care reform in 1994 but failed. By embracing "managed competition," however, the Democrats endorsed market principles, implicitly approving a shake-up of the organization of medical care. The lesson of that failure at reform is that the United States has opted for the market, not government, as a way to address escalating medical costs.

Indeed, the story of medical care since the failure of the Clinton plan could be titled the triumph of the market. Enrollment in managed care is surging; for-profit hospitals and health plans are expanding at a much greater rate than their not-for-profit competitors; and federal, state, and local politicians of both parties promote managed care as the best way to control Medicare and Medicaid costs.

A managed care system has a number of potential advantages. Compared with fee-for-service, capitation theoretically could produce a more rational system, permitting greater flexibility in the range of services provided to sick patients, integrating services for people with chronic illness, and emphasizing prevention. It also curbs the fee-for-service incentives to overuse costly services. Market-based managed care might also succeed at making some needed changes that government is hard pressed to accomplish. For example, in a nation encumbered with excess medical care capacity, the market can force closures, consolidations, and income reductions that would be difficult to get by legislators protecting their hometown interests. A competitive marketplace can also force providers to pay close attention to customer satisfaction.

Pitfalls and perils also loom, however, as managed care becomes our de facto national health policy. The market's relentless pursuit of efficiency leaves consumers concerned that their medical needs will take a backseat to the bottom line. Physicians are experiencing a loss of autonomy as medical decisions increasingly are made by corporate officials with economic priorities. Although there is no question that the health care system could benefit from some greater discipline, it is also important to remember that the practice of medicine is not just another business. Caregivers cannot swap gains in efficiency for losses in compassion.

This new system also has to wrestle with an old and persistent problem—the millions of Americans without health insurance. The number continues to grow. Traditional safety net institutions (such as public hospitals and tax-supported clinics), together with mainstream providers, have thus far subsidized indigent care with fees from paying patients. The system is suboptimal—by many measures, the uninsured fare worse than those with private insurance—but even this level of care could be threatened because providers that increase charges to paying patients risk losing the edge in a competitive marketplace. As a result, access to care for the uninsured is a constantly worsening problem, and one that must be monitored for what may be subtle but important changes over time.

This textbook provides the student of the health care system with the tools to understand and analyze these various changes in the health care system. For years, it has introduced the reader to the basic structure and concepts of United States health care that are a prerequisite to studying or managing aspects of the system. This new revised edition continues to help the reader adjust the focus to take in the new pieces of the health care picture as it adapts to the triumph of the market.

Steven A. Schroeder, M.D.
President
The Robert Wood Johnson Foundation
Princeton, New Jersey

PREFACE

Dramatic changes have occurred in our nation's health care industry in the few years since the last edition of this book was published, changes largely driven by market forces. In the past, public policy initiatives and governmental activity have been the motivating forces for change, primarily centered around Medicare and Medicaid. In recent years, pressure for change has come from the private sector, primarily from employers and other large purchasers of health insurance, as well as from the health insurance industry itself as it has adjusted to changing market conditions. After years of describing the American health care system as being policy driven, it would now have to be said that the system has rapidly become market driven.

These dramatic changes in the dynamics of health care in the United States are reflected in this latest edition of *Introduction to Health Services.* Entirely new chapters from new authors have been written, and all other chapters have been rewritten to reflect very recent changes. Changes in financing patterns and programs have been given added emphasis, and changes in the health care delivery system as a result of managed care pressures have been noted. All in all, this edition reflects an American health care system that is undergoing major change—change that will continue for some time to come.

Part I (Chapter 1) of this book provides an overview of health care in America with a historical focus that sets the stage for all the chapters that follow. This chapter provides a framework for analyzing and dissecting health care in the United States. This chapter also serves to place today's changing system into the context of our nation's long and complex experience in health care. Today's developments do not stand alone; they are merely the latest chapter in a long series of developmental stages.

Part II examines the causes and characteristics of health care utilization in the United States. The first chapter in this section, Chapter 2, presents a medical perspective on the nature of disease occurrence and explores the ways in which illness and disease are defined. Chapter 3, new to this edition, presents a detailed discussion of disease patterns in the United States; this chapter is key to understanding the changing nature of challenges faced by the health care industry in this country. Chapter 4, also new to this edition, presents an overview of the factors associated with the need and demand for health care and also examines the actual utilization of services.

Part III focuses on the financing of health care in the United States and the impact that financial changes are having on the organizational structure of the system. The first chapter in this section, Chapter 5, reviews the sources and uses of financial resources for health care in the United States. Chapter 6 focuses on the increasingly important and rapidly dominant role of managed care in the health care in the United States; although many other chapters include commentaries on managed care, this chapter presents a philosophical and logical overview of the role, structure, and mechanisms inherent in managed care, as well as ethical concerns. Chapter 7 describes the evolution and current status of the private health insurance industry in the United States and addresses the intersection of private health insurance with other key financing and organization trends, such as managed care.

Part IV looks at provider organizations and settings in health care. The first chapter in this section, Chapter 8, addresses the fundamental role of health promotion and disease prevention activities in the health of the public, and stresses the greater public/private partnership for public health that is emerging in the United States. Chapter 9 examines the increasingly central role of ambulatory care services in the provision, coordination, and control of health care; the expansion of group practice and other key ambulatory care providers is also addressed. Chapter 10 looks at the radically changing role of the hospital and the evolution of the hospital from a provider of inpatient services to a coordinator of integrated delivery systems that provide a wide range of services to the public. Chapters 11 and 12 focus on the provision of long-term care and on mental health services, respectively, both key areas in health care that are poised for increasingly rapid change.

Part V addresses the key nonfinancial resources used in the production of health services in the United States. An entirely new chapter, Chapter 13, assesses the pharmaceutical industry and its important role in the future success of health care in diagnosing and curing disease. Chapter 14 looks at human resources in health care, the professional and nonprofessional workers who are necessary to make the health care system function; health care employs millions of people in diverse and often complex roles, so it is vital to have a good understanding of this important resource.

Part VI asks how our health care system can be evaluated, regulated, monitored, and assessed. Chapter 15 examines the role of government in the health care industry and reviews how public policy in health care comes about. Chapter 16, another entirely new chapter, looks at the measurement and evaluation of health care, a key function in determining what our country receives for its immense investment; this chapter also addresses measurement techniques that are gaining prominence among managed care organizations and purchasers of health care. Finally, Chapter 17, another entirely new chapter, looks at ethical issues associated with our nation's health care system in all its various component parts. Ethical issues have always been important issues in health care, but they are becoming even more important as managed care raises new pressures and dilemmas.

Over the last ten years, this country's health care system has increasingly adopted a corporate focus and philosophy, even in the traditional not-for-profit sectors. This market-driven focus has forced our health care system to review its traditional forms of operation and to reduce long-standing redundancies and inefficiencies. At the same time, placing the emphasis on organizational efficiency creates the hazard of forgetting that health care deals with fundamental issues of life and death, not the usual subjects of managerial concern. The new focus has brought needed improvements but has also served to sometimes cloud the reason why the health care system was created in the first place—the protection of a person's ability to live a full and satisfying life.

As a nation, we have much more invested in health care than simply a financial commitment to achieve a profit. This is a complex sector of our economy and it should contribute to our physical and mental well-being first, with its economic contributions coming only after serving the primary purpose of health care. This book tries to take a balanced approach to these issues by addressing both the social and the economic concerns involved in health care in all its aspects. Without a careful balance between the social and economic aspects of health care, a complete understanding of health care cannot be achieved. Our goal, however, should be clearly defined: measurable improvement in the health of our people at a cost that is in keeping with both our social goals and our economic realities.

As in previous editions of this book, a multidisciplinary and empirical approach is used throughout. The emphasis is on practical application of an increasingly sophisticated body of knowledge and research. The challenge is greater for all of us each year, and the complexities continue to compound and confound. We owe a debt of gratitude to the many students and practitioners who provide us with guidance as this book evolves. We are profoundly grateful to our contributors, our editors, our colleagues, and to all others involved in the production of this book. It is our hope that the book itself will continue to contribute to a better health care system for all Americans.

Stephen J. Williams
Paul R. Torrens

CONTRIBUTORS

Ronald M. Andersen, Ph.D.
Wasserman Professor in Health Services
Department of Health Services
School of Public Health
University of California, Los Angeles
Los Angeles, California

A. E. Benjamin, Ph.D.
Professor
Department of Social Welfare
School of Public Policy and Social Research
University of California, Los Angeles
Los Angeles, California

Lester Breslow, M.D., M.P.H.
Professor and Dean Emeritus
School of Public Health
University of California, Los Angeles
Los Angeles, California

William S. Comanor, Ph.D.
Professor of Economics
University of California, Santa Barbara, and
Professor and Director, Research Program on
    Pharmaceutical Economics and Policy
Department of Health Services
School of Public Health
University of California, Los Angeles
Los Angeles, California

Pamela L. Davidson, Ph.D.
Assistant Professor and Chair
Graduate Program in Health Administration
College of Lifelong Learning
Chapman University
Orange, California

William L. Dowling, Ph.D.
Professor of Health Services
Chairman, Department of Health Services
School of Public Health and Community
    Medicine
University of Washington
Seattle, Washington

Connie J. Evashwick, Sc.D., F.A.C.H.E.
Endowed Chair and Professor
Center for Health Care Innovation
California State University, Long Beach
Long Beach, California

Alma L. Koch, Ph.D.
Professor of Public Health
Graduate Program in Health Services
    Administration
Graduate School of Public Health
San Diego State University
San Diego, California

Philip R. Lee, M.D.
Professor Emeritus
Department of Medicine
    and Senior Advisor to the Dean
School of Medicine
University of California, San Francisco
San Francisco, California

Lawrence A. May, M.D., F.A.C.P.
Associate Professor of Medicine
University of California, Los Angeles
Los Angeles, California

Stephen S. Mick, Ph.D.
Professor of Health Policy and Management
Department of Health Management and Policy
School of Public Health
The University of Michigan
Ann Arbor, Michigan

Mary Richardson, Ph.D.
Professor and Director, Graduate Program in
    Health Services Administration
Department of Health Services
School of Public Health and Community
    Medicine
University of Washington
Seattle, Washington

Ruth Roemer, J.D.
Adjunct Professor Emerita
School of Public Health
University of California, Los Angeles
Los Angeles, California

Stuart O. Schweitzer, Ph.D.
Professor of Health Services
School of Public Health
University of California, Los Angeles
Los Angeles, California

Sharyne Shiu-Thornton, M.A.
Lecturer
Department of Health Services
School of Public Health and
    Community Medicine
University of Washington
Seattle, Washington

Paul R. Torrens, M.D., M.P.H.
Professor of Health Services
School of Public Health
University of California, Los Angeles
Los Angeles, California

Pauline Vaillancourt Rosenau, Ph.D.
Associate Professor, Management & Policy
    Sciences, Health Policy Institute
UT-Houston School of Public Health
The University of Texas
Houston Health Science Center
Houston, Texas

Scott Weingarten, M.D., M.P.H.
Director, Health Services Research
Cedars-Sinai Medical Center
Associate Professor of Medicine
University of California, Los Angeles
School of Medicine
Los Angeles, California

Gary Whitted, Ph.D., M.S.
Vice President
United HealthCare
Portland, Oregon

Stephen J. Williams, Sc.D.
Professor of Public Health
Head, Division of Health Services Administration
Graduate School of Public Health
San Diego State University
San Diego, California

PART I

OVERVIEW OF THE HEALTH SERVICES SYSTEM

CHAPTER

Historical Evolution and Overview of Health Services in the United States

Paul R. Torrens

CHAPTER TOPICS

LEARNING OBJECTIVES

Upon completing this chapter, the reader should be able to:

- Understand the major stages in the development of the nation's health care system.
- Appreciate the many forces affecting the development of health services in the United States.
- Realize the key role of technology in shaping health care.
- Understand the social, political, and economic forces affecting health care.
- Follow the development of government's involvement in health services.
- Understand the primary organized delivery systems for health care in the United States.
- Appreciate the principles involved in organizing health services systems.
- Be ready to pursue the detailed content of the remaining chapters of this book.

This chapter provides two fundamental frameworks that are essential for understanding the American health care system. The first framework reviews the historical evolution and development of health care in the United States; this section includes commentary on the most recent changes in the underlying framework for health care in the United States. The second framework presented in this chapter looks at the organization of health care in the United States *as a system;* this second framework attempts to provide a means for understanding how all of the various individual parts of health care fit together. Following the presentation of these two frameworks, the chapter concludes by asking important questions about what might be the best future organization for health care in the United States.

HISTORICAL EVOLUTION OF HEALTH SERVICES IN THE UNITED STATES

The modern American health care system has gone through three important phases in its development and has now entered a fourth (Table 1–1). The first phase began in the mid-nineteenth century *(circa* 1850) when the first large hospitals, such as Bellevue Hospital in New York City and Massachusetts General Hospital in Boston, were established. The development of hospitals symbolized the *institutionalization of health care* for the first time in this country. Before this time, health care in the United States was a loose collection of individual services functioning independently and without much relationship to each other or to anything else. With the development of the first hospitals, health care personnel and technology began to cluster together around the most seriously ill patients, providing for the first time a centralizing, coordinating focus for what had been a dispersed and somewhat random collection of services. The arrival of the first hospitals in the United States brought a sense of order and concentration to health care in this country that had been lacking previously.

The second important phase of development began around the turn of the century *(circa* 1900) with the *introduction of the scientific method into medicine* in this country. Before this time, medicine was not an exact science but was instead a rather informal collection of unproven generalities and good intentions. After 1900, stimulated by the opening of the new medical school at the Johns Hopkins University in Baltimore, medicine acquired a solid scientific base that eventually transformed it from a conscientious but poorly equipped art into a detailed and clearly defined science.

TABLE 1–1   Major trends in the development of health care in the United States, 1850 to present

Trends	1850–1900	1900 to World War II	World War II to Present	Future
Predominant health problems of the American people	Epidemics of acute infections	Acute events, trauma, or infections affecting individuals, not groups	Chronic diseases such as heart disease, cancer, stroke	Chronic diseases, particularly emotional and behaviorally related conditions
Technology available to handle predominant health problems	Virtually none	Beginning and rapid growth of basic medical sciences and technology	Explosive growth of medical science; technology captures the health care system	Continued growth and expansion of technology, with attempts to re-personalize the technology
Social organization for the use of technology	None; individuals left to their own resources or charity	Beginning societal and governmental efforts to care for those who could not care for themselves	Health care as a right; governmental responsibility to organize and monitor health care for everyone	Greater centralization of responsibility and control using information systems; greater use of organized systems of health insurance and financing to shape and control developments within the health care system

With the coming of World War II, the United States underwent a major social, political, and technological upheaval the effect of which was so marked that it ended the second phase of development of health care in this country and signaled the beginning of the third phase, the phase of *growing interest in the social and organizational structure of health care.* During this time, major attention was directed, for the first time, toward the financing of health care with the resulting growth of health insurance plans, such as Blue Cross and Blue Shield, in the nonprofit sector and numerous commercial insurance companies in the for-profit sector. This was also the time of rapidly increasing power in the federal government with regard to health care in the United States, as witnessed by the Hill-Burton Act (Hospital Survey and Construction Act), by the growth of huge research budgets of the National Institutes of Health (NIH), and, in 1965, by the passage and implementation of Medicare and Medicaid. Finally, during this time, largely as a result of the federal "War on Poverty," the principle of health care as a right, not a privilege, was widely discussed and rather widely accepted.

The Fourth Phase

Since the early 1980s, the health care system in this country has moved into a fourth phase of its development, an era of *limited resources, restriction of growth, and reorganization of the methods of financing and delivering care;* it has also been the era of the growth of the *influence of economic market forces* in the shaping of health care in America. Before this phase, it had been presumed that the health care system would always be encouraged to grow and expand, both in size and complexity, and that there would always be sufficient resources to support that expansion. Beginning in the 1980s, it seemed that the limits of our resources were being approached and that the health care system was being forced to consider options or alternatives to unrestricted growth and expansion.

Indeed, reimbursement policies introduced by Medicare and by health insurance plans in general have caused a decrease in the number of inpatient days provided by hospitals each year and an actual reduction in the operating size of most hospitals; the emphasis has been on doing less for patients rather than more. In this vein, expert observers have suggested that the United States is rapidly approaching a major surplus of physicians and has advised that the number of new physicians being produced each year be greatly reduced, at least with regard to specialist physicians and certainly with regard to specialist physicians who are involved in surgical work. On all sides, there are pressures for smaller size, use of fewer services, and reductions in expenditures for health care.

At the same time, the 1990s have witnessed the appearance of many new organizational pressures and models in health care, mostly as a result of forces generated by economic marketplace developments. Indeed, the use of the term *economic markets* with regard to health care would not have been widely accepted prior to the 1990s and certainly not at all prior to the 1980s.

These new economic marketplace forces have spawned the growth of a wide variety of new organizational forms, both for-profit and nonprofit, that was previously unknown. The HMO that existed in relatively few sites in relatively small numbers throughout the country before the 1980s has given way to the broader "managed care plans" that are now present virtually throughout the country in great numbers and involve the majority of the population. (Indeed, "managed care" has become so important that a separate chapter of this book is devoted to that single subject.)

A variety of new enterprises have appeared to provide special services to patients and families at home, not only as a way of providing better services and answering to economic market forces for new products, but also as a way of reducing more expensive alternative services. New intermediary organizations have appeared to provide reviews of quality of patient care and appropriate utilization of services. The term *joint venture* has become an accepted part of our health care language, now used to describe new forms of partnership activities between previously separate components of the health care system: hospitals and physicians; insurance companies and pharmaceutical corporations; hospitals with other hospitals; groups of physicians with other groups of physicians. Virtually no health care organizational model has been untouched by recent trends and changes in this latest phase of historical development in health care in the United States.

In order to fully understand the implications of this historical evolution of health care in the United States, this chapter will look at three separate topics across the time periods of the four phases of development. These topics are (1) the predominant health problems that were the focus of activity of the American health care system, (2) the technology available to the American health care system in each of the time periods, and

(3) the social organization of health care during these time periods.

PREDOMINANT HEALTH PROBLEMS OF THE AMERICAN POPULATION

Since the dawn of recorded history, human beings have repeatedly suffered the sudden and devastating appearance of epidemics of infectious disease. Plague, cholera, typhoid, smallpox, influenza, yellow fever, and a host of other diseases raged almost at will throughout history, creating havoc wherever they struck.

During the period 1850–1900 in this country, these epidemics of acute infectious diseases were the health problem that drew the greatest attention from the then rather rudimentary health care system in the United States. Of particular importance were those diseases related to impure food, contaminated water supply, inadequate sewer disposal, and the generally poor condition of urban housing. During this time, for example, a cholera epidemic occurred throughout the country, resulting in an official death toll of 5,071 in New York City alone and an unofficial toll several times higher. During this same period, yellow fever killed 9,000 in New Orleans in 1853, 2,500 in 1854 and 1855, and another 5,000 in 1858. Abraham Lincoln regularly sent his family away from the White House during the summer months in Washington, D.C., to escape the "fevers," probably malaria, that swept through the city during those months. It can generally be said that the period 1850–1900 was a time in which the American health care system focused on epidemics of acute infectious diseases that were closely related to poor conditions of food, water, and housing.

By 1900, the epidemics of acute infectious disease had generally been brought under control due to improved environmental conditions. In the lat-

ter years of the nineteenth century, cities had begun to develop systems for water purification, for sanitary disposal of sewage, for safeguarding the quality of milk and food, and for monitoring the quality of urban housing. Health departments had begun to grow in number and in strength and had begun to apply the methods of case finding and quarantine with satisfying results. Indeed, by 1990, as Table 1–2 shows, those epidemics that had plagued humanity for centuries were eliminated as major causes of death in the United States.

After 1900, the predominant health problems that attracted the attention of the health care system were those acute events, either infectious or traumatic, that affected individuals one by one. The pendulum had swung away from epidemics of acute infection that affected large numbers of people in epidemics and toward conditions of a personal nature that required individualized treatment.

Relieved from the burden of epidemic illnesses, the newly developed medical sciences turned their attention to better surgical techniques, the discovery of new sera for the treatment of pneumonia, and the development of new tests for more accurate and rapid diagnoses. Hospitals began to grow rapidly, medical schools flourished, and there was a general air of excitement that suggested that the world was on the brink of significant advances in the treatment of individual illnesses.

Significant advances *were* being made. In Baltimore and Boston, the students of William Halsted, the pioneer surgeon at Johns Hopkins Hospital, began to operate on patients whose disease had previously been beyond the ability of surgeons. Advances in obstetrics now made it safer for women to have babies, and for the first time, women did not approach childbirth with a fear of dying in delivery. Research work by two physicians, Banting and Best, in the laboratories of the University of Toronto led to the discovery of insulin in 1922, and for the first time, diabetes could be

TABLE 1–2 Death rates for leading causes of death in the United States, 1900 and 1990

1900		1990	
Causes of Death	*Crude Death Rate per 100,000 Population per Year*	*Causes of Death*	*Crude Death Rate per 100,000 Population per Year*
All causes	1,719.0	All causes	848.4
Pneumonia and influenza	202.2	Diseases of the heart	288.1
Tuberculosis	194.4	Malignant neoplasms	196.4
Diarrhea, enteritis, and		Cerebrovascular accidents	55.2
ulceration of the intestine	142.7	Accidents	36.3
Diseases of the heart	137.4	Chronic obstructive pulmonary	
Senility, ill-defined or unknown	117.5	diseases	35.8
Intracranial lesions of		Pneumonia and influenza	29.8
vascular origin	109.6	Diabetes mellitus	18.9
Nephritis	88.6	Suicide	14.3
All accidents	72.3	Chronic liver disease and	
Cancer and other malignant		cirrhosis	11.4
tumors	64.0	Homicide	9.8
Diphtheria	40.3		

SOURCES: *Vital Statistics of the United States,* 1972, Washington, DC: U.S. National Center for Health Statistics; *Monthly Vital Statistics Report,* (Vol. 39, No. 6), September 27, 1990, Washington, DC: U.S. National Center for Health Statistics.

effectively treated. Other research by Whipple, Minot, and Murphy on the causes of pernicious anemia led to successful medical treatments for that condition and further spurred the rush to find new treatments for other age-old conditions.

There were new discoveries on all fronts, each of which contributed some new advances in medical treatment. In 1928, however, in a cluttered laboratory at St. Mary's Hospital in London, a Scottish researcher, Alexander Fleming, produced the first of several discoveries that were to lead to the treatment of patients with penicillin for the first time in 1941. This discovery absolutely revolutionized medical care and totally changed the patterns of disease that threatened humanity. Within a few years after the treatment of the first patients with penicillin, antibiotics became readily available, and

acute infections that had previously caused various illnesses and possible death now meant nothing more than the discomfort of an injection and a few days of disability. Many older people experienced the incredible effects of the antibiotic era; many of them had contracted pneumonia as children, and their families had admitted them to hospitals and despaired for their lives. Indeed, many of them had died. Now, as older adults, they were told they had a "little pneumonia," given an injection of penicillin, and treated at home.

With the arrival of the antibiotic era in the 1940s and the subsequent conquest of acute infectious disease, the predominant problem for the American health care system became chronic illness. Since acute infections were no longer snuffing out the lives of children, people were living longer and beginning to manifest long-term chronic diseases such as heart disease, cancer, and stroke. As shown in Table 1–2, these three conditions alone now account for two-thirds of all deaths. A similar review of the causes of disability would show arthritis, blindness, arteriosclerosis, and other chronic diseases to be the predominant causes of morbidity and limitation of function.

The American health care system in the 1980s entered a new phase of organization that was accompanied by a sense of new predominant disease concerns. The rather sudden appearance of acquired immune deficiency syndrome (AIDS) in almost epidemic proportions in the early 1980s serves well to highlight the changing patterns of disease in this latest phase of historical development of the American health care system. AIDS is apparently initiated by a viral infection that triggers extensive damage to an individual's immune system, leading to susceptibility to other infections and to various forms of cancer. This combination of viral disease, immune system defects, and cancer as manifest in AIDS is probably only the first of many such new combinations of disease causation we must face.

The Rising Importance of Chronic Illness

Chronic illness will certainly continue to be the predominant health problem of the American people in the future, but increasingly important will be chronic illness related to genetic makeup, personal lifestyles, and environmental hazards. Evidence is accumulating that would suggest that many of the important chronic illnesses now are related to how we live our personal lives, what environmental hazards we subject ourselves to, and what genes we may have received from generations that preceded us. As we move into the twenty-first century, it is clear that chronic illnesses, particularly those related to genetic, environmental, and lifestyle causes, will be increasingly important.

Perhaps equally important, there are several kinds of chronic illnesses that have historically received very little attention and, in many instances, were not even considered "illnesses." The chronic mental illnesses, for example, are now only beginning to receive the attention that they deserve. These illnesses pose an enormous challenge for the health care system of the future. The rapid aging of the American population makes it a certainty that a majority of our population will live for at least eighty years of life, increasing the probability that they will need long-term care services to help them handle the multiple physical and mental challenges of becoming very old. These types of needs must now receive much more attention from the organized health care system.

Chronic illnesses have important characteristics that are different from acute illnesses and that will force a change in the way in which the American health care system deals with them. Chronic illnesses often begin early in life, long before overt symptoms appear and before medical attention is directed toward them. As a result, chronic illnesses have an opportunity to begin and to become firmly implanted before their actual symptoms call attention to their presence. For example, many studies of apparently healthy young people who were victims of automobile accidents or other sudden death have shown that large percentages have already begun to develop early signs of chronic illness detectable by pathological examination, but not yet by clinical tests. If the health care system is to be effective in preventing chronic illness, better methods for early detection need to be developed so that prevention and early treatment can be initiated sooner.

The second major difference between chronic illness and acute illness is that once a chronic illness is present, it usually remains with the patient forever. Chronic illness is not cured by medical treatment, but rather its more prominent symptoms or external manifestations are treated. This means that an acute illness approach with its focus on "cure" over a period of short, intensive treatment no longer provides an appropriate paradigm for the treatment of chronic illness with its long-term and continuing presence. The acute illness treatment model is simply not suitable for much of current chronic illness.

The Importance of Prevention

In the same fashion, our thinking with regard to prevention requires significant change to deal with chronic illnesses. Acute illnesses very conveniently have a clear-cut beginning, middle, and end; as a result, they are often amenable to one-shot solutions. If there is an epidemic caused by the contamination of the water supply, the construction of a sewage treatment facility will eliminate it completely. If there is a threat of polio infection, the use of polio vaccine once or twice will permanently protect a population.

With chronic illnesses, however, prevention cannot be a one-shot affair, even though this is still how our health care system has approached them. Arteriosclerotic heart disease, for example, begins early in life and is probably affected by diet, cigarette smoking, stress, obesity, and several other factors that are directly related to personal habits and lifestyle. Prevention of these conditions cannot be accomplished by giving a person a single lecture on the evils of high cholesterol food or the dangers of heavy cigarette consumption. Rather, prevention must be long-term, continuous, and aimed at bringing about major changes in an individual's knowledge of disease, personal values, and behavioral patterns.

Optimal prevention and treatment for long-term, continuous illness will require a system of health care that is in itself long-term and continu-

ous. Unfortunately, the organization of our health services is still modeled on the disease patterns that were predominant in the 1900–1945 period and concentrates on individual episodes of illness as if they were separate and distinct entities. As a result, the focus of the American health care system is primarily short-term and discontinuous in nature, and it treats chronic illness as if it were merely a series of separate and acute episodes. This trend is further reinforced by the current method of financing health care services, with its great emphasis on paying for and providing individual episodes of care, rendered as individual services, rather than on a long-term, continuous series of services coordinated around the needs of a long-term continuous illness.

It should be noted that the growth of "managed care" with its emphasis on payment for services on a *per capita* basis rather than for individual services may make it easier to develop programs of care that are longer term and continuous. Unfortunately, many of the new "managed care" insurance plans and their providers still have a short-term view of their beneficiaries who typically tend to change health plans frequently, thereby destroying any sense of long-term relationship. The increased emphasis on the use of "managed care" plans for the elderly under Medicare may provide a stronger long-term focus within managed care and may allow managed care plans to develop strategies that are more appropriate for the chronic illness model.

A Challenging Future

It is entirely possible (and, indeed, probable) that the nation's predominant disease patterns will be changing again in the future, creating an entirely different set of conditions that may require an entirely different array of services and interventions. It will be important for future generations of health professionals to watch for changes in the major disease patterns to ensure a health care system that is genuinely appropriate and responsive to the problems of the day.

TECHNOLOGY AVAILABLE TO THE AMERICAN PEOPLE

During the various developmental periods of the American health care system, technology was available in different degrees to handle the diseases that affected the American people and played quite different roles in different time periods.

In the period 1850–1900, only a rudimentary technology was available for the treatment of disease. The scientific base of medicine was still very narrow, and the number of effective medical treatments was very limited. Indeed, a great deal of energy and effort was expended on treatment, but whether a patient recovered from an illness usually depended more on the patient and the disease than on the treatment.

Physicians during this period of time were poorly trained. They usually obtained their skills by serving apprenticeships with physicians already in practice and then taking short courses at unsophisticated medical colleges. What physicians had to offer was usually contained in their black bags that they took with them wherever they went. They spent a good deal of time in patients' homes and almost no time at all in the hospitals. In general, their practice was little different from that of their predecessors for centuries before them.

Nurses during the period 1850–1900 were not much better trained. Generally they were members of religious groups who volunteered to work in the few hospitals that existed, or they were poor, desperate, discarded women who frequented these institutions anyway and were pressed into service. Their work was nonscientific in the extreme and consisted simply of assisting patients with their usual bodily functions in any way possible. Not until the first training program for nurses was

organized at Bellevue Hospital in the 1860s was there any formal preparation anywhere in the country for this important role.

As for hospitals themselves, they were merely places of shelter and repose for the sick poor who could not be cared for at home. Anyone who could stay at home usually did so, since hospitals had little to offer that could not be obtained at home if one had the money. Indeed, the hospitals of those days were often a direct threat to the lives of patients, since they were dirty, crowded, and disease-ridden. Infectious diseases frequently spread rapidly among hospitalized patients; during the typhus epidemics of 1852 in New York City, for example, the highest mortality for the disease was among the patients and staff of the hospitals themselves.

After 1900 conditions began to change, spurred on by the new discoveries that were emerging from the research laboratories in this country and in Europe. In 1912, for example, a Polish chemist, Casimir Funk, published a paper, "The Etiology of Deficiency Diseases," in which he described "vitamines" and opened a whole new field of disease conditions to treatment. In 1908, James MacKenzie, in London, published his famous book, *Diseases of the Heart,* and patients throughout the world were the beneficiaries. In countless medical schools and hospitals throughout this country and Europe, major scientific advances were achieved, each of which contributed to easier and safer diagnosis and treatment of acutely ill patients.

The medical schools led the way in many of these advances as a result of some basic reforms that took place in the early 1900s. Before this time, a large number of small, poorly staffed, free-standing medical colleges existed throughout the country—fourteen in Chicago alone in 1910, and ten each in Missouri and Tennessee. In 1910, Abraham Flexner undertook a study of medical education for the Carnegie Foundation for the Advancement of Teaching and, in his report, *Medical Education in the United States and Canada,* recommended that medical education in this country undergo radical reform. In particular, he strongly urged that the training of physicians be made a university function and that it be based on a firm scientific foundation. On the basis of Flexner's recommendations and the support of the Rockefeller Foundation, many of the small unaffiliated schools began to close and many of the remaining ones became part of universities, with the important result that physicians began to be trained as scientists as well as practitioners.

Gradually, physicians began to have more effective tools with which to work, and the range of their capabilities expanded rapidly. They still continued to spend the majority of their time in their offices or their patients' homes, but they now also began to look to the hospital for the care of their more severely ill patients. The growth of radiology diagnosis during this period of time is a classic example of the new equipment and tools that physicians had available to them; it also emphasizes the new and growing importance of the hospital as the place where this new technology was available.

Hospitals and Technology

Hospitals in the 1900s began to play an increasingly important role in health care. As more technology developed, it tended to be concentrated in hospitals, with the result that patients and physicians began going to hospitals for the technology to be found there. St. Luke's Hospital in New York City, for example, was fifty years old in 1906 when it opened its first private patient pavilion. Before that time, there had been no reason for private patients to go to a hospital because they could usually get the same type of care in their homes. Now, however, hospitals began to offer services and skills that were not available anywhere else.

Although the period 1900–1940 was one of rapid growth in scientific technology, it was nothing compared to what happened with the advent of World War II. With the start of the war, this country mounted a massive effort to organize the best talents available for the care of the wounded and for the solution of health care problems generated by the war. For the first time, relatively large efforts in research were begun under the direction of the federal government, and the results were impressive. The development of antibiotics accelerated rapidly, new surgical techniques for the treatment of trauma and burns were discovered, and new approaches to the transportation of the sick and wounded were developed.

The range and breadth of problems that were subjected to organized investigation were remarkable, opening the way for an even more greatly expanded research effort after the war ended. In 1950, the size of the research commitment begun during World War II had risen to $73 million per year, $35 million of which was distributed through the National Institutes of Health (NIH). By 1974, only twenty-four years later, this expenditure had risen to an annual research budget of $2.5 billion, with $1.6 billion coming from a now greatly expanded NIH.

After World War II, hospitals were no longer the same. Previously, they had been places for the care of patients, with great emphasis being placed on the caring function. Now they became extensions of research laboratories, places where medical science was practiced and where curing was the order of the day. New procedures, new equipment, and new techniques all flourished to such a degree that the hospitals were now captured by their technology. The technology itself became the motivating force for hospitals, and most major decisions were based on that technology and its use.

The operation of these newly complex institutions called for waves of new workers, each more specialized and more highly skilled than the last. Before the war there had been approximately twenty major categories of health care workers; by the 1970s, there were hundreds. With the increasing specialization of services and skills, there was also an increasing interdependence of health care workers on each other and an increasing reliance on the health care system to integrate the work of so many separate groups.

Technology, Physicians, and Medical Care

Physicians were seriously affected by these trends. With the explosive growth of scientific knowledge after World War II, it was impossible for one physician to know everything, and so the trend toward specialization in a particular subarea of medicine had a strong impetus. Before the war, approximately eighty percent of physicians had been general practitioners and twenty percent specialists. In the years after the war, these percentages were reversed. In their training and practice, physicians focused increasingly on the scientific aspects of diagnosis and treatment and, as a result, spent more time in hospitals and less time in patients' homes. The hospital became the emotional center of the physician's life, since it was there that the most important, the most challenging, and most rewarding aspects of training and treatment occurred.

These trends affected nursing and the other health care professions as well. The training of nurses and other health care professionals became increasingly more scientific, more specialized, and more lengthy during the years after World War II. The desire to be recognized as competent in a particular area led to the proliferation of professional groups and to formal accreditation on the basis of scientific training and ability. It also led to university training programs in all of the health care professions.

In the latest period of evolution of the American health care system, the technology available to the American people has advanced to an incredible degree, but this advance has brought serious problems with it. These problems are related to the availability and appropriate use of the new abundant technology. Organ transplantation, gene therapies for various conditions, laser beams, and fiber optic surgical techniques are all accepted as merely the expected developments of the technological age. The merging of technologies from fields other than medicine, such as the development of computerized axial tomographic systems and magnetic resonance imaging systems, has further added to the immense range of technology available to the health care system. This explosion of technology in recent years, however, has not been without its problems. Indeed, the technology itself has *caused* a rather serious set of problems with which present and future generations of health care professionals must grapple.

Complex Issues Involving Technology

One important problem with medical technology is its impact on the form and configuration of the health care system and on the values, patterns, and practice of the professionals in the system. In many ways, the American health services system has been captured by its technology and has been subtly and seductively shaped by its demands. Decisions regarding the design of programs and institutions, the training of personnel, and the distribution of services have been governed by technological considerations that loom larger every year.

A still more profound effect of technology is its ability to insinuate itself into the values of not just the system but also of the people who work in the system. The student entering a health profession rapidly learns that academic success and later professional success comes from mastery of the scientific technology. Increasingly, the student is taught to view excellence as being reached through technical achievements and, as a result, inadvertently taught to give decreasing importance to the more personal, nontechnical aspects of disease. By the time the student becomes a fully accepted member of the profession, a value system may have been established that views illness as a series of technical problems to be solved by the application of specific technical solutions. This value system is then reinforced in practice by the expectations of the public and by the requirements of the regulators, both of whom have come to view quality in terms of technical excellence. The result frequently is professional performance that is excellent in technical terms and occasionally rather poor in human terms.

A quite different problem of technology arises not from its excessiveness but rather from its inequitable distribution to society. There is more technology available than can be provided equitably to all people due to limits on funding. Large portions of society do not benefit as much as they should from technological advances. Marked differences exist, for example, in mortality and morbidity measures for white versus nonwhite segments of society, possibly indicating an unequal access to modern health care technology. The answer obviously is to improve the health services system to ensure adequate distribution of available resources. But there has been relatively little movement in that direction, and the gap in equality of access to modern technology has probably widened rather than narrowed in recent years.

Indeed, the costs of the new technology have been one of the most important and difficult problems for the American health care system to face in this latest phase of its historical development. Expenditures for health care in the United States in the late twentieth century have exceeded fourteen percent of the country's gross domestic product (GDP). A large part of the increase in health care expenditures has been attributed to technology. As attempts are made to control the rising expenditures on health care, attention has naturally turned toward controlling the use of modern technology. The theory here is that if the use of modern technology, which had previously been widely available, could be reduced, the total expenditures for health care would in similar fashion be reduced (or at least would not increase as rapidly). According to this theory, modern technology is seen as extremely expensive, the usage of which should be reduced or at least controlled more closely.

One interesting outcome of the attempts to use technology more carefully has been a growing interest in the evaluation of the various new discoveries and techniques. In the past, many new technologies were adopted without appropriate evaluation of how effective they really were or, even more important, how much *more* effective they would be than already existing technology. Only limited examination of the cost implications of new technology was attempted. Now, the evaluation of new technology and its costs, and the comparison of the benefits of a new technology with the costs attendant to its use, has become much more common. In this latest period of health care evolution, with marketplace forces attempting to reduce (or at least rationalize) the use of services, it is increasingly common to read articles in leading scientific journals on the cost-benefit and cost-effectiveness analyses of new scientific or technical developments.

In summary, virtually no technology was available to treat disease before the 1900s. New technology began to appear and grow rapidly after the turn of the century. World War II fostered an incredible surge of research endeavors that were assisted after the war by major financial support for research provided by the National Institutes of Health. By the 1990s, technology had become such a major driving force in the American health care system, and such a major contributor to rising expenditures for health care, that its use was being challenged, primarily to reduce the use of technology or at least to control its growth. In this latest period of historical development of the American health care system, the emphasis on technology is no longer on unhindered growth and expansion, but rather on careful evaluation and controlled use and availability. At the same time as the use of technology is a subject for control and possible reduction, the number of people in the American population with limited access to technology has continued to grow.

SOCIAL ORGANIZATION OF HEALTH CARE IN THE UNITED STATES

In the four periods of historical evolution of health care in the United States, how has our society organized to use the health resources available to it? What has been the predominant ideology of social organization that has controlled the shaping and the functioning of the health care system? How has that social ideology changed over the various periods of evolution?

During the period 1850–1900, the social organization of health care in the United States was quite loose and simple. Public services were rudimentary and were concentrated on a very narrow range of problems. There were hospitals in a few areas, but they were generally started by religious or charitable groups for the care of those who were obviously and publicly impoverished. The predominant ethic of the time was that people should care for themselves and be self-sufficient. If they were to become dependent, they should take advantage of and be grateful for the various charities established for these purposes. Society did not feel that it had an obligation either to provide health services to the population or to ensure that the population received the services that it needed.

This philosophy of rugged individualism and relative lack of large-scale social organization for health care began to change somewhat in the early 1900s in this country with the development of local efforts to provide care for people through city and county hospitals. Although there was virtually nothing of a national effort to effect the availability and distribution of health services and very little done by individual state governments, city and county governments, particularly those in large cities with large numbers of poor people, realized that something had to be done to provide care for those who otherwise could not obtain it. These local efforts were almost the only social stirrings of policy in the health area until the Great Depression of the 1930s struck with full force.

The Changing Social Role of Government

Prior to the Great Depression, the prevailing social ideology said that health care (and many other matters of social survival) were a concern of individual citizens and that government should intervene as little as possible. When economic forces beyond the comprehension of most Americans struck down many people, destroying their lives and leaving them destitute, the thinking began to change. With the arrival of Franklin Roosevelt in the White House, the New Deal was launched and a wide array of social programs appeared, all aimed at repairing the damage of the Depression. The importance of the New Deal in terms of changing American social ideology cannot be underestimated, since for the first time, the American society created large-scale national programs to assist those who could not assist themselves.

In health care, federal governmental activity was still minimal and limited to a few specific areas of grant-in-aid programs to states to improve certain public health services such as infectious disease control and maternal and child health. Although the services were limited and aimed primarily at the poor, this small start did signify at least a partial assumption of responsibility by the national government for the health of the public, at least in certain specific areas. It is interesting to note that proposals were made to President Roosevelt to develop a universal health insurance system connected with the Social Security program that was actively being developed, but Roosevelt decided that the addition of universal health insurance coverage would arouse too much opposition and would endanger the passage of the entire Social Security effort.

The arrival of World War II brought with it a major change in social organization and social thinking in general in the United States and also planted the seeds for some significant changes in social thinking about health care. As part of the mobilization effort for the war, millions of men and women entered the military service and, as a result, received a wide variety of health services simply by virtue of joining the military. The significance was twofold: (1) for many people in the United States, it was the first time that they had easy accessibility to a wide range of modern health services, and they began to realize the value and the benefits of having such services available; and (2) the services were provided as a right of those in the military—they were clearly not charity for people who could no longer take care of themselves, but rather came as a condition of work or service in the military.

The Growth of Health Insurance

Not only did World War II accustom the country to large-scale health care programs provided by the society to its members, it also encouraged the growth of the health insurance industry. During the war a freeze was imposed on wages and salaries so that very little collective bargaining for increases in salary could occur. Considerable activity did occur in the development of pensions, disability programs, and health insurance plans, however, with the result that the private health insurance industry began to flourish. This industry provided the American public with a new form of social organization—the health insurance company or organization. Before the development of private health insurance, the public had no form of social organization to protect it from a sudden onslaught of medical bills. With the arrival of this new phenomenon, health insurance, the American public began to gain experience in the voluntary cooperative effort of pooling many individual contributions for a common group objective—protection from financial disaster.

The period immediately after World War II witnessed the growth of health insurance plans of both the nonprofit and the for-profit nature. The early Blue Cross and Blue Shield plans were started by voluntary hospital groups (Blue Cross) and state medical societies (Blue Shield). With the success and growth of Blue Cross and Blue Shield, commercial insurance companies also entered the field, offering health insurance plans to employers and industry as part of their life/health/retirement/disability packages. With the rapid advances made by Blue Cross/Blue Shield and the commercial insurance carriers, the percentage of Americans covered by some form of health insurance rose from less than twenty percent at the end of World War II to more than seventy percent by the early 1960s.

The Acceleration of Government in Health Care Funding

In the early 1960s, a major battle was fought and won by those advocating a greater societal role in the organization of health care services. The battle involved the creation of government-sponsored health insurance plans for people over the age of sixty-five and resulted in the passage of legislation that created Medicare. Although Medicare itself was directed primarily to the needs of the country's elderly, its impact was soon felt throughout the entire health care system. The creation of the Medicare program had two immediate major social implications. First, Medicare provided financing for health care for all persons over the age of sixty-five simply on the basis of age; need was not a factor. The American society, in effect, determined that there were certain things that society should do for all its members, regardless of individual needs, since society could ensure equity.

The second major effect of Medicare was the assumption by the federal government of the responsibility for planning, financing, and monitoring a significant portion of the health care services in this country. The society not only wanted social insurance programs for health care, but also wanted the federal government to assume a central role in operating these programs. In one legislative stroke, not only was a massive new program of health insurance coverage developed for an important part of the American people, but the federal government was given direct responsibility for that program and for the financial resources that were made available to it.

Either one of these developments would have been significant alone, but the two together (that is, the creation of a health insurance plan for the elderly in the United States and the assignment of the responsibility for that plan to the federal government) rather suddenly made the federal government a dominant force in shaping the organization and operation of health care in the United States after 1965.

A further significant change in the social organization of health care in this country involving the federal government came in the mid-1960s with the development of the Neighborhood Health Centers program of the United States Office of Economic Opportunity ("War on Poverty"). In this effort a number of health programs were funded for underserved areas of the country by the federal government, each of which were required to have significant participation of consumers through governing boards and committees. This involvement of consumers of health care in the operation of the programs providing them with care was a substantial change from the thinking of the past and soon became standard policy in new governmental programs, awakening people to the possibility of being directly involved in the operation and direction of health programs that had previously been considered the sole prerogative of health care professionals.

This philosophy was vigorously put forward in the National Health Planning and Resources Development Act of 1974, which required a majority of consumers on all local health planning boards. Although the health planning effort in this country has since been dismantled to a large degree, the involvement of consumer advocates in health policy matters was born and continues to be an increasingly important aspect of the United States health care system.

In short, the period from the end of the second world war to the early 1980s was a period of rapid growth of national governmental involvement in the health care system, as a result of the passage of Medicare. It put the federal government in charge of the single largest source for financing of health care in the United States and, almost overnight, completely reversed the complete lack of federal government involvement in the organization and delivery of health services. Indeed, during this period of historical evolution of health care in the United States, it was felt that there was a strong possibility that the United States might develop a national health insurance plan for all of its people, thereby giving the national government even greater control of the health care system and its functioning.

The Move to Limited Resources

In the early 1980s, the health care system of this country entered a fourth phase of its development, an era of resource limitation, restriction of growth, and reorganization of systems of financing for providing care. This was also a period in which general market forces began to play in health care throughout the country and to transform the system of financing and providing services in major ways.

In the early 1980s, with the federal Medicare program experiencing major increases in expenditure every year, interest began to shift toward a possible reduction of benefits, greater cost sharing by the elderly themselves, and a limitation on reimbursements to providers of service. Legislative observers of Medicare now began to fear for its long-term existence, with its present generous reimbursement and financing arrangements, and energy now became focused less on the development of new services or the expansion of coverage than on the control of costs through limitations and reductions. Changes in the manner in which Medicare reimbursed hospitals (by the use of prospective payment and "diagnosis-related groups") were designed to encourage hospitals and doctors to provide less in the way of services and to curtail or limit the number of services provided. This change of policy on the part of Medicare led to a reduction in admissions to hospitals and a great decrease in length of stay within hospitals, both of which led to a gradual shrinkage in the actual supply of operating hospital beds in the United States.

These developments were paralleled in the private sector by the realization of employers that their rapidly rising health care expenditures were a major threat to the long-term existence of their companies. With this understanding, private employers began to look for ways to curtail health benefits and to reduce the rise in their health insurance expenditures. Their efforts have included becoming much more aggressive in seeking lower cost insurance coverage when purchasing insurance as well as moving their employees into new forms of health insurance, such as "managed care," that promise better cost and utilization control. In a very short period of time, the private sector in the United States has taken on a much more aggressive posture with regard to health care and health insurance, demanding lower prices and lower premiums in exchange for its continuing business.

In a remarkable and ironic development, the period since 1980 has seen the federal government and Congress talking about "health care reform" (with a possible objective of expanding benefits and coverage) while the private sector has aggressively carried out its own health care reforms that have rested largely on reduced coverage, reduced choices, and lower prices. The initial success of the private sector in its efforts was demonstrated by national health care expenditures for private health care in 1995, which increased only 2.9% over the previous year, just about equivalent to the rate of inflation, while public sector (particularly Medicare and Medicaid) spending increased by 8.9%. It has become obvious that the private sector's cost containment efforts have worked for the private sector and have not worked for the public sector.

In the period immediately following World War II, the federal government assumed a central role in health care financing, planning, policy, and regulation and seemed to be on its way to being the sole social organizing force for health care in the United States. The federal government controlled a significant portion of the financial support for health care (more than one-third of the total health care expenditures from all sources). By using these massive resources, the federal government set many of the rules by which health care, governmentally funded or not, was provided. It seemed that the health care system of this country, although by no means federally operated, was certainly going to be federally dominated or influenced.

In more recent years, the role of the private sector in reducing health care costs and controlling the use of services has become much more important and in many states, such as California, the predominant force shaping delivery of services. Although the role of the federal government and its programs remains massive, the more aggressive and effective shaping of the health care system in these states (and potentially throughout the country) may now have shifted the focus to the private sector, and particularly to employers who provide health insurance benefits and account for approximately one-third of the health care financing for this country.

In summary, with regard to social organization, the United States entered the twentieth century with a social philosophy that said that people should care for themselves or be satisfied with charity. After 1900, local governments became involved in providing some care for the indigent through local city and county hospitals, but federal and state governments played virtually no role at all. The limited federal role in health care is reflected by the absence of a federal cabinet level health department until 1953 when the Department of Health, Education and Welfare was created.

With the passage and implementation of Medicare in 1965, it seemed as if the federal government would rapidly take on responsibility for the direction and control of health care in the United States, in an almost unchallenged manner. But in the 1980s, private employers began to use their economic power and leverage to reduce health care utilization and costs in ways that the federal government had not imagined. The situation now suggests that the social organization and control of health care in the near future, if not necessarily in the distant future, will be shared between the federal government (operating primarily through its control of the Medicare and Medicaid programs), on the one hand, and the private sector (operating through its control of employer-provided health insurance), on the other.

OVERVIEW OF THE ORGANIZATION OF HEALTH SERVICES IN THE UNITED STATES

In the previous sections of this chapter, the historical evolution of health care in the United States was reviewed in order to gain perspective about how the present structure and organization of our health care has come about. This section of the chapter will describe the overall organizational structure of health services in this country. The remaining chapters of this book explore the components, structure, and operation of the system.

Ways of Looking at the Organization of Health Care

There are several ways of looking at the organization of health care, in this country or any country. The first involves looking at the organization of health services from the point of view of major resources necessary for a system to function. The second looks at the organization of personal health services from the point of view of the consumer and describes the individual service elements that are necessary for a complete health care system. The third looks at the organization of health care from the viewpoint of the major systems of care that exist and how they function.

This overall review of the organization of health care services in the United States will look briefly at health care from the point of view of resource requirements and of the individual service elements. These two perspectives will then be incorporated into a systems view of health care services.

With regard to the major resource needs of a health care system, the basic requirements are rather simple in description but complex in detail. As shown in Figure 1–1, health care delivery requires personnel, financing, technology/pharmaceuticals/equipment, and facilities. Each of these aspects is discussed in detail in subsequent chapters of this book.

With regard to the individual service elements, there are at least ten basic service components that should be included in any complete system of health care, ranging from public health and preventive health services to long-term care and rehabilitation. The correct "mix" of these services in terms of volume, intensity, and availability will vary, depending upon the needs of the population to be served and the resources available to finance these services. In general, however, if one wants to learn how a health care system is organized and functions, one can do so by determining how each of these individual service components is offered.

These individual service elements are presented in Figure 1–2.

Development of Systems of Care

When visitors from abroad come to the United States, they frequently want to know about "the" American health care system and how it works, implying that there is a single "system" that describes all health care organization in this country. They are frequently puzzled when they learn that there is not a single "American health care system," but rather a series of separate subsystems that serve different populations in different ways. Sometimes these subsystems overlap; sometimes they are entirely separate. Sometimes they are supported with private funds, sometimes with public funds, and sometimes with a mixture of both. Sometimes several different subsystems use the same facilities, but sometimes they use facilities and personnel that are entirely separate and distinct.

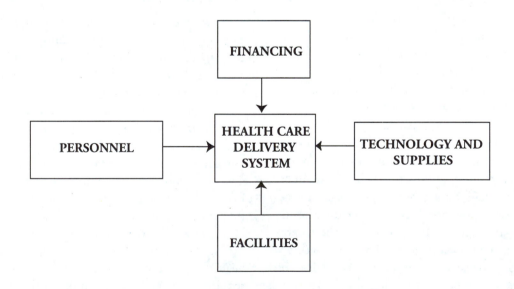

FIGURE 1–1 Resources required to maintain a health care delivery system

- Health promotion and disease prevention services
- Emergency medical services (including transportation)
- Ambulatory care for simple/limited conditions
- Inpatient care for simple/limited inpatient problems
- Inpatient care for complex/multiple inpatient problems
- Long-term care (either in-home or institutional services)
- Services for social/psychological conditions (both inpatient and ambulatory)
- Rehabilitation services (both inpatient and ambulatory)
- Dental services
- Pharmaceuticals/supplies/medical devices and equipment

FIGURE 1–2 Basic service components of a health care system

It should not be surprising that there is a multiplicity of health care systems (or subsystems) in the United States, given the historical development of health services in this country. In the earliest days, health care was entirely a private matter, and people were expected to take care of themselves by obtaining the services of private physicians and nurses when needed, purchasing medications from drugstores and chemist shops, and paying for all these services personally. For those persons who could not take care of themselves, charitable institutions were established as voluntary, nonprofit corporations to provide charity health care. These groups usually centered their efforts on hospitals and usually were located in the larger towns and cities of this country.

In the early twentieth century, a new element was added with the development of city/county hospitals. These hospitals were established by local governments to care for the poor in their area who could not get care either by their own efforts or from the voluntary nonprofit charity hospitals. These public facilities were generally large, acute care general hospitals, with busy clinics and emergency rooms and close connections to local government ambulance services, police departments, and other community services. At the same time, state governments were developing mental hospitals. The cities had previously been responsible for the care of lunatics and the insane, but after the turn of the century, state governments began to assume this burden. Every state soon had at least one mental hospital where the emotionally disturbed were offered what little care was available.

With the explosive growth in the size of the federal government and in the numbers of persons in the armed forces during World War II, separate systems of care developed for active-duty military personnel and their dependents, retired military personnel, and veterans. These were almost entirely self-contained systems, employing salaried physicians and nurses working entirely in military or veterans hospitals directly operated by the federal government.

As the cost of health care began to increase rapidly after World War II, the United States experienced a rather sudden and somewhat bewildering development of a wide variety of health insurance plans. The first to be operated were community-based, nonprofit Blue Cross and Blue Shield plans, developed by hospital and physician associations to spread the cost of health care more widely among the population. These were followed by labor union health and welfare trust funds, established as a consequence of benefit negotiations for union members. At the same time, the private, for-profit commercial insurance companies expanded their efforts on behalf of both individuals and large groups of employees. Finally, several large government-sponsored and publicly supervised health insurance plans evolved, such as Medicare and Medicaid, the latter to aid the medically indigent.

Private medical practitioners, voluntary nonprofit hospitals, city and state government hospitals, military and veterans hospitals, and health insurance plans with a variety of forms and origins all developed in the United States at the same time, separately, and for specific purposes. The resulting picture has been described as having a rich diversity of opportunities and approaches for meeting the health care needs of a population that has in itself a rich diversity of people and situations. It has also been described as chaotic, uncoordinated, overlapping, unplanned, and wasteful of precious personal and financial resources. The reality probably lies somewhere in between.

If there is no single, easily described American health care system, at least some of the subsystems that compose the larger entity can be identified. Although an endless set of variations is possible, it seems appropriate to examine four models or subsystems of health care in the United States, each of which serves a different group. By looking at the components, the system as a whole may be better understood. These systems serve (1) regularly employed, middle-income families with a continuous program of health insurance coverage; (2) poor, unemployed (or underemployed) families without continuous health insurance coverage; (3) active-duty military personnel and their dependents; and (4) veterans of United States military service. For each of these systems, the manner in which basic elements of health care are provided is reviewed.

Employed, Insured, Middle-Income America (Private Practice, Private Insurance)

It is appropriate for two reasons to consider the system of health care used by the typically employed, insured, middle-income individual or family. First, this system is frequently described as *the* American health care system (all others, therefore, immediately becoming somehow secondary to it); second, this system is frequently said to include the best medical care available in the United States and perhaps anywhere in the world.

The most striking feature of the employed, insured, middle-income system of care is the absence of any *formal* system. Each family puts together an *informal* set of services and facilities to meet its own needs. The system, therefore, has no formal structure or organization and is different for each individual or family. Indeed, each family's system may vary widely according to the particular situation in which it is used. The only constant feature of this system is the family itself; all other aspects are transient, changeable, and widely varied.

Two other characteristics are also immediately noteworthy. First, the service aspects of the system focus on and are coordinated by physicians in private practice. Second, the system is financed by personal, nongovernmental funds, whether paid directly by consumers or through private health insurance plans including managed care plans. As the system is described, it will become readily apparent that not only are these two features important descriptively, but they have been important in shaping the system in its present form.

Public health and preventive medicine services for the employed, insured, middle-income system are provided by two different sources. Those services designed to protect large numbers of people, such as water purification, sewage disposal, and air pollution control, are provided by local or state governmental agencies. Frequently these agencies are called *public health departments*. They usually provide their services to the entire population of a region, with no distinction between rich and poor, simple and sophisticated, interested and disinterested. Indeed, these mass public health services are common to all the systems of health care to be discussed. Those public health and preventive medicine services that are aimed at individuals, such as well-baby examinations, cervical cancer smears, vaccinations, and family planning, are provided by individual physicians in private practice. If a middle-income family desires a vaccination in preparation for a foreign trip or wants the blood cholesterol level of its members checked, the family physician is consulted and provides the service. If it is time for the new baby to have its first series of vaccinations, the family pediatrician is usually the one who provides them.

Ambulatory patient services, both simple and complex, are also obtained from private physicians. Many families use a physician who specializes in family practice, while others use an array of specialist physicians such as pediatricians, internists, obstetrician/gynecologists, and psychiatrists who provide both primary care and specialty services. Increasingly these physicians are employed by, or under contract to, a practice management corporation and sometimes a managed care plan. When special laboratory tests are ordered, X-ray films required, or drugs and medications prescribed, private commercial for-profit laboratories or community pharmacies are used. Many of these services, from individual preventive medicine services to complex specialist treatments, are financed by individuals through out-of-pocket payment, since most health insurance plans do not provide complete coverage for their needs. When the middle-income family begins to use institutional services, such as hospital care, the source of payment shifts almost completely from the individual to third-party health insurance plans, including various forms of managed care.

Inpatient hospital services are typically provided to the employed, insured, middle-income family by a local community hospital that is usually voluntary and nonprofit or, increasingly, part of a for-

profit system. The specific hospital to be used is determined by the institution in which the family physician has medical staff privileges or by the managed care plan. Generally, the smaller, less specialized, more local hospitals will be used for simple problems, whereas the larger, more specialized, perhaps more distant, hospitals will be used for more complicated problems. Many of these larger hospitals have active physician training programs, conduct research, and may have significant charity or teaching wards.

The employed, insured, middle-income family obtains its long-term care from a variety of sources, depending on the service required. Some long-term care is provided in hospitals and, as such, is merely an extension of the complex inpatient care the patient has already received. This practice was more common in the past, but utilization review procedures have increased the pressure on hospitals to reduce the length of time people are hospitalized. More commonly, long-term care is obtained at home through the assistance of a visiting nurse or voluntary nonprofit or for-profit community-based nursing service. If institutional long-term care is needed, it is probably obtained in a nursing home or a skilled nursing facility, usually a small (50–100 patients) institution, operated privately, for profit, by a single proprietor or small group of investors. Recently, there has been a general increase in size (100+ patients per facility) and a trend toward absorption of individual facilities into larger multifacility proprietary chains. The employed, insured, middle-income family usually pays for its long-term care with its own funds, since most health insurance plans provide relatively limited coverage for long-term care.

When employed, insured, middle-income families require care for emotional problems, they will again use a variety of mostly private services. As the illness becomes more serious, however, families may, for the first time, rely on government-sponsored service. When emotional problems first begin to appear in the employed, insured, middle-income family, the patient will probably turn to the family physician, who provides simple supportive services such as medication, informal counseling, and perhaps referral for psychological testing. The physician may even arrange for the patient to be hospitalized in a general hospital for some nonpsychiatric diagnosis. If the emotional problems become more severe, the family physician may refer the patient to a private psychiatrist, or to a community mental health center that most likely will be a voluntary nonprofit agency or under the sponsorship of one (such as a voluntary nonprofit hospital). If hospitalization is required, the psychiatrist or the community mental health center is likely to use the psychiatric section of the local voluntary nonprofit hospital if it seems that the stay in a hospital will be a short one. If the hospitalization promises to be a long one, the psychiatrist may use a psychiatric hospital, usually a private or for-profit, nongovernmental community facility. Increasingly both inpatient and ambulatory mental health care will be obtained in a contracted managed care environment.

In those cases in which extended institutional care is required for an emotional problem and the patient's financial resources are relatively limited, the middle-income family may require hospitalization in a state mental hospital. This event usually represents the first use of government health programs by the middle-income family, and as such, it frequently comes as a considerable shock to patient and family alike.

In summary, the employed, insured, middle-income family's system of health care has been an informal, unstructured collection of individual services put together by the patient and the private physician to meet the needs of the moment. The individual services themselves have had little formalized interrelationship, and the only thread of continuity is provided by the family's physician or by the family itself. In general, all of the services are provided by nongovernmental sources and are paid for by private funds, either directly out-of-pocket or by privately financed health insurance plans.

For all of its apparent looseness and lack of structure, the employed, insured, middle-income family's system of health care has allowed for a considerable amount of decision and control by the patient, more than that of the other systems to be discussed. The patient is free to choose the physician, the health insurance plan, and frequently even the hospital. If additional care is required, the patient can seek out and use (sometimes overuse) that care to the limit of the financial resources available. If the patient does not like the particular care being provided, dissatisfaction can be expressed in a more effective manner; the patient can seek care elsewhere from another provider.

On the other hand, the employed, insured, middle-income family's system of care has been a poorly coordinated, unplanned collection of services that frequently have little formal integration with one another. It can be very wasteful of resources, and without central control or monitoring, it is difficult to determine whether it is accomplishing what it should. Each individual service may be of very high quality, but with little evidence of any "linking" taking place to ensure that each service complements the others as effectively as possible.

One special subset of the middle-income model now involves millions of patients in this country. When people reach age sixty-five, they are automatically eligible for Medicare, the federally sponsored and supervised health insurance plan for the elderly. A patient covered by Medicare benefits can utilize the same system of care as the middle-income family, including private practice physicians and voluntary nongovernment hospitals. The main difference now is that the bills are paid by a federal government health insurance plan, rather than the usual private plan in which the typical middle-income family is enrolled. The physicians are the same and the hospitals are the same; only the health insurance plan is different.

Alternatively, these individuals can increasingly elect to enroll in a managed care program. As managed care has become more prevalent, an employed, middle-income insured individual may no longer have an entirely open choice of physician and hospital; rather, the choice now may be limited to only the physicians and the hospitals with which the managed care plan contracts. Also, under managed care, access to specialists may not be as easy to achieve and may not be solely at the choice of the patient, since there may now be a primary care physician who must authorize referral to specialists, and that primary care physician may have incentives to reduce referrals. Since managed care is increasingly the plan of choice for employers and other purchasers of private health insurance, and since Medicare is now strongly advocating the use of managed care by its recipients, the more open, patient-initiated and patient-controlled use of health care services may change very markedly and very rapidly in the near future.

Unemployed, Uninsured, Inner-City, Minority America (Local Government Health Care)

A second major system of health care in the United States serves those people who are not regularly employed, do not have continuous health insurance coverage, and often are minority group members living in the inner city. While the specific details may vary from city to city, the general outline is well known in all major cities of the country. If it is important to study the system of health care for the employed, insured, middle-income population because it represents the *best* health care possible in this country, it is equally important to study the care of the poor, unem-

ployed, and uninsured, since it frequently represents the *worst*.

The most striking feature of the health care system of the poor, inner-city resident is exactly the same as that historically characterizing the middle-income family system: there is no *formal* system. Instead, just as in the middle-income system, each individual or family must put together an *informal* set of services, from whatever source possible, to meet the health care needs of the moment. There is one significant difference, however: the poor do not have the resources to choose where and how they will obtain their health services. Instead, they must take what is offered to them and try to put together a system from whatever they are told they can have.

There are two important characteristics of the system. First, the great majority of services are provided by local government agencies such as the city or county hospital and the local health department. Second, the patients have no real continuity of service with any single provider, such as an employed, insured, middle-income family might have with a family physician. The poor family is faced with an endless stream of health care professionals who treat one specific episode of an illness and then are replaced by someone else for the next episode. While the middle-income system of health care can establish at least some thread of continuity by the ongoing presence of a family physician, the poor family cannot.

The poor obtain their mass public health and preventive medicine services, including a pure water supply, sanitary sewage disposal, and protection of milk and food, from the same local government health departments and health agencies that serve the middle-income system. In contrast to the middle-income system, however, the poor also get their individual public health and preventive medicine services from the local health department. When a poor family's newborn baby needs its vaccinations, that family goes to the district health center of the health department, not to a private physician. When a low-income woman needs a Papanicolaou smear for cervical cancer testing, it is most likely that the local government health department will give the test.

To obtain ambulatory services, the poor family cannot rely on the constant presence of a family physician for advice and routine treatment. Instead, they must turn to neighbors, the local pharmacist, the health department's public health nurse, or the emergency room of the city or county hospital. It has often been said that the city or county hospital's emergency room is the family physician for the poor, and the facts generally support this contention: when the poor need ambulatory patient care, it is quite likely that the first place they will turn is the city or county hospital emergency room.

The emergency room also serves the poor as the point of entry to the rest of the health care system. The poor obtain many of their ambulatory services in the outpatient clinics of the city and county hospitals. To gain admission to these clinics, they must frequently first go to the emergency room and be referred to the appropriate clinic. Once out of the emergency room, they may be cared for in two or three specialty clinics, each of which may handle one particular set of problems but none of which will take responsibility for coordinating all the care the patient is receiving.

When the poor need inpatient hospital services, whether simple or complicated, they again usually turn to the city or county hospital to obtain them. Admission to the inpatient services of these hospitals is usually obtained through the emergency room or the outpatient clinics, thereby forcing the poor family to use these ambulatory patient services if they wish later admission to the inpatient services. The poor may also turn to the emergency room, the outpatient clinics, and the inpatient ward or teaching services of the larger voluntary nonprofit com-

munity hospitals. Since these hospitals are frequently teaching hospitals for the training of physicians, they often maintain special free or lower-priced wards. It is to these wards that the poor are usually admitted. Since the care in the teaching hospitals is generally as good as or better than any that might be obtained at the local city or county hospitals, many poor are willing to become teaching cases in the voluntary nonprofit hospitals in exchange for better care in better surroundings. By and large, however, city and county hospitals carry the largest burden of inpatient care for the poor.

If the long-term care situation of middle-income people is generally inadequate, the long-term care of the poor can only be described as terrible. In contrast to the system of care for middle-income families, most of the long-term care of the poor is provided in the wards of the city and county hospitals, although not by intent or plan. The poor simply remain in hospitals longer because their social and physical conditions are more complicated and because the hospital staffs are reluctant to discharge them until they have some assurance that continuing care will be available after discharge. Since this status is often uncertain, poor patients are likely to be kept longer in the hospital so that they can complete as much of their convalescence as possible before discharge.

Most of the long-term care of the poor is provided in the same types of nursing homes or skilled nursing facilities that are used by middle-income people—either the smaller (50–100 patients) facilities, operated for profit by a single proprietor, or the larger (100+ patients) facilities operated by a proprietary chain. One major difference between the systems used by the poor and the middle-income is the quality of the facility used. The middle-income generally have access to better-equipped and better-staffed nursing homes, while the poor are admitted to less expensive, less well-equipped facilities. Another important difference between the middle-income and the poor is that employed, insured, middle-income patients are more likely to pay for their own care in these institutions, while the poor have their care paid by welfare, Medicaid, or other public funds.

It is interesting to note that the system of health care for the employed, insured, middle-income utilizes entirely private, nongovernmental facilities until long-term care for mental illness is required; at that point, a governmental facility, the state mental hospital, is used. By contrast, the system of health care for the poor is composed almost entirely of public, government-sponsored services until long-term care is required. This care is usually provided in private, profit-making facilities, the first use of such private facilities by the poor.

The convergence of the poor and the middle-income systems of care in the private profit-making nursing homes is important, since it represents an important feature of our multiple subsystems of health care. In many cases, several systems of health care that are otherwise separate and distinct merge in their common use of personnel, equipment, and facilities. The emergency rooms of the city or county and voluntary nonprofit teaching hospitals, for example, serve as the source of emergency medical care for the middle-income family that cannot reach its own family physician. They also serve as the family physician for the poor family that has none of its own. The private, for-profit nursing home serves as the source of long-term care for the middle-income family and may provide the same function for the poor. The radiology department of the voluntary nonprofit teaching hospital provides X-rays for the middle-income patient whose care is supervised by the private family physician, as well as for the poor patient whose care is supervised by a hospital staff physician in training. This does not mean that there is any real, functional integration of the separate systems of care because of their use of the same facility or personnel. Rather, the model

is more like that of a busy harbor in which a variety of ships berth side by side for a short period of time before going their separate ways for separate purposes.

In their use of services for emotional illnesses, the poor return once again to an almost totally public, local government system. Initial signs of emotional difficulties are haphazardly treated in the emergency rooms and outpatient clinics of the city or county hospital. From here, patients may be referred to the crowded inpatient psychiatric wards of these same hospitals, but they are just as likely to be referred to community mental health centers operated by local governmental or voluntary nonprofit community agencies. When long-term care in an institution is required, the poor are sent to the psychiatric wards of the city or county hospital, and from there to the large state governmental mental hospitals, frequently many miles away.

In the past, health services for the poor were usually free, at least to the patients. The local health department, the city or county hospital, or the state mental hospital generally did not charge for its services, regardless of the patient's ability to pay. In the last few years, both local health departments and city and county hospitals have been forced to initiate a system of charges for services that were previously free. They have done this to recapture third-party payments to which the poor patient might be eligible, and patients who are unable to pay are still ordinarily provided the services they need. The imposition of these charges for previously free health services has probably changed the perception of these programs by the poor, but it is still too early to determine the implications of these changes.

As with the employed, insured, middle-income system, there is a subset of the health care system for the poor that requires special comment. Certain persons who are poor enough by virtue of extremely low income or resources may qualify for

Medicaid, the federal-state cooperative health insurance plan for the indigent. Under Medicaid, people whose income and resources are below a level established by the individual states can use a state government-sponsored health insurance program to purchase health care in the private, middle-income marketplace. The purpose of this program is to move the poor out of their usual local government health care system and into the supposedly better private practice health care system of middle-income people. Unfortunately, the ability of Medicaid to move the poor into a better system of care has been limited by the reluctance of private physicians and private hospitals to assume responsibility for many Medicaid patients. This reluctance has been based on what has been seen as a low rate of reimbursement by Medicaid for services provided, an often cumbersome system of paperwork and prior authorizations in order to provide care, and a frequently irrational system of retroactive denials of payment for services already provided.

Just as the situation of the employed, middle-income, insured population is changing to the use of managed care, so too is the situation of the poor, uninsured, Medicaid recipient changing, with somewhat different directions and results.

In many states, some or all of the Medicaid population is being moved out of the standard Medicaid fee-for-service model into a managed care model. Although the models vary from state to state, the central idea is for Medicaid recipients to establish a more permanent relationship with a single primary care physician who will then coordinate ("manage") that patient's use of specialist and hospital services. Just as it does for the employed, insured individual, the use of managed care for Medicaid recipients moves them into a more intentionally organized and monitored system of care, with rigorous standards of service and serious attempts to measure outcomes. Medicaid managed care will significantly change the organizational

form for many of the poor, uninsured patients, probably for the better.

A second subset of the system of care for the poor and uninsured is that for poor people who turn sixty-five. Immediately upon reaching age sixty-five, they are eligible for Medicare and ostensibly should be able to take their new insurance coverage and move into the private, middle-income system of care. Unfortunately, this movement from public to private provider systems by poor people who become sixty-five years of age is limited by the deductible and coinsurance features of Medicare. Under Medicare, everyone (poor included) is expected to spend several hundred dollars for health care first, before Medicare begins to pay bills. Even when this deductible requirement is met, the elderly person is also required to pay a substantial amount for any hospitalization. The level of available cash to pay these deductibles and coinsurance limits the ability of many poor people to take full advantage of the benefits of Medicare when they become eligible at age sixty-five.

In summary, the system of health care for the poor is as unstructured and informal as that for the employed, insured, middle-income, but the poor have to depend upon whatever services the local government offers them. The services are usually provided free of charge or at low cost, but the patient has relatively little opportunity to express a choice and exercise options. Poor patients often cannot move to another set of services if they dislike the one first offered, since those first offered are usually the only services available.

Like the system of health care for the middle-income, the system for the poor is poorly coordinated internally and almost completely unplanned and unmonitored. It is certainly as wasteful of resources as the middle-income system, but because it is a low-cost, poorly financed system, the exact amount of waste is difficult to document. At the same time, the great virtue of the health care system for the poor—its openness and accessibility to all people at all times for all conditions (albeit with considerable delays)—is difficult to evaluate adequately as well, and the introduction of managed care is now seeking to provide some rationalization, as is the case for the middle class.

Military Medical Care System

A person joining one of the uniformed branches of the American military sacrifices many aspects of civilian life that nonmilitary personnel take for granted. At the same time, however, this person receives a variety of fringe benefits that those outside the military do not enjoy. One of the most important of these fringe benefits is a well-organized system of high-quality health care provided at no direct cost to the recipient. Certain features of this military medical care system (the general term used to include the separate systems of the United States Army, Navy, and Air Force) deserve comment. First, the system is all-inclusive and omnipresent. The military medical system has the responsibility of protecting the health of all active-duty military personnel everywhere and of providing them with all the services they may eventually need for any service-connected problem. The military medical system goes where active-duty military personnel go and assumes a responsibility for total care that is unique among American health care systems.

The second important characteristic of the military medical care system is that it goes into effect immediately whether the active-duty soldier or sailor wants it or not. No initiative or action is required by the individual to start the system; indeed, the system frequently provides certain types of health services, such as routine vaccinations or shots, that the soldier or sailor would really rather not have. The individual has little choice regarding who will provide the treatment or where, but at the same time, the services are always there

if needed, without the need to search them out. If a physician's services are needed, they are obtained; if hospitalization is required, it is arranged; if emergency transportation is necessary, it is carried out. There is little that the individual can do to influence how medical care is provided, but at the same time, there is never any worry about its availability.

The third important characteristic of the military health care system is its great emphasis on keeping personnel well, preventing illness or injury, and finding health problems early while they are still amenable to treatment. Great stress is placed on preventive measures such as vaccination, regular physical examinations and testing, and educational efforts toward prevention of accidents and contagious diseases. In an approach that is unique among the health care systems of this country, the military medical system provides health care, and not just sickness care.

In the military medical system, the same mass public health and preventive medicine services that are provided to a locality or a community by a local government health department or health agency may also be provided to the active-duty military personnel. Whenever the personnel are actually within the boundaries of a military reservation or post, however, an additional set of mass public health and preventive medicine services may be provided by the military itself. Sanitary disposal of sewage, protection of food and milk, purification of the water supply, and prevention of vehicular or job-related accidents may be provided for by a local government agency, but each military installation usually has a second, separate system of its own, staffed by its own public health and safety officers. Individual public health and preventive medicine services are also provided by the military medical system according to a well-organized, regularly scheduled routine of yearly examinations, surveys of patient records, vaccinations, and other measures. The persons providing the specific preventive service (for example, a routine tetanus shot) are usually medical corpspersons or other nonphysician personnel; however, their work is carried out according to carefully developed guidelines and is monitored by well-trained supervisory medical personnel.

Routine ambulatory care is usually provided to most active-duty military personnel by the same medics who provide the individual preventive services. These services are usually provided at the dispensary, sick bay, first-aid station, or similar unit that is very close to the military personnel's actual place of work. These ambulatory services may also be provided by physicians or nurses at the same locations, but this is less likely. More complicated ambulatory patient care services are usually provided by physicians, frequently specialists, working at the same dispensary or medical station as the medics or, more likely, in a clinic or outpatient department of a larger facility such as a military hospital. Patients are usually referred by medics or physicians who have first cared for the patients for simpler problems; laboratory tests, X-ray examinations, and medications are obtained at the same military facility to which the patient is referred.

The simplest hospital services are provided using short-stay beds at base dispensaries, in sick bays aboard ship, or at small base hospitals on various military installations around the world. Usually the range of services that can be offered at these installations is limited, and referral to larger institutions is routinely carried out if a more complex problem is suspected. More complicated hospital services are provided to active-duty military personnel in regional hospitals that possess a wide variety of specialized services and facilities. Frequently, these hospitals also have large teaching and training programs, where the atmosphere and the quality of care are similar to what might be expected at a university hospital or a large community teaching hospital.

The military medical system does not pretend to offer the same extensive range of long-term care services that it provides for more acute short-term problems. The military medical system does provide care for potentially long-range problems in military hospitals, as long as there is some reasonable expectation that the patient will someday be able to return to full active duty. Whenever it is determined, however, that the problem is genuinely long-term in nature and that complete return to active duty is not possible, the patient is given a medical discharge from the service and long-term care is provided through the Veterans Administration (VA) facilities.

If military personnel develop emotional difficulties, care is most likely to be provided initially by the medical corpsperson, and then by a physician assigned to that military unit. These personnel provide short-term nonpsychiatric support and counseling, and possibly prescribe certain medications such as tranquilizers. For more severe problems, patients are referred to the psychiatric services of larger military hospitals where the severity of the problem is determined. If the problem is short-term and is not believed to affect the patient's work seriously, an attempt may be made to provide the short-term treatment at the military hospital itself, first on an inpatient and later on an outpatient basis. If there is a significant psychiatric diagnosis, the patient is most likely to be given a medical discharge, with follow-up care to be provided through the psychiatric services of the VA hospitals.

The military medical system is a closely organized, highly integrated, rational, and regionalized approach. A single patient record is used, and the complete record moves from one health care service to another with the patient. Once the need for health care is identified, the system itself arranges for the patient to receive the required care and usually even provides transportation to the services. The patient does not have to search out the necessary service or determine how to use it. This service is provided at no cost to the patient, requires little effort by the patient to initiate it, and generally involves a relatively high-quality product. The system is centrally planned, uses nonmedical and non-nursing personnel to the utmost, and is entirely self-sufficient and self-contained. The services are provided by salaried employees in facilities that are wholly owned and operated by the system itself. The system is not generally available to persons who are not active-duty military personnel or their dependents, although in cases of emergency or pressing local need, it can be. Generally, the patient has little choice regarding the manner in which services will be delivered, but this drawback is counterbalanced by the assurance that high-quality services will be available when needed.

Dependents and families of active-duty military personnel are served by a special subsystem of military medicine that combines the services of the middle-class, middle-income system and the active-duty military system. The dependents and families of active-duty military personnel are covered by an extensive health insurance plan, the Civilian Health and Medical Program of the Uniformed Services (CHAMPUS), provided, financed, and supervised by the military. This health insurance plan allows dependents and families of active-duty personnel to purchase medical care from private practitioners, from health maintenance organizations, and from local community nonmilitary hospitals when similar services cannot be provided at a military installation within a reasonable distance. The dependents and families of active-duty military personnel can also use the same military services that the active-duty personnel use, provided space and resources are available and military authorities determine that this procedure is appropriate. The resulting subsystem of care for military dependents and families generally allows them to participate to some degree in two separate systems of care: the middle-class, middle-

income private practice system and the military medical system. Their participation in either is generally not as clearly focused or as active as it would be for someone firmly planted in either system exclusively, but it still provides them with two viable options for obtaining care.

Veterans Administration Health Care System

Parallel to the system of care for active duty military personnel is another system operated within the continental United States for retired, disabled, and otherwise deserving veterans of previous United States military service. Although the VA system is in many respects larger than the system of care for active-duty military personnel, it is not nearly as complete, well-integrated, or extensive. At the present time, the VA system focuses largely on hospital care, mental health services, and long-term care. It operates 171 hospitals throughout the country that provide most VA care. In recent years, the VA has increasingly provided outpatient services and now maintains more than 200 outpatient clinics. In very recent years, the VA has announced plans to become a much more comprehensive and complete system of care, with major emphasis to be placed on primary care.

A second important characteristic of the VA system is the great preponderance of male patients with multiple-system problems. By and large, the patients using the VA health care system are older, inactive men in whom the occurrence of multiple and chronic physical and emotional illnesses is much higher than in the general population.

A third important feature of the VA system is its existence as only one part of a much larger system of social services and benefits for veterans. Many of the people eligible to use the VA health care system are also receiving other kinds of financial benefits; indeed, access to the VA health care system is sometimes directly dependent on eligibility for financial benefits of various types, including educational assistance grants and disability compensation. Since health care is only one of many VA programs, a great variety of social services interact with and compete for available resources.

A further feature of the VA health care system is its unique relationship with organized consumer groups. Since the VA is organized to provide care exclusively for veterans, and since many of those veterans are members of local and national veterans' clubs and associations, the VA health care system is constantly in direct communication with groups representing the interests of veterans. In a manner that is unparalleled in any other health care system in this country, the interests of the veterans are constantly conveyed to individual VA hospitals, to the VA administrative body in Washington D.C., and to the United States Congress. In no other health care system in this country does organized consumer interest play such a constant, important, and influential role.

Since the VA system is primarily a hospital system, there are few attempts to provide general public health services or routine ambulatory care services. Veterans usually obtain these services from some other system of care, either the middle-income system or the local government system that serves the urban poor. The VA does provide the more complicated ambulatory services, usually through its hospital outpatient clinics. This care is in preparation for possible hospital admission or as follow-up after hospitalization. Many veterans who require these services obtain them from other systems of care and come to the VA system only after a condition is apparent and hospitalization is required. Admission to VA hospitals can be gained through the ambulatory patient care services operated by the VA itself, by direct referrals from physicians in private practice, or by referrals from hospitals in the community. The services in VA hospitals are provided by salaried, full-time medical

and nursing personnel; as in the military medical system, most of the VA hospitals are self-contained, relatively self-sufficient units that require little outside support or staff.

The VA health care system provides a tremendous quantity of long-term care for both physical and emotional illnesses. Indeed, the VA is probably the largest single provider of long-term care in the country, if not the world. In addition to providing considerable long-term care in the acute, short-term care hospitals, the VA also operates a number of domicilaries and nursing homes and pays for care in local community nursing homes and skilled nursing facilities.

The VA system of care is difficult to describe fully for two important reasons. First, it is a system that does not attempt to provide a complete range of services, but instead concentrates on acute hospital services and on long-term care for physical and emotional problems. Second, eligibility for entry into the system is somewhat unclear and sometimes open to variable local interpretation. The system is designed to serve veterans with service-connected disabilities, but offers services to other veterans if they cannot obtain adequate care elsewhere and if adequate VA resources are available. In practice, the actual eligibility requirements and patient mix may vary substantially from one VA hospital to the next.

If the system of health care for active-duty military personnel focuses on preventive, ambulatory, and acute inpatient care, the VA system of care stresses long-term, chronic inpatient care for both physical and emotional problems. Whereas the military medical system offers a complete, well-integrated, well-coordinated package of health care services, the services that the VA offers are primarily hospital-related. In contrast to the military medical system, which actively seeks out and offers services to patients as part of their work environment, the VA provides its services to patients only when they come forward to seek them. Despite these reservations about the VA as a complete system of health care, it should be stressed that the VA serves as the primary source of inpatient hospital care for hundreds of thousands of veterans each year and is a potential source of inpatient care for millions more. As such, it is one of the largest single providers of health care services in this country and must be considered an integral, important component of the American health care scene, both now and in the future.

HEALTH SERVICES: A SUMMARY OF PERSPECTIVES

In reviewing each of these major systems of health care for Americans—the system for employed, insured, middle-income families who use the private sector services; the local government system for the urban poor; the military medical system for active-duty military personnel and their dependents; and the VA system for veterans—it becomes apparent that there are a number of additional systems that could be included as well. Other systems of health care include the one used by rural farming families and the Indian Health Service operated for Native Americans by the federal government. There are also many possible variations within the four systems discussed here. The purpose, however, is not to be exhaustive in describing the systems themselves but rather to point out that there are multiple systems providing services to different populations with different needs. No one system predominates in terms of persons served or benefits provided. Indeed, the purpose here is to point out that there is no one single American health care system but rather a mosaic of subsystems, each with its own characteristics and moving in its own direction.

Is it bad to have so many separate subsystems? Why is it even worth pointing out the obvious fact that many such subsystems exist? There are several pressing reasons for reviewing this country's compartmentalized organization of health care. The first and most important reason is quite simple: in order to improve health service to everyone in the country, an understanding of the component parts of the present health care structure is essential. Without a fundamental understanding of the separate component parts, it is impossible to understand the whole structure. Without an understanding of the interaction among the component parts, one cannot design really appropriate and effective interventions and changes.

The second reason for considering the various separate systems of health care in this country is the vigorous competition for scarce resources of money, people, and facilities. Although the four systems described are separate from one another, they all compete for the same resources, since they are all dependent on the same economy and the same supplies of health personnel and skills.

Whenever there is vigorous competition for resources, two things frequently happen. First, the stronger, more vigorous, more aggressive, or better connected competitors obtain the larger portion of the resources, whether or not this outcome is justified by their needs. In practice, this has meant that the middle-income/private practice system, the military medical system, and the VA system have all done relatively well, while the local government health care system for the poor has always been severely underfinanced and understaffed, a situation that seems to be getting progressively worse.

Second, intense competition for resources frequently results in wasteful duplication and ineffective use of resources. For example, in the same region, a city or county hospital, a private teaching hospital, a military hospital, and a VA hospital may all be operating exactly the same kind of expensive service, although only one facility might be needed, and undoubtedly one large integrated service would provide more efficient use of resources than four smaller ones. Because each institution is part of a separate system, serves a different population, and approaches the resource pool through a different channel, no really purposeful planning or controlled allocation of resources is possible. In the past, this situation might have been acceptable because the resources seemed endless, but in these days of very limited resources, this is no longer acceptable.

In addition to this economic inefficiency, there are other reasons for looking with a critical eye at multiple systems of care, reasons that are related to quality and accessibility of services. Unfortunately, not all of these subsystems of care serve people in the same way with the same results. There is great inequality among the various systems of health care, with the result that different people receive different levels of care simply by accident of birth or membership in a special group. Since all the separate systems of health care in this country ultimately depend on public funds for their continued existence, it is imperative that the inequalities among them be removed as rapidly as possible. This does not necessarily mean eliminating the various separate subsystems of care, but rather requires that all the systems rise to a common high level and equitably share responsibilities and resources.

In the past, there have been various approaches to the question of multiple subsystems of care serving different portions of the American population. All of these approaches have used specific mechanisms of financing, planning, or regulation with the shared purpose of developing a more integrated, more effective, and less costly health care system for the country. Although these proposals have often been limited in nature, their overall purpose generally has been to move the various pieces of the American health care system into a better relationship with each other. These approaches are interesting not only in themselves but also because they tell us more about ourselves and about the possibilities of health care in the United States.

One approach to rationalizing the health care system has been to develop a system of universal health insurance coverage for all people in the United States. Under this type of approach (sometimes referred to as either "national health insurance" or "universal coverage"), the differences in financing disappear and all people are able to approach the delivery system with equal resources and access. Once the differences in health insurance status are removed, it is argued, the system for providing health care will function in a much more rational fashion, with populations approaching individual providers because they chose to do so, not because they must because of their membership in one group or another. Unfortunately, national health insurance and universal coverage have not been easy to develop, and there seems little indication that things will be any different in the near future.

Another proposal that has been considered and actually tried for a short while has been the voluntary (or semivoluntary) health planning approach. With the passage of the original Comprehensive Health Planning legislation and, more important, with the passage of the National Health Planning and Resources Development Act of 1974, it had been thought that providers, consumers, and public officials might come together and develop plans for all states and localities that would then become blueprints for a more rationally organized system of care. This hope did not turn into reality, primarily because of conflicts concerning power and control, and with the demise of the health planning system, this approach toward more rational coordination of health care services has been virtually abandoned. It is doubtful that there will be a return to anything resembling a government-sponsored health planning system again; it is also doubtful that planning without control of subsequent financing of health services (sometimes called "planning without teeth") has any chance of success.

A somewhat different approach to rationalizing the American health care system focuses on the use of financing mechanisms to encourage efficiencies or to force increased coordination of effort throughout the system. The proponents of this line of thought suggest that the power to withhold financial reimbursement to providers who do not comply with efforts to improve the system would be so strong as to be irresistible. Although the argument is used more visibly by many of the proponents of a national health insurance plan, it has also become a major lever by which the Health Care Financing Administration (HCFA) uses Medicare and Medicaid funds to encourage compliance with its long range objectives. It is also evident in the actions of private employers who espouse a return to a more free-market approach to health care; in this approach, purchasers use the power of their economic leverage to force the system to become more efficient and deliver a better product at a lower price. Indeed, it would have to be said that, whatever the specific source, the greatest forces shaping the health care system at present are financial and the greatest power to effect change in the system in the future is in the hands of the large third-party payers for health care: employers, Medicare, and Medicaid.

In the end it should be realized that the American health care system is continuing to evolve not only in response to short-term events and pressures that appear from time to time, but also in response to long-term, strongly held beliefs about our country, our people, and health care. In thinking about the future, the health care professional must keep in mind both the short-term current events, which may seem to be most important on any particular day, and the long-term history, traditions, and values of our people and our system of health care that *are* most important over the years. Our health care system is a product of history and current events, and each professional must be well prepared to deal with both.

PART II

CAUSES AND CHARACTERISTICS OF
HEALTH CARE UTILIZATION

CHAPTER

The Physiologic and Psychological Bases of Health, Disease, and Care-Seeking

Lawrence A. May

CHAPTER TOPICS

LEARNING OBJECTIVES

Upon completing this chapter, the reader should be able to:

- Understand the fundamental nature of disease and illness.
- Assess disease processes and the nature of diagnosis.
- Appreciate the relationship between medicine and social, psychological, and cultural aspects of society.
- Appreciate the relationship between the availability and use of health care services.

In this chapter, the physiological bases of disease and the psychological characteristics of care-seeking behavior are explored. The concepts of illness and disease and the complexities surrounding the exact definitions of diseases are discussed. The orderly relationship among pathologic abnormality, physiologic alteration, and clinical manifestations of disease are presented, especially as they relate to care-seeking behavior. The influence of biologic, pharmacologic, and environmental factors on changing disease patterns is reviewed, and some of the effects of these changing disease patterns on the health services system are demonstrated as a prelude to the remaining chapters of the book.

DEFINING ILLNESS AND DISEASE

The distinction between illness and disease is essential for the understanding of care-seeking behavior. Illness is a lay experience that connotes both a physical and a social state (Apple, 1960). It is an individual's reaction to a biologic alteration and is defined differently by different people according to their state of mind and cultural beliefs. The term *illness,* therefore, is imprecise and represents an individual response to a set of physiologic and psychological stimuli.

By contrast, *disease* is a professional construct. It is perceived as being precise and reflecting the highest state of professional knowledge, particularly that of the physician. The definition of disease is used as the vehicle for informing the patient of the presence of pathology, as a means for deciding on a course of treatment, and as a basis for comparing the results of therapy. It becomes an essential element in the planning and organization of the health care system and in the allocation of resources within that system.

The accurate definition of disease is so important that it is crucial to recognize that considerable imprecision exists in the process of medical diagnosis. An individual physician using the best professional judgment available may diagnose a disease in a particular patient, but this definition may not be shared by other physicians. Even when the definition of a particular disease is similar in different patients, the impact of the diagnosis on those patients may vary widely, depending upon how the definition is applied and on the unique social and biologic characteristics of individual patients.

Attempts to link illness (the individual's perception of loss of functional capacity) with disease (the professional's definition of a pathologic process) is even more complicated. Illness may occur in the absence of real disease, and disease may be present in the absence of perceived illness. It is illness, the individual's perception of impaired function, and not disease that stimulates care-seeking behavior, making the relationship between these two concepts important to understand.

There can be difficulty in defining illness and disease, and significant cognitive dissonance between physician and patient may result. Mitral valve prolapse, a rather common abnormality of a heart valve with a prevalence of five to ten percent of the population, has had an assortment of symptoms attributed to it. Fatigue, irritability, dizziness, and palpitations have all been suggested as symptoms of this condition. A study at Duke University, however, failed to reveal any difference in symptoms in the patients with objectively conformed mitral valve prolapse from a group that had been referred for echocardiographic studies in which no mitral valve prolapse was discovered (Retchin, et al., 1986). Although the control group in this study was not selected randomly, it illustrates that symptoms may exist and be attributable to a medical disease that are, in fact, equally prevalent in a similar population without the disease.

This problem is further illustrated in the case of hypertension, a condition that physicians acknowledge as asymptomatic, but one to which patients attribute a wide variety of symptoms. The generally acknowledged symptoms of headache, ringing in the ears, and nosebleeds failed to be confirmed as having any greater prevalence in those with hypertension than in those without it. The need for patients who perceive themselves as ill to have a disease explanation for their symptoms can pose a major challenge to the physicians; and if a medical explanation for essentially functional symptoms is provided, notable care-seeking behavior can result.

A powerful example of this has been the possible association of chronic fatigue with persistent infection with the Epstein-Barr virus (Tobi & Straus, 1985). This was originally reported in a group of ninety patients who were evaluated for persistent fatigue by several physicians near Lake Tahoe in California (Centers for Disease Control, 1986). The media coverage of this situation created a tremendous interest on the part of patients in determining whether they might be suffering from a disease for which there is admittedly no cure, and for which such poorly defined parameters exist that physicians cannot conclude that the disease actually exists. (A similar historical example was hypoglycemia, which produced numerous physical visits for glucose tolerance tests that are generally felt to

be unnecessary; true hypoglycemia is rare, and symptoms are generally absent in patients with blood sugar levels below the reported normal levels.) The search for an etiologic agent in the well-described syndrome of chronic fatigue has led investigators to consider other etiologic agents, such as herpes virus type 6. Other authors have offered enteroviruses, Borrelia, and a novel retrovirus as possible etiologic agents for chronic fatigue syndrome. The ability of science to establish specific etiology to relatively commonly described and experienced syndromes is apparently limited (Buchwald, et al., 1992).

Examples of Disease Definition

The complexity of defining disease and its interaction with care-seeking behavior is well illustrated by the condition diabetes mellitus. Both the general public and the health care professional understand that diabetes results in an elevated blood sugar level, but the physiologic bases of this metabolic alteration can vary widely (Siperstein, 1975). In one person, the disease may result from impaired secretion of insulin by the pancreas, or it may be caused by a resistance to sufficient amounts of insulin in a patient who is obese. Diabetes mellitus may result from the imposition of a normal physiologic condition such as pregnancy, or it may be due to the use of exogenous drugs such as diuretics or steroids.

Aside from the varying causes of an elevated blood sugar level (referred to as *hyperglycemia),* an important issue is the amount of hyperglycemia that defines a patient as diabetic. Various criteria have been suggested to define who is diabetic, using different numerical measures of elevated blood sugar level, but these criteria do not necessarily separate those who feel healthy, nor do they define a level at which treatment is indicated (O'Sullivan & Mahan, 1968). The myriad criteria that have been applied to diabetes at one time or another would define anywhere between four percent and forty percent of the population over age sixty as having diabetes. In recognition of the fact that even objective measures of disease or health such as blood sugar determination are variable, great effort was expended to reach a consensus on what level of blood sugar elevation defines diabetes. The criteria state that the level must be consistently elevated in the fasting and postprandial states and that this level must be found on two separate occasions. The current criteria for diagnosis of diabetes are a fasting blood sugar level of 140 and a blood sugar level of more than 200 measured two hours after eating on two separate occasions. The previously widely used glucose tolerance test is expensive, unnecessary, and results in an excessive number of false-positive readings in a way that is unacceptable.

The problem illustrated by diabetes extends to many other disease conditions that are defined by an abnormal laboratory measurement or blood test result. Hypertension is a common medical problem resulting from a variety of physiologic bases, including abnormalities in hormone production and use, improper resetting of neurologic control centers, and acquired loss of blood vessel elasticity secondary to atherosclerosis. In view of the variety of causes of hypertension, the selection of an arbitrary number to define individuals or members of a population as having an abnormal condition is a difficult and possibly futile effort. The blood pressure reading of 140/90 has been offered as the boundary of normality, but the meaning of this reading in different persons may vary markedly. A blood pressure of 150/100 in a seventy-two-year-old woman has quite different implications from the same reading in a twenty-six-year-old man. An elevated blood pressure after a half hour of bed rest means something quite different from an elevated blood pressure in a person waiting anxiously for half an hour in a physician's office.

To complicate matters further, as with diabetes, there is no direct relationship between the presence of elevated blood pressure and the development of either perceived symptoms or actual pathologic damage to body organs, at least at the lower ranges of hypertension. Some people with only slight hypertension will attribute a variety of functional complaints to their "blood pressure," whereas others with dangerously elevated levels may not have any symptoms and perceive themselves as being well (Mabry, 1964; Weiss, 1972).

The definition of diabetes or of hypertension is relatively straightforward when compared to diseases that cannot be numerically defined, such as rheumatoid arthritis. The definition of this disease is clinical rather than numerical and is based on the presence of four or more diagnostic characteristics determined by the American Rheumatism Association to be valid criteria for the disease. Even with the use of this symptom aggregation approach, there are still many professionals who confuse rheumatoid arthritis with degenerative joint disease and other forms of arthritis. Further, even with this more orderly approach to the definition of this disease, the ability to measure its impact on a population is comparatively limited.

In summary, the definition of disease is a more imprecise and inexact process than is usually thought. Although it is frequently associated with apparently solid, objective measurements such as blood sugar levels or blood pressure, the implications of these values may vary widely. Finally, the relationship between illness, which is a personal observation by patients, and disease, which is a scientific judgment by professionals, needs to be understood and constantly remembered.

DISEASE PROCESSES

The major pathophysiologic processes involved in disease production are vascular, inflammatory, neoplastic, toxic, metabolic, and degenerative. These processes give rise to disease conditions, but their expression is modified by factors in the host such as age, immunologic status, medication ingestion, concurrent disease, and psychological perceptions. The combination of the pathophysiologic processes and the different host factors creates the various patterns of disease presentation.

Vascular abnormalities may produce disease in a variety of ways in multiple-organ systems. The gradual narrowing and eventual blockage of blood vessels by the deposit of fatty materials in the walls and lumina of the vessels is a characteristic of arteriosclerotic cardiovascular disease. Vascular disease may also be produced by the more rapid occlusion of a blood vessel by an embolus, material from a distant site floating in the bloodstream. Other disease pictures may be produced by bleeding from a ruptured blood vessel in the brain or elsewhere. In some disease conditions, such as stroke, the same clinical picture may result from any one of these three causes. Whatever the initial cause, gradual occlusion, embolus, or rupture, the result is damage to brain tissue and resultant paralysis. It is usually easy to determine that a cerebrovascular accident (stroke) has occurred, but it is frequently impossible to determine whether it was caused by gradual occlusion, embolus, or rupture of a blood vessel.

Inflammation is the basis of disease in many organ systems, but the physiologic basis of that inflammation may be infectious, autoimmune, traumatic, or something else. A single inflamed joint may be due to autoimmune inflammation, the presence of uric acid crystals, or degeneration of cartilage as a consequence of age and use, or it may be due to infection with bacteria or virus. The failure to identify the specific etiologic factor can be highly destructive to the patient, or at least fail to resolve the problem in the appropriate amount of time. Therefore, having defined both the type of

disorder and the mechanism of inflammation, physicians must seek to identify the underlying agent in the process of inflammation.

Neoplastic disease is caused by an abnormal new growth of tissue. Benign neoplasms are abnormal growths that remain localized and do not spread to distant locations in the body. Malignant neoplasms, generally called *cancer,* by contrast, not only grow locally and invade surrounding tissues but also spread to distant sites in the body, producing metastases. Benign neoplasms may cause considerable damage by continued local growth and pressure on surrounding tissues, such as pressure on the brain from a benign growth on its surface. Malignant neoplasms, by contrast, invade the organs directly and disrupt their normal functioning by replacing normal tissue with diseased tissue. Neoplasms may occur spontaneously or may be caused by environmental, toxic, or host factors (Ballard-Barbash, et al., 1990; Farrow & Davis, 1990; Merliss, 1971; Poskanzer & Herbst, 1977; Selikoff, et al., 1964).

Toxic bases for disease involve the presentation to individual organs of chemical materials that are inherently damaging. These materials may originate from environmental pollutants, from the use of potentially damaging materials such as alcohol or cigarettes, or from the ingestion of medications. Alcohol, for example, is toxic to the liver under appropriate conditions, causing hepatitis, fibrosis, and eventual cirrhosis. Cobalt in beer can be toxic to heart muscle cells, bee stings may damage the glomerulus of the kidney, and asbestos may contribute to the development of lung cancer. Cigarette smoking may destroy, inflame, or alter the cells of the lung, producing emphysema, chronic bronchitis, or cancer. Digitalis, an ordinarily useful drug in the treatment of various heart conditions, in excess doses may produce toxicity and life-threatening arrhythmias. In a society with an increasing amount of environmental pollution, drug use, and industrial exposure, toxins are unfortunately becoming a more common cause of disease. The widening hole in the ozone layer is producing precipitous increases in the incidence of cutaneous malignancies (Glass & Hoover, 1989).

Metabolic diseases are caused by chemical disorders within body cells, usually secondary to excess or deficiency of a hormone or nutrient. The excess or deficiency of a thyroid, parathyroid, or adrenal cortical hormone causes clinical disease pictures that are easily recognized by well-trained physicians. A deficiency of insulin, secreted by glands in the pancreas, gives rise to diabetes, as mentioned earlier. Deficiency of important nutrients, caused either by a scarcity of the elements in the diet or by an inability to absorb and use them, results in a wide variety of clinical pictures ranging from anemia to pellagra. The incidence of deficiency states in the developed world is still staggering, and simple supplementation with such minerals as iodine or such vitamins as vitamin A have produced dramatic improvement in health status (Tonglet, et al., 1992).

Degeneration is the final pathophysiologic cause of disease, and may occur as a primary idiopathic disorder or secondary to another process such as aging. Physicians generally resist accepting degeneration as an explanation for disease, but there are many diseases that currently cannot be otherwise explained. For example, many people with senile dementia have a pathologic process of unexplained primary degeneration of brain cells. Degenerative joint disease is usually related to age and may be accelerated by unusual use or trauma, but it remains primarily a degenerative process with no specific vascular, metabolic, or inflammatory explanation.

It should also be clear that a particular disease can be caused or affected by a variety of pathophysiologic mechanisms. Peptic ulcer, for example, is a common disease with a multifactorial physiologic basis. The ulceration of the mucosal lining of the duodenum is caused by gastric acid, may occur in genetically predisposed people, and may be abetted by the toxic effect of drugs such as aspirin or corticosteroids that impair the protective barrier of the mucosa. After all of the insights about ulcer pathogenesis, both psychologic and dietary, the real cause may emerge to be an infectious agent known as Helicobacter pylori (Peterson, 1990). There may be a secondary inflammation producing pain or obstruction, and the ulcer may erode a blood vessel, producing bleeding. To say that any single pathophysiologic process "causes" ulcers would be misleading.

Once the initial pathophysiologic process has given rise to a particular disease entity, its clinical manifestations are modified by a variety of host factors such as age, immunologic status, medication ingestion, concurrent disease, or psychological makeup. For example, in a healthy person with high tolerance for pain, a case of herpes zoster (shingles) may be perceived as a minor discomfort, whereas in a person with a low threshold for pain, it may become a disabling illness for which professional attention and potent analgesics are required. Under the influence of a concurrent disease or the ingestion of drugs such as steroids, which suppress the immunologic response, a usually nonpathogenic fungal infection may produce serious illness. A minor inflammation of the connective tissue such as cellulitis, for example, may become a serious, life-threatening problem in a diabetic with an impaired vascular, sensory, or immunologic status. In a genetically susceptible host, an infectious agent may precipitate an inflammatory response and antibody production leading to systemic lupus erythematosus, whereas in a genetically nonsusceptible host it may not produce any effect.

Thus, there are a variety of pathophysiologic processes that can initiate disease, but the expression of the disease itself may be modified by a variety of factors in the host. Any review of a particular disease entity, therefore, should include consideration of both aspects, so that a complete understanding of the disease can be developed.

Symptom Production and the Pathologic Process

A pathologic process may begin and exist silently for some time without producing any evidence of physiologic alteration. Although the disease is present and active, it may be undiscovered. In many chronic disease situations, it is now well known that the disease condition may be present for a considerable length of time before becoming detectable by current diagnostic procedures. Atherosclerosis, for example, has been detected at autopsy in healthy young eighteen-year-olds dying from accidental causes (Enos, et al., 1958; McNamara, et al., 1971); many prostatic cancers are discovered at autopsy that were never recognized during life.

After a pathologic process has been present for a time, it may not only begin to produce physiologic alterations that can be discovered by appropriate diagnostic tests but may also begin to produce clinical symptoms that are, for the first time, recognized by the patient or the physician. There can be a significant time lag, however, between the onset of the pathologic alteration and the production of symptoms, just as there was between the onset of the pathologic process and the physiologic alteration. A pathologic process may be present and discoverable by diagnostic tests long before it produces sufficient symptoms for a patient to feel its presence. Atherosclerosis and atherosclerotic vascular disease illustrate this continuum of pathologic process, physiologic alteration, and symptom production and are reviewed to provide further insight into the disease process.

Atherosclerosis is a pathologic process characterized by focal accumulation of lipids and complex carbohydrates, producing a secondary narrowing of the arteries. The process affects arterial vessels of the body in the cerebral, coronary, peripheral, and abdominal circulations and is now the leading cause of death in the United States.

As mentioned previously, atherosclerosis without physiologic alteration has been documented in eighteen-year-olds. At this stage, it is a subclinical or presymptomatic process and can be identified only by direct examination of the blood vessels.

Coronary artery disease is a specific manifestation of atherosclerosis in the arteries that provide blood to the heart muscle. As it becomes progressively more serious, it interferes with arterial capability for providing sufficient oxygen to meet the heart muscle's metabolic demands. As the reduction in oxygen supply worsens, ischemia of the heart muscle may occur. With still further progression, any increased demand on the cardiac muscle, as in any kind of exertion, may produce angina pectoris, or chest pain, the cardinal symptoms of coronary artery disease.

Long before the angina is present, coronary artery disease may be identified by an abnormal electrocardiogram (EKG). If an EKG with the patient at rest does not produce evidence of disease, frequently an EKG during controlled exercise will yield the necessary evidence. In these cases, the coronary artery disease may not be sufficiently serious to produce EKG changes during normal demands on the heart, but the increased cardiac demands associated with exercise will provide the necessary diagnostic evidence.

These clinical changes may not evoke any symptoms, but eventually the patient may experience intermittent chest pain on exertion and seek medical care. At this time, the chances of obtaining an abnormal EKG and confirming the presence of coronary artery disease become much greater, but even at this stage a patient may have typical angina pain with an apparently normal EKG. The difficulty of defining the specific relationship between pathology and symptoms may be even greater.

Both resting and exercise EKGs produce a number of false-positive and false-negative results. The absolute criterion for the definition of coronary artery disease becomes arteriography, the injection of dye to outline the coronary artery and the areas of narrowing. It should be understood, however, that many people with no symptoms have demonstrable coronary artery disease, and that many others with classical anginal symptoms and characteristic EKG abnormalities have coronary arteries free of atherosclerosis (Miranda, et al., 1991). It has been well established in the literature that the same objective alterations in the EKG and classic symptoms may be produced by spasm rather that occlusion of the coronary arteries (Fuster, et al., 1992).

In patients with occlusive coronary artery disease, atherosclerosis may eventually occlude a coronary artery completely, causing the heart muscles supplied by the artery to die. This clinical event is known as *myocardial infarction,* commonly called a "heart attack," and is accompanied by prolonged chest pains, nausea, sweating, shortness of breath, and weakness. The arterial occlusion and subsequent tissue death, however, may occur silently and without symptoms, to be discovered by EKG at some later date.

Following the pathologic process a step further, loss of heart muscle function secondary to coronary artery disease may affect the heart's ability to maintain adequate circulation to the rest of the body and may produce a range of secondary signs and symptoms in other organs. As the heart becomes weaker, there may be progressive difficulty in breathing, swelling of the legs and feet, inability to maintain blood supply to the brain and subsequent faintness, and impairment of kidney function with reduction of urinary output. These events are sometimes labeled by the single clinical description of *heart failure.*

Atherosclerosis is a generalized disease and is usually not limited to the coronary arteries; similar events occur in the blood vessels of other organs. This process may produce primary effects in organs that are not related to the secondary effects of heart failure described above. Abdominal pain, bowel necrosis, neurologic deficits, strokes, renal failure, calf pain, and aortic aneurysms may all be produced by atherosclerotic damage to the arteries of various organs. The combination of this primary damage to the organs themselves and the secondary effects of heart failure is complicated and serious, dramatically illustrating why atherosclerosis is such a major cause of morbidity and mortality.

THE PHYSIOLOGIC BASES OF DISEASE

Over the years, the pattern of diseases affecting the United States population has changed profoundly, generally as a result of changes in the environment, in the population's demographic composition, and in medical practice. Infectious diseases as the major cause of mortality have been replaced by chronic diseases associated with aging. At the turn of the century, infectious diseases struck the young and healthy and spread rapidly, often resulting in death. The confluence of improved sanitation, a higher standard of living, antibiotics, and vaccines reduced death and disability from infectious diseases so markedly that they are now a comparatively minor cause of death (see Chapter 1).

The treatability of syphilis, for example, has reduced its incidence and impact markedly, and cases with the secondary or tertiary manifestations of this potentially devastating disorder are now increasingly rare. Smallpox, polio, mumps, diphtheria, measles, pertussis, rubella, tetanus, typhoid, and cholera, all once highly prevalent, have now all but disappeared. Bacterial infections of childhood and infantile diarrheas of all kinds are now effectively treated with antibiotics and intravenous feedings; as a result, they do not present the threat they did at the turn of the twentieth century.

While these disease entities have been diminished or are disappearing, new disease patterns have been emerging to take their place as the most important threat to life and health. Some of these patterns have resulted from the removal of diseases in early life (for example, childhood infections), which has allowed time for disease in later life (for example, atherosclerosis) to appear. Other disease patterns, however, are comparatively new, are far more prevalent than they once were, and are the result of new forces in modern life and environment.

Tuberculosis illustrates how a disease can come under control only to reassert itself with an influx of immigrants from areas where the disease is still endemic, and to emerge in a more virulent form among a vulnerable population such as those with the HIV virus. Tuberculosis, once the scourge of our public hospitals, is again emerging as a major public health crisis (Bloch, et al., 1989).

Changes in the incidence and prevalence of some cancers also provide dramatic evidence of these new patterns. In the early part of the century, cancer of the lung was not a major cause of death, but it began to increase in men as the rate of cigarette smoking in men increased. The incidence of lung cancer in women lagged behind that of men until recently, when it began to rise to a comparable level, probably secondary to the increase in cigarette smoking among women.

In the same vein, there has been a rise in endometrial carcinoma in women, attributed at least in part to the increased use of estrogens by postmenopausal women (Schwarz, 1981; Voigt, et al., 1991). Pancreatic cancer has increased in recent years and is occurring at a younger age than previously, but no clear explanation of this changed disease pattern has been proposed. The etiologic factors contributing to the increased risk of pancreatic cancer have been subject to vigorous epidemiologic debate. Coffee in its caffeinated and decaffeinated forms has been implicated, with considerable refutation of these arguments (Gordis, 1990). Again, recent years have seen a marked rise in mesothelioma, a previously rare type of lung cancer, probably secondary to the markedly increased use of asbestos in manufacturing and construction.

In the same fashion, improvement in our medical technology has changed the patterns of disease, not just by wiping out previously existing scourges, but also by creating new ones. The morbidity and mortality of common diseases such as pneumonia and wound infections have been replaced by serious infections with once nonpathogenic bacteria that are now resistant to antibiotics. Patients whose own defense mechanisms have been compromised by corticosteroids, immunosuppressive agents, and cancer chemotherapy are now susceptible to serious infections with fungi, yeast, protozoa, or bacteria that are not normally harmful (Stamm, 1981).

A dramatic expression of a newer disease pattern is illustrated by acquired immune deficiency syndrome (AIDS), a state of serious impairment in an individual's immune mechanisms, giving rise to greatly increased susceptibility to a variety of infectious and neoplastic diseases (Centers for Disease Control, 1981). The initial descriptions of a series of previously rare infections in young and otherwise healthy homosexual men gave rise to the discovery of a condition with myriad pathologic manifestations as well as profound social and economic implications (Fauci, 1991; Wachtel, et al., 1992).

AIDS Pathogenesis

The human immunodeficiency virus (HIV) infects individuals and, in selected cases, produces a profound alteration and suppression of the host's natural immunity. The entity might therefore be considered an infectious disease because there is a specific infectious agent responsible for initiating the disease process. It must also be acknowledged, however, as an immunologic entity because the virus seems to produce no signs or symptoms but rather alters the immune system. The prevalence of infections seems to be far greater than the development of clinical expression, since there is a large population who have antibodies from the infection but who have no medically defined disease and another large population who have much milder manifestations of infection in a condition termed AIDS-related complex (ARC). Among actual AIDS patients, the manifestation of the illness covers a wide clinical spectrum, including *Pneumocystis carinii* infections of the lung, *Cryptosporidium* infections of the bowel, *Cytomegalovirus* infections of the eye, and Kaposi's sarcoma of a generalized nature.

While AIDS illustrates a fascinating new disease, its impact on care-seeking behavior may be greater than anticipated and, indeed, greater than any previous disease condition. Its existence and rapid spread have markedly changed social and sexual behavior among both the homosexual and heterosexual communities. Many people are voluntarily seeking blood tests for confirmation of possible AIDS, and serious consideration is being given to the imposition of mandatory testing for AIDS in certain special situations of travel or employment. The potential for health care workers to be infected, and conversely the risk that caretakers may transmit the virus to patients, has created considerable concern and debate about testing, as well as fear among health care providers (Centers for Disease Control, 1991). The onset of an unexplained febrile illness in a sexually active person increasingly raises fear of AIDS and stimulates a request for medical care for diseases that may be self-limited and for which no care would have previously been sought or needed. Recognition of the importance of the immune system as a critical link in the body's response to disease has increased society's awareness of possible immunity-related illnesses and has generated greater interest and greater use of health services in this regard.

Other Disease Etiologies

A substantial percentage of hospitalizations are now attributable to drug toxicity and the secondary effects of new surgical procedures such as ileojejunal bypass for morbid obesity or the complications of kidney dialysis for chronic renal disease. A wide spectrum of diseases has been attributed to drug toxicity, but among the most interesting was an epidemic produced by a contaminated, over-the-counter L-tryptophan preparation. A new syndrome called esoinophilia-myalgia was produced by a widely used nonprescription medicine with profound social and scientific implications (Varga, et al., 1992). Cardiac pacemakers prolong life but also produce a new spectrum of morbidity, as do other new prosthetic devices such as cardiac valves, artificial joints, and silicone implants. The lack of prospective studies illustrated by the breast implant controversy suggests how important it is that we monitor new technology and medical procedures from their inception. Organ transplantation has created an entirely new spectrum of biologic diseases based on intentional destruction of the body's immunologic system, its own basic protection from disease. Patients with bone marrow or renal transplants require considerable care and present diseases that are rare if they occur at all in normal, nonimmunosuppressed populations. The potential for transplanting other organs creates considerable flux in the biologic nature of disease and has frightening implications for the ability of persons to provide and pay for these services.

The increased effectiveness of medical intervention is also having a considerable effect on the patterns of disease by changing the gene controlling the incidence of certain diseases. Improvements in prenatal and high-risk obstetric care allow completion of pregnancies in diabetic women who otherwise may not have reproduced. This development may increase the prevalence of an already common disease such as diabetes. The successful introduction of vigorous physical therapy and prophylactic antibiotic use have increased the survival of patients with cystic fibrosis, and a few have successfully reproduced. The impact of the longer-term survival on the gene pool for this disease remains to be seen, but it is a good example of some of the potential hazards caused by new technology.

An additional powerful influence affecting our patterns of disease is environmental change. Motor vehicle accidents are an important cause of morbidity and mortality, and directly reflect our increasing use of the automobile for transportation. Pollution of air and water has already been suggested as at least partially causative in a number of conditions, and toxic aspects of industrial work environments have been suggested as the cause of many more. Indeed, it has been argued that as many as three-fourths of all cancers may be, in part, environmentally determined.

Dietary habits have also been suggested as contributing to changes in disease patterns in recent years. The most obvious result of dietary change is obesity, which is associated with hypertension, heart disease, and diabetes. Diverticulosis, hemorrhoids, appendicitis, and even cancer of the colon may be a consequence of changes in the amount of fiber in the Western diet. Epidemiologists have implicated certain foods as possible causes of atherosclerosis (Turpeinen, 1979). Increased salt intake has already been indicated in certain aspects of hypertension, and increased ingestion of refined sugars has definitely been associated with increased incidence of dental caries and possibly with several other conditions.

In summary, in addition to a wide variety of causes of disease and a wide variety of responses in individual hosts, the overall pattern of disease in a society can change markedly over time. In this country, the pattern of disease has moved from one of acute infectious disease several generations ago to one of chronic disease today. Further, the pattern of disease has been influenced by our ability to wipe out certain diseases, thereby allowing others to be expressed. Finally, many aspects of modern life, such as improved medical technology and environmental pollution, have caused disease patterns that have never existed before.

SOCIAL AND CULTURE INFLUENCES ON DISEASE AND BEHAVIOR

It was once estimated that seventy percent to ninety percent of all self-recognized illness is not generally treated in the conventional medical care delivery system (Dingle, et al., 1964). Conversely, it is reported that more than half of the visits to physicians are related to patient-identified problems for which no ascertainable biologic basis can be determined. It is clear from this finding that seeking medical care may or may not be associated with actual pathologic processes, and that social and cultural values greatly influence an individual's decision to visit a physician (Stoeckle & Barsky, 1980; Zola, 1966).

A large number of physician visits are for complaints in which the physiologic function is well within normal limits, but for which the patient feels that some abnormality exists. Many people seek medical attention, for example, when bowel function is basically normal and no serious pathology can be documented. For some reason, either internally generated or imposed by the prevailing culture, these patients believe that the situation is not quite right and seek medical attention. They have somehow been led to expect bowel function that is different from what they are experiencing, and a medical remedy is sought.

Symptoms of fatigue may be attributed by the patient to a nondisease such as hypoglycemia (Meador, 1965). Conversely, a disease with a well-defined physiologic basis may not produce care-seeking, since it may not be interpreted as a disease. The teenager with acne, for example, has a problem with a well-understood physiologic basis and an obvious clinical manifestation. The potential patient, however, may interpret it as a normal consequence of adolescence that will eventually resolve and for which treatment is either ineffective or unavailable (Ludwig & Gibson, 1969). Seeking care for serious conditions is often delayed because of fear, denial, incorrect knowledge, or financial concerns (Battistella, 1971).

Disease and the perception of illness are not the only reasons people seek medical care. Normal physiologic processes frequently are the occasion for seeking care. Pregnancy or contraception are certainly not pathologic or disease processes, but they usually require professional attention. Heavy menstrual flow, missed or irregular periods, and menopause are basically normal physiologic processes, and yet medical attention is frequently sought concerning them.

An event of modern times illustrates how medicalized normal physiologic processes can become and the interaction of social factors in creating the need for medical care. The increasing rates of infertility and the high incidence of cesarean sections are modern medical problems. Many have attributed the current rates of infertility to the frequent delay in childbearing (DeCherney & Berkowitz, 1982). This decrease in fertility has been well documented and has created substantial medical and psychologic problems and a tremendous base for

care-seeking. The rate of cesarean section is sometimes linked to this phenomenon and to the complex interaction of physician fear of litigation, the presence of monitoring equipment that allows detection of abnormalities that might not have affected the outcome, and the technologic advances that allow cesarean section to be performed with less morbidity than formerly existed. It is not only the perception of illness or the presence of disease, but also the alterations in normal physiological functions and changes in medical practice influenced by social and technologic interventions, that create some of the reasons for care-seeking behavior.

Indeed, in many cases, medical care is sought because the patient is healthy and wants to remain that way. Parents bring infants and small children to the pediatrician for routine evaluations in order to ensure that the child is developing normally. Adults visit their physician periodically for an examination, a chest X-ray film, a Papanicolaou smear, prostrate-specific antigen blood test, or mammogram. Indeed, all care-seeking behavior is carried out in a framework that is intensely affected by current social, cultural, and political values, regardless of the type or severity of the pathologic process. Cultural influences frequently determine what society considers to be a medical problem whereas economic or political realities determine whether medical care is sought. The complex interactions of people and doctors, the personal and cultural influence on disease, and the perception of symptoms have been extensively reviewed in the literature.

Ethnic and Psychosocial Differentials

Zborowsky (1952) studied the differences in attribution between Italian and Jewish patients. Italians were generally satisfied and ceased demanding medical care once pain relief was obtained; Jews were reluctant to take medication and continued to be concerned with the underlying cause of their discomfort rather than simply relief of pain. It can be anticipated that they would continue to seek care until they were reassured that there was no serious underlying pathology.

The deep psychologic meaning of disease was explored by Cassel (1982) in an article on suffering. He argued that suffering was experienced by people. It was not a physical construct, and it was often underappreciated by practicing physicians. He illustrated his point by suggesting that pain in circumstances such as childbirth, in which it is expected, rarely produces suffering and does not call for much care-seeking because of discomfort. In contrast, situations in which pain is unexplained may give rise to considerable suffering and continued care-seeking. He again argues that the physician's failure to appreciate and deal with the bases of suffering may lead to a failure to reassure the patient.

The complex psychologic underpinnings of care-seeking are indicated by the remarkable ability of patients to respond to placebos. Placebos, which have been effective in reducing not only subjective symptoms but also objective test results, are a testament to the importance of symbolic intervention. They argue for a complex interaction between physician and patient on both verbal and nonverbal levels and demonstrate that the encounter itself and the therapeutic relationship have meaning to the individual who seeks medical services (Brody, 1982). Many authors have argued that physicians do not fully recognize the social and cultural determinants of care-seeking. An illuminating article on the couvade syndrome demonstrated failure by physicians in a prepaid practice to recognize the influence of a woman's pregnancy on the husband's medical complaints (Lyokinji & Lamb, 1982). In the couvade syndrome, husbands of pregnant women have symptoms such as nausea, vomiting, anorexia, pain, and bloating—feelings often experienced by their wives—while having no objective organic abnormalities. In this study, husbands of pregnant women had two times the number of physician visits, four times the number of symptoms, and two times the number of prescriptions without any increase in actual pathology during the period of their wives' pregnancy as compared to other periods. The study illustrates the myriad influences on the production of symptoms and the need to seek medical care. It has been argued that consumerism and a critical analysis of health care needs and physician limitations can give rise to a more productive physician-patient relationship (Jensen, 1981). Health care administrators must understand the complex influences on care-seeking and design systems that identify both the physical abnormalities and the cultural determinants that provide the impetus for seeking medical services.

In our society, which is often characterized by an insatiable appetite for the consumption of medical resources, a converse picture exists where appropriate care-seeking is delayed. Investigators have sought to define the basis for delay in care-seeking. It is widely believed that earlier diagnosis of cancer produces a better prognosis. Failure or delay in seeking care is a substantial problem. Social scientists and administrators must determine why women fail to get recommended Pap smears and mammograms, and must consider the reluctance to have such screening procedures as flexible sigmoidoscopies to detect colon cancers. Commonly advanced reasons are time, discomfort, and finances. In addition, the image of cancer as a progressive disease with modest potential benefit from existing therapies persists. Studies have revealed that many people believe the treatment of cancer is often worse than the disease. Several studies that have tried to document the basis for delay in melanoma diagnosis noted that many patients with melanomas visited the physician for reasons other than the suspicious skin lesion (Hennrikus, et al., 1991; Krige, et al., 1991). The educational, psychological, racial, and financial characteristics of the population may have a profound effect on their care-seeking behavior, and consequently the ultimate efficacy of medical care.

As social and cultural values change, the understanding of what constitutes disease and the subsequent care-seeking patterns may change as well (Fuch, 1974; Parsons, 1958). The transference of marital adjustment and childrearing problems from the category of family problems best handled by a member of the clergy to psychologic problems best handled by a physician or psychologist is one example of this trend. The interpretation of poor school performance as a result of a medical problem has received wide attention under the general category of learning disabilities. Dyslexia, a specific process suggesting that intelligent people may have difficulty learning to read, has been considered a disease to be treated by neurologists, psychologists, optometrists, and pediatricians. The medicalization of academic underachievement is a case study worth further investigation (Rosenberg, 1992; Shaywitz, et al., 1992). The recent shift toward the description of alcoholism as a disease requiring medical treatment is another. A further example is the court decision changing abortion from a criminal act to a recognized medical service. The numerous manifestations of psychological problems represent many examples of difficult-to-define illness with a substantial political and value-laden component.

In all of these examples, it should be noted that the underlying pathologic processes have not changed; rather, it is the perception of these processes as disease or not that has been altered. In other circumstances, even our perception of certain conditions as illnesses does not change; instead, external social values change the way we react to them. Psychologic factors may even increase the incidence of the most common diseases (Cohen, et al., 1991).

For example, the increased mobility and weakened family structure of modern American life have made it more difficult to care for elderly and infirm family members at home. Smaller housing units, increased numbers of families in which both adults are employed, and a variety of other social pressures have altered the ability to handle the health problems of the elderly in the fashion of the past. Instead, society has created a new network of health institutions—nursing homes—to provide professional care for pathologic processes that previously were handled at home. The underlying pathologic processes have remained the same. It is the societal response to them that has changed (Somers, 1982).

In other circumstances, the increased availability of information has led to profound changes in the way that patients perceive illness or the ways in which those illnesses are treated. For example, the increase in patient information about asthma has led to dramatic changes in the locus of care for this illness. The focus of treatment of childhood asthma in the home with increasing availability of diagnostic tests and therapy to be self initiated has resulted in great improvement of care and reduction of costs (Lahdensuo, et al., 1996).

Alternative and Traditional Approaches

One of the most ironic developments in the technologic explosions of the 1990s has been a resurgence of interest in older therapies and alternative medicine. A survey conducted by investigators at the Harvard Medical School reported that thirty-four percent of Americans were using at least one type of alternative therapy (Eisenberg, et al., 1993). This is a quintessential example of patient initiated care-seeking. Moreover, the expenditures for these services are largely paid directly "out of pocket": it is estimated that as much out-of-pocket money is expended on alternative therapies as it is for hospital-based care.

The interest in alternative medicine appears to be reaching a crescendo. Many articles have appeared in diverse mass market periodicals, and books on alternative medicine are emerging on best sellers lists in a wide-ranging set of topics (Gordon, 1996; Rosenfeld, 1996; Weil, 1995). Prestigious medical schools, including Columbia, UCLA, and Harvard, are developing small departments instructing medical students, conducting research, and offering continuing medical education in alternative medical procedures to traditionally trained physicians.

The reemergence of ancient and often unproven therapies at a time of medicine's greatest technological achievement perhaps highlights increasing patient dissatisfaction with an impersonal, highly technical, increasingly corporate medical system. This new trend is patient-driven and illustrates the increasing interest of people to play a more important part in selection of medical care. This increased interest in alternative medicine has had two important results: (1) to increase the use of these therapies by patients, and (2) to force traditional practitioners and educational institutions to take these alternative therapies more seriously.

THE INFLUENCE OF SUPPLY

Within the total spectrum of pathologic processes that affect the health of people in this country, it is important to note that some processes receive much more interest and attention from the health care system than others. It is also important to speculate about why this occurs.

The structure and availability of health services contribute significantly to the amount and nature of the care that will be sought. Once the patient makes the initial decision to seek professional attention, much of the additional medical care results directly from the decisions of the physician (Fuch, 1974). The physician usually decides what laboratory tests, X-ray films, treatment procedures, and hospitalizations are necessary and, in so doing, shapes a particular pattern of care for each patient. In some ways, these decisions by the physician also shape the health care system itself by creating a demand for certain services. As long as the demand exists, the institutions, programs, and services will expand to fill the need.

But does the process work this way, or is the reverse true? Do pathologic processes stimulate patients to visit physicians, who, in turn, demand certain services as a result of their decisions? Or do the specialized services become available to physicians, thereby influencing the manner in which they approach disease, and do physicians then shape patients' perceptions and demands on the basis of what they know is available (Stoeckle, et al., 1963)? There is some evidence to suggest that the latter is true, at least in part, and is becoming progressively more important.

Physicians generally do most of their training in hospitals and are introduced early to the use and benefits of sophisticated procedures and tests. The availability of these tests and treatment then influence the physicians' view of disease, since they now make possible the treatment of conditions that were previously beyond consideration. The surgical treatment of degenerative processes, such as hip replacement for osteoarthritis, laser treatment for diabetic retinopathy, and replacement of diseased heart valves with prosthetic devices, has created many new options for the physician. These treatments have also created new reasons for patients to seek care.

Unfortunately, the development of these new approaches is not always in keeping with the real need for care among patients, as determined by the pathologic processes that threaten them. The mere fact that a particular process, such as arthritis or alcoholism, has a major impact on public health does not necessarily mean that sophisticated technology will be developed to deal with it. Instead, the more sophisticated technologies are frequently developed in areas where major technology is available rather than by areas of perhaps greater need.

The influence of supplier on the demand for medical care has increased in the past several years. There has been a significant increase in the offering of specialized "boutique" medical services, which may not be appreciated initially by the public but which are actively marketed and eventually widely used. The proliferation of weight control, substance abuse, eating disorder, and impotence programs are but a few examples of providers generating a perception of need and stimulating care-seeking behavior.

Eating disorder—with its hallmark diseases bulimia and anorexia—illustrates the complex interface between physiology and psychology. How does a normal behavior that results in episodic weight gain and weight loss differ from the behavior of those individuals who binge-eat and use diuretics, laxatives, and enemas as a means of accelerating weight loss? At what point does a natural interest in weight and appearance become a pathologic process in need of costly professional intervention? While physicians and psychologists may debate the definition of disease, the frequent bombardment of radio and television advertising creates the perception of illness in a certain number of individuals who would not previously have labeled themselves as ill. While advertising may make a segment of the population aware of advances, such as intraocular lens implants for the elderly who might otherwise have considered them unaffordable, the consistent interest in generating new sources of income by health care institutions and providers may be creating an unnatural emphasis

on illness for which biologic and behavioral variation are more likely explanations.

It is unclear whether the development of pathologic processes or the availability of services to treat them creates the demand for health care. It is clear, however, that the use of medical services is the result of a unique interaction involving the pathologic processes themselves, the patient's and the physician's perceptions of them, and the availability of services to deal with them (Rosenstock, 1966). Each of these elements must be considered if the use of health services is to be better understood by all concerned.

The most fundamental change in American medicine in the 1990s has been the shift in the relationship between patient and physician (Anders, 1996). The dominant influence is no longer the supply of what providers offer or the demand as reflected in patient preference; rather, the dominant influence is now a complex business relationship dominated by payers. The care-seeking patient has become dissociated from the system, as many lose the critical decision regarding the choice of physician or provider. The changing relationship of financing medical services from out-of-pocket or indemnity insurance to a variety of capitation relationships has made the psychologic and physiologic basis of care-seeking less important. The financial intermediary or health plan provides both a restricted panel of providers and barriers to patient-initiated decisions to seek care.

With an increasing percentage of people in the United States covered under managed care arrangements, there are restricted panels of providers available and a requirement that referral to subspecialists be made by primary care physicians only; this eliminates patient-initiated care-seeking from specialists (Berwick, 1996). The physician is confronted by a different set of financial incentives. It was once argued that excessive and sometimes unnecessary care was provided by health care professionals seeking to maximize their income (Emanuel & Dubler, 1995). It is now feared that access to useful and necessary care may be denied by providers seeking to protect their own income. The myriad of complex ethical and financial relationships that this new form of third-party management creates will dominate the health care debate for the next decade and possibly longer (Bodenheimer, 1996).

SUMMARY

As we enter the new millennium, health care is embroiled in a most complex set of conflicting and paradoxical trends. Diagnostic, pharmacologic, and surgical interventions have reached their zenith of sophistication and efficacy. Through better education and remarkable information technologies, patients and consumers have never been better informed. The supply of practitioners of all stripes is greater than it has ever been, yet access to care is being restricted by institutions and often invisible bureaucracies. The most daunting social decisions such as the place of advanced directives and physician-assisted suicide are colored by fears that managed care organizations will use the new modalities to cut costs (Brode, 1992; Levinsky, 1996). Pharmaceutical companies offer miracles in a bottle that are studied and approved only after extensive testing and review, while at the same time patients spend enormous amounts of money on ancient herbal remedies that are unregulated and unproven. It is the quintessential challenge to rationalize the competing interests and incentives of the care-seeking patient, the often conflicted provider, and the increasingly dominant financial intermediaries.

REFERENCES

Anders, G. (1996). *Health against wealth.* New York: Houghton Mifflin.

Apple, D. (1960). How laymen define illness. *Journal of Health and Human Behavior, 1,* 219–225.

Ballard-Barbash, R., Schatzkin, A., Carter, C. L., et al. (1990). Body fat distribution in breast cancer in the Framingham study. *Journal of the National Cancer Institute, 82,* 286–290.

Battistella, R. M. (1971). Factors associated with delay in the initiation of physicians' care among late adulthood persons. *American Journal of Public Health, 61,* 1348–1361.

Berwick, D. M. (1996). Payment by capitation in the quality of care. *New England Journal of Medicine, 335,* 1227–1231.

Bloch, A. B., Rieder, H. L., Kelly, G. D., et al. (1989). The epidemiology of tuberculosis in the United States. *Seminars in Respiratory Infection, 4,* 157–170.

Bodenheimer, R. (1996). The HMO backlash: Righteous or reactionary? *New England Journal of Medicine, 335,* 1601–1604.

Brode, H. (1992). Assisted death: A compassionate response to a medical failure. *New England Journal of Medicine, 327,* 1384–1388.

Brody, H. (1982). The lie that heals: The ethics of giving placebos. *Annals of Internal Medicine, 97,* 112–118.

Buchwald, D., Cheny, P. R., & Peterson, D. L. (1992). A chronic illness characterized by fatigue, neurologic and immunologic disorders in active herpes virus type 6 infection. *Annals of Internal Medicine, 116,* 103–113.

Cassell, E. J. (1982). The nature of suffering and the goals of medicine. *New England Journal of Medicine, 306,* 639–644.

Centers for Disease Control. (1981). Kaposi's sarcoma and pneumocystis pneumonia among homosexual men—New York City and California. *MMWR (Morbidity, Mortality Weekly Report), 30,* 305–308.

Centers for Disease Control. (1986). Chronic fatigue possibly related to Epstein-Barr virus in Nevada. *MMWR (Mortality, Morbidity Weekly Report), 35,* 350–352.

Centers for Disease Control. (1991). Recommendations for preventing transmission of human immunodeficiency virus and hepatitis B virus to patients during exposure to prone invasive procedures. *MMWR (Morbidity, Mortality Weekly Report), 8,* 1–9.

Cohen, S., Tyrrell, D. A., & Smith, A. P. (1991). Psychological stresses: Susceptibility of the common cold. *New England Journal of Medicine, 325,* 606–612.

DeCherney, A. H., & Berkowitz, G. S. (1982). Female fecundity and age. *New England Journal of Medicine, 306,* 424–426.

Dingle, J. H., Badger, G. F., & Jordan, W. S. (1964). *Illness in the home: A study of 25,000 illnesses in a group of Cleveland families.* Cleveland, OH: Western Reserve University.

Eisenberg, D. M., Kessler, R. C., Foster, C., et al. (1993). Unconventional medicine in the United States. Prevalent costs and patterns of use. *New England Journal of Medicine, 328,* 246–252.

Emanuel, E. J., & Dubler, N. N. (1995). Preserving the physician-patient relationship in the era of managed care. *Journal of the American Medical Association, 273,* 323–329.

Enos, W. F., Beyer, J. C., & Holmes, R. H. (1958). Pathogenesis of coronary disease in American soldiers killed in Korea. *Journal of the American Medical Association, 158,* 912–914.

Farrow, D. C., & Davis, S. (1990). Diet and the risk of pancreatic cancer in men. *American Journal of Epidemiology, 132,* 423–431.

Fauci, A. S. (1991). Immunopathogenetic mechanisms in human immunodeficiency virus (HIV infection). *Annals of Internal Medicine, 114,* 678–693.

Fuch, V. (1974). *Who shall live? Health economics and social choice.* New York: Basic Books.

Fuster, V., Badimon, L., Badimon, J. J., et al. (1992). Mechanisms of disease: The pathogenesis of coronary artery disease in the acute coronary symptoms. *New England Journal of Medicine. Part I, 326,* 242–250. *Part II, 326,* 310–318.

Glass, A. G., & Hoover, R. N. (1989). The emerging epidemic of melanoma and squamous cell skin cancer. *Journal of the American Medical Association, 262,* 2097–2100.

Gordis, L. (1990). Consumption of methylxanthine-containing beverages and risk of pancreatic cancer. *Cancer Letter, 52,* 1–12.

Gordon, J. S. (1996). *Manifesto for a new medicine: Your guide to healing partnerships and the wide use of alternative therapies.* Reading, MA: Addison-Wesley.

Hennrikus, D., et al. (1991). A community study of delay in presenting with signs of melanoma to medical practitioners. *Archives of Dermatology, 127,* 356–361.

Jensen, P. S. (1981). The doctor-patient relationship: Headed for impasse or improvement? *Annals of Internal Medicine, 95,* 769–771.

Krige, J. E., et al. (1991). Delay in the diagnosis of cutaneous melanoma: A prospective study in 250 patients. *Cancer, 68,* 2064–2068.

Lahdensuo, A., Haahtela, T., Herrala, J., et al. (1996). A randomized comparison of guided self management and traditional treatment of asthma over one year. *British Medical Journal, 312,* 745–752.

Levinsky, N. G. (1996). The purpose of advanced medical planning—Autonomy for patients or limitation of care? *New England Journal of Medicine, 335,* 741–743.

Ludwig, E. G., & Gibson, G. (1969). Self perception of sickness and the seeking of medical care. *Journal of Health and Social Behavior, 10,* 125–133.

Lyokinji, M., & Lamb, G. S. (1982). The Couvade symptom: An epidemiologic study. *Annals of Internal Medicine, 96,* 509–511.

Mabry, J. (1964). Lay concepts of etiology. *Journal of Chronic Diseases, 17,* 371–386.

McNamara, J. J., Molot, M. A., Stremple, J. F., et al. (1971). Coronary artery disease of combat casualties in Vietnam. *Journal of the American Medical Association, 216,* 1185–1187.

Meador, C. K. (1965). Art and science of nondisease. *New England Journal of Medicine, 272,* 92–95.

Merliss, R. R. (1971). Talc-treated rice and Japanese stomach cancer. *Science, 173,* 1141–1142.

Miranda, C. P., Lehmann, K. G., & Lachterman, B. (1991). Comparison of silent and symptomatic ischemia during exercise testing in men. *Annals of Internal Medicine, 114,* 649–656.

O'Sullivan, J. B., & Mahan, C. M. (1968). Prospective study of 352 young patients with diabetes. *New England Journal of Medicine, 278,* 1038–1041.

Parsons, T. (1958). Definitions of health and illness in the light of American values and social structure. In E. G. Jaco (Ed.), *Patients, physicians and illness* (pp. 165–187). Glencoe, IL: Free Press of Glencoe.

Peterson, W. J. (1990). Peptic ulcer—An infectious disease? *Western Journal of Medicine, 152,* 167–171.

Poskanzer, D. C., & Herbst, A. L. (1977). Epidemiology of vaginal adenosis and adenocarcinoma association with exposure to stillbestrol in utero. *Cancer, 39* (Suppl.), 1892–1895.

Retchin, S. M., Fletcher, R. H., Earp, J. A., et al. (1986). Mitral valve prolapse: Disease or illness? *Archives of Internal Medicine, 146,* 1081.

Rosenberg, P. B. (1992). Dyslexia—Is it a disease? *New England Journal of Medicine, 326,* 192–193.

Rosenfeld, I. (1996). *Doctor Rosenfeld's guide to alternative medicine: What works, what doesn't, and what's right for you.* New York: Random House.

Rosenstock, I. M. (1966). Why people use health services. *Milbank Memorial Fund Quarterly, 44*(Pt. 2), 94–127.

Schwarz, B. E. (1981). Does estrogen cause adenocarcinoma of the endometrium? *Clinical Obstetrics and Gynecology, 24,* 242–251.

Selikoff, I. J., Churg, J., & Hammond, E. C. (1964). Asbestos exposure and neoplasia. *Journal of the American Medical Association, 188,* 22–26.

Shaywitz, S. E., Escobar, B. A., Shaywitz, J. M., et al. (1992). Evidence that dyslexia may represent the lower tail of a normal distribution of reading ability. *New England Journal of Medicine, 326,* 145–150.

Siperstein, M. D. (1975). The glucose tolerance test: A pitfall in the diagnosis of diabetes mellitus. *Advances in Internal Medicine, 20,* 297–323.

Somers, A. R. (1982). Long term care for the elderly and disabled: A new health priority. *New England Journal of Medicine, 307,* 221–226.

Stamm, W. E. (1981). Nosocomial infections: Etiologic changes, therapeutic challenges. *Hospital Practice, 16,* 75–88.

Stoeckle, J. D., & Barsky, A. J. (1980). Uses of social science knowledge in the doctoring of primary care. In L. Eisenberg & A. Kleinman (Eds.), *The relevance of social science for medicine* (pp. 223–240). Hingham, MA: D. Reidel.

Stoeckle, J. D., Zola, I. K., & Davidson, G. E. (1963). On going to see the doctor, the contributions of the patient to the decision to seek medical aid: A selective review. *Journal of Chronic Diseases, 16,* 975–989.

Tobi, M., & Straus, S. E. (1985). Chronic Epstein-Barr virus disease. A workshop held by the National Institute of Pathology and Infectious Disease. *Annals of Internal Medicine, 103,* 251–254.

Tonglet, R., Bourdoux, P., Minga, T., et al. (1992). Efficacy of low oral doses of iodized oil and the control of iodine deficiency in Zaire. *New England Journal of Medicine, 326,* 236–241.

Turpeinen, O. (1979). Effect of cholesterol-lowering diet on mortality from coronary heart disease and other causes. *Circulation, 59,* 1–7.

Varga, J., Uitto, J., & Jimenez, S. A (1992). The cause and pathogenesis of the eosinophilia-myalgia syndrome. *Annals of Internal Medicine, 116,* 140–147.

Voigt, L. F., Weiss, N. S., Chu, J., et al. (1991). Progestogen supplementation of exogenous estrogens and risk of endometrial cancer. *Lancet, 338,* 274–277.

Wachtel, T., Piette, J., More, V., et al. (1992). Quality of life in persons with immunodeficiency virus infection: Measurement by the medical outcomes study instrument. *Annals of Internal Medicine, 116,* 129–137.

Weil, A. (1995). *Spontaneous healing: How to discover it and enhance your body's natural ability to maintain and heal itself.* New York: Knopf.

Weiss, N. S. (1972). Relation of high blood pressure to headache, epistaxis and selected other symptoms. *New England Journal of Medicine, 287,* 631.

Zborowsky, M. (1952). Cultural components in responses to pain. *Journal of Social Issues, 8,* 16–30.

Zola, L. K. (1966). Culture and symptoms: An analysis of patients' presenting complaints. *American Sociological Review, 31,* 615–630.

CHAPTER

Historical Patterns of Disease in the United States

Stephen J. Williams

Paul R. Torrens

CHAPTER TOPICS

LEARNING OBJECTIVES

Upon completing this chapter, the reader should be able to:

- Trace twentieth century United States demographic trends including births and deaths.
- Understand correlates of mortality, especially with regard to the impact of population trends.
- Understand disease patterns in the United States.
- Relate lifestyle, behavior, and social patterns to health.
- Appreciate cancer survival trends.

Disease patterns throughout history, and the underlying social and demographic characteristics of our population, provide empirical evidence from which to view the need and demand for health care services in the United States. The principal purpose of this chapter is to review the fundamental demographic, social, and economic trends in our nation, principally throughout the twentieth century, and patterns of morbidity, mortality, and other aspects of the measurement of the incidence and prevalence of disease. Analytical, epidemiologic measurement of these patterns illuminate the underlying factors that define the nature of health care services required for our nation.

The analysis presented here first focuses on the underlying demographic trends in our society during the twentieth century. Social and economic trends that define the character of our society and relate to the need and demand for health care services are also discussed.

The next section of the chapter focuses on disease patterns experienced in the twentieth century. Differential mortality and morbidity are presented to emphasize the importance of such variables as age, race, and sex in defining population groups at particular risk for various diseases. Ultimately, identification of risk factors and their association with various personal, sociodemographic, and physiological characteristics, and genetic markers, will greatly heighten our ability to target health services to individuals in greatest need for each category of care.

All aspects of this chapter are integrally related to virtually every other section of this book. The nature of the delivery system itself, including the settings in which services are provided, the nature of services, the technology of our system, and even the financing of care are all directly related to the underlying disease patterns that we experience.

This chapter sets the stage and forms part of the foundation of knowledge necessary for critically assessing how the health care system is structured. Our ability to measure performance within the system itself, including outcomes of care, is related to these fundamental trends as well. Ultimately, the success of the system should be measured against criteria that recognize the true needs of the population with regard to the physiological and psychological manifestations of injury, illness, and disease.

Need, Demand, and Utilization

In discussions of disease patterns and their relation to the utilization of health care services, it is important to differentiate between the concepts of need, demand, and use of health care services. *Need* for health care services is defined as interpretation of an individual's evaluated requirements for obtaining professional care through the health services system. *Demand* for health services is a function of an individual's actually seeking out, but not necessarily obtaining, health services. Demand may be a reflection of professional assessment of an individual's need for services or self-initiated desires for professional services, perhaps triggered by an individual's perceptions of potential illness. Finally, *utilization* is a measure of actual use of services, as discussed in Chapter 4.

The extent to which there is correlation between need, demand, and utilization is the central issue in addressing concerns of appropriateness of care, perceptions of when services should be obtained, and evaluation of access to health care services in our society. Many other issues related to these concepts are addressed throughout this book.

Data Sources and Quality

Morbidity, mortality, and other health status–related data are obtained from a variety of sources (National Center for Health Statistics, 1997). Information presented throughout this chapter and elsewhere in this book is based on such sources as national vital statistics data (National Center for Health Statistics, 1993). National vital statistics data are collected from birth, death, and marriage certificates. Mandatory data collection requirements in the United States provide the most consistent and generally highest-quality data available for determining the health status of our nation's population.

But even mandated vital statistics data collection produces information of inconsistent quality. All data should be viewed with a skeptical eye, recognizing the imperfections of the data collection effort. For primary demographic variables such as age, race, and sex, the quality of data recorded on the primary data source, the vital event certificate, is generally good. However, for more subjective data elements, such as cause of death, the consistency and quality of data reported can vary appreciably, especially in past years, depending on the judgment of the individual, usually a physician, completing the certificate. Vital statistics data collected at the local level are compiled by the states and the federal government, and efforts are directed toward improving quality at each level.

Data on health services utilization, status, attitudes, and other variables are often collected through national probability surveys conducted by the federal government and some private organizations. The National Health Interview Survey collects data from a random probability sample of all Americans, asking questions regarding prior health services utilization, perceived health status, mobility, and other, often somewhat subjective, self-reported variables (Benson & Marano, 1994). Recall ability, response judgments, and other complex factors affect the quality of these types of data.

A third category of data collection for health services use involves the compilation of data from other sources. An example of this is the National Hospital Discharge Survey conducted by the federal government, which compiles the data from a sampling of hospital discharges in the country (McCaig, 1994a, 1994b). Another example is the National Ambulatory Medical Care Survey, also conducted by the federal government, which is based on a sample of physicians who report on the characteristics, diagnoses, and use of services for all patients seen during a two-week interval of time (Shappert, 1994).

Private data collection includes surveys of health services use, attitudes, and costs. National organizations such as the American Medical Association and the Medical Group Management Association conduct surveys on medical groups, physician practices, and hospital services. Various insurance companies, health care systems, and individual facilities also conduct surveys on patient satisfaction and other issues. Finally, data are collected by national voluntary accrediting agencies, health services researchers, and other organizations.

It is important to recognize the sources, quality, and contingencies associated with the data that are analyzed and presented throughout this book. The book's analytical perspective on health services is dependent on the assessment of population-based data, and the best available information is utilized for discussion purposes. Even the relatively solid data available in the United States, however, are subject to numerous limitations. Needless to say, data from many other countries in the world often lag far behind our own in this regard.

THE UNDERLYING DEMOGRAPHIC DETERMINANTS OF HEALTH SERVICES UTILIZATION

The dynamics of population are the most fundamental determinants of the need, demand, and use of health care services. The size and age composition of a population have a tremendous impact on total health services use as well as on the distribution of the use of specific services. Therefore, trends in population dynamics, including population size and demographic characteristics as well as births and deaths, are a basic starting point for assessing the need for health services in a population.

Population Size and Composition

Population size, as reflected in the total number of people in a population, as well as the distribu-

tion of population by age group, defined as the population pyramid, is the appropriate starting point. Table 3–1 presents the age-specific distribution of the United States resident population from 1950 to 1993. These data, obtained from the federal government, are based on national census of population data. The federal government is required by the United States Constitution to conduct a census count of population once every ten years to compile as complete a count as possible of all citizens (U.S. Bureau of the Census, 1990).

Population data between censuses and for future periods are determined through intracensual estimates and projections using prior data and adjusting for estimated population growth and migration (*Current Population Survey*, 1978). Intracensual data estimates are facilitated by using such available statistics as school enrollments, automobile registrations, and utility hookups (U.S. Bureau of the Census, 1992). The original purpose of the census, of course, was to determine representation in the House of Representatives, although these data are now also used for an array of analytical, commercial, and social purposes.

TABLE 3–1   Resident population: United States, selected years

Year	Total Resident Population	Age Group (Population in Thousands)										
		Under 1 year	1–4 years	5–14 years	15–24 years	25–34 years	35–44 years	45–54 years	55–64 years	65–74 years	75–84 years	85 years and over
1950	150,697	3,147	13,017	24,319	22,098	23,759	21,450	17,343	13,370	8,340	3,278	577
1960	179,323	4,112	16,209	35,465	24,020	22,818	24,081	20,485	15,572	10,997	4,633	929
1970	203,212	3,485	13,669	40,746	35,441	24,907	23,088	23,220	18,590	12,435	6,119	1,511
1980	226,546	3,534	12,815	34,942	42,487	37,082	25,635	22,800	21,703	15,581	7,729	2,240
1990	248,710	3,946	14,812	35,095	37,013	43,161	37,435	25,057	21,113	18,045	10,012	3,021
1995	262,755	3,848	15,743	38,134	35,947	40,873	42,468	31,079	21,131	18,759	11,145	3,628

SOURCE: *Health, United States, 1996–97,* National Center for Health Statistics, 1997, Hyattsville, MD: Public Health Service.

The accuracy of the actual census count, of intracensual estimates, and of demographic projections into the future is a subject of considerable debate. The mobility of the population, the lack of tracking for internal migration, and illegal migration into the country complicate the picture. The cost of data collection, analysis, adjustment, and reporting has escalated greatly as the population has grown, as well.

The United States population has grown tremendously during the period presented in Table 3–1. This growth is a result of two principal factors. The first of these is the *rate of natural increase* attributable to the higher number of births as compared to deaths annually in the United States, leading to additions to the total population count. The second factor is the increase in population attributable to net in-migration, which historically has accounted for nearly all of the accumulated population of the country. Current estimated United States population is over 260,000,000 people, which is nearly double the count in 1950. Further detailed data, not presented here, are readily available differentially by sex, ethnic group, and other sociodemographic variables. Depending on the nature of the analysis to be performed, use of the more detailed data can be quite revealing.

The age structure of the population is, as noted above, vitally important for health services purposes. The very young and the older population groups utilize considerably more health care services than other age groups. Table 3–1 also presents the age distribution and hence structure or pyramid of the population.

An important current trend is the aging of the population. On average, the typical American is getting older. This trend is the result of increased longevity and relatively lower fertility than was experienced earlier in the century. The consequences of this trend are reflected in Table 3–2. Projections for the older population groups over the next half century suggest substantial increases in health services utilization, assuming current technology, access to care, and patterns of use. The population aged sixty-five and above uses, on average, approximately twice the health care services as the younger population. This trend in the age structure for the United States is the underlying demographic reason for recent concerns over the future financial viability of the Social Security system and the Medicare program.

Parenthetically, many other countries in the world, especially in Europe, face an even more profound aging of their populations, so that future liabilities for social services, health care, and social security are even more serious than our own. Enhanced longevity as a result of biomedical advances is a two-edged sword leading to longer periods of economic and social dependency, while at the same time enhancing quality of life. As the

TABLE 3–2   Population age group projections, age 65 and above

Age Group	Year (Population in Millions)				
	1995	2000	2025	2050	2075
65 years and over	34.0	35.2	60.6	73.3	83.3
75 years and over	15.0	16.7	25.0	38.9	45.7
85 years and over	3.8	4.4	6.3	14.6	16.9

SOURCE: U.S. Social Security Administration Office of Programs: Office of the Actuary, 1993, Baltimore, MD.

population ages, the burdens on the younger working groups increase. This concept is reflected in the dependency ratio, which measures the proportion of a population that is working to those who are dependent.

FERTILITY TRENDS IN THE UNITED STATES

A key determinant of population that affects health services utilization is fertility. Fertility is a key determinant of the population pyramid, as well as of the use of services for mothers, infants, and children. Fertility eventually influences total population size and has cohort effects in all age groups as a cohort ages.

Fertility behavior is also a socioeconomic characteristic of population. Developing nations, for example, are typically characterized by relatively high fertility rates, while developed, or postindustrial, societies usually experience low fertility rates.

Fertility is a measure of reproduction. Age-specific fertility rates are the primary indicator utilized in measuring this determinant of population. Age-specific fertility rates more accurately reflect differences in fertility patterns based on age groups of mothers than do birth rates, which are a cruder measure of reproduction. Birth rates are computed as the total number of births to total population. Age-specific fertility rates are computed as the number of births to women in a specific reproductive age group. The total fertility rate is the sum of all of the age-specific rates.

Table 3–3 presents age-specific fertility rates for the United States over the past half century. As for many of the other rates discussed in this chapter, age, race, sex, and other characteristics may be utilized to compute more specific rates than those presented.

Fertility, of course, differs greatly by age group, as reflected in Table 3–3. Fertility is highest for women in their twenties and generally declines thereafter as the age of the mother increases. Fertility rates drop off appreciably at the higher reproductive ages, with little fertility in the groups above forty-five years of age.

Recent technological advances have provided an occasional dramatic example of reproduction beyond the historical ranges. Historically, and in most societies, the reproductive ages begin with the physiological marker of menarche. A variety of

TABLE 3–3 Live births and birth rates by age of mother: United States, selected years

Year	Live Births	Age of Mother (Live Births per 1,000 Women)							
		10–14 years	*15–19 years*	*20–24 years*	*25–29 years*	*30–34 years*	*35–39 years*	*40–44 years*	*45–49 years*
1950	3,632,000	1.0	81.6	196.6	166.1	103.7	52.9	15.1	1.2
1960	4,257,850	0.8	89.1	258.1	197.4	112.7	56.2	15.5	0.9
1970	3,731,386	1.2	68.3	167.8	145.1	73.3	31.7	8.1	0.5
1980	3,612,258	1.1	53.0	115.1	112.9	61.9	19.8	3.9	0.2
1990	4,158,212	1.4	59.9	116.5	120.2	80.8	31.7	5.5	0.2
1993	4,000,240	1.4	59.6	112.6	115.5	80.8	32.9	6.1	0.3
1995	3,899,589	1.3	56.8	109.8	112.2	82.5	34.3	6.6	0.3

SOURCE: *Health, United States, 1996–97,* National Center for Health Statistics, 1997, Hyattsville, MD: Public Health Service.

sociological determinants of reproductive behavior such as marriage combine with physiology to produce actual behavior. The reproductive ages usually end with menopause. Other physiological factors, such as voluntary sterilization and infertility, and sociological patterns, such as family dissolution, also have a substantial impact on reproduction. The interaction of these dynamics can be quite complex.

Fertility has declined in most age groups over the past forty years, as reflected in Table 3–3. Reductions in fertility have been rather dramatic in the United States since peak fertility occurred in the mid-1950s.

The dramatic decline in fertility that has occurred in the United States over the past forty years is primarily the result of increases in female labor force participation, marital dissolutions, and other economic and social forces in our society. In recent years our nation has also witnessed delayed average age of first marriage, reduced desired family size, delayed initiation of childbearing due to education and employment prospects, and a number of other important social and economic factors, all of which have further reinforced the primary underlying fertility trends.

Making predictions is a difficult business. Some demographers anticipated a resurgence of fertility to result from delayed childbearing associated with labor force participation by women and subsequent desires to "catch up." This has not occurred, although some slight increase in overall fertility has been experienced in recent years. A substantial change in the now-well-established pattern of United States fertility is unlikely to occur in the foreseeable future.

Other societies have experienced many of the same general changes in fertility experienced by the United States in the twentieth century. The change from a high-fertility, high-mortality environment to a low-fertility, low-mortality environment is typical of most developing countries. This change is termed the demographic transition. Countries that achieve low fertility and low mortality, combined with relatively affluent economic conditions, typically experience substantial social and economic change that results in permanent reversals of the underlying social factors associated with high fertility.

Abortion Trends in the United States

Reproduction may be more appropriately measured in terms of conceptions rather than live births. Conceptions include spontaneous and induced abortions as well as live and dead births. However, the empirical data to accurately count conceptions is considerably weaker than that for live births.

National data are available on therapeutically induced abortions, as reflected in Table 3–4. The United States experiences an estimated 1.2 million abortions annually at the current time, and an unknown number of conceptions result in spontaneous abortions, primarily in the first month of gestation. Abortion practices vary considerably from society to society and over time, and the current acceptance of abortion services in the United States dates back nationally to the 1973 Supreme Court decision to restrict state barriers to such services.

MORTALITY TRENDS IN THE UNITED STATES

Indicators of mortality are often used to measure a society's health status. Trends in mortality indicators over time also reflect a multitude of social, economic, health services, and other underlying trends in a society. Reasonably accurate mortality data are available for the United States population and for many other nations, although in some developing countries the quality of data may be limited.

Mortality data are collected at the time of death through the mechanics of the death certificate, a

TABLE 3–4 Legal abortions, according to selected characteristics: United States, selected years

Characteristic	Year	
	1973	1994
Total number of legal abortions (reported in thousands)		
	616	1,267
Period of gestation (percentage distribution)		
Under 9 weeks	36.1	53.7
9–10 weeks	29.4	23.5
11–12 weeks	17.9	10.9
13–15 weeks	6.9	6.3
16–20 weeks	8.0	4.3
21 weeks and over	1.7	1.3
Type of procedure (percentage distribution)		
Curettage	88.4	99.1
Intrauterine instillation	10.4	0.5
Other	0.6	0.4

SOURCE: *Health, United States, 1996–97,* National Center for Health Statistics, 1997, Hyattsville, MD: Public Health Service.

responsibility of local government. State and federal agencies compile data collected locally to produce, eventually, the vital statistics for the entire country. Since various social and demographic variables are collected on the death certificate, in addition to determinants of the cause of death, mortality data can be analyzed by selected characteristics of population.

Mortality Trends for the United States

This section of the chapter presents quantitative measures of mortality for the total United States population over time. Mortality data for infants and mothers and an analysis of specific causes of death are presented in later sections of this chapter as well. As for fertility, mortality data are generally age-adjusted to control for changes in the population age pyramid. Comparisons over time, in particular, require consideration of any substantial changes in the age structure of a population.

Life Expectancy

A common measure of mortality, particularly popular in the mass media, is life expectancy. Life expectancy is computed from mortality data and reflects a cohort effect for estimated years of life remaining.

Life expectancy can be computed for a population at any specific age, but it is most commonly presented at birth and at age sixty-five. Table 3–5 presents such data for selected countries in the world. Mortality and life expectancy data are typically presented on a sex-specific basis due to the consistent and substantial differences in mortality experienced comparing males and females.

International life expectancy comparisons reveal that for both males and females, life expectancy at birth is greatest in Japan (United Nations, 1992). The United States falls somewhat short in these comparisons, a surprising finding for many people. However, the heterogeneity of our population and our complex social problems associated with violence, accidents, and infectious disease account for much of the cross-cultural deficiencies reflected in our mortality experience. Many Americans are surprised to see that mortality experience measured by life expectancy at birth is lower in the United States than in such countries as Greece and France, perhaps owing a little to the value of red wine, paté, and olive oil!

Life expectancy at age sixty-five is also presented in Table 3–5 for selected countries. By age sixty-five, past the highest-risk periods for mortality attributable

TABLE 3–5 Life expectancy at birth and at 65 years of age, according to sex: Selected countries, 1993

Country	Life Expectancy in Years	
	At birth	*At 65 years*
Male		
Japan	76.5	16.7
Sweden	75.5	15.7
Greece	75.0	16.0
Switzerland	75.0	15.9
Canada	74.9	16.1
England and Wales	73.9	14.6
France	73.8	16.4
Italy	73.7	15.2
Spain	73.4	15.5
Cuba	72.9	15.9
Austria	72.9	14.8
United States	**72.2**	**15.3**
Finland	72.1	14.1
Portugal	70.6	13.9
Female		
Japan	83.1	21.3
France	82.3	21.1
Switzerland	81.7	20.4
Canada	81.4	20.4
Sweden	80.8	19.5
Italy	80.5	19.2
Greece	80.4	18.7
Finland	79.6	18.4
England and Wales	79.6	18.5
United States	**79.1**	**19.2**
Denmark	78.8	18.9
Cuba	76.8	17.8

SOURCE: *Health, United States, 1996–97,* National Center for Health Statistics, 1997, Hyattsville, MD: Public Health Service.

to nonphysiological causes, the differences between sexes are much less, as are the differences between countries. Sex mortality differentials drop by about half by age sixty-five, reflecting the higher risk from violent accidents and lifestyle causes for individuals younger than sixty-five. The remaining differential is probably attributable to physiological factors such as hormones and genetics.

International differences similarly are moderated by age sixty-five, since many of these same causes of mortality in the younger ages have been factored out of the equation. Even at sixty-five, however, life expectancy is greatest in Japan, with females at age sixty-five expecting to live, on average, to about age eighty-six, a truly impressive result.

United States Life Expectancy Data

Table 3–6 presents life expectancy data for selected subgroups of the United States population. Again, mortality experience differs by sociodemographic characteristics such as sex and race. Dramatic differences appear in these data at birth for males as compared to females and for blacks as compared to whites. As noted previously, data are available for numerous subgroups of the population, and only selected illustrative data are presented here.

At birth females have a substantially higher life expectancy than males, a difference of approximately six years of life. An equally dramatic differential is evident for whites as compared to blacks. These differences have been constant throughout modern United States history, as reflected in Table 3–6. At age sixty-five, the differentials continue to exist, but, as for the international comparisons, the differences are much more moderate, indicating that on a biological basis sex differences may be on the order of two to three years. Black/white differentials are also quite moderate at this point.

TABLE 3–6 Life expectancy at birth and at 65 years of age, according to race and sex: United States, selected years

Age Category and Year	White		Black	
	Male	*Female*	*Male*	*Female*
At birth				
1900	46.6	48.7	32.5	35.5
1950	66.5	72.2	58.9	62.7
1960	67.4	74.1	60.7	65.9
1970	68.0	75.6	60.0	68.3
1980	70.7	78.1	63.8	72.5
1990	72.7	79.4	64.5	73.6
1995	73.4	79.6	65.2	73.9
At 65 years				
1900	11.5	12.2	10.4	11.4
1950	12.8	15.1	12.9	14.9
1960	12.9	15.9	12.7	15.1
1970	13.1	17.1	12.5	15.7
1980	14.2	18.4	13.0	16.8
1990	15.2	19.1	13.2	17.2
1995	15.7	19.1	13.6	17.1

SOURCE: *Health, United States, 1996–97,* National Center for Health Statistics, 1997, Hyattsville, MD: Public Health Service.

United States Mortality Rates

Table 3–7 presents age-specific mortality rates for the United States by selected demographic characteristics. These data conform to the life expectancy numbers presented earlier. As expected, mortality rates increase with age. The United States age-specific mortality rates are relatively moderate until the older ages, although notable differentials occur by sex and race. The higher mortality rate for younger black males compared to same-age-group white males is particularly startling; these data are discussed further later in this chapter in the discussion of specific causes of death.

Data on differential mortality help to identify problems in society with regard to causes of illness and disease and barriers to access to health care services. Trends over time reflect progress, or lack thereof, in achieving our goals for greater quality and quantity of life.

Infant and Maternal Mortality

An oft-quoted set of data is mortality experience for infants and mothers. Table 3–8 presents international data on infant mortality. Infant mortality is measured as the number of infants who die in the first year of life per thousand live births. Related measures of mortality for infants include perinatal, postnatal, and other measures, all of which pertain to the time period before or after delivery in which the fetal or infant death occurs.

Once again the United States falls short in international comparisons of infant mortality. Japan leads all nations in having the lowest infant mortality rate. The relatively poor performance of the United States population is again a function of population heterogeneity and such factors as lack of access to prenatal care, high fertility among high-risk young women, poor maternal nutrition, genetic risks, and other complex social, economic, and physiological factors. Differential infant mortality among United States population subgroups indicates that rates are substantially higher for blacks than for whites due to differences in access to health care, nutrition, social factors, and other variables that impact infant viability. These differences reflect underlying social and economic concerns faced by our society. Poor gestational outcomes may result in huge social and economic costs. Implications of inadequate prenatal care, nutrition, and related factors also extend to serious concerns of child intellectual development, social adaptation, and physical maintenance.

Maternal mortality, reflected in Table 3–9, has declined dramatically in the United States since

TABLE 3–7   Death rates for all causes, according to sex and age: United States, selected years

Sex and Age	Year (Deaths per 100,000 Resident Population)					
	1950	1960	1970	1980	1990	1995
White male						
All ages, age adjusted	963.1	917.7	893.4	745.3	644.3	610.5
Under 1 year	3,400.5	2,694.1	2,113.2	1,230.3	896.1	717.5
1–4 years	135.5	104.9	83.6	66.1	45.9	38.8
5–14 years	67.2	52.7	48.0	35.0	26.4	24.5
15–24 years	152.4	143.7	170.8	167.0	131.3	122.3
25–34 years	185.3	163.2	176.6	171.3	176.1	177.7
35–44 years	380.9	332.6	343.5	257.4	268.2	287.7
45–54 years	984.5	932.2	882.9	698.9	548.7	534.6
55–64 years	2,304.4	2,225.2	2,202.6	1,728.5	1,467.2	1,330.8
65–74 years	4,864.9	4,848.4	4,810.1	4,035.7	3,397.7	3,199.0
75–84 years	10,526.3	10,299.6	10,098.8	8,829.8	7,844.9	7,320.6
85 years and over	22,116.3	21,750.0	18,551.7	19,097.3	18,268.3	18,152.9
Black male						
All ages, age adjusted	1,373.1	1,246.1	1,318.6	1,112.8	1,061.3	1,016.7
Under 1 year	—	5,306.8	4,298.9	2,586.7	2,112.4	1,590.8
1–4 years	—	208.5	150.5	110.5	85.8	77.5
5–14 years	95.1	75.1	67.1	47.4	41.2	40.2
15–24 years	289.7	212.0	320.6	209.1	252.2	249.2
25–34 years	503.5	402.5	559.5	407.3	430.8	416.5
35–44 years	878.1	762.0	956.6	689.8	699.6	721.2
45–54 years	1,905.0	1,624.8	1,777.5	1,479.9	1,261.0	1,273.0
55–64 years	3,773.2	3,316.4	3,256.9	2,873.0	2,618.4	2,437.5
65–74 years	5,310.3	5,798.7	5,803.2	5,131.1	4,946.1	4,610.5
75–84 years	—	8,605.1	9,454.9	9,231.6	9,129.5	8,778.8
85 years and over	—	14,844.8	12,222.3	16,098.8	16,954.9	16,728.7
White female						
All ages, age adjusted	645.0	555.0	501.7	411.1	369.9	364.9
Under 1 year	2,566.8	2,007.7	1,614.6	962.5	690.0	571.6
1–4 years	112.2	85.2	66.1	49.3	36.1	31.2
5–14 years	45.1	34.7	29.9	22.9	17.9	16.6
15–24 years	71.5	54.9	61.6	55.5	45.9	44.3
25–34 years	112.8	85.0	84.1	65.4	61.5	64.3
35–44 years	235.8	191.1	193.3	138.2	117.4	125.8
45–54 years	546.4	458.8	462.9	372.7	309.3	294.4
55–64 years	1,293.8	1,078.9	1,014.9	876.2	822.7	788.4
65–74 years	3,242.8	2,779.3	2,470.7	2,066.6	1,923.5	1,924.5
75–84 years	8,481.5	7,696.6	6,698.7	5,401.7	4,839.1	4,831.1
85 years and over	19,679.5	19,477.7	15,980.2	14,979.6	14,400.6	14,639.1

TABLE 3–7 *continued*

Sex and Age	Year (Deaths per 100,000 Resident Population)					
	1950	*1960*	*1970*	*1980*	*1990*	*1995*
Black female						
All ages, age adjusted	1,106.7	916.9	814.4	631.1	581.6	571.0
Under 1 year	—	4,162.2	3,368.8	2,123.7	1,735.5	1,342.0
1–4 years	—	173.3	129.4	84.4	67.6	62.9
5–14 years	72.8	53.8	43.8	30.5	27.5	26.5
15–24 years	213.1	107.5	111.9	70.5	68.7	70.3
25–34 years	393.3	273.2	231.0	150.0	159.5	166.6
35–44 years	758.1	568.5	533.0	323.9	298.6	327.7
45–54 years	1,576.4	1,177.0	1,043.9	768.2	639.4	619.0
55–64 years	3,089.4	2,510.9	1,986.2	1,561.0	1,452.6	1,350.3
65–74 years	4,000.2	4,064.2	3,860.9	3,057.4	2,865.7	2,823.7
75–84 years	—	6,730.0	6,691.5	6,212.1	5,688.3	5,840.3
85 years and over	—	13,052.6	10,706.6	12,367.2	13,309.5	13,472.2

SOURCE: *Health, United States, 1996–97,* National Center for Health Statistics, 1997, Hyattsville, MD: Public Health Service.

TABLE 3–8 Infant mortality rates: Selected countries, 1993

Country	Deaths to Infants under One Year (per 1,000 Live Births)
Cuba	9.40
United States	**8.37**
Greece	8.30
Spain	7.19
Italy	7.16
France	6.50
Canada	6.30
England and Wales	6.24
Australia	6.11
Switzerland	5.55
Denmark	5.40
Sweden	4.84
Finland	4.40
Japan	4.35

SOURCE: *Health, United States, 1996–97,* National Center for Health Statistics, 1997, Hyattsville, MD: Public Health Service.

1950. In addition to the overall decline in these rates, the reduction in maternal mortality for the higher age groups is quite notable.

Again, a very significant differential exists by race. Black women have experienced a significant decline in maternal mortality since 1950, but they still have rates that are much higher than those of white women. The reductions in infant and maternal mortality discussed in this chapter represent a real success in our national efforts to improve the quality and quantity of life. But much remains to be done to achieve more optimal results for all Americans and to fully invest in the future of our children.

SPECIFIC CAUSES OF DEATH FOR THE UNITED STATES POPULATION

Age-adjusted death rates for selected causes of death for the United States population from 1950

TABLE 3–9 Maternal mortality rates for complications of pregnancy, childbirth, and the puerperium, according to race and age: United States, selected years

Race and Age	Year (Deaths per 100,000 Live Births)					
	1950	*1960*	*1970*	*1980*	*1990*	*1995*
White						
All ages, age adjusted	53.1	22.4	14.4	6.7	5.1	3.6
Under 20 years	44.9	14.8	13.8	5.8	N/A	N/A
20–24 years	35.7	15.3	8.4	4.2	3.9	3.5
25–29 years	45.0	20.3	11.1	5.4	4.8	4.0
30–34 years	75.9	34.3	18.7	9.3	5.0	4.0
35 years and over	174.1	73.9	59.3	25.5	12.6	9.1
Black						
All ages, age adjusted	—	92.0	65.5	24.9	21.7	20.9
Under 20 years	—	54.8	32.3	13.1	N/A	N/A
20–24 years	—	56.9	41.9	13.9	14.7	15.3
25–29 years	—	92.8	65.2	22.4	14.9	21.0
30–34 years	—	150.6	117.8	44.0	44.2	31.2
35 years and over	—	299.5	207.5	100.6	79.7	61.4

SOURCE: *Health, United States, 1996–97*, National Center for Health Statistics, 1997, Hyattsville, MD: Public Health Service.

to the present are presented in Table 3–10. Heart disease, cancer, and stroke are, of course, the three leading causes of death in the United States and have been for quite some time. Interestingly, examination of the equivalent data at the turn of the twentieth century would reveal a much greater prevalence of infectious as opposed to chronic diseases for the leading causes of death. Mortality attributable to such causes as nephritis and tuberculosis, which accounted for many deaths at the turn of the century, is far less common today. Influenza and pneumonia were also very important causes of death in the early 1900s. A dramatic outbreak of influenza occurred in 1918, causing considerable mortality.

Figure 3–1 illustrates the predominance of infectious diseases early in the twentieth century and the rise of chronic disease since midcentury. Chronic diseases, of course, are more prevalent because people are living longer and not dying early from infectious diseases. The control of many infectious diseases has been one of the most important successes in public health during the twentieth century. It is notable that the dramatic decline in infectious disease mortality had already occurred prior to the introduction of modern medical technologies such as antibiotic therapy.

Although the predominant challenges for mortality are now focused on chronic diseases, our nation must remain vigilant against outbreaks of infectious disease. Morbidity and mortality associated with the epidemic of human immunodeficiency virus illustrate the constant threat of infectious disease that we face even today. In many developing countries, infectious disease remains a principal cause of mortality, particularly among the very young and the very old. Such diseases as the Ebola virus and other startlingly virulent infectious

TABLE 3–10 Age-adjusted death rates for selected causes of death: United States, selected years

Causes of Death	Year (Deaths per 100,000 Resident Population)					
	1950	*1960*	*1970*	*1980*	*1990*	*1995*
All causes	840.5	760.9	714.3	585.8	520.2	503.9
Natural causes	766.6	695.2	636.9	519.7	465.1	451.7
Diseases of heart	307.2	286.2	253.6	202.0	152.0	138.3
Ischemic heart disease	—	—	—	149.8	102.6	89.5
Cerebrovascular diseases	88.6	79.7	66.3	40.8	27.7	26.7
Malignant neoplasms	125.3	125.8	129.8	132.8	135.0	129.9
Respiratory system	12.8	19.2	28.4	36.4	41.4	39.7
Colorectal	19.0	17.7	16.8	15.5	13.6	12.7
Prostate	13.4	13.1	13.3	14.4	16.7	15.4
Breast	22.2	22.3	23.1	22.7	23.1	21.0
Chronic obstructive pulmonary diseases	4.4	8.2	13.2	15.9	19.7	20.8
Pneumonia and influenza	26.2	28.0	22.1	12.9	14.0	12.9
Chronic liver disease and cirrhosis	8.5	10.5	14.7	12.2	8.6	7.6
Diabetes mellitus	14.3	13.6	14.1	10.1	11.7	13.3
Human immunodeficiency virus infection	—	—	—	—	9.8	15.6
External causes	73.9	65.7	77.4	66.1	55.1	52.2
Unintentional injuries	57.5	49.9	53.7	42.3	32.5	30.5
Motor vehicle crashes	23.3	22.5	27.4	22.9	18.5	16.3
Suicide	11.0	10.6	11.8	11.4	11.5	11.2
Homicide and legal intervention	5.4	5.2	9.1	10.8	10.2	9.4

SOURCE: *Health, United States, 1996–97,* National Center for Health Statistics, 1997, Hyattsville, MD: Public Health Service.

diseases could become a threat to developed nations' populations at any time. Increased international mobility provides vectors of transmission for infectious disease that were not common years ago.

Number of Deaths for Specific Causes

Table 3–11 presents actual numbers of deaths for selected subgroups and causes for the United States population. The leading causes of death for each subgroup are listed. Although much more extensive analysis is available, these data sets dramatically demonstrate the tragic involvement of economic, social, and lifestyle factors in causing mortality in the United States. The high ranking for such causes as injuries, violence, and human immunodeficiency virus infection is quite striking in the younger age groups. Data for the older ages present a picture more common to our typical characterization of mortality causes in the United States.

Mortality attributable to selected causes is presented in the next few tables. Again only limited data sets can be presented here, and much more extensive statistical information is available from a variety of official governmental sources. Table 3–12 presents data for cardiovascular mortality in the United States. The data illustrate the dramatic

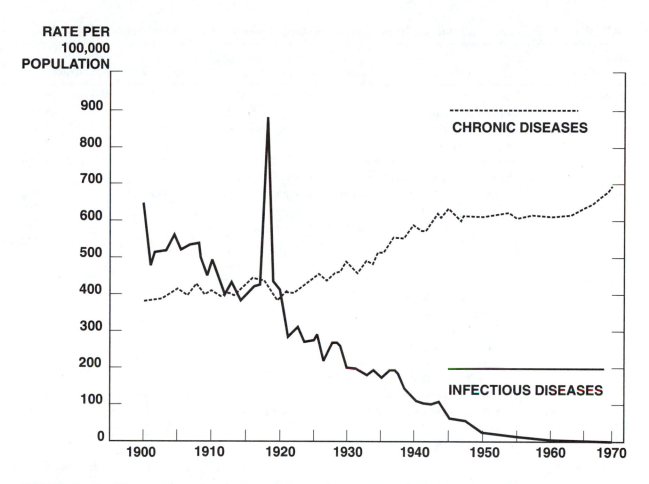

SOURCE: Reprinted by permission of Appleton-Lange from *Dynamics of Health and Disease,* by C. L. Marshall and D. Pearson, 1972, Appleton-Century Crofts, Inc.

FIGURE 3–1   Infectious and chronic disease death rates, 1900–1970

and generally consistent decline in mortality from this cause over time and across age groups. Data for various population subgroups based on age, sex, race, and certain other variables would reflect similar patterns. As is typical in illness and mortality data, declines have occurred for many population subgroups, but the results lead to numbers for blacks, American Indians, and some other population groups that are not nearly as low as for whites. The reduction in cardiovascular mortality is attrib-

utable to improvements in living conditions, diet, and health care services, particularly interventions for such events as myocardial infarction and coronary occlusion.

Data for cerebrovascular disease–related mortality are presented in Table 3–13 and reflect a consistent decline over time and across age groups. Racial- and sex-specific data show similar declines as for cardiovascular mortality. Rates for whites are at lower levels at all points in time as compared to blacks.

TABLE 3–11   Leading causes of death and number of deaths, selected ages: United States, 1995

Age and Rank Order	Cause of Death	Deaths
Under 1 year		All causes 29,583
1	Congenital anomalies	6,554
2	Disorders relating to short gestation and unspecified low birth weight	3,933
3	Sudden infant death syndrome	3,397
4	Respiratory distress syndrome	1,454
5	Newborn affected by maternal complications of pregnancy	1,309
6	Newborn affected by complications of placenta, cord, and membranes	962
7	Unintentional injuries	788
8	Infections specific to the perinatal period	787
9	Intrauterine hypoxia and birth asphyxia	492
10	Pneumonia and influenza	475
1–4 years		All causes 6,393
1	Unintentional injuries	2,280
2	Congenital anomalies	695
3	Malignant neoplasms	488
4	Homicide and legal intervention	452
5	Diseases of heart	251
6	Human immunodeficiency virus infection	210
7	Pneumonia and influenza	156
8	Certain conditions originating in the perinatal period	87
9	Septicemia	80
10	Benign neoplasms	57
5–14 years		All causes 8,596
1	Unintentional injuries	3,544
2	Malignant neoplasms	1,026
3	Homicide and legal intervention	562
4	Congenital anomalies	449
5	Suicide	337
6	Diseases of heart	294
7	Human immunodeficiency virus infection	189
8	Chronic obstructive pulmonary diseases	143
9	Pneumonia and influenza	128
10	Cerebrovascular diseases	105
15–24 years		All causes 34,244
1	Unintentional injuries	13,842
2	Homicide and legal intervention	7,284
3	Suicide	4,784
4	Malignant neoplasms	1,642
5	Diseases of heart	1,039
6	Human immunodeficiency virus infection	629

TABLE 3–11 *continued*

Age and Rank Order	Cause of Death	Deaths
7	Congenital anomalies	452
8	Chronic obstructive pulmonary diseases	246
9	Pneumonia and influenza	207
10	Cerebrovascular diseases	172
25–44 years		All causes 160,015
1	Human immunodeficiency virus infection	30,754
2	Unintentional injuries	27,660
3	Malignant neoplasms	21,985
4	Diseases of heart	17,064
5	Suicide	12,759
6	Homicide and legal intervention	10,280
7	Chronic liver disease and cirrhosis	4,309
8	Cerebrovascular diseases	3,492
9	Diabetes mellitus	2,458
10	Pneumonia and influenza	2,102
45–64 years		All causes 378,512
1	Malignant neoplasms	132,084
2	Diseases of heart	102,738
3	Unintentional injuries	16,004
4	Cerebrovascular diseases	15,208
5	Chronic obstructive pulmonary diseases	12,744
6	Diabetes mellitus	12,184
7	Chronic liver disease and cirrhosis	10,603
8	Human immunodeficiency virus infection	10,499
9	Suicide	7,336
10	Pneumonia and influenza	5,537
65 years and over		All causes 1,694,326
1	Diseases of heart	615,426
2	Malignant neoplasms	381,142
3	Cerebrovascular diseases	138,762
4	Chronic obstructive pulmonary diseases	88,478
5	Pneumonia and influenza	74,297
6	Diabetes mellitus	44,452
7	Unintentional injuries	29,099
8	Alzheimer's disease	20,230
9	Nephritis, nephrotic syndrome, and nephrosis	20,182
10	Septicemia	16,899

SOURCE: *Health, United States, 1996–97,* National Center for Health Statistics, 1997, Hyattsville, MD: Public Health Service.

Cancer Mortality in the United States

Among those disease categories where our morbidity and mortality experience has been especially disappointing over the course of the last fifty years are various types of cancer (Ries, et al., 1993). Mortality attributable to various cancers has remained fairly constant, in contrast to the dramatic declines experienced for cardiovascular and cerebrovascular disease. Furthermore, cancer survival rates after diagnosis generally have not improved very dramatically thus far.

Table 3–14 presents cancer mortality experience for the United States since 1950 by age group. As is evident from the data in this table, cancer mortality has actually increased over time. Increasing cancer mortality may be partially attributable to greater overall longevity, to genetic and environmental factors, to increased case-finding, to declines in other causes of death, leaving people more susceptible to cancer mortality, and to lifestyle issues.

Tables 3–15 and 3–16 present cancer mortality for two major categories of malignant neoplasms, breast cancer in women and lung cancer. The dramatic increases in mortality attributable to lung cancer are, of course, primarily a function of exposure to tobacco products. Breast cancer mortality trends are more difficult to explain, particularly in light of current controversy regarding the etiology of this cancer.

Cancer Survival Rates

Cancer survival rates, presented in Table 3–17, are disturbing in that, for most categories of cancer, survival rates have not improved appreciably in recent years. Cancer survival is highly dependent on early detection and effective therapeutic intervention. Mass screening for various types of cancer, such as breast, cervical, testicular, and colorectal, can be beneficial for high-risk population sub-groups. Population screening has complex cost-benefit trade-offs and other considerations regarding test accuracy, identification of population subgroups appropriate for screening, and other concerns. Our nation is now entering an era of medicine that will probably include much more effective screening techniques and more definitive interventions for cancer.

Survival rates relate to access to medical care, cancer staging at the time of detection, the availability of therapeutic interventions, patient compliance, and numerous other factors. The absence of dramatic improvement in cancer survival rates reflects the lack of definitive new therapies for most cancers. Current biomedical and clinical research holds the hope of much greater improvement in these survival rates in the future. Data for the newest era of detection and treatment, when available, will likely show greater progress than for these past time periods. Numerous issues remain to be addressed regarding appropriateness of various screening efforts, selection of alternative therapies, and preventive strategies for populations.

Cancer Incidence Rates

Table 3–18 presents cancer incidence rates for selected sites for white males and white females in the United States over the latter part of the twentieth century. For many categories of cancer, particularly lung, prostate, and breast, incidence rates have increased, in some cases sharply. The extent to which increases in cancer incidence are the result of increased case-finding and greater patient awareness is difficult to elucidate. There is also controversy regarding the fundamental causes of cancer and the extent to which genetic, environmental, behavioral, and dietary factors trigger its development. Further clarification of the causation and biological mechanisms of various cancers will be a

TABLE 3–12   Death rates for diseases of heart, according to sex and age: United States, selected years

Sex and Age Group	Year (Deaths per 100,000 Resident Population)			
	1950	1970	1990	1995
Male				
All ages, age adjusted	383.8	348.5	206.7	184.9
Under 1 year	4.0	15.1	21.9	17.5
1–4 years	1.4	1.9	1.9	1.7
5–14 years	2.0	0.9	0.9	0.8
15–24 years	6.8	3.7	3.1	3.6
25–34 years	22.9	15.2	10.3	11.4
35–44 years	118.4	103.2	48.1	47.2
45–54 years	440.5	376.4	183.0	168.6
55–64 years	1,104.5	987.2	537.3	465.4
65–74 years	2,292.3	2,170.3	1,250.0	1,102.3
75–84 years	4,825.0	4,534.8	2,968.2	2,615.0
85 years and over	9,659.8	8,426.2	7,418.4	7,039.6
Female				
All ages, age adjusted	233.9	175.2	108.9	100.4
Under 1 year	2.9	10.9	18.3	16.7
1–4 years	1.2	1.6	1.9	1.5
5–14 years	2.2	0.8	0.8	0.7
15–24 years	6.7	2.3	1.8	2.2
25–34 years	16.2	7.7	5.0	5.6
35–44 years	55.1	32.2	15.1	17.1
45–54 years	177.2	109.9	61.0	56.0
55–64 years	510.0	351.6	215.7	193.9
65–74 years	1,419.3	1,082.7	616.8	557.8
75–84 years	3,872.0	3,120.8	1,893.8	1,715.2
85 years and over	8,796.1	7,591.8	6,478.1	6,267.8

SOURCE: *Health, United States, 1996–97*, National Center for Health Statistics, 1997, Hyattsville, MD: Public Health Service.

TABLE 3–13   Death rates for cerebrovascular diseases, according to age: United States, selected years

Age Group	Year (Deaths per 100,000 Resident Population)			
	1950	1970	1990	1995
All ages, age adjusted	88.6	66.3	27.7	26.6
Under 1 year	5.1	5.0	3.8	5.4
1–4 years	0.9	1.0	0.3	0.3
5–14 years	0.5	0.7	0.2	0.2
15–24 years	1.6	1.6	0.6	0.5
25–34 years	4.2	4.5	2.2	1.9
35–44 years	18.7	15.6	6.5	6.4
45–54 years	70.4	41.6	18.7	17.7
55–64 years	195.3	115.8	48.0	45.9
65–74 years	549.7	384.1	144.4	136.2
75–84 years	1,499.6	1,254.2	499.3	480.3
85 years and over	2,990.1	3,014.3	1,633.9	1,616.4

SOURCE: *Health, United States, 1996–97*, National Center for Health Statistics, 1997, Hyattsville, MD: Public Health Service.

product of ongoing epidemiologic and biomedical research.

Cancer remains one of the most challenging categories of disease with respect to detection and successful therapeutic intervention. Biomedical researchers are successfully elucidating the causes and mechanisms of various cancers, although the challenges from this complex category of disease remain great. Future therapeutic interventions hold great promise. The biomedical research pipeline is producing discoveries daily. However, cancer incidence rates continue to climb, and survival rates remain little improved from earlier years.

TABLE 3–14 Death rates for malignant neoplasms, according to age: United States, selected years

Age Group	Year (Deaths per 100,000 Resident Population)			
	1950	1970	1990	1995
All ages, age adjusted	125.3	129.8	135.0	129.9
Under 1 year	8.7	4.7	2.3	1.8
1–4 years	11.7	7.5	3.5	3.1
5–14 years	6.7	6.0	3.1	2.7
15–24 years	8.6	8.3	4.9	4.6
25–34 years	20.0	16.5	12.6	11.9
35–44 years	62.7	59.5	43.3	40.3
45–54 years	175.1	182.5	158.9	142.2
55–64 years	392.9	423.0	449.6	416.0
65–74 years	692.5	751.2	872.3	868.2
75–84 years	1,153.3	1,169.2	1,348.5	1,364.8
85 years and over	1,451.0	1,320.7	1,752.9	1,823.8

SOURCE: *Health, United States, 1996–97,* National Center for Health Statistics, 1997, Hyattsville, MD: Public Health Service.

TABLE 3–15 Death rates for malignant neoplasm of breast for females, according to age: United States, selected years

Age Group	Year (Deaths per 100,000 Resident Population)			
	1950	1970	1990	1995
All ages, age adjusted	22.2	23.1	23.1	21.0
Under 25 years	*	*	*	*
25–34 years	3.8	3.9	2.9	2.7
35–44 years	20.8	20.4	17.8	15.0
45–54 years	46.9	52.6	45.4	41.4
55–64 years	70.4	77.6	78.6	69.8
65–74 years	94.0	93.8	111.7	103.3
75–84 years	139.8	127.4	146.3	142.0
85 years and over	195.5	157.1	196.8	203.7

SOURCE: *Health, United States, 1996–97,* National Center for Health Statistics, 1997. Hyattsville, MD: Public Health Service.

Human Immunodeficiency Virus Mortality

The epidemic of AIDS can be traced back to the late 1970s with rapid progression throughout the 1980s (Centers for Disease Control, n.d.). Mortality attributable to AIDS is reflected in Table 3–19. High-risk groups include male intravenous drug users and gays. Life expectancy after diagnosis has increased significantly in recent years, although the epidemic is still extracting a terrible toll from the nation.

However, to put this disease in perspective, more people die annually from many other causes, including accidents and violence. Parenthetically, it should be kept in mind that AIDS is an international epidemic with over 40,000,000 infected individuals worldwide and is virtually endemic in certain areas and population groups.

Other Causes of Mortality

Perhaps one of the most tragic causes of mortality and morbidity in our society is vehicular-related accidents. An estimated 40,000 people are killed and approximately 2,000,000 people are injured annually in vehicle-related accidents, a national tragedy. Safer roads and vehicles and a lower driving speed have led to reductions in vehicular mortality over the past twenty years. The tragic toll of motor vehicle accidents is reflected in Table 3–20. Those at highest risk are young adult male drivers and the oldest age groups.

Mortality attributable to firearms is another inexcusable national tragedy. Table 3–21 reflects mortality rates by age group due to firearms-related

TABLE 3–16 Death rates for malignant neoplasms of respiratory system, according to sex and age: United States, selected years

Sex and Age	Year (Deaths per 100,000 Resident Population)			
	1950	1970	1990	1995
Male				
All ages, age adjusted	21.3	50.6	61.0	55.3
Under 25 years	0.2	0.1	0.1	0.1
25–34 years	1.3	1.5	1.0	0.8
35–44 years	8.1	17.0	9.1	7.6
45–54 years	39.3	72.1	63.0	49.9
55–64 years	94.2	202.3	232.6	196.1
65–74 years	116.3	340.7	447.3	432.4
75–84 years	105.1	354.2	594.4	573.4
85 years and over	95.4	215.3	538.0	567.6
Female				
All ages, age adjusted	4.6	10.1	26.2	27.5
Under 25 years	0.1	0.1	0.0	0.0
25–34 years	0.6	0.6	0.6	0.7
35–44 years	2.3	6.5	5.4	5.1
45–54 years	6.7	22.2	35.3	30.1
55–64 years	15.4	38.9	107.6	104.8
65–74 years	26.7	45.6	181.7	205.0
75–84 years	38.8	56.5	194.5	245.1
85 years and over	42.0	56.5	142.8	187.5

SOURCE: *Health, United States, 1996–97,* National Center for Health Statistics, 1997, Hyattsville, MD: Public Health Service.

accidents and violence. This includes mortality associated with suicide, homicide, police intervention, and accidents. Approximately 20,000 Americans are killed annually in firearms-related situations, with numerous others sustaining various injuries.

The violent nature of our society is also reflected in Table 3–22, which presents selected data on mortality attributable to homicide and legal intervention. These data partially overlap with firearms mortality when firearms are involved in the homicide or legal intervention

As we seek to improve the quality and quantity of life in this country, we have to constantly appreciate the considerable morbidity and mortality attributable to social, economic, lifestyle, and other non-physiological causes. Finding answers to problems of unhealthy diets and personal practices, consumption of alcohol, cigarettes, drugs, and other unhealthy substances, and the prevalence of social problems leading to violence in our society must be a high priority as we also seek biomedical solutions to our physiological problems. At the same time, we also face a wide range of psychological and mental health problems that cause tremendous disruption in our lives and our society; these, too, must be addressed from both biomedical and social perspectives.

INCIDENCE OF INFECTIOUS DISEASES

From an international perspective, our nation is now largely spared the tragedies of many of the infectious diseases that are still prevalent throughout the world (World Health Organization, 1993). However, not all infectious disease has been eradicated in this nation, and new challenges continue to surface.

Table 3–23 presents the incidence of infectious disease over the latter half of the twentieth century for the United States (Centers for Disease Control, 1993). The decline of many infectious diseases that are now avoidable through immunization and vaccination is evident in this table. At the same time, the table illustrates the continuing challenge of many infectious diseases that remain, especially those associated with sexual activity.

Likely further declines in reportable infectious diseases will occur in the future with the introduction of new immunizations for such diseases as

TABLE 3–17 Five-year relative cancer survival rates for selected sites, according to race and sex: Selected geographic areas, 1974–1976 and 1986–1991

| Sex and Site | Percent of Patients Surviving More than Five Years | | | |
| | White | | Black | |
	1974–1976	1986–1993	1974–1976	1986–1993
Male				
All sites	41.9	56.5	31.3	41.1
Oral cavity and pharynx	54.3	51.8	31.2	28.4
Esophagus	4.3	12.1	2.1	7.5
Stomach	13.2	16.6	15.5	16.9
Colon	49.8	64.2	44.1	51.6
Rectum	47.8	60.4	34.1	51.0
Pancreas	3.1	3.6	1.4	4.5
Lung, bronchus	11.0	12.7	11.0	10.5
Prostate gland	67.7	90.2	58.0	75.3
Urinary bladder	74.5	85.1	54.1	65.0
Non-Hodgkin's lymphoma	47.7	48.7	43.1	40.0
Leukemia	33.5	43.8	32.6	31.4
Female				
All sites	57.4	62.3	46.8	47.9
Colon	50.8	62.1	46.6	53.3
Rectum	49.7	60.8	49.3	53.0
Pancreas	2.1	3.9	3.1	5.7
Lung, bronchus	15.8	16.1	13.1	12.2
Melanoma of skin	84.8	91.1	—	78.7
Breast	74.9	85.5	62.9	70.0
Cervix uteri	69.2	71.4	63.5	57.1
Corpus uteri	88.6	85.9	60.4	55.3
Ovary	36.3	46.5	40.1	41.9
Non-Hodgkin's lymphoma	47.3	56.6	54.1	49.0

SOURCE: *Health, United States, 1996–97,* National Center for Health Statistics, 1997, Hyattsville, MD: Public Health Service.

chicken pox. For other diseases, such as gonorrhea, the challenge continues, particularly with physiologic resistance to many current drug treatments. And, of course, the AIDS epidemic dramatically illustrates the potential threat from new infectious diseases. Other particularly gruesome infectious diseases, such as the Ebola virus, have come to the forefront in recent years, clearly demonstrating how we can be challenged by disease, even with the advancing state of our knowledge.

TABLE 3–18 Age-adjusted cancer incidence rates for selected cancer sites, white males and white females, selected geographic areas and years

Race, Sex, and Site	Year (Number of New Cases per 100,000 Population)	
	1973	1994
White male		
All sites	364.3	462.0
Oral cavity and pharynx	17.6	14.4
Esophagus	4.8	5.9
Stomach	14.0	9.3
Colon and rectum	54.3	52.2
Colon	34.8	36.6
Rectum	19.5	15.7
Pancreas	12.8	9.6
Lung and bronchus	72.4	72.6
Prostate gland	62.6	135.3
Urinary bladder	27.3	31.2
Non-Hodgkin's lymphoma	10.3	19.8
Leukemia	14.3	12.4
White female		
All sites	295.0	347.1
Colon and rectum	41.7	36.4
Colon	30.3	27.3
Rectum	11.5	9.1
Pancreas	7.5	7.4
Lung and bronchus	17.8	43.3
Melanoma of skin	5.9	11.6
Breast	84.4	112.8
Cervix uteri	12.8	7.1
Corpus uteri	29.5	22.4
Ovary	14.7	14.4
Non-Hodgkin's lymphoma	7.5	13.3

SOURCE: *Health, United States, 1996–97,* National Center for Health Statistics, 1997, Hyattsville, MD: Public Health Service.

TABLE 3–19 Death rates for human immuno-deficiency virus (HIV) infection, according to age: United States, selected years

Age Group	Year (Deaths per 100,000 Resident Population)	
	1987	1995
All ages, age adjusted	5.5	15.6
Under 1 year	2.3	1.5
1–4 years	0.7	1.3
5–14 years	0.1	0.5
15–24 years	1.3	1.7
25–34 years	11.7	29.1
35–44 years	14.0	44.4
45–54 years	8.0	26.3
50–64 years	3.5	11.0
65–74 years	1.3	3.6
75–84 years	0.8	0.7

SOURCE: *Health, United States, 1996–97,* National Center for Health Statistics, 1997, Hyattsville, MD: Public Health Service.

LIFESTYLE PATTERNS AND DISEASE

Numerous behaviors and lifestyle patterns affect our health. Examples discussed previously in this chapter include exposure to violence, vehicular accidents, alcohol, drugs, and infectious agents.

An excellent example of the association between disease and behavior is the consumption of tobacco products. Cigarette consumption has been associated with numerous illnesses including cardiovascular disease, lung cancer, and oral cancer. Reduction in cigarette and other tobacco product consumption has been a national goal for thirty years.

TABLE 3–20 Death rates for motor vehicle crashes by age: United States, selected years

Age Group	Year (Deaths per 100,000 Resident Population)		
	1950	1970	1995
All ages, age adjusted	23.3	27.4	16.1
Under 1 year	8.4	9.8	4.8
1–4 years	11.5	11.5	5.4
5–14 years	8.8	10.2	5.6
15–24 years	34.4	47.2	29.4
25–34 years	24.6	30.9	19.4
35–44 years	20.3	24.9	15.0
45–54 years	22.2	25.5	13.7
55–64 years	29.2	27.9	14.2
65–74 years	38.8	32.8	17.5
75–84 years	52.7	43.5	29.2
85 years and over	45.1	34.2	30.1

SOURCE: *Health, United States, 1996–97,* National Center for Health Statistics, 1997, Hyattsville, MD: Public Health Service.

TABLE 3–21 Death rates for firearm-related injuries, according to selected sex, race, and age: United States, 1995

Sex, Race, and Age	Deaths per 100,000 Resident Population	
	White male	Black male
All ages, age adjusted	19.3	55.6
1–14 years	1.9	4.6
15–24 years	31.4	140.2
25–34 years	26.1	94.4
35–44 years	21.2	46.6
45–64 years	19.7	29.1
65 years and over	32.3	21.4

SOURCE: *Health, United States, 1996–97,* National Center for Health Statistics, 1997, Hyattsville, MD: Public Health Service.

Government policy has been directed toward reducing morbidity and mortality by intervening in people's destructive behavior. Interventions include the use of taxation, public education, and restrictions on product production and distribution.

A reduction in cigarette consumption in the United States has occurred during the period of aggressive intervention, as reflected in Table 3–24. Many current smokers may be consuming greater quantities of tobacco products than the typical smoker did in past years. Many of those giving up tobacco products were casual users.

The net effect on morbidity and mortality from tobacco product consumption is difficult to estimate. However, any reduction in use of these products is positive for the nation's health overall, probably substantially so.

HEALTH, LIFESTYLE, AND SOCIAL STRUCTURE

The relationship between lifestyle and health is well established with regard to practices such as tobacco products consumption, as discussed previously. Numerous other lifestyle issues also significantly impact health. Alcohol consumption and illicit drug use are examples of personal decision making and patterns of behavior that have tremendous adverse effects on health and on the nation's economy.

Alcohol consumption, beyond a very moderate level, is associated with numerous physiological complications including cirrhosis of the liver, various cancers, intestinal disorders, and brain function deterioration. Equally severe psychological and social complications ranging from divorce to poor job performance are also common. Alcohol abuse results in illness and injury to others, including, but certainly not limited to, vehicular accidents, job-place injuries, poor fetal outcomes associated

TABLE 3–22 Death rates for homicide and legal intervention, according to selected sex, race, and age: United States, 1995

Sex, Race, and Age	Deaths per 100,000 Resident Population	
	White male	Black male
All ages, age adjusted	8.2	57.6
Under 1 year	7.1	22.4
1–14 years	1.5	6.7
15–24 years	16.5	152.1
25–34 years	12.9	109.0
35–44 years	9.2	65.3
45–64 years	5.8	34.6
65 years and over	3.0	19.9

SOURCE: *Health, United States, 1996–97,* National Center for Health Statistics, 1997, Hyattsville, MD: Public Health Service.

TABLE 3–23 Selected notifiable disease cases: United States, selected years

Disease	Year (Number of Cases)	
	1950	1995
Diphtheria	5,796	0
Hepatitis A	—	31,582
Hepatitis B	—	10,805
Mumps	—	906
Pertussis (whooping cough)	120,718	5,137
Poliomyelitis, total	33,300	2
Rubella (German measles)	—	128
Rubeola (measles)	319,124	281
Tuberculosis	121,742	22,860
Varicella (chickenpox)	—	120,624
Syphilis	217,558	68,953
Gonorrhea	286,746	392,848

SOURCE: *Health, United States, 1996–97,* National Center for Health Statistics, 1997, Hyattsville, MD: Public Health Service.

with fetal alcohol syndrome, and spousal and child abuse.

Like alcohol abuse, illicit drug use results in a spectrum of adverse consequences for our society. In addition to many of the adverse consequences already mentioned for alcohol abuse, illicit drug use leads to high levels of violent crime, general social dysfunction, and many other untoward consequences.

The implications of tobacco, alcohol, and drug abuse alone are wide-ranging and contribute to the destruction of the fabric of our society and of individuals' lives. And these three areas constitute only a portion of dysfunctional behavior that impinges on health, with consequent increased morbidity and mortality.

The range of other behaviors that adversely affect health is tremendous. Enhanced morbidity and mortality have been associated with various complications of dietary behaviors such as elevated consumption of fat, sodium, and sugar. Sexual behaviors are associated with the spread of communicable diseases such as AIDS, gonorrhea, syphilis, and other sexually transmitted diseases, leading to increased levels of infertility, cancer, and other complications. Societal stress is associated with deterioration of the immune system and consequent morbidity and mortality, workplace violence, marital difficulties, spousal abuse, and other problems.

Thus, the etiology of much of our morbidity and mortality can be traced to behavior, social interaction, lifestyle, and other nonphysiological determinants. Solving the primary physiological causes of illness and disease may be easier than adequately addressing these social and behavioral ones. The challenges to modify behavior are great, and the complications introduced by our modern society make the task ever more difficult. As we move into the new century, the failure of our society in

TABLE 3–24   Current cigarette smoking by persons 18 years of age and over, according to sex and age: United States, 1965 and 1994

Sex and Age	Percent of Persons 18 Years of Age and Over	
	1965	*1994*
Males		
18 years,		
age adjusted	51.6	27.8
18–24 years	54.1	29.8
25–34 years	60.7	31.4
35–44 years	58.2	33.2
45–64 years	51.9	28.3
65 years and over	28.5	13.2
Females		
18 years,		
age adjusted	34.0	23.3
18–24 years	38.1	25.2
25–34 years	43.7	28.8
35–44 years	43.7	26.8
45–64 years	32.0	22.8
65 years and over	9.6	11.1

SOURCE: *Health, United States, 1996–97,* National Center for Health Statistics, 1997, Hyattsville, MD: Public Health Service.

the twentieth century to adequately address the social, behavioral, and economic causes of disease and illness will continue to haunt us.

SUMMARY

This chapter has traced many of the primary patterns of population dynamics and illness in our society during the twentieth century. A fundamental understanding of these trends is essential in interpreting the optimal structure of health services delivery systems as discussed in the remainder of this book. Understanding the relationships between these epidemiological trends and the physiological and psychological nature of the human body and of the determinants of health services utilization is important in defining the overall nature of a population's use of health care and, in turn, forms the basis for the organization and financing, and eventually evaluation, of that system.

REFERENCES

Benson, V., & Marano, M. (1994). *Current estimates from the National Health Interview Survey,* 1993.

(Vital Health Stat 10, 190). National Center for Health Statistics.

Centers for Disease Control and Prevention. (n.d.). *HIV/AIDS surveillance report* (published quarterly). Surveillance and Evaluation Branch, AIDS Program, National Center for Infectious Diseases. Atlanta, GA: Author.

Centers for Disease Control and Prevention. (1993). Summary of notifiable diseases. *U.S. Morbidity and Mortality Weekly Report, 42*(53) (1994, Oct.). Atlanta, GA: Public Health Service, DHHS.

McCaig, L. (1994a). National Ambulatory Medical Care Survey: 1992 emergency department summary. *Advance data from vital and health statistics* (No. 245). Hyattsville, MD: National Center for Health Statistics.

McCaig, L. (1994b). National Hospital Ambulatory Medical Care Survey: 1992 outpatient department summary. *Advance data from vital and health statistics* (No. 248). Hyattsville, MD: National Center for Health Statistics.

National Center for Health Statistics. (1993). *Vital statistics of the United States, 1989* (Vol. I, Natality, DHHS Pub. No. (PHS) 93-1100 and Vol. II, Mortality, Pt. A, DHHS Pub. No. (PHS) 93-1101). Washington, DC: Public Health Service, U.S. Government Printing Office.

National Center for Health Statistics. (1997). *Health, United States, 1996–97.* Hyattsville, MD: Public Health Service.

Ries, L. G., et al. (1993). *Cancer statistics review, 1973–90.* National Cancer Institute (NIH Pub. No. 93-2789). Bethesda, MD: Public Health Service.

Shappert, S. (1994). 1992 summary: National Ambulatory Medical Care Survey. *Advance data from vital and health statistics* (No. 253). Hyattsville, MD: National Center for Health Statistics.

United Nations. (1992). *Demographic yearbook* (United Nations Pub. No. ST/ESA/STAT/SER.R/20). New York: Author.

U.S. Bureau of the Census. (1990). *1990 census of the population, general population characteristics* (Series 1990, CP-1). Washington, DC: Author.

U.S. Bureau of the Census. (1992). U.S. population estimates by age, sex, race and Hispanic origin: 1980–1991. *Current Population Reports* (Series P-25, No. 1095). Washington, DC: U.S. Government Printing Office.

World Health Organization. (1993). *World health statistics annual 1993.* Geneva, Switzerland: Author.

CHAPTER

Measuring Access and Trends*

Ronald M. Andersen

Pamela L. Davidson

CHAPTER TOPICS

* Reprinted with permission from *Changing the U.S. Health Care System,* edited by Ronald M. Andersen, Thomas H. Rice, and Gerald F. Komnski, 1996, San Francisco, CA: Jossey-Bass.

LEARNING OBJECTIVES

Upon completing this chapter, the reader should be able to:

- Understand how access is measured for each type of access.
- Understand the measurement of utilization and relate these indicators to health services management.
- Appreciate differentials in utilization between various population groups.
- Relate access measures to health policy.

The purpose of this chapter is to present basic trends as well as research and policy issues related to health care access. Access is the actual use of personal health services and everything that facilitates or impedes the use of personal health services. It is the link between health services systems and the populations they serve. The conceptualization and measurement of access is key to the understanding and formulating of health policy because it predicts health services use, can be used to promote social justice, and can be used to promote health outcomes.

This chapter presents a conceptual framework for understanding access to medical care. The various types of access are considered and related to their policy purposes. Examples of key access measures are provided and trend data are used to track changes that have occurred over time. Findings from various national studies are synthesized to determine whether access is improving or declining in the United States—for whom and according to what measures. The chapter concludes by discussing future access indicators and research directions.

UNDERSTANDING ACCESS TO HEALTH CARE

This section provides a conceptual framework for understanding access to medical care based on a systems perspective. The framework is a potentially powerful analytical tool that can be applied by policy analysts and health services managers to describe, predict, and explain population-based health services utilization and health outcomes. Also reviewed are the types of access measures and their definitions according to components of the framework.

Conceptual Framework

Figure 4–1 presents a behavioral model of health services use, which is helpful in understanding access to medical care. The conceptual framework presents a systems approach to understanding a population's access to health care and consists of four major components: environmental factors, population characteristics, health behaviors, and health outcomes.

External environmental factors affect the health status of individuals within the community. Environmental factors reflect the economic climate, relative wealth, politics, level of stress and violence, and prevailing norms of the society that may affect the way society views health and whether access to health care is considered the responsibility of the individual or the state.

Health care system characteristics are the policies, resources, organization, and financial arrangements influencing the accessibility, availability, and acceptability of medical care services.

Personal characteristics of the population at risk, conceptualized as predisposing characteristics, enabling resources, and need, influence personal health practices and utilization of health services, which in turn influence health status and consumer satisfaction. Among the predisposing characteristics,

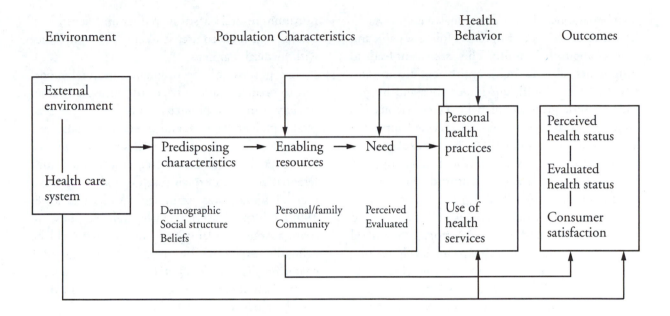

FIGURE 4–1   A behavorial model of health service use

demographic factors such as age and gender represent biological imperatives suggesting the likelihood that people will need health services. Social structure is measured by a broad array of factors that determine the status of a person in the community, his or her ability to cope with presenting problems and to command resources to deal with these problems, and how healthy or unhealthy the physical environment is likely to be. Traditional measures used to represent social structure include education, occupation, and ethnicity. Expanded measures of social structure might include social networks, social interactions, and culture (Bass & Noelker, 1987; Guendelman, 1985; Portes, et al., 1993).

Health beliefs are attitudes, values, and knowledge that people have about health and health services that influence their subsequent perceptions of need and use of health services. Health beliefs provide one means of explaining how social structure

might influence enabling resources, perceived need, and subsequent use.

Both community and personal enabling resources must be present for use to take place. Community resources include supply factors, such as physician and hospital bed population ratios. Health personnel and facilities must be available where people live and work. Then people must have the personal means and know-how to obtain those services. Income, health insurance, a regular source of care, transportation, and acceptable travel and waiting times are some of the important measures of enabling resources. More detailed organizational measures, such as utilization control mechanisms, managed care gatekeepers, certification for emergency room use, second opinions for surgery, and coordination of services, can also be included as enabling factors.

Any comprehensive effort to model access to health care must consider how people view their own general health and functional state, as well as how they experience symptoms of illness, pain, and worries about their health. This assessment leads to judgments about their health condition and whether it is of sufficient importance and magnitude to seek professional help. Perceived need is largely a social phenomenon that, when appropriately modeled, should itself be largely explained by social factors (such as ethnicity and education) and health beliefs (such as health attitudes and knowledge of health care).

However, within rather broad limits established by predisposing and enabling factors, a biological imperative accounts for some people's help seeking and consumption of health services (Hulka & Wheat, 1985). This imperative is better represented by the evaluated component of need (Andersen, et al., 1975). Evaluated need represents professional judgment and objective measurement about a patient's physical status and need for medical care (for example, blood pressure readings, temperature, blood cell count). Of course, evaluated need is not simply, or even primarily, a valid and reliable measurement from biological science. It also has a social component and varies with the changing state of the art and science of medicine as well as the training and competency of the professional expert doing the assessment. Logical expectations of the model are that perceived need will help us to better understand the care-seeking process and adherence to a medical regimen, while evaluated need will be more closely related to the kind and amount of treatment that will be provided after a patient has contacted a medical care provider.

The environment and population characteristics may have direct effects but also work through health behaviors to influence outcomes. Health behavior includes personal health practices as well as use of formal health services. Personal health practices performed by the individual to maintain or improve health can include appropriate diet and nutrition, exercise, stress reduction, control of alcohol and tobacco use, self-care, and compliance with medical regimens.

The purpose of the original behavioral model was to predict health services use measured rather broadly as units of physician ambulatory care, hospital inpatient services, and dental care consumed during a given year. We hypothesized that predisposing, enabling, and need factors would have differential ability to explain use depending on what type of service was examined (Andersen, 1968, 1995). Hospital services utilized in response to more serious problems and conditions would be primarily explained by need and demographic characteristics, while dental services, considered more discretionary, would likely be explained by social structure, health beliefs, and enabling resources. We expected all the components of the model to explain ambulatory physician use because the conditions stimulating care-seeking would generally be viewed as less serious and demanding than those resulting in inpatient care, but more serious than those leading to dental care.

More specific measures of health services use could be used to describe a particular medical condition or type of service or practitioner or could be linked to an episode of illness. For example, a longitudinal study of rheumatoid arthritis patients could measure visits to different types of providers, treatment provided, level of patient compliance to treatment, and associated changes in functional status and pain over time. While such linked analyses are in many ways likely to be more informative, the more global ones (for example, number of physician visits and self-rated general health status) still have a role to play. Global measures provide needed comprehensive indicators of the overall effects of policy changes over time.

Outcomes include people's perception of their health status and clinical assessment by health care professionals as well as their general satisfaction with the care they receive. Perceived health status relies on the judgment and values of the individual or others responsible for the individual's welfare. It indicates the extent to which a person can live a functional, comfortable, and pain-free existence within society. Evaluated outcomes are dependent on the judgment of the professional, based on established clinical standards and state-of-the-art practices. Consumer satisfaction describes how individuals feel about the health care they receive and can be judged by ratings of waiting time, travel time, communications with providers, and technical care received.

The model also includes feedback. We expect health behavior to alter people's need for services. Outcomes (health status and satisfaction) might also result in changes—in both health behavior and population characteristics (such as predisposing beliefs or perceived need).

Types of Access

A major goal of the behavioral model is to provide measures of access to medical care. Access is a relatively complex health policy measure and can be reasonably defined in multidimensional terms. Figure 4–2 presents the types of access to health

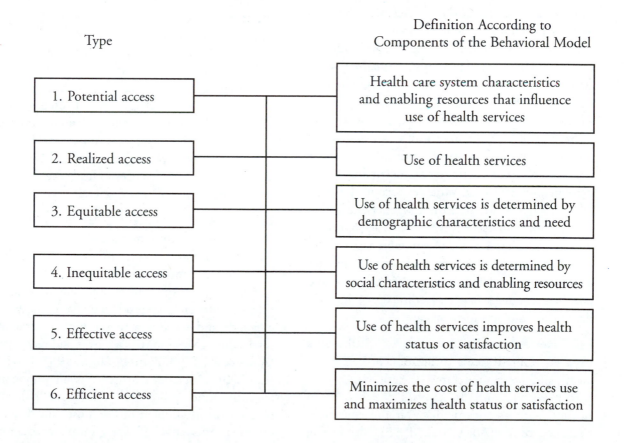

FIGURE 4–2 Types of access to health services

care and their definitions according to components of the behavioral model.

Potential Access. Potential access may be described in terms of structural indicators such as characteristics of the health care delivery system and enabling resources that influence potential care-seekers' use of health services. More enabling resources provide the means for, and increase the likelihood that, use will take place.

Realized Access. Realized access is the actual use of services. Realized access indicators include actual utilization of physician, hospital, and other health services.

Equitable and Inequitable Access. Access is defined as equitable or inequitable according to what determinants (for example, age, ethnicity, insurance status, or symptoms) of realized access are dominant in predicting utilization. Equity is in the eyes of the beholder. Value judgments about which components of the model should explain utilization in an equitable health care system are crucial to the definition. Traditionally, equitable access has been defined as occurring when demographic and need variables account for most of the variance in utilization (Andersen, 1968). Demographic characteristics (such as age or gender differences) are indicators of equitable access to the extent that they are precursors of need. Inequitable access occurs when social characteristics and enabling resources (such as ethnicity or income) determine who gets medical care.

Effective Access. Effective access is the link between realized access (utilization of health services) and health outcomes (health status, consumer satisfaction). It assesses the benefit of medical care as measured by improvements in health outcomes (Aday, et al., 1993). Measures of effectiveness examine the relative impact of health services utilization within the context of other pre-

disposing, enabling, need, and health behavior variables. Predisposing variables, such as age, gender, and social support, can influence the patient's health status following treatment. Access to personal enabling resources (health insurance, income, regular source of care) can result in expeditious medical treatment with highly trained practitioners using state-of-the-art medical technology. Conversely, lack of enabling resources can lead to delays in seeking medical advice and episodic, fragmented treatment with a potential negative impact on health outcomes and satisfaction with medical care. Researchers conducting effectiveness and outcomes research have developed strategies for risk adjustment to control for the effects of medical need (for example, severity of illness, number of symptoms, and comorbidities) before intervention. Personal health practices (diet, exercise, stress management) and compliance with medical regimens prior to and subsequent to treatment can also influence health outcomes. Analytical models used to determine the effectiveness of alternative medical treatments on health outcomes must consider the influence of these varying personal and behavioral factors as well as differences in health care delivery systems and external environment.

Efficient Access. Efficient access links resources consumed to health services and associated health outcomes. Efficient access minimizes the cost of health services and maximizes health status or consumer satisfaction. Aday and her colleagues describe efficiency as producing the combination of goods and services with the highest attainable total value, given limited resources and technology (Aday, et al., 1993; Byrns & Stone, 1987; Davis, et al., 1990). Efficiency consists of two components, allocative and productive. Allocative efficiency requires the attainment of the most valued mix of outputs. Productive efficiency means producing a given level of output at minimum cost. Efficiency attempts to quantify the cost-effectiveness or cost-benefit of health services in assessing the extent to which finite private, public, or personal resources should be invested in assuring access to those services (Aday, 1993a).

POLICY PURPOSES OF ACCESS MEASURES

Earlier policies were designed to increase health services use and promote social justice. The cost containment movement resulted in the design of strategies to control utilization. Eventually, policy analysts linked medical services use to health out-

comes to measure the actual benefit of medical care. Resource management efforts now identify the most cost-effective interventions to promote health outcomes and minimize cost. Figure 4–3 summarizes the major policy uses of access measures and how the emphasis has changed from one policy goal to another with the passage of time.

To Change or Monitor Utilization

Historically, the United States has experienced improving trends in access to health care as measured by increasing health services utilization rates. Access to health services was considered an end goal

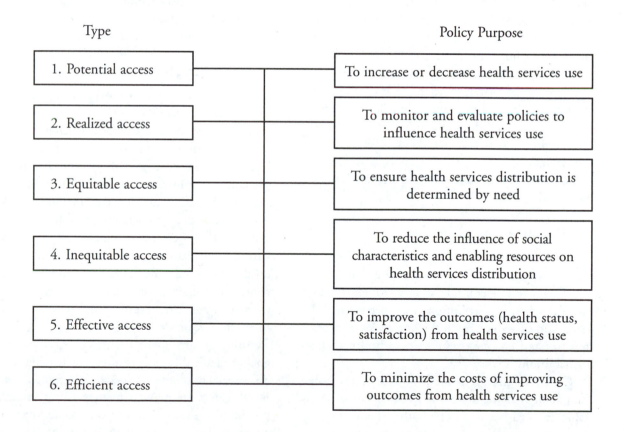

FIGURE 4–3   Policy purposes of access measures

of policy change. Potential access measures were used as indicators of increasing access to medical care services. Realized access measures were used to monitor and evaluate policies to influence health services use. Policies were implemented in the 1950s and 1960s to increase the numbers of physicians, to supply hospital beds in rural communities, and to create federal programs to increase access including Medicare and Medicaid legislation.

The United States health care system evolved from decision making grounded in altruism through increasing the access and supply of resources to a position of caution and financial prudence (McManus & Pohl, 1994). The predominant focus on increasing medical care utilization shifted in the 1970s to concern for health care cost containment and creation of mechanisms to limit access to health care, including HMO legislation, coinsurance, deductibles, utilization review, and the genesis of managed care. In the 1980s and 1990s, HMOs competing with fee-for-service organizations enjoyed double-digit growth in profit margins (Coyne & Meadows, 1991; Kenkel, 1989; Larkin, 1989). HMO growth, however, may be slowing as the managed care market becomes saturated.

To Promote Social Justice

The social justice movement, dominant in the 1960s and early 1970s with the passage of Medicare and Medicaid, sought to ensure that health services distribution was determined by need and to reduce the influence of social characteristics and enabling resources on health services distribution.

Equity of access to medical care is the value judgment that the system is deemed fair or equitable if need-based criteria rather than enabling resources (insurance coverage or income) are the main determinants of whether or not, or how much, care is sought. Subgroup disparities in the utilization of health services (for example, according to race/ethnicity or health insurance coverage) would be minimized in a fair and equitable system, while underlying need for preventive or illness-related health care would be the principal factor determining utilization. In reality, social and economic factors are related in varying degrees to health risk and health outcomes in countries with all types of political, economic, and health care systems (Aday, et al., 1993).

This dominant emphasis on social justice declined in the 1970s and 1980s with increasing concern for cost containment. The 1990s are turbulent times in health care, and significant portions of high-risk vulnerable subgroups in the nation are uninsured and unable to pay for health care services (McManus & Pohl, 1994).

To Promote Health Outcomes

The cost containment movement became more sophisticated in the late 1980s and 1990s. The next generation of health services research began to measure the impact of health services utilization on health outcomes. Accordingly, the Institute of Medicine Committee on Monitoring Access to Personal Health Care Services defined access as "the timely use of personal health services to achieve the best possible health outcomes" (Institute of Medicine, 1993). This definition relies on the use of both health services and health outcomes as yardsticks for judging whether access has been achieved. The resulting measures are referred to as effective access.

Although improving health status is an essential goal of medical care, it is often challenging to link differential outcomes to specific components of the health care system. Weissman and Epstein (1994) provide this example of our limited ability to link access to health care to health status outcomes. One group of patients suffers higher rates of complications several weeks after discharge from the hospital. It is difficult to determine whether the causes of the poor outcomes were initiated during the hospital stay or postdischarge in the ambulatory setting, by differences in the home environment or individual health behaviors, or by measured differences between the groups in severity of illness. In spite of these measurement challenges, health outcomes are important ultimate indicators of access to health care.

To Promote Health Outcomes and Minimize Cost

In recent years, concerns about cost containment have been combined with those directed to improving health outcomes. The results are measures of efficient access. These measures are similar to measures of effective access with the added emphasis on measuring resources used to influence outcome. The policy purpose is to promote health outcomes while minimizing the resources required to attain improved outcomes.

EXAMPLES OF KEY ACCESS MEASURES

This section discusses the kinds of measures used to describe the various types of access. Data are collected and analyzed from multiple sources to measure access to health care, including hospitals and other health organizations at the national, state, or regional level, or within a single health services organization or community clinic. Tables 4–1 and 4–2 provide visual summaries of the material.

Potential Access Measures

Potential access measures are the structural characteristics of the health care delivery system and enabling resources. The first section of Table 4–1 presents these measures. Structural characteristics include measures of capacity (for example, physi-

cian/population ratio or hospital bed/population ratio), organization (percentage of the population enrolled in managed care programs), and financing (per capita expenditures for health services or percentage of population with health insurance). Enabling characteristics are personal resources (regular source of care, income, health insurance coverage) and community resources (urban or rural community, region of residence) that may be associated with potential access.

Realized Access Measures

Realized access is measured by number, type, site, and purpose of services, as shown in Table 4–1. Type of services utilized can be ambulatory, inpatient, prescriptions, or dental care services. The site of service utilization can be the physician's office, hospital, or community clinic. Service purpose can be primary (preventive or early treatment), secondary (more complex treatment for acute or chronic conditions), or tertiary (rehabilitative or custodial) care.

Equitable Access Measures

The test of equity of access involved determining whether there are systematic differences in use and outcomes among groups in United States society and whether these differences are associated with financial or other barriers to care (Institute of Medicine, 1993). Equitable access is indicated when services are distributed according to need for care, as shown in the third section of Table 4–1. Perceived need is captured by patient self-reporting of symptoms, pain, and general health status. Evaluated need is documented in medical records and test results recorded by medical professionals. Inequitable access (the fourth section of Table 4–1) is indicated when services are distributed according to predisposing social characteristics (such as race/ethnicity, education, or occupation) and

TABLE 4–1 Potential, realized, equitable, and inequitable access measures

Type	Measures	Examples
Potential access		
Health care system characteristics	Capacity	Physician/population ratio Hospital bed/population ratio
	Organization	Percentage of population in managed care
	Financing	Per capita expenditures for health services Percentage of population with health insurance
Enabling characteristics	Personal resources	Regular source of care Income Health insurance coverage
	Community resources	Urban or rural community Region of residence
Realized access	Type of service	Ambulatory Inpatient Prescription Dental
	Site of service	Physician office Hospital Community clinic
	Purpose of service	Primary care Secondary care Tertiary care
Equitable access	Services distributed according to perceived patient need	Symptoms Pain General health status Functional status
	Services distributed according to evaluated need	Medical history Test results
Inequitable access	Services distributed according to predisposing social characteristics	Race/ethnicity Education Occupation
	Services distributed according to enabling characteristics	Regular source of care Income Health insurance coverage

TABLE 4–2 Effectiveness and efficiency access measures

Objective	Realized Access Measures (Use of Services)	Outcome Measures
Primary prevention		
1. Promoting successful birth outcomes	Percentage of women obtaining adequate care based on Kessner index (trimester in which care first sought, number of visits, gestational age)	Infant mortality rate Low birth weight Congenital syphilis
2. Reducing the incidence of vaccine-preventable childhood diseases	Percentage of preschool-age children (ages 1 to 4 years) who have been vaccinated	Incidence of preventable childhood communicable diseases (diphtheria, measles, mumps, pertussis, polio, rubella, and tetanus)—cases per 1,000 population
3. Early detection and diagnosis of treatable diseases	Breast and cervical cancer screening—percentage of women undergoing selected procedures (clinical breast exam, mammography, Pap test in given period)	Percentage of (breast, cervical cancer) tumors diagnosed at early stages
4. Promoting functional dentition status	Percentage of population with a dental visit in the past year	Percentage of children with untreated decayed teeth Percentage of adults with no teeth
Illness-related care		
1. Reducing the effects of chronic diseases and prolonging life	Average number of annual physician contacts for those in poor health Use of high-cost, high-tech procedures	Avoidable hospitalization for chronic diseases Number of deaths per 100,000 population estimated to be due to access problems
2. Reducing morbidity and pain through timely and appropriate treatment	Percentage of individuals with acute illness who have no physician contact	Avoidable hospitalization for acute conditions

enabling resources (such as regular sources of care, income, or health insurance coverage).

Effective and Efficient Access Measures

Table 4–2 presents examples of objectives for primary prevention and illness-related care linked to measures of realized access (use of services) and health outcomes.

Measures of effectiveness link utilization to health outcomes. Efficiency measures are measures of effectiveness with a valuation of resources expended (such as cost per unit of improved health) to attain effectiveness. The particular objectives listed are based on those selected by the Institute of Medicine Committee on Monitoring Access and the Robert Wood Johnson report, "Key Indicators for Policy" (Center for Health Economics Research, 1993; Institute of Medicine, 1993).

Promoting Successful Birth Outcomes. A realized access measure expected to be associated with successful birth outcomes is the Kessner index, which is based on trimester of initiation, frequency of prenatal care, and gestational age. Outcome measures of effectiveness assumed to be affected by prenatal care include rates of infant mortality, low birth weight, and congenital syphilis. Efficiency might measure the relative impact on infant mortality of resource allocation for prenatal care services compared to neonatal intensive care services.

Reducing Vaccine-Preventable Childhood Diseases. The relevant realized access measure here is percentage of children vaccinated. The outcome measures of effectiveness would be the incidence of preventable childhood communicable diseases, and related efficiency measures would be estimates of the costs of reducing incidence through vaccinations.

Promoting Early Detection and Diagnosis. Examples of realized access measures are breast and cervical cancer screening rates for women. Important outcomes measures, in this case, are the stages at which tumors are diagnosed. An increased proportion of tumors diagnosed in early stages would suggest more effective and, perhaps, more efficient access. Efficiency measures would help providers determine the optimal age for allocating fixed resources to provide mammography screening in the adult female population (Eddy, et al., 1988; Mushlin & Fintor, 1992; O'Grady, 1988).

Promoting Functional Dentition Status. A realized access measure is the proportion of people who see a dentist. Among the relevant outcome measures of effectiveness are reduced proportions of children with untreated decayed teeth and adults who experience total tooth loss. Efficiency measures might compare the relative time, cost, and personnel mix required to provide dental services in alternative practice settings (Marcus, et al., 1990).

In addition to the primary prevention objectives already discussed, realized access may influence the course of a current illness. Illness-related objectives include the following.

Reducing the Effects of Chronic Diseases and Prolonging Life. Realized access measures selected here include number of physician contacts for people reporting poor health. The related outcome measure is avoidable hospitalizations for chronic disease through physician contact. Another realized access measure is the use of high-cost, high-tech procedures such as open heart surgeries or transplants, with the related outcomes being reduced chronic disease or prolonged life. Efficiency measures might compare the cost for routine physician monitoring of chronic disease to the cost of avoidable hospitalizations.

Reducing Morbidity and Pain. A realized access measure in response to acute illness is the proportion of individuals who do not see a physician. A related effectiveness outcome measure is an estimate of hospitalizations for acute conditions that might have been avoided with appropriate physician monitoring. Efficiency measures might compare the cost of visits for acute illness to the cost of hospitalizations for acute conditions that might have been avoided.

TRENDS IN ACCESS

In this section, the trends in access are examined according to different types of access measures. We consider changes over time in potential access (health insurance coverage), realized access (use of hospital, physician, and dental services) and equitable access (health insurance availability and health services use according to income and race).

We also examine some key research findings concerning effective and efficient access.

Potential Access

Table 4–3 reports critical potential access measure—health care coverage—for persons under sixty-five years of age from 1980 to 1994. The uninsured proportion of the population increased from 13% to 18% in that time period. While

TABLE 4–3   Health care coverage by age, race/ethnicity, and income

	Private Insurance[c]			Medicaid[c]			Not Covered[c]		
				Percentage of population					
	1980	*1989*	*1994*	*1980*	*1989*	*1994*	*1980*	*1989*	*1994*
Age									
Under 15 years	75	72	63	10	11	20	13	16	16
15–44 years	79	77	70	4	4	7	14	18	22
44–64 years	84	83	81	3	3	4	9	11	12
Race/ethnicity									
White	82	80	74	3	4	8	11	14	17
Black	60	59	52	18	17	24	19	22	22
Hispanic origin[a]	–	51	49	–	10	17	–	31	33
Income[b]									
Less than $14,000	39	35	25	28	27	38	38	37	35
$14,000–$24,999	61	71	54	9	5	12	26	21	30
$25,000–$34,999	79	88	78	3	1	4	15	9	16
$35,000–$49,999	90	92	89	1	1	1	6	6	9
$50,000 or more	94	96	93	1	*	1	4	3	6
Total	79	77	70	6	6	10	13	16	18

– Not available

* Less than 0.5%

a Hispanic origin based on self-report; may include persons classified as either white or black according to race.

b Family income categories for 1989 and 1993. Family income categories for 1980 are less than $7,000, $7,000–$9,999, $10,000–$14,999, $15,000–$24,999, $25,000 or more.

c The sum of the percentages for private insurance, Medicaid, and no coverage may not come to 100% because other types of health insurance (such as Medicare or military policies) do not appear in the table and because persons with both private insurance and Medicaid are counted in both columns.

SOURCE: *Health, United States, 1995,* (p. 260), National Center for Health Statistics, 1996, Hyattsville, MD: Public Health Service.

Medicaid coverage increased (from 6% to 10%), the overall decline in coverage resulted from a drop in the proportion covered by private insurance from 79% to 70%.

The proportion of the uninsured population increased for adults aged fifteen to forty-four years since 1980, reaching 22% in 1994. The proportion covered by private insurance decreased for every age group, but the decline was especially noticeable for children under fifteen, declining from 75% to 63%. Since 1980, however, Medicaid has covered an increasing proportion of children, reaching 20% in 1994. This increase reflects the expanded Medicaid income eligibility enacted by Congress in the mid-1980s. Even for children, however, the proportion uninsured was greater in 1994 (16%) than in 1980 (13%). The results overall leave little doubt that a significant decline in potential access has occurred for the United States population, particularly for people aged fifteen to forty-four years, because of a decline in health insurance coverage.

Realized Access

Table 4–4 presents an historical perspective of personal health care use for the United States population from 1930 to 1993. It provides trend data on realized access for three types of services: services in response to more serious illness (hospital admissions), services provided for a combination of primary and secondary care (physician visits), and services for conditions that are rarely life-threatening and generally considered discretionary but still have an important bearing on people's functional status and quality of life (dental visits).

The hospital admission rate for the United States population doubled between 1930 (six admissions per hundred persons per year) and the early 1950s (twelve admissions). A rising standard of living, the advent of voluntary health insurance, the increasing legitimacy of the modern hospital as

a place to have babies and treat acute illness, and the requirements necessary for developing more sophisticated medical technology all contributed to expanded use of the acute care hospital. Hospital admissions further increased in the 1960s and early 1970s (reaching fourteen admissions per hundred in 1974), reflecting continued growth in medical technology, private health insurance, and the advent of Medicare coverage for the elderly and Medicaid coverage for the low-income population in 1965.

Beginning in the mid-1970s, however, use of the acute care hospital began to decline, dropping to ten admissions per hundred population by 1987 and nine in 1993. Those declines accompanied increasing efforts to contain health care costs by a shift in care from the more expensive inpatient setting to less expensive outpatient settings, a shift from fee-for-service to prospective payments by Medicare, reduced coverage and benefits with increasing coinsurance and deductibles for health insurance, and a shift in certain medical technology and styles of practice reducing reliance on the inpatient settings.

Physician visits (Table 4–4) also increased substantially from the 1930s (2.6 visits per person per year) to the early 1950s (4.2 visits), for many of the same reasons that hospital admissions were increasing in this period. However, unlike hospital admissions, number of physician visits continued to increase, reaching 4.9 visits in 1974 and 6.0 visits in 1993. In part, the relative deemphasis of the inpatient setting and the shift to outpatient settings may account for the divergence in trends of these basic realized access measures.

Trends in dentist visits (Table 4–4) for the total United States population paralleled those for physician visits. Twenty-one percent of the population visited a dentist in 1930. The proportion increased consistently, reaching one-half of the population in 1974. Further increases in the last twenty years

TABLE 4–4   Personal health care use by income

	1928–1931[a]	1952–1953[a]	1963–1964[a]	1974[a]	1987[b,g]	1993[c]
Hospital admissions						
(admissions per 100 persons per year)						
Low income[d]	6	12	14	19	14	14
Middle income[e]	6	12	14	14	11	9
High income[f]	8	11	11	11	8	7
Total	6	12	13	14	10	9
Physician visits						
(visits per person per year)						
Low income[d]	2.2	3.7	4.3	5.3	6.8	7.6
Middle income[e]	2.5	3.8	4.5	4.8	5.4	5.9
High income[f]	4.3	6.5	5.1	4.9	5.3	5.9
Total	2.6	4.2	4.5	4.9	5.4	6.1
Dentist visits						
(percentage seeing a dentist within year)						
Below poverty[h]					33%	36%
Low income[d]	10%	17%	21%	35%	42%	
At or above poverty[h]					52%	64%
Middle income[e]	20%	33%	36%	48%	60%	
High income[f]	46%	56%	58%	64%	76%	
Total	21%	34%	38%	49%	58%	61%

a   *Source:* Various surveys reported in "Trends in the Use of Health Services," by R. Andersen and O. Anderson, in *Handbook of Medical Sociology* (3rd ed., pp. 374, 378, 379), H. E. Freeman, S. Levine, and L. G. Reeder, 1979, Englewood Cliffs, NJ: Prentice Hall.

b   *Source: Health, United States, 1994* (pp. 171, 179, 180), National Center for Health Statistics, 1995, Hyattsville, MD: Public Health Service.

c   *Source: Health, United States, 1994* (pp. 169, 177, 178), Hyattsville, MD: Public Health Service.

d   Low income = lowest 15% to 27% of family income distribution

e   Middle income = middle 51% to 73% of family income distribution

f   High income = highest 12% to 32% of family income distribution

g   1989 for dental visits

h   Dental visit data from National Center for Health Statistics, unpublished data from the National Health Interview Survey, persons aged twenty-five years or older

resulted in sixty-one percent of the population visiting a dentist in 1993.

Equitable Access

Table 4–5 completes the picture begun in Tables 4–3 and 4–4 of health insurance coverage and personal health care use among the United States population. Equitable access is indicated by similar levels of insurance coverage and use by different income and ethnic groups. Inequitable access is suggested by discrepancies in coverage and use for these groups.

TABLE 4–5 Personal health care use by race

	1964[a]	1981–1983[b]	1987–1989[a,c]	1993[d]
Hospital admissions				
(admissions per 100 persons per year)				
Black[e]	8	14	12	11
White	11	12	10	9
Total	11	12	10	9
Physician visits				
(percentage with physician visit within year)				
Black[e]	58%	75%	75%	79%
White	68%	76%	77%	79%
Total	67%	76%	77%	79%
Dental visits				
(percentage seeing a dentist within year)				
Black[e]	22%	36%	44%	47%
White	45%	53%	60%	64%
Total	43%	50%	58%	61%

a *Source: Health, United States, 1993* (pp. 174, 179, 180), National Center for Health Statistics, 1994, Hyattsville, MD: Public Health Service.
b *Source: Health, United States, 1988* (pp. 107, 111), National Center for Health Statistics, 1989, Hyattsville, MD: Public Health Service.
c 1989 for dental visits
d *Source: Health, United States, 1994* (pp. 172, 178), National Center for Health Statistics, 1995, Hyattsville, MD: Public Health Service.
e For 1964, the total given as "black" actually includes all non-Caucasians.

Health Insurance. Table 4–3 suggests considerable inequity in insurance coverage in 1980, continuing to the present time. Minorities and low-income people are least likely to have private health insurance. Medicaid compensates for some of this inequity but still leaves high proportions of blacks (23%), Hispanics (34%), and low-income persons (35%) uninsured in 1993.

The trends in Table 4–3 provide a somewhat mixed picture as to whether inequities in health insurance coverage are increasing over time. Between 1980 and 1993, coverage through private health insurance declined for all ethnic groups while the proportions covered by Medicaid or without coverage increased for all of them.

Although potential access as measured by insurance coverage declined for all ethnic groups and inequities existed over the entire period (whites were less likely to be uninsured than minorities), there is no clear trend toward greater or less inequity according to ethnicity.

Trends in equity according to income level are even more complex. Between 1980 and 1993, private health insurance coverage of the lowest income group declined consistently, with the rate of decline apparently increasing in recent years. For the lower-middle income groups, private insurance coverage increased during the early 1980s but then declined considerably in the early 1990s, so that by 1993 the coverage was similar to what it was in

1980. Most of the highest-income groups had private health insurance coverage throughout the period. Increases in Medicaid coverage more than compensated for decline in private insurance coverage for the lowest-income group, so that the proportion uninsured has been increasing (21% to 27%). Consequently, it appears that inequities in insurance coverage have been increasing for the lower-middle income groups.

Hospital Admissions. Tables 4–4 and 4–5 suggest increasing equity according to income and race for hospital admissions. In 1928–1931, the highest-income group had the highest admission rate (Table 4–4). By the 1950s, the rates had equalized. In subsequent years, the rates by income diverged. Hospitalization for the lowest-income group increased relative to those with higher incomes, so that by 1993 the lowest-income group had a rate (fourteen per hundred) twice that of the highest-income group (seven). Does this indicate that inequity exists in favor of the low-income group? Probably not. Studies taking into account need for medical care suggest that the greater hospital use for low-income persons can be largely accounted for by their higher rates of disease and disability (Davis & Rowland, 1983). The hospital admission rate in 1964 for whites (eleven) was still considerably higher than the rate for blacks (eight), as shown in Table 4–5. By the 1980s, however, the rate for blacks exceeded the rate for whites, and the higher rate for blacks continued into the 1990s. The higher hospital admission rates for blacks, similar to the higher rates for low-income people, can be largely accounted for by higher levels of medical need (Manton, et al., 1987).

Physician Visits. The trends in Tables 4–4 and 4–5 also suggest increasing equity for physician visits according to income level and ethnicity. In 1928–1931, the lowest-income group averaged only one-half as many visits to the doctor (2.2 vis-

its) as the highest group (4.3 visits), as shown in Table 4–4. Over time the gap narrowed. By 1974, the lowest-income group was actually visiting a physician more frequently than the higher-income groups, and the difference increased in the 1980s and early 1990s. Again, research results suggest that the apparent excess for the low-income population can be accounted for by their greater levels of medical need (Davis & Rowland, 1983). Similar trends have taken place for the black population, as shown in Table 4–5, but parity with the white population in proportions seeing doctors have remained the same for blacks and whites into the early 1990s. The physician use rate for the growing Latino population remains considerably below that for both blacks and whites (Andersen, et al., 1981; Burciaga, et al., 1993).

Dental Visits. Tables 4–4 and 4–5 tell a story of major inequities according to income and race in dental visit rates that existed in 1928–1931 and continue to exist into the 1990s. The proportion seeing a dentist has increased considerably for all income and racial groups. Still, by 1993, only 36% of the below-poverty group saw a dentist compared to 64% of those at or above poverty, as shown in Table 4–4. Similarly, Table 4–5 shows that 47% of blacks saw a dentist compared to 64% of whites.

Key Findings for Effective Access

The effectiveness and outcomes movement initiated in the late 1980s was in response to several major developments converging on the national scene (Heithoff & Lohr, 1993). The Health Care Financing Administration proposed a research program called the Effectiveness Initiative, stimulated by their need to ensure quality of care for the thirty million Medicare beneficiaries, to determine which medical practices worked best and to aid policy makers in allocating Medicare resources. At about the same time, an Outcomes Research Program was authorized by Congress, largely inspired by the work of John Wennberg and associates in small-area variations in the utilization and outcomes of medical interventions. A third major development stimulating the effectiveness movement stemmed from efforts led by Robert H. Brook and associates to determine whether medical interventions used in the normal practice setting were being used appropriately. Within the same time period, the Agency for Health Care Policy and Research was created, with a responsibility for developing medical practice guidelines. The guidelines represent the practical application of the outcomes and effectiveness research movement.

Prior to the effectiveness initiative, research was limited by weak study designs (observational and cross-sectional) that were not capable of determining the clear direction of effects and their potential causality (Aday, et al., 1993). Most studies used mortality as the outcome variable, which was shown to be more sensitive to environmental and socioeconomic factors than to medical care utilization (Martini, et al., 1977). Moreover, the appropriate risk adjustments were usually not available in mortality data sets.

The Medical Outcomes Study (MOS) was undertaken in response to these methodological limitations. The MOS sampled physicians and patients from different health care systems, including traditional fee-for-service (FFS) plans, independent practice associations (IPAs), and health maintenance organizations (HMOs), and health care settings to investigate the relationships between structure, process, and medical outcomes. Specifically, the MOS was designed to determine whether variations in medical outcomes were explained by differences in the system of care (structure and process) and medical specialty, and to develop instruments to assess and monitor medical outcomes (such as clinical endpoints, functioning, perceived general health status and well-being, and satisfaction with treatment (Stewart, et al.,

1989; Tarlov, et al., 1989; Ware, 1990). Results from the MOS indicated that patient mix was related to utilization, that is, increasing levels of severity were associated with decreasing levels of functional status and well-being and increasing levels of utilization (hospitalizations, physician visits, prescription drugs), and differed significantly across systems of care and medical specialties (Kravitz, et al., 1992). Variations in resource use, while related to patient mix, were significantly influenced by specialty training, payment system, and practice organization (Greenfield, et al., 1992). The MOS also compared indicators of primary care quality across the various health care systems, controlling for patient and physician characteristics (Safran, et al., 1994). Performance indicators in the three payment settings revealed notable differences in primary care quality: financial access was highest in prepaid systems; organization access, continuity, and accountability were highest in the FFS system; and coordination was highest and comprehensiveness lowest in HMOs. Ultimately, research results demonstrated that multiple factors—patient mix, medical specialty, and system of care—influence patient outcomes, and when patient and physician characteristics are controlled, quality indicators of primary care vary across systems of care.

Key Findings for Efficient Access

Efficiency studies have been conducted at multiple levels including the macroeconomic level, the health plan system level, and the consumer behavior level. At the macroeconomic level, comprehensive data available on major, industrialized countries have been used to compare health services utilization, health resources and expenditures, and health outcomes. The Organization for Economic Cooperation and Development study comparing per capita health care expenditures in seven major industrialized countries found that the United States spent about forty percent more than

Canada and almost three times more than the country with the lowest expenditures, the United Kingdom. The large expenditure gap for the United States was not offset by health outcome advantages, which raised concerns that resources were being misallocated to services with low benefit relative to cost (Aday, 1993a).

Efficiency analyses conducted at the health plan system level usually compare traditional indemnity plans with FFS providers to HMOs. Results from the randomized RAND Health Insurance Study (HIS) indicated that the HMO provided care at twenty-five percent less expense with no adverse health effects on the general population. The change in financial incentives and better resource management (for example, fewer hospital admissions) were seen as strategies to reduce inefficiencies (Aday, et al., 1993). Other studies have conducted production efficiency analyses concentrating on the size and personnel mix of physician practices and other medical care delivery settings, and results indicate that physicians could raise the productivity of their practices and lower the total cost per office visit by employing more aides (Brown, 1988; Reinhardt, 1972; Smith, et al., 1972).

Efficiency analyses focusing on the consumer population have investigated whether health services were being utilized in the most efficient way. Cost sharing is portrayed as a mechanism to decrease inappropriate utilization and therefore produce more efficient health services delivery. Participants in the HIS were randomly assigned to a free-care group or to insurance plans requiring them to pay part of the cost (cost sharing). A physician panel judged whether symptoms were minor (not warranting a physician visit) or serious (warranting a physician visit). No significant differences were reported between the free-care and cost-sharing groups in visiting the physician for serious symptoms. Utilization for minor symptoms, how-

ever, was decreased by more than thirty percent in the cost-sharing group compared to the free-care group. These findings provided empirical evidence demonstrating that efficient utilization management could be achieved by modifying patient behavior through cost sharing, without compromising health outcomes (Shapiro, et al., 1986).

SUMMARY: TRENDS IN ACCESS

Is access improving or declining in the United States? For whom and according to what measures? Although we have documented continuing increases in some realized access measures, including physician and dental visits, inpatient hospital use has been declining for twenty years. And a key potential access measure, health insurance, reveals that while increasing numbers of persons are being covered by Medicaid (although the program is currently under severe threat), there has been a decline in the numbers covered by private insurance in the last fifteen years and an overall increase in the proportion without any health insurance coverage. Low-income and black populations appear to have achieved equity of access according to gross measures of hospital and physician utilization (not adjusting for their greater need for medical care) but continue to lag considerably in receipt of dental care. Equity has certainly not been achieved according to health insurance coverage, as the proportion uninsured is fifty percent higher for blacks and more than twice as high for Latinos and the low-income population as for whites.

A number of recent national investigations of access considering effectiveness and efficiency as well as potential and realized measures provide rather discouraging conclusions about trends, particularly those regarding equity of access. The Commonwealth Fund, citing "serious health problems," "shorter life spans," and "high infant mortality" of minority Americans compared to white Americans, sponsored a national health access survey of more than 3,700 African American, Hispanic, Asian, and white adults in 1994. Two-fifths of Hispanics and Asians reported no regular doctor or provider compared to one-fifth of white adults. Waiting too long to seek care is a major problem for 27% of minority adults (46% for those of Chinese descent) compared with 16% of white adults. Of Americans who visited a doctor in the last year, the proportion that did *not* receive preventive care services such as blood pressure tests, Pap smears, and cholesterol readings was considerably larger for some minorities (Vietnamese, 47%; Mexican, 39%; and Puerto Rican, 38%) than for white (26%). Karen Davis, president of the Commonwealth Fund, thus asks, "if minority Americans already face problems obtaining care . . . how will they be affected by changes in health care financing and practice, the competitive pressures under managed care, and future curbs in Medicaid and public health programs?" (The Commonwealth Fund, 1995).

The Center for Health Economics Research, commissioned by the Robert Wood Johnson Foundation to investigate access to health care in the United States, notes that while "in the last few decades the United States has made notable improvements in health status attributable in part to improved access, for example, striking declines in deaths from heart attacks and strokes (linked to better control of high blood pressure and cardiovascular treatments) and greater survival among low birth weight white infants (linked to neonatal intensive care) . . . *the access picture has worsened for many, particularly the poor*" (Center for Health Economics Research, 1993). The study concludes that even though people in the United States are spending more on health care than on food and housing combined, pressures to curtail costs threat-

en to further erode access to care. Supporting evidence includes:

- The proportion of unattended births (associated with insufficient prenatal care and low birth weight infants) is rising.
- Neonatal death rates for blacks are twice the rates for whites.
- Rates of early prenatal care, a service that may save three dollars for every dollar spent, show almost no progress.
- United States immunization rates are lower than those for most other developed countries.
- Breast and cervical cancer screening rates have increased, but poor and black women are less likely to be screened and more likely to be diagnosed late (after metastasis).
- Even though hospitalizations can be avoided by regular physician visits, the poor are not reaping such benefits, for example, residents of low-income areas have four and one-half times the rate of hospitalization for asthma as do persons in higher-income communities.
- Primary care physicians and dentists tend to practice in wealthier communities (Center for Health Economics Research, 1993).

The Committee on Monitoring Access to Personal Health Care Services of the Institute of Medicine (1993) concludes that *there is little evidence of progress over the last decade.* Although there have been some advances, for example, in the rates of breast cancer screening, they have been counterbalanced by the return of diseases that can be avoided, such as tuberculosis and congenital syphilis. Further, with respect to the AIDS epidemic, it appears that access to medical care helps with respect to longevity and quality of life but is not less costly. Particularly disturbing is the growing division between the haves and the have-nots. Even when improvements in access are noted for all, they are generally less for blacks and other minorities. The committee notes growing discrepancies in infant mortality and proportion of low birth weights and suggests that one-third to one-half of the mortality gap between middle-aged blacks and whites might be attributable to access problems.

In summary, trends according to the various measures of access provide a mixed picture. Although some trends in realized access (physician and dental visits) suggest continued improvement, other trends in potential access (health insurance coverage) and equity of access according to ethnicity and income show declines. Further, while access to care has apparently been effective in improving some outcomes (deaths from heart attacks, strokes, and low birth weights), we continue to pay increasingly higher prices for medical care, suggesting trends in efficiency leave much to be desired.

SUMMARY: FUTURE ACCESS INDICATORS AND NEEDED RESEARCH

The question underlying the design of a new generation of access indicators is to what extent does medical care contribute to people's health (Aday, 1993a)? Issues of effectiveness, efficiency, and equity will all become guiding norms in the development of these indicators (Aday, et al., 1993).

New measures of realized access should have "a fairly well-recognized service intervention with clear guidelines regarding who should receive the services" and closely linked outcomes (Institute of Medicine, 1993). Good examples would be the ratio between the proportion of children vaccinated for a preventable disease such as measles and the incidence of the disease. Further, there should be a source of routine data for the new measures, or one should be developed.

The Committee on Monitoring Access to Personal Health Care Services has noted the need to develop access measures concerning HIV/AIDS, substance abuse, migrants, homeless people, people with disabilities, family violence, emergency services, postacute care for the elderly, and prescription drugs (Institute of Medicine, 1993). Development of access measures for vulnerable populations is especially important because many of them have interrelated needs (Aday, 1993b). "For instance, the broad group of alcohol and substance abusers can include high risk mothers with fetal alcohol syndrome, intravenous drug users with AIDS, mentally ill substance abusers, drug users who attempt suicide, addictive families suffering domestic abuse, homeless people with substance abuse problems, and substance abusing refugees" (Institute of Medicine, 1993).

Considerably more research is also needed to further develop the link between realized access measures and outcome measures outlined in Table 4–2. Some of the most important work to improve the effectiveness and efficiency of access will include efforts:

- *To promote successful birth outcomes.* We need additional research on the relationships among medical risk factors, the content of prenatal care, and birth outcomes. We also need continued research on the increasing disparity between black and white infant mortality.
- *To reduce the incidence of vaccine-preventable childhood diseases.* We need research on the relationships among race, barriers to vaccination access, and infectious disease.
- *To promote early detection and diagnosis of treatable diseases.* We need exploration in more depth of why women do not seek breast and cervical cancer screening. We also need research to determine why improvements in the rates of cancer screening among blacks are not reflected in

improvements in early diagnosis, mortality rates, and survival compared with rates for whites.

- *To promote functional dentition status.* We need further examination of the continuing differences in use of dental services according to income and ethnicity and the impact of these differences on functional status.
- *To reduce the effects of chronic diseases and prolong life.* We need further attention to the differences in use of high-cost discretionary care according to gender, ethnicity, income, and insurance status and attention to whether these differences represent overuse or underuse of these services.
- *To reduce morbidity and pain through timely and appropriate treatment.* We need to explore methods to better define what constitutes timely and appropriate use of physician services during episodes of acute illness, and research on factors that lead to the hospitalization of people with acute diseases.

REFERENCES

Aday, L. A. (1993a). *Access to what and why? Towards a new generation of access indicators.* Proceedings of the Public Health Conference on Records and Statistics (DHHS Pub. No. 941214, pp. 410–415). Washington, DC: U.S. Government Printing Office.

Aday, L. A. (1993b). *At risk in America: The health and health care needs of vulnerable populations in the United States.* San Francisco: Jossey-Bass.

Aday, L. A., Begley, C. E., Lairson, D. R., & Slater, C. H. (1993). *Evaluating the medical care system: Effectiveness, efficiency, and equity.* Ann Arbor, MI: Health Administration Press.

Andersen, R. M. (1968). *Behavioral model of families' use of health services* (Research Series No. 25). Chicago: Center for Health Administration Studies, University of Chicago.

Andersen, R. M. (1995). Revisiting the behavioral model and access to medical care: Does it matter? *Journal of Health and Social Behavior, 36,* 1–10.

Andersen, R. M., Kravits, J., & Anderson, O. (1975). *Equity in health services: Empirical analysis in social policy.* Boston: Ballinger.

Andersen, R. M., Lewis, S. Z., Giachello, A. L., Aday, L. A., & Chiu, G. (1981). Access to medical care among the Hispanic population of the southwestern United States. *Journal of Health and Social Behavior, 22,* 78–89.

Bass, D. M., & Noelker, L. S. (1987). The influence of family caregivers on elders' use of in-home services: An expanded conceptual framework. *Journal of Health and Social Behavior, 28,* 184–196.

Brown, D. M. (1988). Do physicians underutilize aides? *Journal of Human Resources, 23,* 342–355.

Burciaga, V. R., Giachello, A., Rodriguez-Trias, H., Gomez, P., & De La Rocha, C. (1993). Improving access to health care in Latino communities. *Public Health Reports, 108,* 535–539.

Byrns, R. T., & Stone, G. W. (1987). *Economics.* Glenview, IL: Scott, Foresman.

Center for Health Economics Research. (1993). *Access to health care: Key indicators for policy.* Chestnut Hill, MA. Prepared for the Robert Wood Johnson Foundation, Princeton, NJ.

The Commonwealth Fund. (1995). *Managed care: The patient's perspective: A briefing note—Karen Davis, President.* New York: Harkness House.

Coyne, J. S., & Meadows, D. M. (1991). California HMOs may provide national forecast. *Healthcare Financial Management, 45,* 36–39.

Davis, K., Anderson, G. F., Rowland, D., & Steinberg, E. P. (1990). *Health care cost containment.* Baltimore: Johns Hopkins University Press.

Davis, K., & Rowland, D. (1983). Uninsured and underserved: Inequities in health care in the United States. *Milbank Quarterly, 61,* 149–176.

Eddy, D. M., Hasselblad, V., McGivney, W., & Hendee, W. (1988). The value of mammography screening in women under 50 years. *Journal of the American Medical Association, 259,* 1512–1519.

Greenfield, S., Nelson, E. C., Zubkoff, M., Manning, W. G., Rogers, W., Kravitz, R. L., Keller, A., Tarlov, A. R., & Ware, J. E. (1992). Variations in resource utilization among medical specialties and systems of care: Results from the medical outcomes study.

Journal of the American Medical Association, 267, 1624–1630.

Guendelman, S. (1985). Health care users residing on the Mexican border: What factors determine choice of the U.S. or Mexican health system? *Medical Care, 23,* 438–460.

Heithoff, K. A., & Lohr, K. N. (Eds.). (1993). *Effectiveness and outcomes in health care.* Washington, DC: National Academy Press.

Hulka, B. S., & Wheat, J. R. (1985). Patterns of utilization: The patient perspective. *Medical Care, 23,* 438–460.

Institute of Medicine (U.S.). (1993). Committee on Monitoring Access to Personal Health Care Services. *Access to health care in America* (Millman, M., ed., p. 4). Washington, DC: National Academy Press.

Kenkel, P. J. (1989). HMO profit outlook begins to brighten. *Modern Healthcare, 19,* 98.

Kravitz, R. L., Greenfield, S., Rogers, W., Manning, W. G., Zubkoff, M. Nelson, E. C., Tarlov, A. R., & Ware, J. E. (1992). Differences in the mix of patients among medical specialties and systems of care: Results from the medical outcomes study. *Journal of the American Medical Association, 267,* 1617–1623.

Larkin, H. (1989). Law and money spur HMO profit status changes. *Hospitals, 63,* 68–69.

Manning, W. G., Liebowitz, A., & Goldberg, G. A. (1984). A controlled trial of the effect of a prepaid group practice on use of services. *New England Journal of Medicine, 310,* 1505–1510.

Manton, K., Patrick, C., & Johnson, K. (1987). Health differentials between blacks and whites: Recent trends in mortality and morbidity. *Milbank Quarterly, 65*(1), 129–199.

Marcus, M., Koch, A. L., Schoen, M. H., & Tuominen, R. (1990). A proposed new system for valuing dental procedures: The relative time-cost unit. *Medical Care, 28*(10), 943–951.

Martini, C., Allen, J. B., Davidson, J., & Backett, E. M. (1977). Health indexes sensitive to medical care variation. *International Journal of Health Services, 7,* 293–309.

McManus, S. M., & Pohl, C. M. (1994). Ethics and financing: Overview of the U.S. health care system. *Journal of Health and Human Resources Administration, 16*(3), 332–349.

Mushlin, A. I., & Fintor, L. (1992). Is screening for breast cancer cost-effective? *Cancer, 69,* 1957–1962.

O'Grady, L. F. (1988). Breast cancer. In T. W. Hudson, M. A. Reinhart, S. D. Rose, & G. K. Stewart (Eds.), *Clinical Preventive Medicine.* Boston: Little, Brown.

Portes, A., Kyle, D., & Eaton, W. W. (1993). Mental illness and help-seeking behavior among Mariel Cuban and Haitian refugees in South Florida. *Journal of Health and Social Behavior, 33,* 283–298.

Reinhardt, E. (1972). A production function for physician services. *Review of Economics and Statistics, 54,* 55–66.

Safran, D. G., Tarlov, A. R., & Rogers, W. H. (1994). Primary care performance in fee-for-service and prepaid health care systems: Results from the medical outcomes study. *Journal of the American Medical Association, 271,* 1579–1586.

Shapiro, M. F., Ware, J. E., & Sherbourne, C. D. (1986). Effects of cost sharing on seeking care for serious and minor symptoms: Results of a randomized controlled trial. *Annals of Internal Medicine, 104,* 246–251.

Smith, K. R., Miller, M., & Golladay, F. L. (1972). An analysis of the optimal use of inputs in the production of medical services. *Journal of Human Resources, 7,* 208–255.

Stewart, A. L., Greenfield, S., Hays, R. D., et al. (1989). Functional status and well-being of patients with chronic conditions: Results from the medical outcomes study. *Journal of the American Medical Association, 262,* 907–913.

Tarlov, A., Ware, J., Greenfield, S., Nelson, E. C., Perrin, E., & Zubkoff, M. (1989). The medical outcomes study: An application of methods for monitoring the results of medical care. *Journal of the American Medical Association, 262,* 925–930.

Ware, J. E. (1990). Measuring patient function and well-being: Some lessons from the medical outcomes study. In K. A. Heithoff & K. N. Lohr (Eds.), *Effectiveness and Outcomes in Health Care* (pp. 107–119). Proceedings of the invitational conference by the Institute of Medicine, Division of Health Care Services. Washington, DC: National Academy Press.

Weissman, J. S., & Epstein, A. M. (1994). *Tears in the safety net: The impact of insurance status on access to care.* New York: Oxford University Press.

PART III

FINANCING AND STRUCTURING HEALTH CARE

CHAPTER

Financing Health Services

Alma L. Koch

CHAPTER TOPICS

Health Expenditures
Health Insurance
Medicare
Medicaid
Physician Reimbursement
Initiatives in Health Care Finance
Health Care Reform
Summary

LEARNING OBJECTIVES

Upon completing this chapter, the reader should be able to:

- Differentiate among types of health insurance—voluntary, social, and welfare.
- Distinguish among various health financing schemes for provision of care and postulate future changes in these systems.
- Understand and elaborate upon provider incentives and disincentives stemming from the financing system for health care.
- Intelligently discuss major health care financing issues of the day.
- Compare the United States health care financing system with that of other advanced nations.
- Describe the principles of insurance and apply them in evaluating health insurance plans.

The system for financing health services in the United States reflects the fragmentation of health care as a whole. It is a patchwork of loosely connected financing mechanisms varying by sponsorship and provider type. It also reflects the age, health, and economic status of the specific patient groups that are being served. In view of the growing number of Americans who are uninsured for health care, one may say that it is a disappointing financing system. These observations, however, do provide a touchpoint for studying the financing apparatus as it now exists. If one looks at the "system" in light of the role of tradition and the values of the American people, as well as the political philosophy of the times, the organization of health finance in the United States comes into better focus.

This chapter will examine the size and scope of the health care financing system in the United States. Where possible, comparisons will be drawn between the United States and other countries. Special attention will be paid to differences and similarities in the public and private financing components of the system, reimbursement of various provider categories, and trends that we may expect to see in the future. The role of health insurance as a financial conduit will be explored, and monetary business objectives will be contrasted with the altruistic goals of health care as a human service.

HEALTH EXPENDITURES

Size of the United States Health Care Industry

The health care industry is by far the largest service industry in the country. In dollar volume, the health care industry ranks second after total durable goods manufacturing (U.S. Bureau of the Census, 1996). In 1995, Americans spent $989 billion on health care, comprising 13.6% of the gross domestic product (GDP) and amounting to $3,621 per capita (Levit, et al., 1996). The United States spends far more on health care than other industrialized democracies. For example, in 1994, the United Kingdom and Japan fell at the lower end of the spectrum, spending 6.9 and 7.3% of their respective GDPs on health care. Canada, France, Switzerland, and Germany came closer to the United States figures with 9.8, 9.7, 9.6, and 8.6% of their respective GDPs spent on health care, with most other industrialized nations falling in the established range (U.S. Bureau of the Census, 1996).

Growth in Health Expenditures. Since 1940, national health expenditures have grown at a rate substantially outpacing the GDP. Table 5–1 shows that, prior to World War II, only 4.0% of the GDP was devoted to health care, both public and private. By 1995, the proportion of the GDP expended for health care increased by almost ten percentage points. Since the onset of Medicare and Medicaid

TABLE 5–1 Aggregate and per capita national health expenditures, United States, selected years

Year	Total (Billions)	Per Capita	GDP (Billions)	Percent of GDP
1940	$4.0	$30	$100	4.0
1950	12.7	82	287	4.4
1960	26.9	141	527	5.1
1970	73.2	341	1,036	7.1
1980	247.2	1,052	2,784	8.9
1990	697.5	2,683	5,744	12.1
1995	988.5	3,621	7,254	13.6

SOURCE: Adapted from "National Health Expenditures, 1995," by K. R. Levit, et al., Fall 1996, *Health Care Financing Review*, *18*(1), pp. 175–214.

in mid-1966, national health expenditures have grown particularly rapidly, from about 6.3% of the GDP to the present figure. Most of this growth is quantitatively explained by economywide inflation, excess medical inflation, and increased intensity in the provision of health care services, in that order. Only a small fraction of growth in health care can be attributed to the growth in the United States population. From 1993 to 1995, however, health care spending exhibited no change, stabilizing between 13.5 and 13.6% of the GDP. This stability was precipitated by a slowdown in the rate of growth of health care spending, rather than an upswing in overall economic growth (Levit, et al., 1996).

A variety of qualitative factors is believed to have contributed to the disproportionate growth in health care spending relative to the growth in GDP. These include (1) rising expectations about the value of health care services, (2) the rapid development and dissemination of medical technology that has expanded the treatment of disease, (3) government financing of health care services, (4) the nature of third-party reimbursement, (5) the growth in the proportion of the elderly, (6) the lack of competitive forces in the health care system to increase efficiency and productivity in the delivery

of services, and (7) the maldistribution of physicians and other providers of health services.

Monetary Flow

Payment Sources. Figure 5–1 contrasts the monetary inflow and outflow in the United States for total health spending in 1995. Private health insurance finances less than one-third of all health expenditures; direct patient payment finances about one-fifth. These payment sources, together with other private sources (mostly philanthropy), account for the 54% of all health care expenditures that are privately financed in the United States. The other 46% is financed publicly by federal, state, or local government sources. The largest single public program is Medicare (the federal social security health insurance plan for the elderly, the disabled, and other groups), followed by Medicaid (the federal/state welfare program for health care) and other government programs (Levit, et al., 1996).

Spending for Medicare and Medicaid has been increasing even more rapidly than total national health expenditures. In 1995, Medicare and Medicaid together comprised 33% of the total health care bill; in 1967, the two programs represented only 15% of the total health care bill.

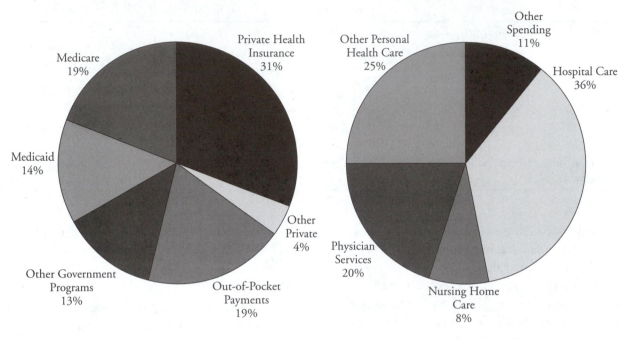

Where It Came From

Where It Went

SOURCE: "National Health Expenditures, 1995," by K. R. Levit, et al., Fall 1996, *Health Care Financing Review, 18*(1), p. 200.

FIGURE 5–1   The nation's health dollar, 1995

Out of approximately 273 million people in the United States in 1995, over one-quarter (74 million people) were enrolled in either or both programs. Medicare's role was clearly most substantial for hospital care, while Medicaid's role was most prominent for nursing home care; the growth in these two services has indubitably been spurred on by the two public programs (U.S. Department of Health and Human Services, 1996).

Outlays. In terms of outlays, 4% of the money spent for health in 1995 was used to purchase hospital and nursing home services, although hospital expenditures, which totaled $350 billion, have dropped substantially as a proportion of health care expenditures in recent years. Another 45 cents of the health care dollar was divided among physi-

cians' services and other personal care items (that is, dental services, other professional services, vision services, home health care, drugs, eyeglasses and appliances, and other miscellaneous health care services and products). Research and construction, program administration, and public health activities comprised the final 11 cents of the health care dollar for 1995 (Levit, et al., 1996).

Personal Health Care. Figure 5–2 shows financing trends since 1950 for personal health care expenditures (PHCE), which include total health expenditures minus program administration, public health activities, research, and construction (Levit, et al., 1996). Government plus private insurance have grown enormously in the postwar era, funding more than three-quarters of all PHCE. Direct

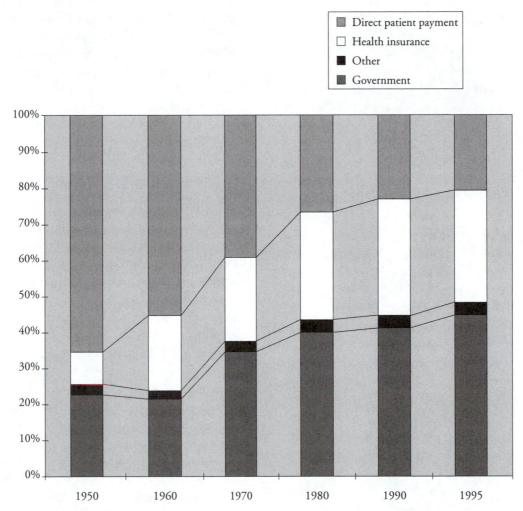

SOURCE: "National Health Expenditures, 1995," by K. R. Levit, et al., Fall 1996, *Health Care Financing Review, 18*(1), p. 205.

FIGURE 5–2 Percentage distribution of U.S. personal health care expenditures by source of funds, selected years

payments by patients have dropped commensurately to just over one-fifth of PHCE.

Sources of funding for major providers of personal health care are depicted in Figure 5–3. Government funding dominates hospital reimbursement, with over 60% financed by Medicare, other government programs, and Medicaid, in that order. Another 32% of the national hospital bill is footed by private health insurance. Physician outlays are clearly dominated by the private sector. Private insurance and direct patient payments account for more than 65% of physician funding; Medicare, which in recent years has diminished as a financier of physicians' services, picks up another 20%. Nursing home funding reflects the "rich man, poor man" dichotomy of the long-term care

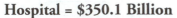

Hospital = $350.1 Billion

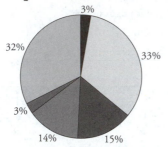

Physician = $201.6 Billion

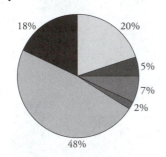

Nursing = $77.9 Billion

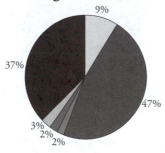

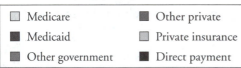

☐ Medicare   ■ Other private

■ Medicaid   ☐ Private insurance

■ Other government   ■ Direct payment

SOURCE: "National Health Expenditures, 1995," by K. R. Levit, et al., Fall 1996, *Health Care Financing Review, 18*(1), pp. 206–208.

FIGURE 5–3 Personal health care expenditures for total U.S. population by type of service and source of funds, 1995

industry, wherein patients must "spend down" their assets in order to qualify for government assistance. Eighty-three percent of nursing home revenues are funded by direct patient payment and Medicaid. Medicare's share of funding for nursing homes has nearly tripled since 1990.

HEALTH INSURANCE

Origins of Health Insurance

Health insurance originated in Europe in the early 1800s when mutual benefit societies arose to lighten the financial burden for those stricken with illness. The focus was on low-skilled, low-income workers who were industrially employed. (Providers in Europe wanted to keep highly skilled employees in the private medical market.) The first government health insurance program arose in Germany in 1840, mandating workers below a certain income level to belong to a "sickness fund." The concept of health insurance as linked to employment in the industrial sector persists internationally to this day. The health insurance networks of many nations grew out of this linkage and still reflect an emphasis on nonagricultural employment and coverage of the worker, irrespective of dependents (Roemer, 1977, 1978).

Today in the United States, the framework of health insurance stems clearly from its European antecedents and breaks down into three categories that, in some sense, reflect employment status. *Voluntary health insurance* (VHI) is private insurance, usually denoting current industrial employment; *social health insurance* (SHI) reflects participation in a government entitlement program linked to previous (or current) employment; and *public welfare* health care programs connote lack of employment, low-income employment, or the inability to gain employment stemming from a disabling condition.

Distributing Risk

Insurance is a way of pooling or distributing risk. Risk is the probability of incurring a loss. Risk stems from two kinds of occurrences: (1) unanticipated events such as fires, car accidents, or airplane crashes; and (2) anticipated events such as death, old age, and sickness. Health or, more correctly, illness is an anticipated event associated with old age and death. Thus, we know that illness is a likely event, but we do not know when it will strike, to whom it will happen, or how severe it will be. Therefore, health is uncertain for the individual, but not for a group. Groups are actuarially (that is, statistically) predictable.

Moral Hazard. In the theory of insurance, it is assumed that risks are independent of each other: (1) that what befalls one person does not affect another, and (2) that for a single individual, risks are independent. Neither assumption is true in health insurance because one person's sickness may spread contagiously, and illness in one part of the body may weaken another part. These phenomena, together with the *moral hazard* inherent in medical care, make health insurance and health costs, in general, extremely volatile. Moral hazard means that, to the extent that the event insured against can be controlled, there exists a temptation to use the insurance. (The classic example of moral hazard is setting fire to a failing business in order to collect the insurance.) Health insurance usage is highly discretionary; doctors and patients can conspire (intentionally or not) to use the insurance. An example is where a private patient with a traditional type of policy is kept in the hospital an extra day because it would be difficult or inconvenient for the family to receive the patient back home on the earliest possible discharge day. In this example, the insured extra day in the hospital, at a cost of $700 or more to the carrier, saves a loss in earnings for the family, and the expense is borne by purchasers of the policy, as reflected in the price of the premium.

Benefit Structure. Because of moral hazard, health insurance usually pays less than the total loss incurred by levying out-of-pocket or direct costs on the patient. In fee-for-service provider reimbursement, these take the form of deductibles and copayments. A *deductible* is a sum of money that must be paid, typically every year, before the insurance policy becomes active. Deductibles have long been criticized in health insurance for posing an impediment to first-contact care, discouraging the patient from seeking care until the condition becomes severe. Since higher costs may be incurred for more severe illness, deductibles have been postulated to contribute to health cost inflation, rather than stimulating parsimonious consumer utilization. A *copayment* is paid as the beneficiary uses the insurance. For example, in a policy with a traditional *indemnity benefit,* a fixed cash amount is paid to the beneficiary per procedure or per day in the hospital (for example, $800 for a one-night stay in the hospital following a hernia repair). If the hospital charges $1,100, then the patient must pay a copayment of $300. Thus the patient is liable for any amount in excess of the indemnity payment. An insurance plan with a *service benefit* reimburses on a percentage basis and the patient pays *coinsurance.* Using the previous example, the insurance plan would pay 80%, or $880, of the surgeon's charges, leaving only $220 in coinsurance to be paid by the patient. Thus, if the percentage rate is high, the reimbursement structure of service benefits usually works to the patient's advantage when compared to indemnity benefits.

Pure types of indemnity or service benefits are becoming increasingly rare. Nowadays, to control health cost inflation, there is a growing trend toward hybrid benefit structures, combining both service and indemnity features. A plan may, for example, pay a percentage of charges up to a specified limit, beyond which point the patient becomes responsible for the balance. Preferred provider organizations (PPOs) utilize this technique, often in concert with low price ceilings, to reimburse nonparticipating providers. Using the previous example, the PPO might pay 80% up to an $800 limit on charges for a nonparticipating hospital. The plan would pay $640, and the patient would thus incur a $460 copayment. However, if the patient utilizes a hospital participating in the PPO, the plan might pay 90% of the discounted fee of $1,000 (that is, a contractually determined "allowed amount" of $900), resulting in a copayment of only $100 for the patient.

Premium Determination. Because of the financial implications of choosing one type of health insurance plan over another, and because the possibility of moral hazard is a real one in health care utilization, health insurance plans are particularly vulnerable to the phenomenon of *adverse selection.* Adverse selection may be at work when an insurance policy experiences a higher number of claims from sickness than would be probable on a random basis. If an employee is offered an alternate choice of plans, for example, a "sicker" person or a potentially higher utilizer of health care services is likely to elect the plan with more generous provisions (that is, lower deductible and copayments, and fewer limitations or exclusions), even if the employee's share of the premium is higher. Therefore, more liberal fee-for-service plans may experience an adverse selection of sicker enrollees compared to a more restrictive managed care plan, such as a PPO or a health maintenance organization (HMO). This may result in ever-spiraling claims for the liberal plan as costlier people join and as healthier individuals defect to the lower-cost alternative plans.

Because of adverse selection, most health insurance plans today are *experience rated;* the premiums are based upon the demographic characteristics,

such as age and sexual composition, of the employer group or upon the actual experience of the group in that plan in prior years. *Community rating,* originated by Blue Cross and Blue Shield, bases premiums upon the wider utilization of the defined geographic area (for example, census tracts, city, county, and so on). Today, most fee-for-service plans are experience rated, as are the Blues, which must contend with stiff price competition from commercial carriers. HMOs, on the other hand, more widely use community ratings for their enrolled groups, but even this is fading as HMOs face price competition or enter the for-profit arena.

Voluntary Health Insurance

Voluntary or private health insurance in the United States can be subdivided into three distinct categories: (1) Blue Cross and Blue Shield, (2) private or commercial insurance companies, and (3) health maintenance organizations. The respective sponsorships of these types of VHI may be providers, third parties or middlemen, and patients or independent carriers. Nowadays, it is common for the Blues and commercials to own and operate HMOs and other managed care plans.

Growth and Development. The year 1929 was a landmark year for VHI. In spite of active opposition from the American Medical Association (AMA) to any type of health insurance from 1920 onward, both Blue Cross and the HMO movement got their start in this last pre-Depression year. Blue Cross was initiated by Baylor teachers in Dallas, Texas, who organized to provide hospital care for three cents a day. Michigan and New Jersey were next in the movement for hospital insurance. In 1934, the depths of the revenue depression for hospitals, the American Hospital Association (AHA) united these plans into the Blue Cross network. Today Blue Cross has broken away from its original AHA sponsorship, but the hospital-sponsored underpinnings remain strong in many locales (Roemer, 1977, 1978).

In Oklahoma also in 1929, the Farmer's Union started their Cooperative Health Association, the first HMO. Independently, in the same year in Los Angeles, two Canadian physicians founded the Ross-Loos group practice and sold the first doctor-sponsored health insurance plan with prepayment to the Department of Water and Power and Los Angeles City workers.

As these and other plans grew during the 1930s, the AMA reversed its opposition to VHI in response to dwindling physician and hospital incomes, and in 1939, the California Medical Society developed and sponsored a plan known as Blue Shield to pay doctor's bills in a hospitalized environment (Roemer, 1977, 1978).

By 1946, private health insurance plans were experiencing astronomical growth as wage and price restrictions in the post–World War II period spurred the growth of fringe benefits, especially in unionized industries. Insurance companies, already having the inside track in sales and actuarial information in life insurance, went headlong into the health insurance business in competition with Blue Cross and Blue Shield.

Although voluntary health insurance plans were initiated by consumer cooperatives or employers, followed by provider-sponsored plans in the 1920s and 1930s, and supplemented by commercial insurance companies in the 1940s, the rate of growth in VHI programs has been in the reverse order. Most programs in the United States today are sponsored by insurance companies, then providers, with consumers lagging far behind. Blue Cross and Blue Shield currently administer a total of 58 member plans, 48 of which combine the Blues into one association. About 650 commercial insurance companies offer health insurance plans, and at least 550 HMOs of varying sponsorship have been organized (Levit, et al., 1996).

Population Coverage. About 70% of the entire United States population in 1995 was covered by private health insurance. About 85% of this group obtained health insurance as an employment benefit, either as the primary insured member or as a dependent. In addition, almost 70% of the elderly, who with few exceptions are covered by Medicare, hold private insurance coverage (known as "Medigap" insurance) to supplement their Medicare benefits. In 1994, about 70% of the United States population under sixty-five had some form of VHI, over 80% of whom had their health insurance linked to current employment. Firms that do not offer any health benefits at all tend to be small and nonunionized, hire seasonal workers, and employ relatively large numbers of low-wage employees with no college education (U.S. Bureau of the Census, 1996).

An unfortunate effect of employment-linked private health insurance is that people who are least able to pay for health care have the least insurance due to lack of employment (or full-time employment). The alternatives for these people are to purchase a nongroup or individual plan, usually a less generous and more expensive option in terms of out-of-pocket premiums, or to accept the risk of doing without any health insurance. Estimates vary, but according to the United States Census Bureau, about 15.2% of the total United States population in 1994 (39.7 million people), had no health insurance coverage at all, either public or private (U.S. Bureau of the Census, 1996).

Benefits. Private health insurance coverage varies widely in terms of benefits provided, the extent of reimbursement for covered services, and exclusions or limitations. *Basic insurance plans* are designed to provide limited protection for the most expensive services and usually cover inpatient hospital and physician services, and outpatient hospital services, including laboratory procedures. Limits may apply to a group of related services such as those provided during the course of a hospitalization. The most commonly covered services for the privately insured are linked to inpatient hospitalization: room and board, surgeons' and other physicians' fees, and outpatient diagnostic services.

Major medical insurance extends basic benefits to such services as physician office visits, outpatient mental health care, prescribed medicines, durable equipment and supplies, ambulance services, and the like. Thus, these plans are designed to protect against large medical bills as well as many expenses associated with routine types of medical care. For a traditional indemnity claim, the insurer typically pays a specified share of total covered expenses (for example, 80 to 90%) in excess of a deductible (usually $100 to $200 per year for an individual), with a high maximum allowance. The beneficiary pays the deductible and coinsurance, which comprise the share of the incremental expenses not covered by the plan, subject to a limited amount known as the "out-of-pocket limit" or "stop-loss provision." A limit of this kind may range from $1,500 to $3,000. Many major medical plans limit deductibles for family members to a specified amount (typically $300 to $500 per family) or waive the deductible for the rest of the family once two or three members have met their deductibles.

Comprehensive plans combine the features of both basic insurance and major medical plans. The deductible and other provisions apply to all expenses for all covered services. In contrast, "Medigap" plans are designed to reimburse only the deductibles and coinsurance associated with Medicare-covered services.

Hospital indemnity plans are another type of private insurance coverage that is noteworthy. Hospital indemnity plans offer specified cash payments (for example, $100 per day) for each day of inpatient hospitalization, regardless of the expenses actually incurred. Thus, the hospital indemnity plan is a type of disability insurance wherein the payment is not linked to the amount or type of medical services provided, but rather to the length of the hospital stay, and the payment is not generous in relation to the actual hospital expenses.

Prepaid Plans. HMOs and other similar plans provide fairly comprehensive coverage in return for a prepaid fee, usually without deductibles and coinsurance for most services, and therefore offer coverage against the risk of large health care financial losses. Prepaid health plans are the most rapidly growing segment of the private health insurance market. Today, there are about 550 HMOs in the United States, covering about 46 million people (U.S. Bureau of the Census, 1996). This compares to about 50 HMOs in 1973, prior to the passage of the HMO Act, which requires employers with over twenty-five employees to offer a dual choice of health plans including one HMO, if one is available locally.

It was anticipated that the HMO concept would foster incentives toward prevention and cost-consciousness on the part of physicians who are encouraged to be frugal in the use of secondary services, particularly hospitalization. However, because the prepayment of premium does not necessarily translate into capitated provider reimbursement and tight prospective budgeting, cost-containment experience is mixed due to legislative and economic incentives that are sometimes perverse (Hillman, Welch, & Pauly, 1992).

Social Health Insurance

The United States government sponsors two major mandatory social health insurance programs: (1) Worker's Compensation for the costs and pain of suffering job-related accidents, and (2) Medicare for the elderly, disabled, and other special groups. Several states sponsor social insurance programs in the areas of temporary disability (California) or health insurance (Hawaii).

Worker's Compensation is offered in all fifty states to some extent. It is usually the first type of social insurance enacted in a nation, and the vast majority of nations worldwide have some form of industrial accident insurance. The first worker's compensation law in the United States was passed by New York State in 1914 in response to the tragic Triangle Shirt factory fire in which 146 women lost their lives. In 1950, Mississippi became the last state to enact workers' compensation. In recent years, over 80% of the United States workforce is covered to some extent by workers' compensation, leaving the remaining workers, many of whom are agricultural, casual, and domestic workers, without coverage. Unfortunately, it is often these same people who are not covered by any type of health insurance (Roemer, 1978).

Worker's Compensation provides two basic benefits: (1) cash replacement of a portion of wages lost from disability, and (2) payment for all or part of the medical care necessary. Workers' compensation may be underwritten by a private insurance company, a state government insurance fund, or a corporate contingency fund. Premiums are usually determined by experience rating. In 1993, Worker's Compensation paid out about $43 billion in hospital and medical expense claims, comprising about 1.7% of covered payroll (U.S. Bureau of the Census, 1996).

Medicare. In 1935, national health insurance almost became a reality as part of the Social Security Act. Because of strong opposition from the AMA and conservative members of Congress, national health insurance was scrapped from the act by President Roosevelt who did not want to risk passage by Congress. In 1939, and every two years for several Congresses thereafter, the Wagner, Murray, Dingell national health insurance bill was proposed in Congress. The timing of this bill coincided with the growth curve of private health insurance enrollment, which precluded a pressing interest in national health insurance. Private health insurance, however, was largely sponsored by employers and thus did not serve the nonworking population, particularly the aged. Nonetheless, about 50% of the elderly enrolled in voluntary health insurance programs during the 1957–1964 pre-Medicare period (Roemer, 1978).

In 1957, Representative Forand of Rhode Island introduced the bill that was the precursor of Medicare (Title XVIII of the Social Security Act). On July 30, 1965, Medicare became the first entry of the federal government into the provision of social health insurance rather than medical assistance (public welfare medicine) such as that offered by the Kerr-Mills Act of 1960—"Medical Assistance for the Aged."

Strictly speaking, only Medicare Part A— Hospital Insurance (HI)—is social health insurance (see Figure 5–4). Part B—Supplementary Medical Insurance (SMI)—is neither compulsory nor funded by a trust fund. Sixty-four percent of the funds for SMI comes from the general treasury, and the other 36% comes from Medicare Part A recipients who elect that Part B premiums be deducted from their monthly Social Security check (U.S. Department of Health and Human Services, 1997).

Medicare utilizes an *indirect pattern* of finance and delivery, wherein the Health Care Financing Administration (HCFA), a branch of the United States Department of Health and Human Services, contracts with independent providers. Medicare recipients also access providers independently. The HCFA sees to it that the provider is paid, but the providers are neither owned nor hired by the government, as in SHI systems utilizing the *direct pattern* of delivery. Generally speaking, if the private medical market is strong at the time when SHI is enacted, an indirect pattern of delivery emerges. If the market is weak, a direct financing route emerges.

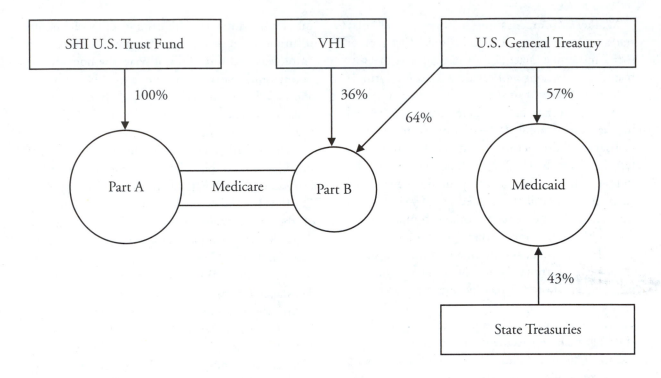

Each circle reflects the relative size of the program.

FIGURE 5–4   Flow of federal and state financing for Medicare and Medicaid

Welfare Medicine

Public Assistance. *Public assistance* or *welfare medicine* is sponsored by a plethora of federal, state, and local government programs, but the most far-reaching program is Medicaid (Title XIX of the Social Security Act). Administered at the federal level by the HCFA, Medicaid is financed by an average federal contribution from the general treasury of 55% and from state treasuries at an average contribution of 45% (see Figure 5–4). Federal matching varies from 50 to 77%, depending on the income of the individual state (U.S. Department of Health and Human Services, 1996). General treasury funds are generated from personal income tax, corporate income tax, and various excise taxes, and to the extent that these taxes are borne by higher-income individuals and organizations, Medicaid represents a type of transfer payment to the poor.

The distinction between welfare medicine and social health insurance, both of which are public programs, is an important one and rests on the philosophical difference between a transfer payment and entitlement. Medicaid is a *transfer payment* "in kind," meaning that medical services are provided as a welfare benefit in lieu of cash. Welfare recipients also receive cash subsidies to pay for their living expenses, but medical benefits are paid directly to the provider so that the recipients will not be tempted to spend the money on expense items other than health care. (Food stamps are another "in kind" benefit, providing vouchers solely for the purpose of purchasing food and groceries.) Thus, the transfer payment is a type of "relief" that government bestows upon the poor; it is a form of charity.

Social health insurance is an *entitlement* program, not charity. It is a right earned by individuals in the course of their employment. The funds for SHI programs are contributed by a payroll tax (for 1997, 2.9% of total wages), which, in the case of Social Security, is divided equally between the worker and the employer. Workers' Compensation, too, is financed, at least in part, by worker contributions. When the worker retires or suffers a temporary or sustaining injury related to employment, SHI becomes active for the worker and dependents. The fundamental aim of a compulsory, government-provided or -supervised SHI program is social adequacy—to provide members of society with protection against hazards so widespread as to be considered risks that individuals cannot afford to deal with themselves. Eligibility in SHI is derived from contributions having been made in the program, and benefits are a statutory right not based on need. Recipients are thus entitled to the benefits of SHI. About half the countries in the world have an SHI system for financing health care (Roemer, 1978; U.S. Department of Health and Human Services, 1996).

In reference to Figure 5–4, it is interesting to note that the federal share of funding (coming from the United States General Treasury) for Medicare Part B and Medicaid has been growing in recent years.

MEDICARE

Medicare, the principal SHI program in the United States, provides a variety of hospital, physician, and other medical services for (1) persons sixty-five and over, (2) disabled individuals who are entitled to Social Security benefits, and (3) end-stage renal disease victims. In 1995, Medicare financed

$193.9 billion in health services, comprising 42.5% of all publicly financed health expenditures and 22.1% of personal health care expenditures. Medicare reimbursed 32.2% of all hospital expenditures and 19.8% of all physician expenditures in 1995 (Levit, et al., 1996).

Hospital Insurance

Ninety-eight percent of the aged population of the United States is enrolled in Part A of Medicare, Hospital Insurance (HI). Part A finances four basic benefits for the covered population:

1. Ninety days of inpatient care in a "benefit period" (A benefit period is a spell of illness beginning with hospitalization and ending when a beneficiary has not been an inpatient in a hospital or skilled nursing facility for sixty continuous days. There is no limit to the number of benefit periods a beneficiary can use.)
2. A lifetime reserve of sixty days of inpatient care, once the ninety days are exhausted
3. One hundred days of posthospitalization care in a skilled nursing facility
4. Home health agency visits

Since the inception of the Medicare program, Hospital Insurance has required the beneficiary to participate in cost sharing. The patient is required to pay an inpatient hospital deductible in each benefit period, which approximates the cost of one day of hospital care ($736 in 1996). Coinsurance based on the inpatient hospital deductible is required for days 61 to 90 of inpatient hospitalization and is always equal to one-fourth of the deductible ($184 in 1996). For days 21 to 100 of skilled nursing facility (SNF) care, the coinsurance equals one-eighth of the deductible ($92), and for the sixty-day lifetime reserve, the patient pays one-half of the deductible ($368) for each day of inpatient hospitalization. About 70% of Medicare enrollees have private "Medigap" policies, which primarily cover some or all of the deductibles and coinsurance under Medicare. About 11% of the aged and 38% of the disabled have Medicaid coverage also (a group known as "crossovers"), and Medicaid usually assumes responsibility for the cost sharing under Medicare (U.S. Department of Health and Human Services, 1996).

While hospital expenditures have grown at a rapid rate since the inception of Medicare, skilled nursing facility, home health agency, and outpatient benefits have all shifted significantly as a percent of total Medicare benefit payments. Skilled nursing facility payments have dropped from 6.5% of payments in 1967 to 5.2% in 1995. Currently the fastest growing component of Medicare, home health agency payments, totaled 8.4% of Medicare outlays in 1995, and outpatient outlays comprised 8.2% (U.S. Department of Health and Human Services, 1996).

Catastrophic Coverage. In 1988, amendments to Medicare were enacted to shield Medicare beneficiaries from catastrophic hospital and doctors' bills related to acute illnesses. Although the bill provided no new benefits for long-term care, it did provide for the first broad coverage of outpatient prescription drugs. Because of pressure from organized groups of elderly who objected to the additional income taxes and substantial premium increases targeted at them, Congress repealed the bill in 1989. Only a few minor provisions in the amendment were subsequently incorporated into the regular Medicare benefit structure.

Supplementary Medical Insurance

Ninety-five percent of Part A beneficiaries are enrolled in Part B, Supplementary Medical Insurance (SMI). Part B is the third largest federal domestic program, exceeded only by the Social Security cash benefit program and Medicare's Part A program. SMI was designed to complement the HI program. It provides payments for physicians, physician-ordered supplies and services, outpatient hospital services, rural health clinic visits, and home health visits for persons without Part A.

SMI requires the beneficiary to meet a deductible (currently $100) each year, in addition to paying a monthly premium ($43.80 in 1997). Under "buy-in" agreements, most state Medicaid programs pay the premiums for Medicaid enrollees who qualify to participate in SMI (U.S. Department of Health and Human Services, 1997).

Drugs on an outpatient basis, dental care, routine eye examinations and eyeglasses, preventive services, and long-term institutional services are not covered by either part of Medicare. Hospice benefits, however, became available for persons who are terminally ill in 1983. Enrollees in Medicare can elect the hospice benefit for two ninety-day periods and one thirty-day period, with a subsequent extension period during the individual's lifetime.

From 1967 to 1992, Part B of Medicare grew faster than Part A—at an average annual rate of 15.2% as compared to 13.9%. Therefore, although Part B represented only 36% of Medicare expenditures in 1995, Part B has increased as a proportion of Medicare expenditures since 1967, whereas Part A has shrunk commensurately (U.S. Department of Health and Human Services, 1995, 1996). To constrain SMI inflation, the Deficit Reduction Act of 1984 placed a freeze on Medicare maximum payment levels (originally slated for fifteen months, but continuing for several years) and introduced the concept of "participating physicians," who are those who "accept assignments" for all services. Incentives to participate were introduced and resulted in substantial increases in assignment. Nationally, the annual assignment rate increased from 51% in 1983, to 96% in 1995 (U.S. Department of Health and Human Services, 1997).

Provider Reimbursement

Hospitals. Medicare has operated primarily on a fee-for-service basis for physicians and related services and, until 1983, on a cost-based retrospective basis for hospital services. Hospitals were reimbursed for any reasonable costs incurred in the provision of covered care to Medicare patients. Commencing in 1983, payment rates were prospectively determined on a per-case basis. The Medicare hospital Prospective Payment System (PPS), discussed in detail later in this chapter, uses diagnosis-related groups (DRGs) to classify cases for payment. Except for four major classes of specialty hospitals (children's, psychiatric, rehabilitation, and long-term), all hospitals must participate in PPS to qualify for Medicare reimbursement, billing Medicare directly.

Physicians. Under Medicare Part B, physicians may elect one of two reimbursement strategies. The first is to accept the Medicare Fee Schedule (MFS) as payment in full (that is, accepting the assignment), billing Medicare directly, and receiving 80% payment from the Medicare intermediary. The beneficiaries are liable for the remaining 20% coinsurance, also according to the MFS. On unassigned claims, the beneficiary is additionally liable for the difference between the physician's charge and the Medicare allowed charge.

The Deficit Reduction Act of 1984 thus created two classes of physicians: participating and nonparticipating. A participating physician must accept assignment for all claims for all Medicare patients, with no exceptions. Several incentives of a pecuniary and marketing nature have been employed by Medicare to entice physicians to participate. A nonparticipating physician can continue to treat Medicare patients, accepting assignments or not on a claim-by-claim basis, but Medicare will reimburse only 95% of the MFS amount.

Claims are processed by intermediaries or fiscal agents, such as Blue Cross or a commercial insurance company, contracted by the Medicare program to review and pay the bills. Enrollees can also join HMOs and similar forms of prepaid health care, and special reimbursement provisions apply to these organizations. The Tax Equity and Fiscal Responsibility Act of 1982 (TEFRA) included major revisions to the Medicare law to encourage growth in the number of HMOs and other comprehensive medical plans enrolling Medicare beneficiaries. By 1995, 274 managed care plans, with 3.8 million members, held contracts with Medicare (U.S. Department of Health and Human Services, 1996). TEFRA also set limits on Medicare reimbursements for hospital costs at the per-case level— the harbinger of DRGs under PPS.

Utilization. The average Medicare enrollee spent over $4,750 in 1995. As in any insurance program, however, utilization is uneven. A study of 1995 data showed that less than one-third of the enrolled population had small claims of $500 or less, and about 20% had no claims at all. The highest 14.4% of users had reimbursements of $10,000 or more, and these enrollees consumed 51.5% of program payments (U.S. Department of Health and Human Services, 1997). Other studies have demonstrated that high Medicare reimbursements are related to terminal illness. A seminal study by Lubitz and Prihoda (1984) found that reimbursements for decedents averaged $4,527 for the last year of life, whereas reimbursements averaged $729 for a comparison group who survived the period under study. Fuchs (1984) showed that the greatest proportion of medical care costs are incurred in the year prior to death, regardless of the age of natural death. For Medicare enrollees in 1976, the average reimbursement for those in their last year of life was 6.6 times as large as for those who survived at least two years. Thus, one may surmise that the principal reason why health expenditures rise with age is that the proportion of persons near death increases with age. Other studies have found a great deal of consistency over time in the utilization of health expenditures by the highest users, the top one percent accounting for twenty or more percent of health care dollars (Gornick, et al., 1985).

MEDICAID

Program Structure

Medicaid was enacted into law on July 30, 1965, as Title XIX of the Social Security Act and became part of the existing federal-state welfare structure to assist the poor. Until 1956, there had been no federal participation in health care for the poor. This public obligation was delegated to the states as part of their *police powers*. Prior to Medicaid, many doctors donated their services or used a sliding scale of fees in treating the poor, and as a rule, hospitals admitted charity cases. Under the purview of the states, however, health care for the poor varied widely from state to state and manifested all the forms of discrimination tolerated in each locale. The Kerr-Mills Act of 1960, Medical Assistance for the Aged, was the forerunner of the Medicaid model and was later subsumed under Title XIX.

Eligibility. Supported by federal grants and administered by the states, Medicaid is limited to specific groups of low-income individuals and families. Medicaid is welfare medicine and thus has no strict entitlement features (although lately the word *entitlement* has been used indiscriminately, particularly by politicians and the media, in reference to Medicaid and other welfare programs). Recipients must prove their eligibility for Medicaid according to their income, and prior to 1976, states were even permitted to put a lien on a recipient's home or other personal property.

The program was designed to cover those groups who are eligible to receive cash payments under one of the two existing welfare programs established under Social Security—Aid to Families with Dependent Children (AFDC) and Supplemental Security Income (SSI). In most instances, receipt of a welfare payment under one of these programs means automatic eligibility for Medicaid. The mandatory eligibility groups covered by Medicaid include (1) families with children which receive AFDC; (2) pregnant and postpartum women with children under six years of age, whose incomes do not exceed 133% of the Federal Poverty Level (FPL); (3) aged, blind, and disabled individuals who receive SSI; and (4) certain other specifically defined groups.

Figure 5–5 compares the distribution of Medicaid recipients to that of expenditures by eligibility category. AFDC families were the largest group of recipients (70.1%) in 1995 but accounted for a relatively small part of the Medicaid budget (26.5%), which is a reflection of the relatively good health of most Medicaid children. Due largely to high utilization of nursing home services, 30.7% of total Medicaid outlays was attributable to the aged, who comprise only 11.6% of the Medicaid population. Outlays for the disabled totaled 41.6% of Medicaid expenditures, a disproportionately large amount as compared to the number of recipients (116.6%), largely reflecting the high rate of expenditures ($68,613 per person) for the 151,000 persons in intermediate-care facilities for the mentally retarded (U.S. Department of Health and Human Services, 1996, 1997). These facts serve to dispel the conventional wisdom that AFDC families incur the lion's share of Medicaid expense. The impoverished aged and the disabled (which includes the mentally retarded) have no alternative but to expend large per capita amounts in the Medicaid program.

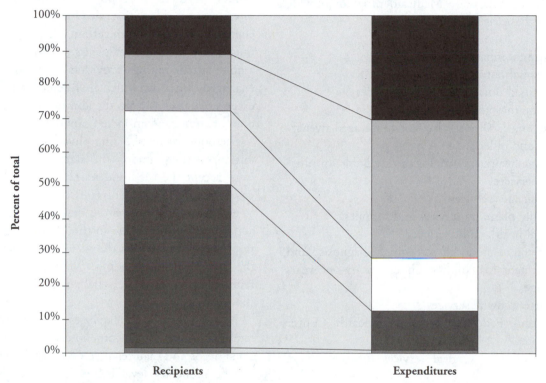

SOURCE: *1996 HCFA Statistics* (HCFA Pub. No. 03394, pp. 211–229), U.S. Department of Health and Human Services, Health Care Financing Administration Bureau of Data Management and Strategy, September 1996.

FIGURE 5–5   Distribution of Medicaid recipients and expenditures by eligibility category, 1995

States may choose to provide Medicaid to certain "optional eligibility groups." Most of these optional groups share characteristics of the mandatory groups (parents and children, aged, blind, and disabled), but the income eligibility ceilings are higher (for example, 1.33 to 1.85 times the federal poverty level—$11,569 for a family of three in 1995).

"Medically needy" persons comprise another optional group—those who spend down their income and wealth, due to medical bills, to the medically needy standard. Under federal guidelines, states set income and asset levels for cash assistance and medical eligibility. Because there is considerable variation in the coverage of optional groups by the states and in income standards across Medicaid jurisdictions, the degree to which programs cover the poverty population varies considerably.

Benefits Provided

Services. Title XIX of the Social Security Act mandates that every state Medicaid program provide specific basic health services:

- Hospital inpatient care
- Hospital outpatient services
- Certified nurse practitioner services
- Laboratory and X-ray services
- Nursing facility services for those aged twenty-one and older
- Home health services for those eligible for nursing services
- Physicians' services
- Family planning services and supplies
- Rural health clinic services
- Early and periodic screening, diagnosis, and treatment for children under twenty-one years of age
- Nurse midwife services
- Certain Federally Qualified Health Center services
- Medical and surgical services furnished by a dentist

States may determine the scope of services offered (for example, limit the days of hospital care or the number of physician visits covered) and provide a number of other elective services. The most commonly covered optional services include:

- Clinic services
- Nursing services in a care facility for the aged and disabled
- Intermediate care facility services for the mentally retarded
- Inpatient psychiatric services

- Optometrist services and eyeglasses
- Prescribed drugs
- Prosthetic devices
- Dental care

Administration. Medicaid operates primarily as a vendor payment program. Payments are made directly to providers of service for care rendered to eligible individuals. With certain exceptions, a state must allow Medicaid recipients freedom of choice among participating providers of health care. Managed care plans, which are foremost among the exceptions, usually hold the ability to restrict freedom of choice to contracted providers.

Methods for reimbursing physicians and hospitals vary widely among the states, but providers must accept the Medicaid reimbursement level as payment in full. Payment rates must be sufficient to enlist enough providers so that comparable care and services are available to the Medicaid population as are available to the general population in the area. Notwithstanding, Medicaid physician reimbursement rates are usually less generous than those of Medicare.

In long-term care facilities, individuals are required to turn over income in excess of their personal needs and maintenance needs of their spouses (the monetary level being determined by the state) to help pay for their care. States may require cost sharing by Medicaid recipients, but they may not require the mandatory eligible to share costs for mandatory services. As noted previously, most state Medicaid programs have buy-in agreements with Medicare in which Medicaid assumes the responsibility for the Medicare cost sharing for persons covered under both programs (Gornick, et al., 1985; Waldo, 1990).

States participate in the Medicaid program at their option. All states except Arizona (which has a demonstration project of capitated health delivery that excludes long-term care services) currently have

Medicaid programs. The District of Columbia, Puerto Rico, Guam, the Northern Marianas, and the Virgin Islands also provide Medicaid coverage.

The states administer their Medicaid programs within broad federal requirements and guidelines. These requirements allow states considerable discretion in determining not only eligibility but also covered benefits and provider payment mechanisms. Some states also include in the Medicaid program persons known as "state-only" enrollees, who do not meet federal requirements and hence do not qualify for federal matching funds. As a result of state options and policy decisions, the characteristics of Medicaid programs vary considerably from state to state. Medicaid expenditures also vary widely across the states, and states' benefit mix offerings change frequently.

Growth of Medicaid

From 1980 to 1995, growth in Medicaid expenditures (561%) exceeded that of Medicare, which grew by 526% over the same period. A disproportionately large share of this growth took place in the 1990 to 1995 period. During this time, Medicaid recipients as a percentage of the total civilian population have risen from 10.2% to 13.8%, an increase of 35%. This rise in the Medicaid population is principally attributable, in turn, to an expansion of those covered in the mandatory eligible groups and to the economic ravages of the early-1990s' recession on family income.

Providers. Hospital care (inpatient and outpatient) accounted for a much smaller proportion of 1995 Medicaid expenditures (34%) than Medicare hospital outlays (50% in 1995). Nursing home care, including skilled nursing, intermediate care, and intermediate care facilities for the mentally retarded (ICF/MR), commanded the same amount as the hospital component of the Medicaid budget (U.S. Department of Health and Human Services, 1996, 1997).

Medicaid continues to be the largest payer of long-term care services, financing 47% of nursing home care in 1995. Although growth in spending for nursing facility care has slowed considerably in recent years, since the early 1970s, Medicaid has funded at least 80% of all public spending for nursing home care. Compared with other services that Medicaid provides, Medicaid payments for long-term care are also the most costly per user. Health Care Financing Administration statistics from 1995 showed that the average Medicaid payment for nursing facility services was $17,424. From 1993 to 1995, however, the highest growth rates in Medicaid payments occurred for ICF/MR care and for prescription drugs (U.S. Department of Health and Human Services, 1997).

State Spending. Since 1975, Medicaid is the fastest growing component of aggregate state spending. In 1995, Medicaid spent $120.1 billion of combined federal and state funds for vendor payments for personal health care. Program spending for Medicaid recipients accelerated in the 1990s. Spending grew by 286% for the entire decade of the 1980s, whereas from 1990 to 1995, Medicaid spending grew by 218%. As a result, Medicaid's share of personal health care expenditures grew from 11.3% in 1989 to 12.2% in 1995 (Levit, et al., 1996; U.S. Department of Health and Human Services, 1995, 1996).

In order to curtail Medicaid growth, cost-containment initiatives began in the early 1980s. During this time, important experiments were launched in prepaid managed health care, utilization review, case management, reimbursement via diagnosis-related group (DRGs), and new services for the elderly, disabled, and persons with AIDS. In 1990, Congress enacted careful and selective expansion of Medicaid coverage, particularly for low-income (and pregnant) women and children. Currently, the focus is on shifting Medicaid funding from the federal coffers to state budgets and encouraging states to model their systems on HMOs (U.S. Department of Health and Human Services, 1995).

PHYSICIAN REIMBURSEMENT

Paying the doctor traditionally calls upon one of three reimbursement mechanisms: fee-for-service, prepayment, or salary. Health insurance plans, either public or private, may utilize any or all of the three reimbursement types. According to Reinhardt (1985), there is no optimal system for paying the doctor.

Fee for Service. Fee for service (FFS) is widely used throughout the world for paying the doctor and is typically the physician's preferred mode of payment. In FFS, the unit of remuneration is the medical act, either a service or a procedure. In the days before health insurance for physician reimbursement was widespread, most physicians had a sliding-fee scale wherein the poor paid lower fees than wealthier patients. With the advent of health insurance in both the public and private sectors, physician payment became more regulated, and physicians adopted one schedule of charges used for all payers, whether they were individuals or third parties. By the 1980s, however, fees schedules began to vary widely by the type of health plan or insurance organization, public or private.

Among the advantages to fee-for-service reimbursement is that the remuneration adjusts automatically for case complexity, linking the provider's reward closely to the output of services. The billing system, in turn, provides a great deal of "transparency" of the physician's profile of practice. The ease with which patients may change physicians in a traditional fee-for-service system enables them to directly exercise considerable economic clout over practitioners (Reinhardt, 1985).

Indemnity. Insurance policies that reimburse on a fee-for-service basis offer payment either by indemnity or service benefits or by fixed fees. *Indemnity payment* stipulates a certain dollar value per procedure, usually according to a "table of allowances." These allowances may vary widely among insurance plans. In traditional indemnity, the provider can charge anything above the stipulated allowed amount and collect the remainder directly from the patient. Often, the table of allowances is based upon a "relative value scale," in which each procedure is rated according to a point system—relative value units (RVUs) that reflect the relative technical difficulty and time cost of the procedure, and each point is worth so many dollars. The dollars amount per RVU may vary widely among insurance plans. This type of system is easy to administer and update for inflation and changing practice patterns, but no provision is made by the insurer to protect the patient from outlandish charges.

Service Benefits. Service benefits pay a percentage per procedure, usually 80% of "usual, customary, and reasonable" (UCR) fees. In this scheme, the UCR fee schedule protects the carrier from unlimited liability in the wake of high charges and also may give the patient information about reasonable fee norms. UCR means that the fee is "usual" in that doctor's practice, "customary" in that community, and "reasonable" in terms of the distribution of all physician charges for that service in the community. The latter is commonly expressed as a percentile (for example, the policy will pay up to the seventy-fifth percentile). Until 1992, Medicare Part B used a similar standard of "customary, prevailing, and reasonable fees."

Hybrid Fee-Based Systems. Hybrid systems came into vogue with the advent of PPOs, combining features of both indemnity and service reimbursement for cost containment. In a hybrid system, the intermediary contracts with the participating physician (or hospital) to accept a discounted version of the UCR table of allowances. The plan considers these "allowed amounts" to be the maximum covered expenses. For a participating provider, the PPO will typically pay 90% of the allowed amount for most procedures, with the remaining 10% paid by the patient as coinsurance. This arrangement protects both the intermediary by effectively capping the reimbursement (as in an indemnity payment) and the patient by limiting the liability for the difference beyond 10% of the allowed amount.

Fixed Fees. In some reimbursement plans, physicians can only charge, and will only be paid, according to fixed fees, usually with little cost sharing (for example, $5.00 per physician office visit) or none at all on the part of the patient. If the provider accepts the plan, then the fee schedule must be accepted. This arrangement exists in Medicaid, and many private plans also stipulate fixed fees in order to protect the patient and to contain costs. Many HMO plans also mandate fixed fees, especially for specialists contracted with the health plan.

Prepayment

In prepayment or capitation, the person served, rather than the medical act, is the unit of remuneration. The capitation payment takes care of reimbursement for a stipulated length of time, usually a year. Using capitation as a reimbursement methodology, HMOs have encouraged physicians to form networks linked to hospitals and have spurred the popularity of Independent Practice Associations (IPAs), in which the participating physicians actually sponsor and administer the HMO. Advantages to prepayment are that it is administratively simple; it facilitates advance global budgeting; and it gives physicians incentive to control the cost of medical treatments. If patients are allowed to switch primary care physicians from time to time, they still retain some economic clout over physicians (Reinhardt, 1985).

Salary

Salary is payment to the doctor for time consumption, irrespective of the units of service or the number of patients. On a large scale, salaried practice almost always takes place in a highly organized network like the National Health Service in Great Britain. On a smaller scale in the United States, urban public hospitals that serve indigent populations often have large attending staffs which are salaried. Countries in which salaried practices are common rarely include specialists in this payment mechanism. Instead, general practitioners or primary care providers have a "panel" of patients in the community. Advantages to salaried reimbursement for physicians are that it is administratively simple; the medical treatments selected are not influenced by relative profitability; and it encourages cooperation among physicians. Furthermore, salaries facilitate budgeting for health expenditures *ex ante* (Reinhardt, 1985).

Monitoring

All payment mechanisms have faults, and each must be monitored for abuses. In FFS, the incentives are for overwork by the physician and overutilization by the patients. FFS fosters unnecessary or duplicative service to the point where the high volume of services may actually affect the quality of care adversely. Unfortunately, in the United States, malpractice suits have encouraged defensive medicine, wherein overutilization and extra fees are simply passed on to the consumer in higher insurance rates. Also, if fees for all procedures do not stand in constant proportion to costs incurred, the choice of treatment may favor more profitable procedures. For these and other reasons which foster inflation, fee-for-service reimbursement is very difficult to budget in advance.

In prepayment, on the other hand, underutilization must be monitored because the incentives are to decrease costs and services provided vis-à-vis the capitation payment. In many prepayment schemes, any cost savings realized are distributed to the participating physicians, which may be an inducement to cut costs too far. In HMOs where only the primary care physicians are capitated, there also exists the incentive to excessively refer patients to specialists. Likewise, capitation gives physicians incentives for "dumping" patients with complex, costly conditions onto other providers. Finally, the administrative system for prepayment yields little insight into the transparency physician's practice profile. Of late, many HMOs mandate that physicians submit monthly *encounter data* on patient visits and/or procedures delivered as a condition of participation in the health plan.

In salaried practice, incentives favor underwork or seeing too few patients. Doctors literally "get paid by the hour," resulting in no inducement toward higher volume. According to Reinhardt (1985), unless the salary is linked to output and patient satisfaction, patients lose economic clout over the physician, who, in turn, may render care as an act of *noblesse oblige*. Like capitation, salaried practice gives little transparency as to the physician's practice profile.

INITIATIVES IN HEALTH CARE FINANCE

Factors in Health Care Inflation

The implementation of Medicare and Medicaid in 1966 heralded a twenty-five year era of unprecedented health care cost inflation. Aaron (1993/94) attributes the continually rising costs of health care to three main factors:

1. The technological transformation of medical care, including new diagnostic techniques and new methods of treatment
2. The demand of consumers for low-benefit care
3. The lack of budget limits on hospitals and fee controls on physicians

He also notes that high administrative costs, compensation for medical malpractice, and bad health habits of the populace are not important factors in the rising costs of care.

Cost Containment Measures. In the 1970s, the federal government experimented with a number of programs and reimbursement methods to contain health care costs. Major programs included (1) the establishment of reasonable cost limits for hospitals; (2) the initiation of state and local networks of health planning agencies along with the "certificate-of-need" procedure for augmenting capital plant and equipment; (3) the establishment of the Professional Standards Review Organization (PSRO) program to review care and to eliminate unnecessary hospital days for federally funded patients; and (4) the encouragement of the growth of HMOs to promote the use of preventive services and to decrease the utilization of hospital inpatient care. It can be safely said that the programs of the 1970s were unsuccessful in containing health care costs.

Early in the 1980s, during the Reagan administration, legislative efforts to change the monetary incentive system in health care began in earnest. While the 1980s and 1990s have witnessed considerable flux in health care financing, along with inducements to reduce overutilization, cost-containment efforts have shown mixed results (Rice, 1992). Furthermore, they have held painful consequences for many groups of people. The balance between reasonable costs and equitable access has not yet been struck, but what is clear is that the traditional health care market has no apparatus to reflect social or economic rationing decisions regarding the provision of health care which might help to stem inflation. Managed care, particularly capitated prepaid care, holds better incentives for efficiency, productivity, and management coordination. Yet, even with more closely managed utilization, better quality management, and the continual expansion of government programs, universal access to health services remains elusive.

Procompetition. Early in the 1980s, Enthoven (1981) and other health economists exposited strategies of *procompetition* that were meant to restrain health care costs by creating competitive market conditions via direct incentives both for consumers and for employers who purchase group health insurance policies. Among these strategies was the imposition of a "tax cap" on employer income tax deductions for health insurance expenses, raising the threshold for individual income tax deductions, and offering multiple choices by employers in health insurance plans. While the threshold for personal income tax deductions for medical out-of-pocket expense was raised to 7.5% of gross income, the other strategies, while not formally enacted, had a profound effect on the thinking of health policy makers. The programs of the 1980s reflect this conservative philosophy, and in most cases, the scorecards for their success are mixed, at best.

The Tax Equity and Fiscal Responsibility Act (TEFRA)

The Tax Equity and Fiscal Responsibility Act (TEFRA), signed into law on September 30, 1982, and enacted the next day, set limits on Medicare reimbursements on a per-case basis for hospital costs and also placed a limit on the annual rate of increase for Medicare's reasonable costs per discharge. TEFRA was expected to reduce Medicare reimbursement by 4.5% in real dollars over the ensuing three years, during which time reimbursement increases, based on projected inflation rates, would be in effect. Because of the fast enactment of the Prospective Payment System one year later, it was difficult to evaluate the impact of TEFRA. However, the act was the harbinger of prospective payment, and a number of features of the latter program were borrowed from it. These features were part of the *section 223 limits* on hospital costs. They included (1) grouping hospitals by bed size and size of locale, (2) wage adjustments by locality, and (3) an adjustment for case-mix index (Deloitte Haskins & Sells, 1982a).

Today, most hospitals that are excluded from the Medicare Prospective Payment System are reimbursed according to TEFRA regulations.

The section 223 limits were calculated according to a complicated formula whereby the labor-related component for the hospital region, adjusted by a geographic wage index, was added to a regional nonlabor component. The product was then multiplied by a case-mix index, specific to each hospital. These figures were all specified by the Health Care Financing Administraiton (HCFA) and published in the *Federal Register*. The formula used to calculate the section 223 limits was substantially retained for figuring reimbursement rates for the Prospective Payment System.

The HCFA developed institutional-specific case-mix indexes based on a diagnosis-related group (DRG) system designed at Yale University. The DRG classification system sorts patients into uniform, clinically compatible groups that have been categorized on the basis of traditional resource use by patients with similar diagnoses. The original Yale DRGs were modified to reflect variation solely in Medicare cases. For each hospital, the HCFA used a 20% sample of the Medicare billing forms submitted for calendar year 1980. Using the 10,167 ICD-9-CM diagnosis codes from these claims and each hospital's Medicare cost report, the HCFA developed the case-mix index. In essence, this case-mix index was intended to compare a particular hospital's case mix with that of all other hospitals in the nation. Table 5–2 shows how five hypothetical hospitals with five DRGs, each varying in volume by hospital, can calculate their case-mix indexes, which reflect the relative severity of each hospital's caseload. Hospital D, with 46% of its cases in the high-weighted DRG 3, claims the highest case-mix index of 1.6031. This contrasts with Hospital A, which, with almost 70% of its cases in the low-paying DRGs 2 and 4, holds a case mix index of 0.8900. Extending this calculation to all cases in all hospitals participating in PPS, the national average case-mix index always equals 1.0000. The dollar amount ascribed to a DRG of 1.0000 is recalculated on a yearly basis.

Target Rates. Another ceiling established by the HCFA, concurrent with the section 223 limits, was the *target rate ceiling*. This target rate limited the

allowable amount of growth in Medicare reimbursable inpatient operating costs limits. In essence, TEFRA reimbursement gave bonuses to hospitals whose inpatient operating costs per discharge were less than the target rate ceiling, providing that the target rate was below the section 223 limit. Today, although the section 223 limits have been abandoned, the target rates have been retained for Medicare reimbursement for hospital categories exempt from PPS. If a hospital's per-discharge costs fall below the target rate, the hospital is given 50% of the difference. On the other hand, if a hospital's per-discharge costs are above the target, the hospital is reimbursed at the target rate plus 50% of the costs in excess of it, so long as the excess is limited to 10% of the target rate. In this way, TEFRA provides an incentive system for hospitals to lower their costs on Medicare discharges rather than to incur spiraling excesses year after year.

TABLE 5–2 Calculation of Medicare case-mix index[a]

Hospital	DRG 1	DRG 2	DRG 3	DRG 4	DRG 5	Total (Percent)	DRG Weighted Expected Cost Per Case ($)[b]	Case-Mix Index[c]
A	2.5	27.3	10.5	41.5	18.2	100	1660.40	0.8900
B	21.0	.9	30.1	2.0	46.0	100	2401.30	1.2872
C	40.6	5.0	2.3	47.2	4.9	100	1346.30	0.7227
D	5.1	18.4	62.5	10.0	4.0	100	2990.70	1.6031
E	30.4	65.0	1.0	1.6	2.0	100	929.00	0.4980
Average Proportion for all hospitals	19.92	23.32	21.28	20.46	15.02	100	1865.54	—
DRG cost weight	$1000	$800	$4100	$1500	$2000	—	—	—

a   Adjusted to make these 5 DRGs hypothetically represent all 356 Medicare DRGs
b   For hospital A, calculated as follows:
   $0.025(1000) + 0.273(800) + 0.105(4100) + 0.415(1500) + 0.182(2000) = \$1660.40$
c   For hospital A, calculated as $1660.40 divided by $1865.54 = 0.8900

SOURCE: *Tax Equity and Fiscal Responsibility Act of 1982: Management Strategies for Health Care Providers*, Deloitte, Haskins & Sells, 1982, New York: Author.

The Prospective Payment System

The Prospective Payment System (PPS) was enacted on October 1, 1983, two years ahead of schedule. The Social Security Amendments of 1983 (PL 98-21) initiated the new system and contained provisions to base payment for hospital inpatient services on predetermined rates per DRG. Today, 5,233 hospitals participate in PPS, representing 82% of all short-stay hospitals in the United States. Of the remaining hospitals, 95% still participate in Medicare under different reimbursement arrangements (Deloitte, Haskins & Sells, 1982b; Guterman & Dobson, 1986). Excluded from PPS are psychiatric, rehabilitation, and children's hospitals, long-term care hospitals, and other special medical facilities that have an approved waiver. Except for children's hospitals, which are still reimbursed according to costs, these facilities remain on TEFRA regulations.

PPS is a major departure from the preceding reimbursement system—cost-based reimbursement—in that payment bears no direct relationship to length of stay, services rendered, or costs of care. For a given discharge, a hospital with actual costs below the designated PPS rate for a given DRG is permitted to keep the difference in payment. If discharge costs exceed the payment level, the hospital is required to absorb the loss. Certain costs, such as capital depreciation and direct medical education costs, are exempt from PPS provisions and have their own payment formulas. Payment for hospital-based physician services (for example, radiology, anesthesiology, pathology, and so on), which previous to enactment of PPS were reimbursed on the basis of reasonable costs under Medicare Part A, is included in the hospital's PPS rate. As a result, many such physicians have defected to Part B of Medicare, billing patients directly for their services.

Standardized Payment Amount. PPS pays a standardized amount for each DRG. Standardized amounts are updated each year by the HCFA according to region of the country (for example, New England, Middle Atlantic, and so on) and by urbanization of the area (large urban or other areas). This amount is further divided into two components—a labor-related amount and a nonlabor-related amount. To compute the payment amount for a DRG of 1.0000, the labor-related amount is multiplied by a wage index, specific to each locality, and the product is added to the nonlabor-related amount. Proposed for the 1998 fiscal year (beginning October 1, 1997), for example, a hospital in San Diego is subject to a large urban labor-related amount of $2,857.85, times a wage index of 1.2266, plus a nonlabor-related amount of $1,161.63. Thus, the DRG payment for a hospital in San Diego is $4,667.07. This "final" figure is adjusted upward by an area-specific capital factor ($504.23 for San Diego) and other hospital-specific adjustments for indirect medical education and disproportionate share of low-income patients.

DRG Weights. The DRG weight classifications used in TEFRA were updated for use in PPS using a stratified sample of 400,000 medical records drawn from patient discharges in 332 hospitals during the last half of 1979. To date, 503 DRGs have been developed, expanding on the original 468 principal diagnoses. A contracted fiscal intermediary, such as Blue Cross or a commercial insurer, assigns a DRG from a bill submitted by the hospital for each case. Using classifications and terminology consistent with the ICD-9-CM and the Uniform Hospital Discharge Data Set (UHDDS), the intermediary assigns the DRG using the Grouper Program (an automated classification algorithm), which compares information contained in the bill with appropriate DRG criteria. Criteria include the patient's age, sex, principal and secondary diagnoses, procedures performed, and discharge status (American Medical Association, 1984). (Figure 5–6 presents a schematic diagram of the Grouper Program.) For all but a few DRGs that require clarification by the hospital before the payment amount is determined, the intermediary determines the payment amount and pays the hospital.

Outliers. Bills for "outliers," which result in extra payment for the hospital above the standard DRG rate, require special consideration. About four percent of the pool of total PPS payments is reserved for outliers. Length-of-stay or day outliers, though

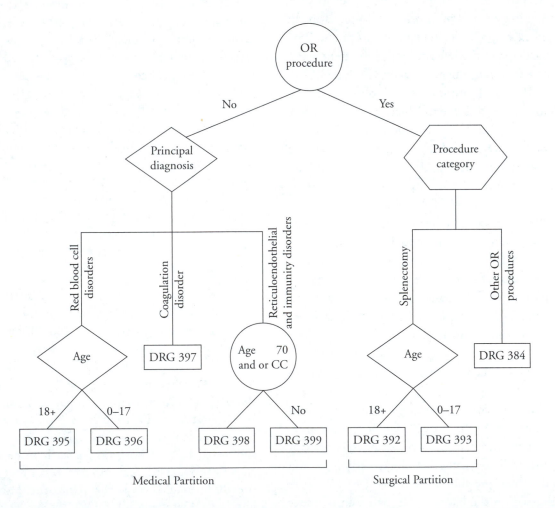

SOURCE: Reprinted with permission of American Medical Association, *Diagnosis-Related Groups (DRGs),* 1984, Chicago: Author.

FIGURE 5–6   Flowchart of the Grouper Program for major diagnostic category 16: Disease and Disorders of the Blood and Blood-Forming Organs and Immunological Disorders. (OR, operating room; CC, comorbidity and/or complication.)

slated to be eliminated in 1998, are identified by the intermediary, and after appropriate review, payment is made to the hospital. Fixed-loss or cost outliers, however, are not identified by the intermediary. The hospital must identify cost outliers and request payment. (It is important to note that the classification of DRGs depends largely on the principal diagnosis, which may not be the diagnosis consuming the most resources.)

For a discharge to be considered as an outlier, the rules are very stringent. In 1992, the threshold for a day outlier expanded to thirty-four days beyond the geometric mean length of stay for a specific DRG or three standard deviations above the mean, whichever is less. A simple appendectomy (DRG 167) with a mean length of stay of four days, for example, would not be considered an outlier until the inpatient episode reached fifteen days. Cost outliers are calculated using a fixed-loss threshold equal to the PPS rate for the DRG plus $7,600.

Quality Indicators. A clear incentive in the PPS system is for hospitals to expand services still qualifying for cost-based Medicare reimbursement. Opportunities for marketing expansion include specific ambulatory programs, satellite clinics, and health-related services such as family planning, chemical dependency treatment, and laboratory or other ancillary services used by physicians. Hospital-sponsored skilled nursing, rehabilitation, home health services, and other services that may facilitate earlier discharge of patients and provide additional sources of revenue for hospitals have experienced marked growth since the inception of PPS. Many of these programs may be accomplished by conversion of acute care beds, replacing services eliminated by PPS-induced financial considerations or making use of excess capacity.

The major deleterious incentives anticipated in the enactment of PPS included: (1) multiple, unnecessary admissions of the same patient for a set of related procedures resulting in more discreet DRG payments, a practice known as *churning;* (2) *skimming* more profitable, less severely ill patients in each DRG, or *dumping* high-cost patients; and (3) reducing length of stay, tests, and procedures per admission to dangerously low levels, increasing mortality and morbidity.

Empirical findings as to the validity of these assertions have shown few ill effects of PPS or are inconclusive due to the rapidly changing nature of the health care sector (Guterman & Dobson, 1986; DesHarnais, et al., 1987; Guterman, et al., 1988). Prior to PPS, hospital admissions had been falling for all payers for a number of years; once PPS was enacted, Medicare admissions went down as well. The figures for the fiscal year 1984 (the first full year of PPS) indicated an 11.3% decrease in admissions, resulting in a per Medicare enrollee decline of 15.9%, which was counter to the steady rise in Medicare admissions during the 1978–1984 period. While anecdotal evidence of skimming and dumping did surface, widespread usage of these practices by hospitals were largely documented for the uninsured and, in some states in particular, for Medicaid patients, rather than for Medicare patients. From 1990 to 1995, hospital admissions per 1,000 enrollees remained steady at about 315 (Guterman & Dobson, 1986; Guterman, et al., 1988; U.S. Department of Health and Human Services, 1996).

Length of stay has been falling for Medicare since the inception of the act. Under the PPS system, an even steeper decline in average length of stay (down 17% for the first three years of PPS), combined with reduced admissions, has resulted in declining patient volumes. This reduced length of stay has been achieved through shorter stays across the board, rather than through efforts aimed specifically at patients who have the longest stays (that is, the most severely ill). From 1990 to 1995, length of stay continued to decline from 9.0 days per admission to 7.1 days. These phenomena indicate that PPS has been effective in encouraging hospitals to improve efficiency in the provision of inpatient care (Guterman, et al., 1988).

The Medicare case-mix index increased sharply and the percentage of hospital days spent in special care units increased in the first three years after the implementation of PPS, possibly due to more judicious selections of candidates for inpatient hospitalization. Other studies of severity of illness at admission and discharge also show increases in the post-PPS period. The discharge of patients "quicker and sicker" has fostered rapid growth in the use of skilled nursing facilities and home health agency services by Medicare enrollees. Research indicates a tendency under PPS to increase the care provided to patients in other than inpatient settings. A survey of two hundred physicians in five states shows that under prospective payment, hospitals encourage physicians to reduce ancillary services, shorten hospital stays, and increase outpatient testing (Guterman & Dobson, 1986; Guterman, et al., 1988).

Hospital mortality rates for the Medicare population have increased under PPS, but studies have explained this movement in terms of changing case mix and heightened severity of illness of patients. All in all, there is no systematic evidence that access to needed care has been hampered by PPS (DesHarnais, et al., 1987; Guterman, et al., 1988).

Criticisms of PPS. A number of criticisms have been levied against the incentives inherent in the DRG system. First, speculation exists that DRGs may not be "economically neutral" in that a hospital may be rewarded or penalized for performing an activity. To the extent that individual DRGs reflect procedures actually performed (for example, types of surgery) as well as diagnosis, the choice of treatment may vary according to the "profitability" of that DRG, and treatment decisions may not be made on purely clinical grounds. In a similar vein, physicians, in their clinical notes, and medical records adminis-

trators, in abstracting data for the DRG grouper program, might call upon *gaming* strategies to assure *DRG creep* to higher-level, revenue-enhancing diagnoses (Jencks, et al., 1984).

Other criticisms involve the structure and mathematical integrity of DRGs. Several methods for changing PPS to a severity-based, rather than diagnosis-based, case-mix system have been postulated along with schemes for refining DRG coding to reflect the severity of the condition. Research has demonstrated that the mathematical constructs of the DRGs lend themselves to "compression" in DRG prices; the prices of the truly high-cost DRGs are set low relative to their actual costs, whereas the prices of truly low-cost DRGs are set high relative to their costs. Recent research has confirmed the persistence of this phenomenon. Compression could create a situation in which hospitals may want to discriminate against providing service to patients in the high-cost DRGs, or on a positive note, it could encourage a few hospitals in competitive markets to specialize in efficiently providing "high-cost" services, such as coronary bypass surgery, at more profitable rates (Horn & Horn, 1986; Jencks, et al., 1984; Keeler, et al., 1990; Lave, 1985; Smits, et al., 1984).

Financial Performance. Hospitals have generally fared well financially under PPS, but the distribution of results is uneven. On average, hospitals received Medicare reimbursements that were considerably higher than their corresponding costs. In the first three years of PPS, urban hospitals, large hospitals, and teaching hospitals experienced wider payment margins than their rural, small, and nonteaching counterparts. In terms of overall financial performance, urban and proprietary hospitals, as well as regional referral centers, have manifested large margins, and sole community hospitals are disproportionately represented at the lower end of the range (Guterman, et al., 1988). The spate of hospital bankruptcies that were predicted at the inception of PPS has not taken place, but acquisitions and mergers have been rampant in the health care industry in recent years.

PPS appears to have decelerated the rate of increase in Medicare inpatient hospital expenditures. Although outpatient payments, which are excluded from PPS, have mushroomed, total Medicare benefit payments are increasing at a slower rate due to the sharp decline in growth of Part A payments. From 1974 (which marked the end of wage and price controls under the Nixon administration) through 1983 (the enactment of PPS), Medicare inpatient hospital benefit payments increased at an annual rate of 18.3%. From 1983 to 1995, program payments for hospital services dropped to 7.7% per year. For the first three years of PPS, the slowdown was even more dramatic—a real annual rate of increase of 3.5% (Guterman & Dobson, 1986; Guterman, et al., 1988; U.S. Department of Health and Human Services, 1997).

It is interesting to note that prospective payment for hospitals based on DRGs has become an export item for the United States health care industry. As of 1992, nine other industrialized nations were already using or proposing to use DRGs, or a modification thereof, for hospital reimbursement. Nations in the process of phasing in DRGs include England, Australia, Belgium, Norway, Portugal, and Sweden (Wiley, 1992).

Medicare Physician Reimbursement

From 1975 to 1995, Medicare's total payments for physician services grew at a faster rate than payments for hospital services. By 1990, physician services reached 22.6% of total Medicare spending, up from 21.4% in 1975. Over the same period, hospital care dropped as a share of total Medicare expenditures from 74.4 to 63.7%. Although the Reagan administration had intended to reform physician reimbursement for Medicare, these plans were postponed until 1990 because of pressures from opponents of government regulation in the private sector. Nonetheless, there was general agreement that physician payment under Medicare needed to be revised (U.S. Department of Health and Human Services, 1995).

Congress directed the administration to study physician payment reform when it established Medicare's DRG-based prospective payment system for hospital care. One of the favored options was to develop a national fee schedule that would set a price for each type of service with adjustments for local wage costs. Another possible reform alternative was to establish physician DRGs. Research into this option, however, disclosed thorny problems in (1) applying DRGs to outpatient care, which is typified by a large number of encounters at a relatively small price per visit; (2) dividing the DRG payment among a number of doctors who may be involved in one illness episode; (3) marked geographic variations in practice patterns; and (4) cost variability in DRGs used to reimburse the medical versus the surgical specialties, the latter of which are more homogeneous and lend themselves better to DRG-based payment (Culler & Ehrenfried, 1986; Mitchell, 1985).

Resource-Based Relative Values. On January 1, 1992, Medicare initiated a new system for reimbursing physicians using a resource-based relative-value (RBRV) scale. The new payment method divides resources needed to produce physician services into three components: physician work, practice expenses, and malpractice insurance costs. For each procedure, each of the three components is characterized by a numerical value representing its relative contribution to the expenses incurred in delivering the service (Table 5–3). In addition, as shown in Table 5–4, the relative values of the three components are each adjusted for geographic cost/price variations. The total units drive the fee, which is derived by multiplying the total units by a

TABLE 5–3   Resource-based relative value units (RBRVs), Medicare 1992: Selected procedures

Description	Physician Work	Practice Expense	Malpractice Insurance	Total Units
Repair of inguinal hernia, age 5 years or older	5.12	4.75	0.98	10.85
Cholecystectomy without cholangiography	9.81	8.03	1.70	19.54
Replacement of aortic valve	25.25	32.30	5.66	63.21
Coronary arteries bypass	25.63	38.90	6.81	71.34
Insertion of intraocular lens subsequent to cataract removal	8.39	13.16	0.69	22.24
Repair of retinal detachment, schleral buckling, with or without implant	14.87	22.15	1.16	38.18
Arthroscopy, knee, surgical; with meniscectomy (medial or lateral, including meniscal shaving)	7.93	12.02	1.94	21.89
Interpretation of computerized axial tomography scan of the brain with and without contrast	1.23	0.60	0.09	1.92
Vasectomy, unilateral or bilateral, including postoperative semen examination(s)	3.40	2.74	0.29	6.43
Transurethral resection of prostate, including control of postoperative bleeding, complete	12.23	12.65	1.23	26.11

SOURCE: Adapted from "RBRVs: How New Physician Fee Schedule Will Work," by P. L. Grimaldi, 1991, *Healthcare Financial Management, 45*(9), p. 64.

conversion factor. The conversion factor is a set of national values: $35.77 for each unit of primary care services, $40.96 per unit of surgical services, and $33.85 for other nonsurgical services. The final fee is thus a geographically weighted summation of the three components of the RBRVs times the conversion factor (Grimaldi, 1991; Hsiao, et al., 1988a, 1988b).

For surgery, the RBRV payment schedule also establishes a uniform definition of "global surgery" to ensure that identical payments are made for the same amount of work and resources expended in furnishing specific surgical services on a nationwide basis. The initial evaluation or consultation by a surgeon is paid separately from the global surgery package. The global fee includes all preoperative visits and all medical and surgical services related to a procedure, covering a ninety-day postoperative period for all visits by the primary surgeon.

Simulations done by the Harvard University developers of the new reimbursement system (Hsiao, et al., 1988a), showed that certain types of physicians would be financial winners and losers under RBRVs in comparison to what they would have earned under the old fee schedule. Pathologists, radiologists, thoracic surgeons, cardiovascular surgeons, and opthalmologists stood to lose from 25 to 45% of their former Medicare fees. Physicians specializing in evaluation and management, such as internists, family practitioners, and immunologists, on the other hand, would be likely to gain from 35 to 65% over their previous Medicare earnings. Recent quantitative and qualitative evidence supports the accuracy of these

TABLE 5–4 Geographic practice cost indexes used to weight components of RBRVs: Selected cities, 1992

Locality	Physician Work	Practice Expense	Malpractice Insurance
Birmingham, AL	0.981	0.913	0.824
Los Angeles, CA	1.060	1.196	1.370
San Francisco, CA	1.038	1.303	1.370
Colorado	0.999	0.988	0.683
Washington, DC, area	1.059	1.168	0.947
Miami, FL	1.034	1.025	1.641
Atlanta, GA	0.975	1.022	0.752
Lexington and Louisville, KY	0.984	0.917	0.667
New Orleans, LA	0.994	1.003	1.185
Detroit, MI	1.059	1.091	1.763
St. Paul–Minneapolis, MN	1.014	1.024	0.748
Montana	0.967	0.926	0.718
New York, NY (Manhattan)	1.059	1.255	1.647
Dallas, TX	0.996	0.971	0.504
Vermont	0.942	0.942	0.533
Urban Massachusetts	1.002	1.131	0.855
Chicago, IL	1.004	1.114	1.773
North-central Iowa	0.971	0.916	0.666

SOURCE: Adapted from "RBRVs: How New Physician Fee Schedule Will Work," by P. L. Grimaldi, 1991, *Healthcare Financial Management, 45*(9), p. 66.

predictions. Other benefactors of the changes include chiropractors, psychiatrists, and hematologists/oncologists.

Hsiao et al. (1992) later published an article criticizing the HCFA for setting the monetary conversion factors at unreasonably low levels and claiming that Medicare continued to reimburse invasive services with more units than research justified, according to the RBRVs actually assigned in the Medicare fee schedule.

Selective Contracting

In 1982, the California legislature cleared the way for the state Medicaid program (Medi-Cal) and private insurers to enable payers to draw up contracts for the delivery of health services to their beneficiaries, selecting only hospitals and physi-

cians that agreed to accept a negotiated price for their services. This practice of *selective contracting* was first embraced by the Medi-Cal program to contract hospitals at low per diem rates. The selection rule was uncomplicated: if the price was right and other specified conditions were met, a contract would be secured.

Not all hospitals competing for contracts, including large traditional Medi-Cal providers, gained them, and as a result of these shockwaves in the health care marketplace, the contracting process was enormously successful, with 67% of California hospitals, accounting for 72% of the Medi-Cal patients, awarded contracts by the end of the first year of negotiations. Furthermore, for the first two years of selective contracting, there was no evidence of reduced access to health resources for

Medi-Cal patients or any change in the quality of care they received. Savings to the state were estimated at $165 million for the first year of the program and $235 million for the second year (Johns, et al., 1985a, 1985b).

Cost cutting on an unprecedented scale was reported by hospitals receiving Medi-Cal contracts, demonstrating that competitive bidding shifts the burden of proof in hospital rate setting and encourages an active search for economies of operation. For contracted hospitals, total payments (in constant dollars) fell 9.6% in the first year of the program; average payments per day fell 18.4%, and payments per admission fell 19.7%. Teaching hospitals, nonprofit hospitals, and investor-owned hospitals absorbed the largest reductions in average payment per day. Even though the per diem rates held incentives for increasing inpatient stays, length of stay fell 1.5%. Hospital financial analyses showed that contractors were, on the whole, not adversely impacted by selective contracting in the first two years (Mennemeyer & Olinger, 1989). Anecdotal evidence, often citing the moneys supplied by federal legislation for hospitals serving a "disproportionate share" of Medicaid patients, supports the continued cost-saving effects of selective contracting by Medi-Cal.

Zwanziger & Melnick (1996) confirm that in competitive managed care markets in California, where selective contracting is the norm, hospitals showed far slower growth and lower relative costs since 1982.

Preferred Provider Organizations. The entry of private insurers and firms into selective contracting began in earnest in 1984 and quickly became known as "preferred provider organizations" (PPOs). PPOs have become a rapid growth area in health insurance. By 1993, enrollment in PPOs had increased to 26% of health plan participants, as compared to 23% in HMOs.

A PPO is an arrangement or contract between a panel of health care providers, usually hospitals and physicians, and purchasers of health care services; the providers agree to supply services to a defined group of patients on a discounted fee-for-service basis. The exclusive provider organization (EPO) is the extreme form of a PPO, wherein services provided by nonparticipating providers are not reimbursed at all (forcing the patient to pay the entire cost out-of-pocket unless care is rendered by an affiliated provider). Many PPO plans are sponsored by health insurance companies or self-insured employers.

PPOs generally have five key elements: (1) a limited number of physicians and hospitals, (2) negotiated fee schedules, (3) utilization review, (4) consumer choice of provider with lower out-of-pocket costs as an incentive to use participating providers, and (5) expedient settlement of claims (de Lissovoy, et al., 1986).

Utilization review is the principal mechanism used by PPOs for controlling costs via reducing inappropriate use of services. Typical methods of utilization review include preadmission certification for hospital stays and certain types of high-cost outpatient procedures. Other mechanisms utilized by PPOs for cost control are contracting with low-cost providers and establishing a reimbursement system that realizes saving through discounted provider charges or incentives for reduced utilization. Discounts are generally in the range from 10 to 13% below usual charges, and insurers are reporting premiums at 10 to 20% below standard indemnity plans (Gabel, et al., 1986).

HEALTH CARE REFORM

National Health Insurance

National health insurance (NHI) is a concept that has been espoused by many for over sixty years for containing health care costs and for providing universal access for the United States population. NHI came close to becoming part of the Social Security Act of 1935, and numerous bills, representing a spectrum of schemes, have been introduced and seriously debated by most congressional sessions ever since then. In the mid-1970s, the issue of NHI became so heated that both political parties introduced some bills that were strikingly similar. NHI bills ran the gamut from expanding Medicare to new population groups (for example, children under five years of age) to a national health service (NHS) concept like that of Sweden or Great Britain where the government owns the hospitals and the doctors are paid on the basis of capitation or salary by the NHS.

When President Carter was elected in 1976, many in the health arena assumed that NHI would be an eventuality in a Democratic administration, but early on, it was evident that Carter took little interest in health issues. In the 1980s and early 1990s, the Reagan and Bush administrations were active in introducing cost-containment measures, such as PPS and RBRVs for Medicare, but no serious consideration was given to sweeping reform of the entire system.

Recent Strategies for Reform

American Medical Association. An unprecedented issue of the *Journal of the American Medical Association (JAMA)* appeared in May 1991. The entire issue was devoted to health system reform proposals, a subject traditionally anathema to organized medicine. Thirteen articles, by authors spanning a plethora of special interests, detailed a variety of strategies for achieving a new system.

Most proposals called for a revised system administered by private insurers with employer/employee premium sharing, supplemented by some form of government financing for nonworking individuals and families. With few exceptions, the proposals called for universal access to health care and for the provision of health insurance to all employees. Looking to the political left, it was interesting that no plan advocated a national health service model. On the right, only one of the plans called for increased privatization and freedom of choice.

In what can only be called a courageous editorial, Lundberg (1991, p. 2566), then the editor of the *JAMA,* summed up the findings :

> Although there may be consensus that our society must provide basic medical/health care for all of our people, we seem not to be close to a consensus on how to do it. Virtually all comprehensive health care proposals involve major legislation of some sort. Since consensus means "general agreement or unanimity; group solidarity in sentiment or belief," it is unlikely that, either as a society or as a profession, we will ever reach a true consensus on how to proceed, so we must not wait for one. To pass federal legislation requires only a simple majority in both houses of Congress plus presidential approval.

Bush Proposal. In 1992, President Bush unveiled his proposal for health care reform. Calling upon conservative principles, he advocated a type of voucher system, whereby needy families would be allowed to take up to a $3,750 family tax credit, inversely related to income, for the purchase of private health insurance. With the goal of providing better access to the poor, states would be financially induced to capitate and expand Medicaid programs.

Critics of the proposal noted that the tax credit voucher approach, linked to income taxes, might bypass many nonworking poor. Further, they held that it would take as much as $100 billion in additional government revenues to compensate for taxes lost to the credits, and the president gave no indication as to how such a shortfall in revenues would be avoided. Finally, the plan did not elucidate on how cost controls would be achieved in the market-based approach. Needless to say, the Bush proposal was cast to oblivion.

The Clinton Plan. Health care reform has become one of the hottest domestic political issues of the 1990s. Pressures for such reform have come from a wide variety of groups including providers, the elderly and disabled, labor unions, state and local governments, and insiders within the Washington establishment. Even the health insurers and managed care organizations have called for change. The two main targets of discontent are (1) the growing numbers and financial burden of uninsured and underinsured Americans, and (2) the ever-spiraling costs of health care which serve to erode American competitiveness in the international marketplace.

In response to these pressures, President Clinton introduced *The President's Health Security Plan* (The White House Domestic Policy Council, 1993), which was largely the work of a task force headed by the First Lady Hillary Rodham Clinton. The plan was subject to a great deal of criticism (and negative television advertising) from a large number of wealthy special interest groups, with the result that the plan died in Congress within a few months.

The essence of the plan was to create regional health alliances (that is, health insurance purchasing cooperatives), wherein various competing insurance plans would be offered, at various premium supplements, to all participating employers and thus their employees. The model was based, in part, upon the California Public Employees Retirement Program (CalPERS) health insurance, which has been quite successful for a number of years in containing costs, maintaining quality, and offering a wide range of comprehensive traditional and managed care plans to its members. The Health Security Plan also would have created a separate risk pool for the uninsured.

Perhaps the ultimate reason that the Health Security Plan failed was that its implementation depended on global prospective budgeting for health care at a national level, the moneys from which would be dispersed to state budgeting agencies and then on to the regional alliances. Many influential opinion makers maintained that the United States had no viable administrative apparatus whereby such complex *ex ante* budgeting could take place. They predicted that a large and costly new government bureaucracy would emerge at a time when the electorate was seeking to curtail the size of government and its possible intrusion into peoples' personal lives.

The irony of the failed outcome of the Clinton plan is that, in many regions of the country, such health alliances are emerging within the private sector, spurred by consolidation of health plans and providers into large health systems and managed care plans. Government purchasers are also mimicking the CalPERS marketing formula.

President Clinton, in the face of his defeated plan, has been active in pushing health reform legislation incrementally, based upon the research conducted for the Health Security Plan. Among areas of federal legislative reform enacted in 1996 are (1) increasing the portability of health benefits from one employer to another, (2) encouraging growth for Medicare managed care plans which, in 1995, enrolled only about 10% of Medicare members, (3) expanding mental health benefits in health plans so that they are comparable to physical health benefits, and (4) providing incentives to form Medical Savings Accounts (MSAs). MSAs, drawing the greatest amount of political attention, are similar in concept to Individual Retirement Accounts, offering upscale "savings accounts" with comprehensive benefits subject to high yearly deductibles (for example, $6,000 per year). To date, MSAs have attracted only a few thousand people.

Medicaid Reform

The Welfare Reform Act of 1996 placed new restrictions on eligibility for AFDC, SSI, and other federally funded welfare programs, including Medicaid. Furthermore, greater discretion was given to the states as to how to organize and enact welfare programs. Chief among the new provisions is that Medicaid will be delinked from cash assistance programs and states will be required to re-determine Medicaid eligibility for all welfare recipients. Another new federal provision is that states may deny Medicaid and cash assistance to current legal immigrants. Legal immigrants who arrive after the bill is enacted are subject to a five-year waiting period before they become eligible for means-tested programs. (This provision holds great cost-cutting opportunities for states with high rates of immigration, like California and Texas, but may hold dire consequences for public health and communicable disease.) Finally, new criteria for SSI will result in about 50,000 children, most with behavioral disorders, losing Medicaid coverage. As of this writing, states are working out the logistics of implementing welfare and Medicaid reform without much guidance from the federal government. It remains to be seen whether certain progressive programs initiated by several states will be successful at containing Medicaid costs without reducing access for needy populations or to medical treatment alternatives.

The Uninsured

Health reform cannot be discussed without addressing the growing plight of the uninsured. In 1994, approximately 15.2% of the United States population, comprising about 40 million people, was not covered by health insurance, either public or private. This percentage is up from 1987, when about 12.9% of the population was uninsured for health care. Groups that predominate among the uninsured are Hispanics and, to a lesser extent, African Americans, those from eighteen to thirty-four years old, and those with low educational attainment. Males are more likely than females to be uninsured. The South and the West are also disproportionately represented among the uninsured, with the highest rates in Arkansas, California, New Mexico, and Texas (U.S. Department of Health and Human Services, 1996). Needless to say, the majority of the uninsured are poor or hovering close to the poverty level.

In addition to the growing ranks of the uninsured, anecdotal evidence attests to the transience of private insurance coverage for all Americans, linked as it is to employment status and subject to fluctuations in the economy. Constantly changing eligibility requirements for Medicaid and other public programs also adds to the problem of frictional uninsurance for many of the nation's low-income population.

The problem of uninsurance impinges on the health care of all Americans for several reasons. First, it results in reduced access to care for the uninsured themselves, who are likely to postpone needed care to a time when their medical conditions have escalated in severity. Thus, the heightened intensity of caring for sicker people increases the cost of their care. Second, providers must recoup the costs of serving the uninsured from their paying customers—private insurers or the government. Insurance premiums go up commensurately, and the taxpayer's burden enlarges. Third, this cost shifting imposes yet another pressure on the efficient production of American goods and services, many of which stand to lose their competitive advantage in the world economy. Finally, in a spiral effect, uninsurance feeds on itself. With health insurance premiums constantly escalating, many businesses, especially small businesses, cannot afford to initiate or continue health insurance, thus adding to the problem.

International Comparisons

A great deal of interest in recent years has been focused on the health care systems of other industrialized nations, particularly Canada and Germany (Hurst, 1991; Iglehart, 1986a, 1986b; Neuschler, 1990; Reinhardt, 1990). Although each system has its flaws, comparable countries have achieved universal access, ostensibly high-quality, high-volume care, and significant cost controls. The Canadian system is financed equally by federal and provincial government general revenues in most provinces; Germany relies primarily on social health insurance linked to employment, supplemented by public general revenue funds. In both systems, global budgets are prospectively determined on an annual basis. In both systems, providers are predominantly private, independent contractors with the relevant health ministry acting as third party payer—the sole purchaser and reimburser of health services. Many assert that it is this monopsony purchasing power that fosters coalition building around issues of cost control, negotiated rate setting, and sustained quality of care. It is also argued that a universal reimbursement system promotes efficiencies that vastly reduce administrative costs.

In contrast to the Canadian and German national health insurance systems, the national health service (NHS) model has been a growing movement in Europe (Abel-Smith, 1985). Among twelve nations in the European Community, six now have an NHS model: the United Kingdom, Denmark, Spain, Italy, Greece, and Portugal. France, West Germany, Belgium, Luxembourg, Ireland, and the Netherlands remain without an NHS. Increasing regulation of health care is also notable in Western Europe.

SUMMARY

Financing health services in the United States includes a plethora of institutions and activities. The growth of employer-based private health insurance has stimulated unprecedented growth in health expenditures and biomedical advancement for the nation in the post–World War II era. The advent of Medicare and Medicaid in 1966 heralded a period of even more rapid growth, along with unbridled inflation, that persists to this day.

Inequities in access to health care, thought to be alleviated by Medicare and Medicaid, and the extensive provision of voluntary health insurance for employed groups have not been resolved. Universal health coverage has not been realized, and a substantial and growing percentage of the United States population are uninsured. State revenues have grown at rates slower than health care costs, inducing across-the-board reductions and more restrictive eligibility requirements for state Medicaid programs. Very recently, the Prospective Payment System, the new Medicare fee schedule for physicians, selective contracting, and managed care plans have shown some success in ameliorating uncontrolled inflation in health care spending. However, effective means for identifying and monitoring the adequacy and appropriateness of health care, in an environment of either overutilization or underutilization, have not been developed.

The cry for health care reform resounds in all sectors of the United States economy. Although most policy makers agree upon universal access, they are far from an agreement on how to finance the system, reimburse the providers, and impose cost controls. Whatever transpires in the future is likely to revolve around the fundamental politic of health finance: private versus public, entitlement versus social welfare, monopsony purchasing versus competitive concessions, fee for service versus prepayment.

This chapter has provided an historical and methodological framework for understanding and analyzing health care finance in the United States today. The principles that have been presented will apply to health finance, no matter how dynamic the future of the health care sector proves to be.

REFERENCES

Aaron, H. J. (1993/94). Paying for health care. *Domestic Affairs, 23,* 23–78.

Abel-Smith, B. (1985). Who is the odd man out?: The experience of western Europe in containing the costs of health care. *Milbank Mem Fund Quarterly, 63,* 1–7.

American Medical Association. (1984). *Diagnosis-related groups (DRGs) and the prospective payment system.* Chicago: American Medical Association.

Culler, S., & Ehrenfried, D. (1986). On the feasibility of physician DRGs. *Inquiry, 23,* 40–55.

de Lissovoy, G., Rice, T., Ermann, D., et al. (1986). Preferred providers organizations: Today's models and tomorrow's prospects. *Inquiry, 23,* 7–15.

Deloitte, Haskins & Sells. (1982a). *Tax Equity and Fiscal Responsibility Act of 1982: Management strategies for health care providers.* New York: Author.

Deloitte, Haskins & Sells. (1982b). *Medicare prospective payment system—1983: Strategies for health care providers.* New York: Author.

DesHarnais, S., Kobrinski, E., Chesney, J., et al. (1987). The early effects of the Prospective Payment System on inpatient utilization and the quality of care. *Inquiry, 24,* 7–16.

Enthoven, A. (1981). The competition strategy; status and prospects. *New England Journal of Medicine, 304,* 109–112.

Fuchs, V. R. (1984). "Though much is taken": Reflections on aging, health, and medical care. *Milbank Mem Fund Quarterly, 6,* 143–166.

Gabel, J., Ermann, D., Rice, T., et al. (1986). The emergence and future of PPOs. *Journal of Health Politics, Policy, Law, 11,* 305–322.

Gornick, M., Greenberg, N. J., Eggers, P. W., et al. (1985). Twenty years of Medicare and Medicaid: Covered populations, use of benefits, and program expenditures. *Health Care Financing Review* (Ann. Suppl.), 13–59.

Grimaldi, P. L. (1991). RBRVs: How new physician fee schedule will work. *Healthcare Financial Management, 45*(9), 58–75.

Guterman, S., & Dobson, A. (1986). Impact of the Medicare prospective payment system for hospitals. *Health Care Financing Review, 7,* 97–114.

Guterman, S., Eggers, P. W., Riley, G., Greene, T. F., & Terrell, S. A. (1988). The first 3 years of Medicare prospective payment: An overview. *Health Care Financing Review, 9*(3), 67–77.

Hillman, A. L., Welch, W. P., & Pauly, M. V. (1992). Contractual arrangements between HMOs and primary care physicians: Three-tiered HMOs and risk pools. *Medical Care, 30*(2), 136–148.

Horn, S. D., & Horn, R. A. (1986). Reliability and validity of the Severity of Illness Index. *Medical Care, 24,* 159–178.

Hsiao, W. C., Braun, P., Becker, E. R., et al. (1992). Results and impacts of the resource-based relative value scale. *Medical Care, 30*(11), NS61–NS79.

Hsiao, W. C., Braun, P., Dunn, D., Becker, E. R., DeNicola, M., & Ketcham, T. R. (1988a). Results and policy impications of the resource-based relative-value study. *New England Journal of Medicine, 319*(13), 881–888.

Hsiao, W. C., Braun, P., Yntema, D., & Becker, E. R. (1988b). Estimating physicians' work for a resource-based relative-value scale. *New England Journal of Medicine, 319*(13), 835–841.

Hurst, J. W. (1991). Reform of health care in Germany. *Health Care Financing Review, 12*(3), 73–101.

Iglehart, J. K. (1986a). Canada's health care system: Part one. *New England Journal of Medicine, 315*(3), 202–208.

Iglehart, J. K. (1986b). Canada's health care system: Part two. *New England Journal of Medicine, 315*(12), 778–784.

Jencks, S. F., Dobson, A., Willis, P., et al. (1984). Evaluating and improving the measurement of hospital case mix. *Health Care Financing Review* (Ann. Suppl.), 1–11.

Johns, L., Derzon, R. A., & Anderson, M. D. (1985a). Selective contracting in California: Early effects and policy implications. *Inquiry, 22,* 24–32.

Johns, L., Anderson, M. D., & Derzon, R. A. (1985b). Selective contracting in California: Experience in the second year. *Inquiry, 22,* 335–347.

Journal of the American Medical Association. (1991, May 15). *265*(19).

Keeler, E. B., Kahn, K. L., Draper, D., Sherwood, M. J., et al. (1990). Changes in sickness at admission following the introduction of the prospective payment system. *Journal of the American Medical Association, 264*(15), 1962–1968.

Lave, J. R. (1985). Is compression occurring in DRG prices? *Inquiry, 22,* 142–147.

Levit, K. R., Lazenby, H. C., Braden, B. R., Cowan, C. A., McDonnell, P. A., Sivarajan, L., Stiller, J. M., Won, D. K., Donham, C. S., Long, A. M., & Stewart, M. W. (1996). National health expenditures, 1995. *Health Care Financing Review, 18*(1), 175–214.

Lubitz, J., & Prihoda, R. (1984). Use and costs of Medicare services in the last two years of life. *Health Care Financing Review, 5,* 117–131.

Lundberg, G. D. (1991). National health care reform: An aura of inevitability is upon us. *Journal of the American Medical Association, 265*(19), 2566–2567.

Mennemeyer, S. T., & Olinger, L. (1989). Selective contracting in California: Its effect on hospital finances. *Inquiry, 26,* 442–457.

Mitchell, J. B. (1985). Physician DRGs. *New England Journal of Medicine, 313,* 670–675.

Neuschler, E. (1990). *Canadian health care: The implications of public health insurance.* Washington, DC: Health Insurance Association of America.

Reinhardt, U. E. (1985). The compensation of physicians: Approaches used in foreign countries. *Quality Review Bulletin, 11,* 366–377.

Reinhardt, U. E. (1990, September). West Germany's health-care and health-insurance system: Combining universal access with cost control. In The Pepper Commission, *A call for action: Final report of the U.S. Bipartisan Commission on Comprehensive Health Care.* Washington, DC: U.S. Government Printing Office.

Rice, T. (1992). Containing health care costs in the United States. *Medical Care Review, 49*(1), 19–65.

Roemer, M. I. (1977). *Comparative national policies on health care.* New York: Dekker.

Roemer, M. I. (1978). *Social medicine: The advance of organized health services in America.* New York: Springer.

Smits, H. L., Fetter, R. B., & McMahon, L. F., Jr. (1984). Variation in resource use within diagnosis-related groups: The severity issue. *Health Care Financing Review* (Ann. Suppl.), 71–78.

U.S. Bureau of the Census. (1996). *Statistical Abstract of the United States: 1996* (116th ed.). Washington, DC: U.S. Government Printing Office.

U.S. Department of Health and Human Services, Health Care Financing Administration, Bureau of Data Management and Strategy. (1996, September). *1996 HCFA Statistics* (HCFA Pub. No. 03394).

U.S. Department of Health and Human Services, Health Care Financing Administration, Office of Research and Demonstrations. (1995, February). Medicare and Medicaid statistical supplement. *Health Care Financing Review* (HCFA Pub. No. 03348).

U.S. Department of Health and Human Services, Office of Strategic Planning. (1997, October). Medicare and Medicaid Statistical Supplement. *Health Care Financing Review.* (HCFA Pub. No. 03399).

Waldo, M. O. (1990). Addendum: A brief summary of the Medicaid program. *Health Care Financing Review* (Ann. Suppl.), 171–172.

The White House Domestic Policy Council. (1993). *The president's health security plan.* New York: Times Books.

Wiley, M. M. (1992). Hospital financing reform and case-mix measurement: An international review. *Health Care Financing Review, 13*(4), 119–133.

Zwanziger, J., & Melnick, G. A. (1996). Can managed care plans control health care costs? *Health Affairs, 15*(2), 185–199.

CHAPTER

Managed Care: Restructuring the System

Paul R. Torrens

Stephen J. Williams

CHAPTER TOPICS

LEARNING OBJECTIVES

Upon completing this chapter, the reader should be able to:

- Understand the variety of arrangements included under the term *managed care.*
- Appreciate the roles of all key players, especially the consumer, in managed care.
- Understand the underlying mechanisms of managed care.
- Appreciate the complex challenges involved in the future of managed care.
- Analyze the appropriate role of managed care in the nation's health care system.

Although the term *managed care* has become increasingly familiar to anyone involved with health care in the United States in the last few years, there are two major misunderstandings with regard to the term and its use. First, the term *managed care* is sometimes used as though all forms of managed care are the same and managed care were a single organizational structure that functions like a tightly unified entity. Unfortunately, nothing could be further from the truth on both counts; *managed care* covers a wide variety of organizational forms, and in any one of the organizational forms, there are three or four separate subunits that make up the whole.

The second misunderstanding with regard to managed care is often a misunderstanding of the impact of the arrival of managed care on the American health care system. Sometimes, managed care is discussed as if it were merely one more change in the way health insurance is organized and in the way that providers of health services are paid. Frequently, managed care is described as yet one more technical innovation in what has become an increasingly specialized field of insurance.

Unfortunately, viewing managed care as merely a new set of technical changes misses the point that managed care has brought about a major change in the way in which health care in the United States is delivered by providers and utilized by patients. It should be understood that although the technical changes included in managed care are very interesting, it is much more important to realize the structural and policy changes in American health care that are currently being wrought by the increasing presence of managed care.

This chapter examines both aspects of managed care: the technical and descriptive aspects of managed care itself, and the impact on the American health care system. The implication for changing objectives and incentives is emphasized.

WHAT IS MANAGED CARE?

It is virtually impossible to provide a definition of *managed care* that satisfies all participants in all circumstances, since the applications of the term are so wide and varied (Fox, 1997; Miller & Luft, 1994). One definition might be: "managed care is an organized effort by health insurance plans and providers to use financial incentives and organizational arrangements to alter provider and patient behavior so that health care services are delivered and utilized in a more efficient and lower-cost manner." This definition includes the central principles of managed care: it is an organized effort that involves both insurers and providers of health care; it uses financial incentives and organizational structures in reaching its goal; and its purpose is to increase efficiency and reduce health care costs (Table 6–1) (Drake, 1997).

THE COMPONENT PARTS OF MANAGED CARE

Managed care includes at least four basic component parts (Figure 6–1). These parts are: the purchaser/ultimate payer for health care; the health

TABLE 6–1 Objectives of managed care

- Enhanced cost containment
- Some forms of rationing
- Promote administrative and clinical efficiency
- Reduce duplication of services
- Enhance appropriateness of care
- Promote comprehensive contracting mechanisms
- Manage care processes by managing provider and consumer behavior

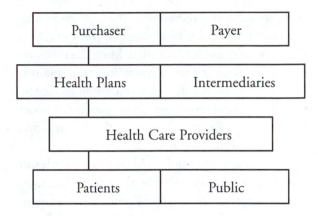

FIGURE 6–1 Component parts of managed care

insurance plans/intermediaries; the providers of care (that is, hospitals, physicians, and others involved in the direct delivery of personal health care); and the patients/public receiving care.

The *purchaser/payer* of managed care is generally one of three large groups: employers who purchase health insurance for their employees, the federal Medicare program, or state Medicaid programs. The *health insurance* plans are organizations licensed by their individual states to offer health insurance coverage that is bought by the purchasers/payers. Health insurance plans create the benefit packages, market the plans, enroll the beneficiaries, arrange for the provision of health care services to these beneficiaries, and monitor the results. The *providers of care* are licensed health care professionals, organizations, and institutions that actually deliver the needed health care services to the individual beneficiaries, under the terms of the health insurance plans' benefit packages. The *patients/public* are the individual people covered by the health insurance plans who receive individual health care services from the providers. In recent years, it has been suggested that a fifth important component part of the managed care structure might be the health insurance *brokers,* since an increasingly high percentage of health insurance (particularly that provided by employers) is arranged through the technical and organizational assistance of the brokers.

In most instances of managed care, these four (or five) component parts are separate organizational units, linked together by negotiated contracts. In some forms of managed care, such as the Health Insurance Plan of New York and the Kaiser-Permanente Health Plan, the insurance and provision of care functions are seemingly joined together in a single organization that appears to be both the insurer and the entity providing services. In most other managed care arrangements in the United States today, this is not the case, and it is perhaps better to consider the insurance and the provision of services functions as separate organizational subunits that can be either more loosely or more tightly linked together.

HOW MANAGED CARE WORKS

The process of making the managed care system work begins with certain important decisions made by the purchaser/payer (Enthoven & Singer, 1996). With these decisions, the purchaser must decide how many and what type of health insurance plans are to be offered and how much the purchaser/payer will pay for each premium. In the past, purchasers frequently selected a wide range of plans and paid different amounts for each plan. More recently, purchasers are selecting fewer health insurance plans to offer and are paying the same amount of money for their health insurance premium, regardless of which plan the beneficiary chooses, with the employee paying any difference.

Specifically, purchasers/payers must decide whether they wish to give their beneficiaries a wide-open range of choices of providers or whether they wish to limit, in some fashion, the choices available to the beneficiaries. The more restrictive plans offer fewer choices of provider and greater restrictions on consumer behavior but may yield lower costs (Figure 6–2). In the same fashion, the purchasers/payers must decide whether they want to have their beneficiaries enrolled in health insurance plans that pay providers on a fee-for-service or capitation (that is, a fixed amount per person per month covered) basis. In this set of choices, the

purchaser/payers usually find themselves choosing between a preferred provider organization (PPO) or a health maintenance organization (HMO). The PPO allows the recipient of health insurance a wider choice of providers and pays those providers on a modified fee-for-service basis; the HMO offers a more constrained range of choices among providers and usually pays the provider organization on a *per capita* (a fixed amount per person) basis.

A survey of employer-sponsored health insurance provided in 1995 showed that 80% of the firms surveyed offered health insurance benefits of some kind. Of the health insurance benefits offered, 73% of the plans included some type of managed care; this was a significant increase from 51% only two years earlier. The types of managed care plans offered to employees were HMOs (28%), PPOs (25%), and "point-of-service" (POS) plans (20%). Point-of-service plans combine elements of both HMOs and PPOs, allowing an

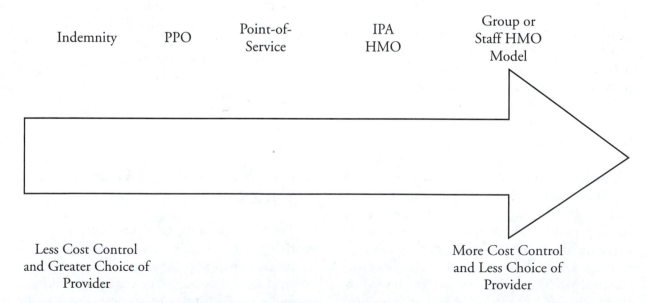

FIGURE 6–2 Continuum of cost control in the U.S. health care system

enrollee to obtain care from providers outside the PPO network but with a substantially higher copayment, as discussed in more detail later. This survey also showed that the premiums paid for employer-sponsored health insurance increased by only 2.3% in 1995, which was less than the rate of general inflation during that year; as recently as six years earlier in 1989, employer health insurance premiums had increased by 17% in a single year (Jensen, et al., 1997). More recent evidence suggests that the rate of increase is rising again.

Types of Managed Care Plans

The two main representative types of managed care health plans now offered to purchasers/payers by insurance organizations, preferred provider organizations (PPOs) and health maintenance organizations (HMOs), are both types of managed care. But these plans differ significantly in their major characteristics.

The PPO is essentially a fee-for-service type of health plan that allows a beneficiary to either use a wide-open range of providers or select from a narrower list of providers who have agreed to give the health insurance plan a discount. If the beneficiary chooses to use a provider on the narrower list, the plan, the provider, and the beneficiary all benefit. The health plan generally has negotiated a discounted rate for the provider's services (sometimes a very significant discount), so the plan uses its purchasing power to get a lower price. The providers agree to take a lower price but, in return, hope that the health insurance plan's members will choose them more frequently because they are now put on a special list of "preferred providers" that are made available to the health plan's members.

The health plan members benefit by choosing a preferred provider because, if they do, the member's share of the cost (as expressed by the plan's deductibles and coinsurance) is reduced, so the member may actually pay nothing at all to use the preferred provider. In other words, financial incentives are used to create a buyer/seller/user network that benefits all three parties.

For purchasers/payers, the PPO is a very attractive option, since it means that the purchaser/payer is not forcing the beneficiaries to limit their choices or change their behaviors if they do not want to. However, if they do wish to save some money and choose the preferred provider, they benefit, and the purchaser/payer has not coerced them to do something that they would rather not do.

The HMO type of managed care plan, now covering over fifty million Americans (Table 6–2), has many significant differences when compared with the PPO type of managed care. Indeed, the differences in the two types are so major that it is confusing to describe them under the same general heading of managed care, as though both are closely related and are only minor variants of each other.

The HMO type of managed care plan offered to purchasers/payers of health insurance plans has a number of important premises built into its framework. First, the HMO form of managed care depends upon the fact that the health plan has developed a contract with a group of physicians to take on total responsibility for a list of enrolled patients. The HMO form of managed care depends upon an individual patient/person choosing to sign up with one particular group of physicians and then to receive virtually all of their medical care, both primary and specialty, through that group of physicians, either directly or by referral. That particular group of physicians, in return, is paid a fixed fee per patient (capitation rate) that the group agrees to take on for total responsibility. This *per capita* form of reimbursement to the medical provider and the continuing, comprehensive responsibility for total patient care of the enrolled population is what makes the HMO form of managed care significantly different from the PPO form of managed care.

TABLE 6–2 Health maintenance organization enrollment: United States, selected years

Plans and Enrollment	1980	1996
Plans	*Number*	
All plans	235	628
Model type		
Individual practice association	97	366
Group	138	122
Geographic region		
Northeast	55	111
Midwest	72	181
South	45	217
West	63	119
Enrollment	*Persons in millions*	
Total	9.1	52.5
Model type		
Individual practice association	6.4	21.7
Group	14.6	13.5
Mixed	—	17.2
Federal program		
Medicaid	0.6	8.5
Medicare	1.1	3.7
	Percent of population enrolled in HMOs	
Geographic region		
Northeast	3.1	23.8
Midwest	2.8	16.2
South	0.8	13.2
West	12.2	30.7

SOURCE: *Health, United States, 1996–97* (DHHS Pub. No. PHS 97-1232, 1997), Washington, DC: U.S. Government Printing Office.

In the HMO form of managed care, the linkages are tighter and more formal, and the payment is on a *per capita* basis rather than on a fee-for-service basis, modified or not. In this form of managed care, just as in the PPO form, the three participants (health plan, providers, and patients) form a network of mutual benefit, but it is much tighter and based on different principles. The health plan benefits because it is able to limit its financial exposure by paying the provider group a fixed amount for taking care of the enrolled population. The plan knows that no matter how much care the provider is required to give patients to handle their medical problems, the health plan will not be asked for any additional financial payments. From the provider's point of view, these plan contractual arrangements provide a steady stream of revenue, whether individual patients seek care or not. The provider organizations are able to plan on a more stable and long-term basis than they could if they were in the situation of a company's fee-for-service plan, dependent as it is on individuals' choices; the providers' contracts with the plan guarantee financial stability, at least to some degree. The patient benefits as well, since there are usually few or no copayments, deductibles, or other payments in an HMO form of managed care. The patient knows, therefore, that once the premium is paid each month, there will be little or no additional financial claims directed at the patient for covered services.

Providers have a wide variety of possible ways in which they may relate to managed care plans. Hospitals, for example, may agree to contract with PPOs and offer substantial discounts when PPO members are actually hospitalized at a contracting hospital. Hospitals also may contract with HMOs to provide hospital care for an enrolled population on a *per capita* basis, although this type of *per capita* contract with hospitals is less common. Hospitals may also agree to take part in joint contracting efforts involving physician groups/organizations/individual practice associations (IPAs) which agree to take on an enrolled population for a *per capita* payment, with the *per capita* later being divided by mutual agreement between the physician group and the hospital.

For their part, physicians have a variety of ways to take part in managed care health plans, either singly or in larger groups and organizations. With regard to PPOs, physicians working alone or in groups can simply agree to take members of PPOs on a fee-for-service basis, the fee usually being a decrease or discount from the physician's usual fee. This type of arrangement is organized around individual patients making individual visits to a doctor and implies no long-term commitment to a relationship between the physician and the health plan, or between the physician and an individual patient.

By contrast, when physicians are faced with HMOs, their decisions are more critical, since they have much broader and much longer-term implications. In the IPA, the physician in practice voluntarily joins a collaborative group of physicians, all of whom are in independent practice and all of whom join the IPA in order to be able to take part in large contracts with HMOs. In the IPA, the physician remains in independent practice and agrees to care for those patients that the IPA attracts and assigns to that physician. The physician in practice usually has many other patients that come from other sources, some of whom may be paid for on a fee-for-service basis and others for whom payment may be from other managed care arrangements, including HMOs. The IPA allows individual physicians the benefits of independence, multiple sources of patients, and involvement in other contracting arrangements. The individual physician may also be an owner of the IPA, but that is not usually a necessary condition of the physician's involvement with the IPA as a provider of care.

When IPAs first began to appear, it was felt that they might be merely a transitional form of medical organization that might gradually give way to tighter forms of group practice and staff model

HMOs, but that has not been the case. The IPA model of physician involvement has many advantages to physicians, as well as to health plans, and probably will be a permanent feature on the health care scene. The longer they are in existence, the more tightly IPAs are organized and managed, but the fundamental model of physicians in independent private practice who voluntarily join a collaborative contracting group remains the same.

Physicians can also participate in HMO managed care by joining organized medical groups and having the medical groups contract with HMOs to provide care to an enrolled population. In this form of involvement in managed care, a physician chooses to become a formal member of an organized medical group that practices together, shares premises, and may share patients and revenues. The formal contract with the HMO is between the medical group and the HMO, not necessarily with individual physicians. The HMOs may prefer this type of arrangement, since the internal discipline of an organized medical group is usually, though not necessarily, much tighter than the internal discipline of an IPA (made up as it is of large numbers of doctors who work in separate locations). The physician selection process here is that a physician first must decide to join an organized medical group and practice medicine actively together with other physicians. Then the physician is a member of an organized medical group that contracts with an HMO to care for patients enrolled in that HMO.

In relatively few circumstances, a physician may decide not to go into independent practice and not to join a medical group that is separate from an HMO, but may instead decide to join a "staff" model HMO that actually employs its own physicians. In this model, the doctor decides to become directly associated with the HMO itself, rather than to become a part of a contracting medical group that is separate from the HMO. In this type of an organization, the physician is in effect becoming a salaried member of a larger corporation that may actually have its own hospitals and clinics in a number of locations and that markets its own HMO under its own name. In some instances, due to state medical practice laws, the physicians may actually form a partnership that then exclusively contracts with the HMO.

There are other types of physician relationships with managed care plans, but these three—the IPA model, the medical group, and the staff model—are the most common forms of physician–managed care collaboration.

In summary, it can be seen from this brief review that *managed care* is not a single monolith organization, nor is it characterized by a single form of operation. Managed care involves a variety of choices in a variety of organizational relationships on the purchaser/payer level, on the health insurance plan level, and on the provider level. In considering any issues related to managed care, therefore, it is important for the health care professional to first identify which level of the managed care structure is actually being discussed and which issue is under review.

Depending upon the level of the managed care system or structure and depending upon the issue being discussed, the details and outcomes of such discussions may vary greatly. Managed care is not a single, all-encompassing, unified structure but, rather, a series of separate subunits, linked together by a series of decisions, contracts, and administrative structures. The result is a wide variety of managed care activities and operations.

KEY CONCEPTS AND PRINCIPLES OF MANAGED CARE

In the previous section, it has been stressed that managed care is more of a concept and a process than a specific, single entity; it is a series of various organizational subunits that are linked together in different ways to achieve certain outcomes. A managed care program serving any one particular person may be quite different in the details of its organization from a managed care program serving another. In the same fashion, an individual physician or a hospital may participate in many different types of managed care programs at the same time, each having some significant variation from the rest.

Having said this, however, there are some important concepts and principles that are common in a general sense to all types of managed care programs. It is important to understand these key principles, since they apply in a general way across the entire spectrum of managed care.

The Need for Education/Preparation of the Insured in Managed Care

One of the most important principles of managed care is the need for careful preparation and education of the insured about the way in which managed care works. If managed care is to succeed in its goals, it is important that the insured be told very specifically what managed care is and what it is not. Since the use of health care under a managed care arrangement may be quite different from previous patterns of utilization and behavior, it is important that patients be instructed about what services are covered, how care can be obtained, and how care might be different from previous ways of behaving under more conventional fee-for-service coverage.

Unfortunately, there is very little preparation carried out by the purchasers/payers when they make a decision to use managed care plans for the provision of health insurance coverage to their beneficiaries. Often the purchasers/payers leave it to the health plans to inform the enrolled members that there are certain new procedures that they must follow and new behaviors that they must assume, since the purchasers/payers may actually wish to stay away from passing on the bad news themselves.

Unfortunately, many of the health insurance plans do not do a very good job of instructing their members in detail about how the plans function. It is clear that if managed care is to succeed in the future and is to be accepted by patients/people, a better job of information exchange and education must be done by the purchasers/payers at the time of the decision to enroll beneficiaries in a managed care plan.

The Importance of an Information System and the Insistence on Quality and Outcome Measures

One of the central characteristics of all forms of managed care is the absolutely central necessity of much more advanced information systems that will provide more accurate and timely data on the utilization of services and on the quality and outcomes of those services (*How Good Is Your Health Plan?*, 1996). In the past, under fee-for-service forms of health insurance, the key information that was collected came from claims data (that is, data from requests for payment for the provision of specific items of services). Under an HMO type of managed care, claims data are no longer gathered, since payment is based on a *per capita* rather than fee-for-service basis. In addition, the previous claims data usually revealed very little about the quality of the services provided or the effect/outcomes of those services on the health status of the insured.

The importance of these new information systems is further heightened by the requirement of the purchasers/payers of care to the health plans that they be able to report to the purchasers on the quality of services provided, often using standardized data sets such as the HEDIS (Health Care Employee Data Information Systems) format. In the same manner, the plans themselves are requiring the provider groups and systems to gather and report more sophisticated utilization and quality/data outcomes to enable the plans to better evaluate the services of the providers and also to make it possible for the plans to report back to the purchasers/payers on the quality of services for which they are paying.

It is felt that only a small portion of the data being gathered at the present time is being utilized to its maximum potential. However, it is clear that this situation will change very quickly, given the increasing demands for better data and for better use of the data that is being generated.

Plan/Provider Control of Utilization

Control of costs, utilization, and, to an extent, consumer behavior depend heavily on influencing provider, and especially physician, behavior (Table 6–3). There are numerous considerations involved in influencing physicians, ranging from careful selection of efficient participating providers (economic credentialing) to overt utilization reviews and controls. Enhanced controls on both providers and consumers, sometimes using highly restrictive mechanisms, are a central hallmark of managed care.

TABLE 6–3 Influencing physician behavior in managed care practices

- Provide feedback and comparisons to the norm using quantitative data
- Physician recruitment and selective contracting policies
- Socialization to group goals and philosophy
- Positive rewards such as money, benefits, on-call preference, and leave time
- Promote teamwork and quality management
- Financing and reimbursement incentives
- Promote efficiency and productivity enhancements

Since one of the main objectives of managed care is to reduce unnecessary use of services and to provide health care in a more efficient fashion, the review and control of the utilization of health services is central to the idea of managed care. The control of the utilization of services begins with decisions that are made by the purchaser/payer with regard to what services should be included in the benefits package. Increasingly, the range of services to be included as a benefit of managed care is being narrowed by the purchasers, who are ever more anxious to limit their financial exposure. Many times, the health plans find themselves blamed for not paying for certain health care services when the actual decision to limit services has been made by the purchaser/payer in designing the benefit package.

The health plans themselves also have methods for reviewing the utilization of services and frequently require the provider to report on the use of expensive services such as inpatient care and high-technology diagnostic and treatment services. The basic contract between the insurance organization and the providers frequently stipulates the nature and extent to which providers must review their own utilization of services and provide summary data.

Most utilization review and control occurs at the level of the provider organization itself, however, which is usually in the IPA or medical group providing medical services. Since these medical groups are increasingly being paid on a *per capita* basis and are, therefore, at risk for the financial consequences of any high utilization, it is logical that the most active and aggressive control of utilization occurs within the medical group or IPA itself (Kerr, 1996). Indeed, as IPAs and medical groups learn that their financial futures now depend upon the medical group providing less rather than more services, the utilization control processes used within the medical group or IPA can become increasingly stringent. In some instances recently, IPAs and medical groups have begun using hospital-based physicians to handle all of their admissions ("hospitalists"), thereby reducing variation on inpatient admissions and length-of-stay patterns (Moore, 1997).

At the heart of any utilization control system is the concept of the primary care physician (PCP) as a "gate-keeper." The gate-keeper concept rests on the idea that one individual physician, usually a PCP in family practice, internal medicine, pediatrics, or, less often, obstetrics/gynecology, is responsible for providing all of the primary care for the patient. The PCP also determines when referral to specialists is needed and then provides oversight and coordination for the use of the specialist on an ongoing basis. The gate-keeper concept is designed to control the patient's use of expensive resources, to reduce the self-initiated use of specialty physicians, and to ensure overall coordination of care.

Placing the primary care physician in the position of gate-keeper is increasingly being seen as a potential source of conflict of interest for physicians playing this role. If the primary care physician aggressively seeks to ensure that the patient has all possible diagnostic procedures and specialists opinions, that PCP may also be draining the IPA or medical group's total financial pool under capitation. The PCP realizes very quickly that the more aggressively the patient's best interests are pursued, the less advantageous it may be to the physician personally. Generally little empirical data is available to determine the impact of this potential conflict of interest. The subject is one of serious concern to physicians and medical organizations and will clearly become a more important issue as more experience is gained with managed care.

Capitation

Central to the HMO type of managed care program is the concept of capitation, the payment of a fixed fee per person to physicians or hospitals in exchange for their willingness to assume responsibility to provide a complete range of services as needed (Bader & Matheny, 1994). In contrast to the fee-for-service form of reimbursement for the provision of health services, capitation provides entirely different incentives to those providing care. Under fee-for-service, the more services that are provided, the more the provider is paid. Under capitation, the fewer services that are provided, the more funds there are left over for the provider. The incentives, therefore, are for the provider to be more careful and frugal in the use of health services resources and in the referral of specialists, since the provider is rewarded for doing less rather than more.

The use of *per capita* payments for coverage of services exists throughout the entire managed care structure. The purchaser/payer pays the health plan on a *per capita* basis, providing a fixed amount in exchange for a guarantee of a range of services by the health insurance plan. The HMO type of managed care health insurance plans, in turn, generally use *per capita* payments to medical groups or combined hospital/medical group joint enterprises, also in exchange for a guarantee that the providers will offer a wide range of services to those covered by the health insurance plan.

Within the IPAs or medical groups, capitation can also be used to reimburse individual physicians in different ways. For example, it is quite common for an IPA to reimburse primary care physicians on a *per capita* basis, but then reimburse specialists within the IPA or medical group on a modified fee-for-service basis. In recent years, various IPAs and medical groups have begun to experiment with the use of capitation in exactly the reverse fashion: primary care physicians are now occasionally being paid on a fee-for-service basis and specialists are occasionally being paid on a *per capita* basis. The point remains that capitation is a powerful tool in managed care, is central to the concept of managed

care, and can be used in different ways throughout the entire managed care structure.

Risk Sharing

Of increasing importance and interest in managed care is the use of risk-sharing pools of various sorts. These vary widely, but in general, they involve the establishment of a pool of money from which certain services are paid throughout the year. Funds remaining at year end are then divided, either between the providers and the health insurance plan or between the physicians and a hospital with whom those physicians have joined in a collaborative effort.

The general concept of the risk pools is to provide an incentive to reduce use, particularly with regard to hospitalization, specialty referrals, and high-technology diagnostic and treatment services. The extent to which risk pools are effective in reducing use and saving money is not clear. It is also not clear whether risk pools (and the previously mentioned use of capitation payments) result in underuse of needed services. The greatest fear in managed care, both on the part of patients and of providers, is that the incentives to control overuse of health services that have been so common in the past under fee-for-service forms of reimbursement will now lead to serious underuse and denial of needed services, with a resulting negative impact on the health status of the covered population. Indeed, of all of the questions involved in managed care, this is probably the most critical one to continuously examine over the next few years.

The Importance of Contracts in Managed Care

With the exception of staff model HMOs that employ their own physicians, managed care consists of a series of separate subunits that are linked together by legal contracts. Indeed, managed care can be seen as a series of separate entities whose only connection is through legally negotiated systems of contracts.

Unfortunately, many clinical professionals in health care are very unused to the negotiating and contracting process and, as a result, pay less attention to it than they should. In effect, managed care consists of a series of legally binding contracts and documents that set the terms and boundaries for everything that happens within the managed care structure. Therefore, the negotiation of proper contracts and the clear understanding of all the details in the contracts, by all parties to those contracts, is essential for the long-term success of managed care. At the present time, the negotiation and creation of contracts between the various parties in managed care is probably one of the most challenging and uncertain areas of managed care.

It should also be pointed out that probably the least informed and prepared party in the managed care structure is the patient or person covered by the health insurance policy. If the health insurance policy is considered a contract between the health plan and the patient/person, it is very important that the patient/person understand better what is in that contract, even if they have no part in the actual negotiations. There is growing interest in and concern for methods of better education and preparation of patients/public in the interpretation of their health insurance contracts, as well as a growing interest in discovering ways in which patients/public can take a more active part in the actual negotiation of better contracts for themselves, either with the purchasers/payers or with the health plans. One of the most interesting and potentially important areas of future activity in managed care is the possible increase in the power of groups of patients/public as members of the managed care structure.

ISSUES FOR THE FUTURE OF MANAGED CARE

Looking into the future, there are a number of important issues to be considered with regard to the development of managed care programs and their services to patients. Among the important issues are: consolidation among health plans, the impact of managed care on the provider system, Medicare and Medicaid managed care, managed behavioral health care, conflicts of interest, and protection of the public.

Consolidation Among Health Insurance Plans

As managed care matures, one phenomenon that is developing rapidly is consolidation among the health insurance plans. Every year sees more and more of the nation's health insurers merging with or acquiring other health insurers in what can only be described as a major change in the health care financing landscape. This consolidation of health insurance providers and plans is a concern for several reasons.

The first concern about consolidation of the health insurance industry is the tendency of plans to become so large that they have an unfair advantage in dealing both with purchasers/payers and with providers. The larger a health insurance plan becomes, the more financial assets it has and the more enrolled lives it controls. This means that the leverage among the plans may become unduly strong and make it difficult to have an even balance among purchasers/payers, health plans, and providers. In their defense, the health plans very frequently say that they must consolidate, since the purchasers/payers and the providers are themselves consolidating into larger bargaining units; the plans must consolidate if they are not to be overwhelmed by the larger size and strength of their negotiating partners.

The second reason why consolidation among the health plans may be a concern in the future is the potential reduction of variation among health plans and their products. At a time when everyone is still trying to learn about managed care and when there still seems to be considerable experimentation about the insurance products being offered, consolidation among the health plans may reduce this variability significantly. The opportunity to learn exactly what are the best forms of managed care insurance products for our various subpopulations may be prematurely ended before we have had a chance to learn the lessons that should be learned.

Consolidation that leads to a reduction in the number of health plans also reduces the competitive nature of the marketplace, which in itself may be a bad outcome for purchasers/payers and the public. Healthy competition among providers of any service is critically important to the success of any market-oriented industry, and this is no less true when considering the managed care health insurance industry. A purchaser/payer who goes into the marketplace seeking health insurance and is confronted with a small choice of competing health insurance plans is less able to engage these plans in a marketplace dialogue on price and quality of services than that purchaser/payer would be if there were a wide variety of plans competing amongst themselves for the business.

There are obviously major antitrust and monopoly issues to be considered in regard to consolidation. The formal legal and regulatory mechanisms in this area move so slowly that significant reshaping of the managed care health insurance industry may take place before the formal governmental protections are able to come into effect (Kuttner, 1997). Also, since there are very few legal or regulatory precedents in this area in the health care industry, those formal governmental protections may be even slower to come into effect than in a well-established industry.

Impact of Managed Care on the Provider System

It has been stressed in this chapter that managed care is really a series of subunits that are linked together by a series of legal, contractual, and organizational mechanisms. Therefore, a change in any one subunit tends to bring about changes in other subunits that are linked to it. This means that any change in the methods for financing health care through health insurance (such as the growth of *per capita* HMO insurance mechanisms) will cause changes in the provider system as well.

In practice, what has happened among provider systems has been a growth of new organizational forms and new operating principles with regard to the provision of care, in response to change on the financing side (Table 6–4). This has led to the growth of larger groups of physicians working together, groups of physicians entering into joint ventures of one kind or another with hospitals, a drive for increased efficiency of operation, and an overall rethinking about the most appropriate

TABLE 6–4 Provider concerns under managed care

- Carefully enter into contracts
- Know practice strengths and weaknesses
- Use clinical protocols and other control guidelines
- Establish performance goals and measures of success or failure
- Ensure that management information systems are adequate
- Continually monitor results and respond to information
- Reduce inpatient utilization
- Be cost conscientious
- Emphasize primary care
- Monitor and manage risk
- Maintain provider relationships
- Enhance consumer controls and satisfaction

organizational structure for the delivery of personal health care services.

The rethinking may have both positive and negative effects. On the positive side, the reorganization of the provider system may lead to greater efficiency and better effectiveness of that system and, therefore, to better patient care with improved outcomes. This scenario suggests that the previous organizational structure of health care under a fee-for-service stimulus may not have been the most efficient or effective and that managed care–driven changes in the delivery system are a distinct improvement.

On the negative side, the drive for increased efficiency of operation, the emphasis on providing fewer services rather than more, and the overwhelming concern about economic issues may all serve to dampen or reduce the humane and compassionate personal aspects of health care as it was previously delivered in the United States. Under this scenario, the provider system for health services in the United States may become more coldly efficient and effective in an organizational sense, but it may be less satisfying in a personal and psychological sense to the people receiving services.

A point to remember here is that changes in the way in which health care providers are paid are not merely financial or economic changes. They also drive organizational changes, and those organizational changes may be either for the better or the worse, depending upon how they are developed.

Medicare/Medicaid in Managed Care

Although much has been said about the impact of managed care in reducing the health care expenditures for employers and the private sector, the major impact of managed care may actually be felt on the two major public sector financing programs in health care, Medicare and Medicaid. The impact on each of these programs may be quite different, given the different nature of the constituencies they serve and the specifics of their financing. They have in common the fact that they will both be impacted in a major way by the use of managed care.

With regard to the Medicare program, the tentative goal of the federal Health Care Financing Administration (HCFA) is to have approximately half of all Medicare beneficiaries enrolled in managed risk/managed care programs by the year 2007 (Table 6–2). With the Medicare program in deep financial trouble and with its expenditures increasing at a rate of approximately eight percent per year, the HCFA has determined that managed care will play a major part in the long-term solution of Medicare's financial woes.

The implications for patients served under Medicare are potentially both good and bad (Wagner, 1996). On the positive side, Medicare beneficiaries may actually be able to receive more benefits and services (particularly a much wider range of pharmaceutical benefits than are now available to them) and may also have their patterns of care and the outcomes of that care more closely monitored and controlled. Medicare beneficiaries may actually get better services and may have more confidence in the care that they are receiving from their providers, since that care may be more closely observed and measured.

On the negative side for Medicare beneficiaries is the effect of consolidation among the provider health care systems mentioned earlier. Medicare beneficiaries that may previously have been treated personally, warmly, and humanely by an individual solo-practice physician with whom they have had a very close personal relationship may find that solo-practice physicians are becoming a thing of the past, replaced by comparative supermarkets of physicians whose hallmarks are efficiency of a less warm kind. Moving into a Medicare managed risk/managed care program may mean that elderly Medicare patients have less time to talk with their physicians, less personal connection, and less personal involvement than they had under the previous fee-for-service arrangement. Only time will tell whether individual physicians and the organization of medical practice is able to remain user-friendly for Medicare recipients in the future.

In the same fashion, the Medicaid programs around the country are moving very rapidly to use managed care for their recipients' care, and it seems clear that the impact on Medicaid recipients will also be quite marked, if different from the impact on Medicare beneficiaries (Table 6–2) (*Medicaid Makeovers,* 1996). In the case of Medicaid, the changes from the increased use of managed care are more likely to be positive than negative.

In the past, Medicaid recipients generally received their care in a somewhat random and scattered fashion from local governmental hospitals, clinics, and emergency rooms, interested physicians, and a wide variety of free clinics and other community organizations. There usually was very little cohesion among the providers and very little coordination of the patterns of care that was being given.

Under a managed care structure, Medicaid recipients will have a firm and formal connection with a medical group or medical provider and will be required to have a designated primary care physician as the coordinator of all of their services. There will be a formal set of required services that must be provided on a regular basis, and there will be an organized method for determining whether these services were actually provided to Medicaid recipients. This will mean that, perhaps for the first time, Medicaid recipients will develop longer-term relationships with a primary care physician, will be mandated to receive a predetermined package of services, and will have outcomes that are measured in a formal fashion. In a very real sense, managed care presents a great opportunity to improve the quality of care received by Medicaid recipients across the country.

Mental Health and Managed Care

One of the most interesting areas of application of managed care, and also one of the most rapidly expanding, is the implementation of managed care for mental and behavioral health services. If the use of managed care is increasing in general health services across the country, it can only be said that managed mental health services are increasing at an almost explosive rate.

The reasons for the increased use of managed care mechanisms to organize mental health benefits are fairly obvious to any student of the provision of mental health services in the past. The general criticism has been made of mental health services over the years that they were relatively unstandardized, poorly supervised, and without any meaningful measures of results or outcomes. It was also generally felt that there was an excessive use of expensive inpatient mental health services, the utilization of which was governed by the availability of health insurance payments for inpatient services.

The shift to managed care in mental health services is causing significant concern among both patients and providers of mental health services and is also forcing patients and providers to learn a new set of procedures and policies in obtaining and in providing mental health services. Rather than a wide-open patient-initiated selection of mental health practitioners, the managed behavioral health plans require beneficiaries to first use a "triage" process, which attempts to determine the severity of the problem and the most appropriate form of treatment. The triage process usually also arranges the connection for the patient with what is felt to be that most appropriate form of treatment. This means that an individual patient may no longer be free to pick the psychiatrist of their choice, call and make an appointment, and begin therapy for what may be an indefinite period of time. Now all of those previous forms of behavior are organized and managed by the managed mental health organization itself. That organization then also attempts to monitor results of treatment and determine outcomes.

From the patient's point of view, this means that there will be much more formal and supervised systems of determining the severity of the initial problem and a much more standardized process for obtaining care; there also will be a very deliberate attempt on the part of the managed care organization to determine the credentials of the mental health practitioners before they are accepted as providers by the plan. For their part, providers of mental health services may now find themselves dependent upon the managed care plan for a flow of initial patients to their practices and may find their ability to provide care limited by the number of encounters that are authorized by some other seemingly artificial time constraints. For mental health practitioners, this is seen as an imposition on their independence and on their clinical judgment, and for the most part, mental health professionals are not very positive or supportive in their views about managed mental health programs. Unfortunately, there is presently insufficient research evidence to determine exactly the positive or negative impacts of managed mental health programs on the quality of patient care and the outcomes of that care.

Conflict of Interest in Managed Care

One of the most important issues facing managed care in the future is the question of conflict of interest among and between the various participants in any type of managed care system (Gray, 1997). The conflict is centered around the need to reduce the use of various health services, products, and procedures. The economic survival and prosperity of all of the major players in managed care depends upon the imposition of tight controls on the use of health services, with the implication that

services have been overused in the past and that this overusage must be eliminated.

Although there is general agreement that many types of health services have been overused in the past and that unnecessary health services have been provided, it is not always clear exactly which of those services have been used in excess (and, therefore, need reduction) and which services have not. The application of across-the-board methods to reduce the use of health services in general will affect both those services that may have been overused and overprovided in the past as well as those services that may not have been overused and overprovided. The net result may be that *all* health services utilization may be reduced, both those services that needed reduction and those that did not. The end result *may* be that patients who need some services may not get them in the future.

For the most part, purchasers/payers and the health insurance plans have been unwilling to concede or even discuss the possibility of a conflict of interest affecting their participation in managed care, but increasingly physicians have been more vocal about the difficult situation in which they find themselves. Indeed, since physicians are directly involved with their patients on a face-to-face basis, it is very likely that the issues of conflict of interest will be most apparent in this part of any managed care system. It is also very obvious that the discussion of conflict of interest in managed care will most likely be led by physicians, since it is here that the stresses and strains are felt most acutely (Kerr, 1996). As ethical principles and economic pressures begin to impede on each other more actively around the provision of physician services, that is where the most active discussion of this important issue will start; it will certainly not end there, however, because there is a fundamental conflict of interest throughout the entire managed health care structure.

Protection of the Public

A final issue of importance to the future of managed care is the development of better mechanisms for the protection of patients and the public interest. At the present time, it appears that individual patients and the public in general are somewhat at the mercy of a managed care structure that is consolidating very rapidly, from purchasers/payers, through health insurance plans, to provider systems (Bodenheimer, 1996). The only part of the managed care structure that is not consolidating itself (and, therefore, is better able to exert itself in the new economic marketplace) is the area of individual patients and the public in general.

For most individual people/patients who must make their way through the managed care structure in a relatively unaided fashion, the complexities of managed care leave them very vulnerable and relatively unprotected. From the time when purchasers/payers select a health insurance plan under which the employees will be covered (sometimes without choice or options and other times with options that are not clearly explained), the individual is at a significant disadvantage because of the relative lack of information, experience, and sophistication. Later, in dealing with the individual health insurance plans and their consumer relations departments, which are established ostensibly for the purpose of service to plan enrollees, the individual person/patient is also at a disadvantage, since they are dealing with a health plan staff member who is much more experienced and knowledgeable about the details of the plan's operation; the plan employee may also have been given the specific direction to constrain or reduce the utilization of services and may have the best interest of the health plan uppermost in mind, and not necessarily the best interest of the patient (as seen by the patient).

Finally, when an individual person/patient must deal with a physician or a medical group in an attempt to get additional services, the group's process for approving or denying services may not be clearly described and may be implemented in widely varying forms, and with different effects, depending upon the patient and/or the physician involved. All of these circumstances tend to make many members of managed health care plans suspicious and distrustful even when the plans and the physicians are actually doing as much as they can to provide appropriate service. The sense of vulnerability among individuals when they are confronted with the various aspects of the machinery of managed care may tend to make the individual person/patient feel that they have fewer options and less power than they may really have.

One response to this sense of isolation and vulnerability among members of managed care plans has been the passage of a series of legislative and regulatory efforts by the Congress, state legislatures, and state departments of insurance/corporations/industry to "protect" the interests of the public. Legislation mandating the number of days that a woman may remain in the hospital after a normal delivery and legislation prohibiting the performance of outpatient surgery for a specific condition (for example, mastectomy for breast cancer) are certainly well-intentioned but raise a serious question about their wisdom. Nevertheless, until patients/people organize themselves to more strongly protect themselves from the apparent imbalance of power, and until purchasers/payers and managed care health insurance plans do much more in the way of direct communication and assistance to patients and the public, the only channel of recourse available to the patients/public will be through laws or regulation. It is in the best interest of patients and the public to organize themselves into aggressive consumer protection organizations, and it is equally in the best interest of purchasers/payers and health plans to better serve the members of managed care health plans to prevent further legislative or legal overreaction.

Until that time comes (and it probably will take some time), one can expect to see much more in the way of legal, legislative, or regulator solutions governing the organization and the conduct of managed care.

SUMMARY: MANAGED CARE AND THE FUTURE OF HEALTH CARE

Managed care represents an array of arrangements and mechanisms designed in one form or another to organize health care services. New forms of managed care are still emerging, and the conflicting political, economic, and social currents in our society are constantly influencing our assessments of the nature and ramifications of managed care. These are dynamic, not static, currents, and the pendulum of change will always be in motion.

Some of the complex issues faced in assessing the role of managed care are listed in Table 6–5. These concerns include the most fundamental factors involved in designing health care systems. How do we influence, and limit, provider and consumer behavior? Where do we draw the lines in rationing services? How do we collect information to moni-

TABLE 6–5 Complex issues in managed care

- Controlling physician behavior
- Controlling consumer behavior
- Rationing/caps on care
- Monitoring care and reacting
- Information collection and use
- Administrative and medical leadership
- Encouraging competitive markets
- Protecting against underutilization
- Measuring costs and ensuring access
- Enhancing provider, payor, and consumer satisfaction

tor and control behavior? How do we provide leadership in the system? How do we assess costs? How do we promote both provider and consumer satisfaction while controlling use and costs? These are difficult, complex questions that require us to address the most basic issues and moral concerns in providing health care.

The future of managed care will be different from the past. Experimentation is ongoing. Some paths may prove politically, socially, or economically unacceptable. The use of information technology, in particular, will radically change our ability to measure, monitor, control, compare, and influence the behavior of all participants in health care. Dramatic technological change will also radically affect the incentives, alternatives, and costs of nearly all aspects of health care, and increasing recognition of the need for more prevention, combined with greater ability to actually prevent illness, will challenge the focus on individuals versus populations.

The ultimate forms of managed care arrangements that are implemented and, perhaps, new alternative health care systems in the future remain to be determined. But there is little likelihood that the payers of health care will allow any return to the open-ended systems and plans of the past. The challenge for managed care is to find the balance between choices and control that promotes efficiency, contains costs, enhances satisfaction, and assures quality.

REFERENCES

Bader, B., & Matheny, M. (1994). Understanding capitation and at-risk contracting. *Health Systems Leader.*

Bodenheimer, T. (1996). The HMO backlash . . . righteous or reactionary? *New England Journal of Medicine, 335,* 1601–1604.

Drake, D. (1997). Managed care: A product of market dynamics. *Journal of the American Medical Association, 277,* 311–314.

Enthoven, A., & Singer, S. (1996). Managed competition and California's health care economy. *Health Affairs, 15,* 40–57.

Fox, P. (1997). An overview of managed care. In P. Kongstvedt (Ed.), *Essentials of managed health care,* Aspen Publishers.

Gray, B. (1997). Trust and trustworthy care in the managed care era. *Health Affairs, 16,* 34–49.

How good is your health plan? (1996). *Consumer Reports.*

Jensen, G., Morrisey, M., Gaffney, S., & Liston, D. (1997). The new dominance of managed care: Insurance trends in the 1990s. *Health Affairs, 16,* 125–136.

Kerr, E. (1996). Quality assurance in capitated physician groups. *Journal of the American Medical Association, 276,* 1236–1239.

Kuttner, R. (1997). Physician-operated networks and the new anti-trust guidelines. *New England Journal of Medicine, 336,* 386–391.

Medicaid makeovers. (1996). *Modern Healthcare.*

Miller, R., & Luft, H. (1994). Managed care plans: Characteristics, growth, and premium performance. *Annual Review of Public Health, 15,* 437–459.

Moore, J. (1997). The inpatient's best friend. *Modern Healthcare.*

Wagner, E. (1996). The promise and performance of HMOs in improving outcomes in older adults. *Journal of the American Geriatrics Society, 44,* 1251–1257.

CHAPTER

Private Health Insurance and Employee Benefits

Gary Whitted

CHAPTER TOPICS

Insurance Concepts
A Brief History of United States Health Insurance
Alternate Health Insurance Taxonomies
The Commercial Health Insurance Industry
Blue Cross and Blue Shield Plans
Health Maintenance Organizations
Private Health Insurance as a Financing Mechanism
Health-Related Insurance Programs
Funding Alternative for Group Health-Related Insurance
"Core" Medical Employee Benefits
Changes Facing the Health Insurance Industry

LEARNING OBJECTIVES

Upon completing this chapter, the reader should be able to:

- Understand the history, structure, and role of health insurance.
- Appreciate the commercial health insurance industry's size, objectives, products, and marketplace.
- Identify the impact of managed care on private health insurance.
- Differentiate various health insurance provisions, terms, conditions, and product types.
- Understand related insurance products.
- Appreciate the challenges facing this industry in the future.

After Medicare, private health insurance is the most prevalent source of financing for the United States health care system. Few other industrialized countries maintain systems of private medical insurance programs that even approximate those established in the United States. Private health insurance coverage is by far the most comprehensive source of medical care financing for Americans, and it continues to play a pivotal role in influencing the direction and structure of the United States medical care system.

The term *health insurance* often is employed to mean a wide array of health care financing mechanisms—the social insurance of Medicare, the public assistance of Medicaid, the "self-insurance" techniques adopted by large employers, and the managed care programs of health maintenance organizations (HMOs) and preferred provider organizations (PPOs). This chapter expands on the concepts in Chapter 5 focusing extensively on the private sector since the subjects of Medicare, Medicaid, and other government-sponsored medical care financing programs are covered in Chapter 5. Since health insurance and employee medical benefits are inextricably linked for most American families, this chapter will often look at these two concepts together, even though many medical benefits programs are not "insurance" in the technical or legal sense.

INSURANCE CONCEPTS

Central to any definition of *insurance* is the notion of "risk." One standard insurance text defines *risk* as "the possibility of an adverse deviation from a desired outcome that is expected or hoped for," or more simply as a "possibility of loss" (Vaughn & Elliott, 1978). Insurance is a mechanism for managing or controlling the financial exposure to this risk through two basic principles: (1) transferring or shifting risk from an individual to a group, and (2) sharing losses on some equitable basis by all members of the group (Vaughn & Elliott, 1978). Depending on individuals' or employers' preferences about how much risk they want to assume, as well as their various abilities to withstand the economic consequences of the losses, the amount and type of insurance required can vary substantially.

When health insurance began in the United States, conceptually it was similar to most other types of insurance—for example, auto insurance. In both cases, insurance was purchased to protect an individual from an expensive loss—hospital care or a badly damaged automobile. As private health insurance evolved to cover more people and a wider variety of medical expenses, however, it began to assume characteristics very dissimilar from traditional forms of insurance, by violating certain implied rules such as:

1. A "loss" is supposed to be something out of the ordinary, as well as something to be avoided. However, ill health is not a substantially abnormal event for most people, and in many cases,

the "loss" being indemnified (for example, a physician office visit) is not necessarily an event to be dreaded.

2. "Losses" are intended to be fairly independent events. In contrast, the very nature of infectious illness (or, in the extreme, an epidemic) implies a great degree of dependency among insureds' losses.

3. The "loss" should be of such financial magnitude that it is realistically unbudgetable for most insureds. The growth of so-called "first-dollar" base/major medical health plans (prominent in the 1970s and early 1980s) directly violated this tenet. Even today, providing insurance coverage for items such as pharmaceuticals or vision care stretches the limits of the "insurance" principle.

Thus, it is not surprising that health insurance has become a fundamentally different product from most other forms of insurance. And many health care observers have noted that these unique characteristics of health insurance, when added to the economic structures of the medical care marketplace, have made health insurance a chief contributor to the continued rapid growth of health expenditures in the United States. Ironically, the presence and growth of health insurance in the 1950s and 1960s provided a financial foundation for much of the medical-industrial complex that now fuels medical expenses. And the presence of health insurance creates a "catch-22" situation in which the existence of the insurance mechanism (often distorted to include first-dollar coverage of noncatastrophic expenses) stimulates demand and increases medical care prices, thereby raising the cost of health care and encouraging even greater insistence on more comprehensive coverage.

A BRIEF HISTORY OF UNITED STATES HEALTH INSURANCE

The history of medical expense insurance in the United States, discussed briefly in the previous chapter, goes back to the middle of the nineteenth century, when in 1850 the Franklin Health Insurance Company of Massachusetts offered coverage for bodily injuries that did not result in death (Health Insurance Association of America, 1991). Ten years later, the Travelers Insurance Companies first extended health coverage in a form similar to today's insurance. By 1866, sixty other insurance companies were writing forms of such coverage. At the end of the century, accident and life insurers were writing health insurance policies, primarily to indemnify against loss of income and for certain acute illnesses. The real beginning of modern private health insurance took place in 1929, however, when a group of teachers made a contract with Baylor Hospital in Dallas, Texas, to provide coverage against certain hospital expenses, thereby starting the first "Blue Cross" plan.

During the 1930s and until the wartime period of the 1940s, health insurance coverage grew rather slowly, in terms of both the insured population and the types of coverage offered. In 1940, insurers provided some form of medical expense protection to 12 million people, 9% of the total United States population (Table 7–1). A series of legal and tax developments in the mid-1940s and early 1950s provided nontrivial inducements for both employers and employees to purchase comprehensive health insurance benefits (Congressional Budget Office, Congress of the United States, 1980, 1991; Feldstein & Friedman, 1977; Greenspan & Vogel, 1980; "In the Future, Employee Health May Tax Employer," 1979). In 1942, only 37 insurers wrote group health insurance coverage; by 1951, this number had climbed to 212 (Congressional Budget Office, Congress of the United States,

1991). By 1950, the number of people covered by the nation's health insurers had climbed to nearly 77 million, 53% of the United States population. Fueled by the strong union gains of the 1950s and 1960s, collectively bargained employee benefits packages quickly became the norm throughout industrial America.

In 1960, 123 million Americans held some type of health insurance protection, generating about $5 billion in payments and accounting for nearly 21% of the financing for personal health care expenditures (see Tables 7–1 and 7–2). During the 1960s, health insurance coverage was expanded to an additional 36 million Americans, while health insurance payments tripled to $15 billion, representing more than 23% of total United States personal health care expenditures. The inauguration in 1965 of Medicare and Medicaid greatly expanded

Americans' protection against catastrophic medical expenses for our most vulnerable citizens, the elderly and indigent. But these two programs also gave substantial impetus to the notion that affordable access to the health care system was a right for Americans.

The decade of the 1970s witnessed another 29 million Americans added to the roster of the health insured population, as the health insurance industry plateaued in terms of the depth of medical coverage, while introducing new forms of health insurance protection (principally dental and prescription drug insurance). By 1980, health insurance paid 29% of the nation's personal health care bill, more than $62 billion. Although the 1980s saw proportionately slower growth in the number of Americans with private health insurance protection than did earlier decades, private health

TABLE 7–1   Distribution of covered persons, by type of private health insurance

Year	Net Number of Persons with Private Health Insurance (Millions)	Percentage Distribution		
		Commercial Insurance Companies	Blue Cross/ Blue Shield Plans	HMOs and Self-Funded Plans
1940	12.0	31%	50%	19%
1945	32.0	33%	59%	8%
1950	76.6	46%	48%	5%
1955	101.4	48%	46%	6%
1960	122.5	56%	47%	5%
1965	138.7	52%	44%	5%
1970	158.8	52%	43%	5%
1975	178.2	50%	43%	7%
1980	187.4	47%	38%	15%
1985	181.3	43%	34%	24%
1990	181.7	35%	30%	36%
1994	182.2	30%	26%	44%

Note: Percentages may not sum to 100%, as persons with duplicate coverages are counted multiple times.

SOURCE: *Source Book of Health Insurance Data, 1996* (p. 41), Health Insurance Association of America, 1997, Washington, DC: Author.

insurance expenditures more than tripled to $202 billion by 1990, even though neither the depth nor breadth of coverage increased nearly as dramatically as in previous eras. By 1995, private health insurance and employee benefit programs were responsible for financing nearly one-third of all personal medical care expenditures (see Table 7–2).

Despite an increase from 12 million people protected by private health insurance in 1940 to 182 million in 1994 (about two-thirds of the total United States population), political concern escalated in the early 1990s about the number of individuals without any financial protection for health care expenses. Perhaps the best evidence of concern over the uninsured was demonstrated by the normally staid American Medical Association, which devoted an entire issue of its journal (and subsequent articles in later issues) to this topic (*Journal of the American Medical Association,* 1991).

The National Center for Health Statistics estimated at this time that 34 million people in the civilian, noninstitutionalized population (nearly 14%) lacked health care coverage of any type (private health insurance, Medicare, Medicaid, or military and VA) (National Center for Health Statistics, 1991). This substantial number of Americans made vulnerable to the economic consequences serious

medical illness (or for low-income individuals, even relatively routine medical care) has become a potent political cause as the United States enters the last decade of the twentieth century. Lack of health insurance protection was greatest for the unemployed, minority, younger-age, and low-income/moderate-income segments of the United States population (Congressional Budget Office, Congress of the United States, 1991; Health Insurance Association of America, 1997; National Center for Health Statistics, 1991).

Yet even among the employed population under age sixty-five, more than 14% were without health insurance protection, due principally to lapses of coverage between jobs, the preexisting condition clauses of most employee benefits programs, and lack of employee benefits for employees in many small businesses and the self-employed. Indeed, two-thirds of the uninsured population are in families of full-year, steadily employed workers, most of whom are employed full-time. Nearly half of uninsured workers are self-employed or are employed in small concerns with fewer than twenty-five employees (Health Insurance Association of America, 1997). Employees working in small establishments are particularly vulnerable to

TABLE 7–2 Private health insurance as a health care financing vehicle

Year	Private Health Insurance Expenditures (Billions)	Per Capita Health Insurance Expenditures	Private Health Insurance as a Percent of Total Personal Health Care Expenditures
1960	$5.0	$26	21%
1970	$14.8	$69	23%
1980	$62.0	$264	29%
1985	$113.8	$460	30%
1990	$201.8	$776	33%
1995	$276.8	$1,014	31%

SOURCE: "National Health Expenditures, 1995," by K. R. Levit, et al., 1996, *Health Care Financing Review, 18*(1), Table II, p. 205.

inadequate or nonexistent health insurance coverage (Table 7–3). Contrary to popular opinion, most Americans are not employed by Fortune 500 corporations, as Table 7–4 clearly depicts.

ALTERNATE HEALTH INSURANCE TAXONOMIES

Most of what falls into the category "health insurance" is a combination of true insurance and employee benefits. One methodology for gaining an overview of health insurance is to subdivide the general area using different criteria. First, the principal insurance vehicles provide benefits associated with ill health: (1) basic employee benefits (primarily medical, dental, vision, and prescription drug coverage); (2) disability (short- and long-term insurance offered as part of many employee benefits programs, as well as compulsory temporary disability insurance mandated by five states); and (3) workers' compensation. Employers pay for some or all of each category of insurance, with the first type of insurance reimbursing most of the expenditures attributed to "health insurance."

A second major categorization of health insurance is by the type of organization furnishing the coverage. First and foremost among such organizations are the approximately eight hundred insurance carriers that comprise the "commercial" health insurance industry (*National Underwriter Profiles,* 1990). Second, as of 1996 there were sixty-six Blue Cross and Blue Shield plans. While technically offering insurance, the "Blues" historically maintained a different tax status from that of the "commercials." (The Tax Reform Act of 1986, PL 99514, removed the federal tax exemption for Blue Cross and Blue Shield organizations engaged in providing commercial-type insurance.) Third, health maintenance organizations (HMOs) offer a form of health insurance, although not in the same legal definition as either the Blues or the commercials. HMOs, in addition to retaining different tax and regulatory structures from those of either the Blues or commercials, differ from those two entities in one very fundamental sense: HMOs are not guaranteeing to *reimburse* the insured for medical expenses; rather, their obligation to the insured is more direct—to actually provide medical services to them. A fourth major entity in furnishing health insurance is employers (primarily large corporations) that self-fund or partially

TABLE 7–3 Percentage of companies offering group health insurance coverage to employees, by size of firm

Year	Number of Employees in Firm			
	1–24	*25–99*	*100–499*	*500+*
1979	36%	65%	77%	86%
1988	39%	66%	74%	81%

SOURCE: *Wall Street Journal,* November 22, 1991; data are from the U.S. Small Business Administration.

TABLE 7–4 Distribution of employees at U.S. business establishments, by size of establishment, 1991

Number of Employees	Percentage of Total Employees
1–24	30%
25–99	13%
100–499	14%
500–999	5%
1,000+	37%

Note: Figures may not sum to 100%, due to rounding.

SOURCE: "Americans' Health Insurance Coverage, 1980–91," by K. R. Levit, et al., 1992, *Health Care Financing Review, 14*(1), Table 7, p. 40.

self-fund employee benefits for workers and their families. Although declining in importance, unions are a fifth type of health insurance sponsor. Finally, corporations and unions sometimes jointly sponsor and administer "Taft-Hartley" health and welfare funds.

A third taxonomy of health insurance is by funding mechanism: (1) fully insured, (2) partially insured, and (3) self-funded or self-insured. The funding mechanisms of health insurance should not be confused with the three principal administrative intermediaries: (1) insurers, (2) third-party administrators (TPAs), and (3) self-administration. The market shares for these types of intermediaries have changed drastically in past time frames (Figure 7–1).

THE COMMERCIAL HEALTH INSURANCE INDUSTRY

There are several ways to describe the "commercial" health insurance industry. Perhaps the most fundamental distinction is between "mutual" and "stock" insurers. Mutual insurance companies (examples are Prudential and Metropolitan) essentially are owned by their policyholders, in contrast to stock insurance companies (for example, Aetna/U.S. Healthcare, CIGNA, and United HealthCare), which are owned in the more traditional corporate fashion by stockholders. Within each type of insurer are so-called "multiline" carriers and "single-line" insurers. Multiline insurers, such as CIGNA, offer life insurance and accident

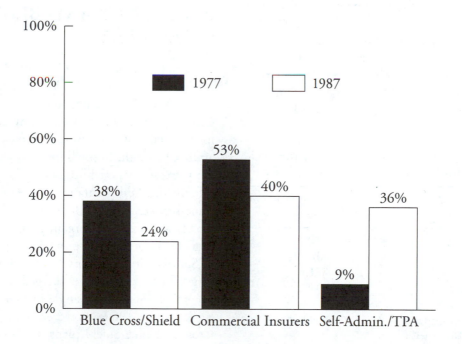

SOURCE: "Conventional Health Insurance: A Decade Later," by S. DiCarlo & J. Gabel, 1989, *Health Care Financing Review, 10*(3), p. 82.

FIGURE 7–1 Market shares for "conventional" health insurance, by type of intermediary. "Conventional" is non-HMO and non-PPO.

and health insurance, as well as "property/casualty" insurance (for example, auto, homeowners, workers' compensation, comprehensive general liability, and so on). Many multiline insurers also operate businesses that offer a range of financial products and services, particularly in the pension and investment areas. In contrast, single-line insurers usually offer the majority of their insurance products in the life insurance, property/casualty, or health insurance/employee benefits arena. Examples of single-line insurers are State Farm and Allstate ("Accident and Health Premiums," 1990).

Despite the approximately eight hundred companies that participate in writing health insurance and/or providing employee benefit programs, the commercial health insurance industry is moderately concentrated. As Table 7–5 depicts, about one-quarter of the $79 billion in total net accident and health premiums written by accident and health insurers in 1994 was contributed by only five large insurers, with the top ten insurers maintaining 37% of the premium volume and the top fifty insurers responsible for 73% of total premiums. In 1994, seventeen large commercial accident and

TABLE 7–5 Market concentration in the accident and health insurance industry, 1994

	Percent of Total Premiums Written
Top 5 insurers	24%
Top 10 insurers	37%
Top 50 insurers	73%
Top 300 insurers	98%
Total net premiums written	79 billion
Number of insurers with greater than $1 billion in premiums	17

SOURCE: *Best's Review* (Life/Health Edition), December 1995, copyright A.M. Best Company, used with permission.

health insurers each wrote more than $1 billion in premiums ("Accident and Health Premiums," 1995). (Use of the word *premium* generally refers only to true "insured" products, not to partially insured or self-funded medical payments that flow through insurance companies via other administrative arrangements. These latter moneys often are described as "premium-equivalents" and usually are several times the size of true premiums.) Because most of the major United States self-funded employee benefits programs are administered by the largest accident and health insurers, the concentration of the total generic health insurance/employee benefits industry is even more pronounced than indicated by accident and health insurance premium volume alone.

BLUE CROSS AND BLUE SHIELD PLANS

As noted earlier, Blue Cross plans initiated the modern era of private health insurance in 1929. Throughout the early portion of their history, Blue Cross plans focused attention on medical insurance for hospital costs, and Blue Cross itself was closely affiliated with the hospital industry. Approximately ten years after its establishment, Blue Shield began offering medical insurance protection for physicians' services. As with Blue Cross, Blue Shield was loosely affiliated with organized medicine because of its focus on insuring physician expenditures.

Since their inceptions, many Blue Cross and Blue Shield plans have merged their activities, becoming essentially a single insurance entity in a state. By the 1980s, however, a number of Blue Cross and Blue Shield plans reversed this posture and divorced themselves from each other, in a few cases becoming bitter rivals. In 1996, there were sixty-six Blue Cross and Blue Shield plans throughout the United States. In recent years, the national Blue Cross and Blue Shield Association, which heretofore had provided only a minimal amount of integration among its member constituents, has become more aggressive in attempting to marshal the resources of individual plans (for example, in the area of centralized claims processing). This cooperation has been necessary in order to compete effectively with large national commercial insurance companies for the business of employers operating in more than one state. The Blue Cross and Blue Shield Association also developed a national HMO network, for the same reason.

Unlike commercial insurance companies, which are regulated in most states by a state insurance department, most Blue Cross and Blue Shield plans are subject to special enabling state legislation. In addition to the close affiliations of the Blues with hospital and physician providers, the Blues have differentiated themselves historically from commercial insurers by establishing premium levels using a "community" rating methodology (in contrast to the "experience" rating most often used by commercial insurers).

Another key area of differentiation historically between the Blues and commercial insurers is the former's adoption of "service" benefits (that is, reimbursement for the total costs of covered benefits), rather than the "indemnity" benefits (that is, payment of a fixed sum for a covered benefit) of commercial insurers. Today, however, particularly for group insurance, commercial insurers offer service benefits; major exceptions are some individual and supplementary policies, as well as specialty insurance (for example, cancer insurance).

One final point of distinction for the Blues is their traditional reluctance to underwrite quite as rigidly as commercial carriers, particularly with respect to refusing coverage for entire industry groups or for individuals. In some states, for some populations, the Blues are the only health insurer of any significant size. All of these historical differences between the Blues and commercial insurers, however, are rapidly disappearing.

Due in part to these unique historical roles and unconventional insurance financial practices, a number of large Blues plans have been chronicled as teetering on financial instability ("Blue Cross Beset by Financial Problems," 1991). Most notably, during 1990 Blue Cross of West Virginia essentially became insolvent, leaving behind $50 million in unpaid medical bills. Its financial obligations and territory were assumed by Blue Cross and Blue Shield of Northern Ohio.

The mid-1990s have witnessed profound changes in the structure and organization of Blue Cross and Blue Shield plans. First, the number of Blues plans has been decreasing steadily, from eighty-six plans in 1985 to sixty-six plans in 1996. This consolidation has occurred primarily due to mergers between Blue Cross and Blue Shield plans (for example, the creation of Highmark Blue Cross/Blue Shield in Pennsylvania, from the combination of Pennsylvania Blue Shield and Blue Cross of Western Pennsylvania) and between Blues plans in different states (for example, the proposed merger of the Blue Cross/Blue Shield plans in Texas and Illinois). Second, pseudoconsolidation is occurring on a marketing or administrative basis, as Blues plans collaborate formally (but without legal mergers), usually on a regional basis (examples are The Regence Group of Blues plans in Oregon, Washington, and Idaho, and an affiliation of six Blues plans in the Northeast). Third, in an attempt to compete effectively for the business of multistate employers, Blues plans throughout the country are cooperating to market and administer their services jointly. One example of this trend is the "Blues Connect" product announced in 1997, where several dozen Blues plans will be working with two independent benefits outsourcing firms to offer multistate medical benefits programs. Fourth, many Blues plans have converted, or are seriously planning to convert, to for-profit status (in some cases, Blues plans are only creating separate for-profit subsidiaries). The rationale for this conversion is primarily to gain access to capital markets for the extensive investments needed to pursue managed care initiatives. Fifth, Blues plans will continue to emphasize managed care with greater zeal than historically has been the case. In 1996, for the first time in history, Blues plans nationwide enrolled more than half of their members in HMO, PPO, or "point-of-service" (POS) plans.

HEALTH MAINTENANCE ORGANIZATIONS

Although coining of the term *health maintenance organizations (HMO)* was attributed to Dr. Paul Ellwood in the early 1970s, these insurance-like organizations have been in existence for over a half-century. In 1929, the Ross-Loos Clinic in Los Angeles was the first generally recognized HMO (or prepaid group practice, to use the pre-Ellwood term); however, one can argue that the true roots of prepaid group practice began at the Mayo Clinic in the late 1800s.

Beginning with Kaiser's coverage of the health needs associated with workers building the Grand Coulee Dam in the 1930s, HMOs grew relatively slowly until the Nixon administration sparked new interest in these providers of predominantly group medical benefits. Enrollment has been strongest since the mid-1980s (Table 7–6), fueled by employers' dissatisfaction with the escalating costs of their employee medical benefits programs and the concomitant published research demonstrating the cost-containment success of many HMOs. Growth of HMOs was also stimulated by the HMO Act of 1973 (PL 93-222) and its subsequent amendments. These statutes required employers with more than twenty-five employees to offer an HMO option if a local, federally qualified HMO so "mandated." The

TABLE 7–6 HMO growth, 1970–1996

Year	Number of Plans	Enrollment (Millions)
1970	N/A	2.9
1975	N/A	5.7
1980	235	9.1
1985	391	18.8
1990	553	33.6
1996	628	52.5

SOURCE: *Health, United States, 1996–97,* National Center for Health Statistics, 1997, Hyattsville, MD: Public Health Service.

legislation also required employers to contribute toward the HMO premium of its employees an amount equal to that contributed toward indemnity plan premiums—the so-called "equal contribution" rule.

By mid-1995, the Health Insurance Association of America (HIAA) indicated that more than 53 million Americans were covered by HMOs, about 20% of the total United States population (Health Insurance Association of America, 1997). In 1995, InterStudy counted 593 HMOs in operation. Data from HIAA shows that five states (California, Pennsylvania, New York, Florida, and Oregon) accounted for 44% of total HMO enrollment. In ten states, HMO enrollment exceeded 25% of the state's residents (Health Insurance Association of America, 1997).

In the 1990s, HMO growth has slowed somewhat, due to several factors. First, the emergence of competing "alternative delivery systems," such as preferred provider organizations and, more recently, point-of-service managed care options, has provided employers with cost-effective, middle-of-the-road medical benefit plan options. Principal among the attractions to employers of these non-HMO options is the enhanced employee freedom of choice regarding providers, particularly physicians. Second, the wave of enthusiasm for HMOs regarding their potential cost-containment prowess was tempered during the late 1980s, when many HMOs' premium increases reached levels nearly as great as those of indemnity insurers and the Blues (Shellenbarger, 1991). In addition, research findings (aided by the "gut" feelings of many large employers) indicted HMOs for "cream skimming" the healthier risks toward the HMO, supposedly leaving the remaining indemnity medical plan options saddled with the "sicker" insured ("HMOs: Employers Shed Casual Attitudes," 1988; Scanlon & Austin, 1987). Finally, for reasons of administrative ease and fear of the financial and liability consequences of dealing with potentially insolvent HMOs, some employers have substantially trimmed the numbers of HMOs offered to employees. This trend continued during the 1990s, particularly beginning in 1995 when the dual-choice "mandating" provision of the 1973 HMO Act no longer applied to employers due to legislative amendments enacted in 1988. This same legislation, updated by the Department of Health and Human Services in 1991, also permitted greater employer flexibility in determining their required contributions to HMO premiums (Geisel, 1991).

As discussed in detail in Chapter 6, HMOs generally are characterized by their form of organization, according to one of our principal structures: (1) group, (2) staff, (3) independent practice association (IPA), and (4) network (see Figure 7–2). In group plans (Kaiser is the most prominent one), a physician medical group contracts with an entity that is financially responsible for covering enrollees. For example, the Kaiser Permanente Medical Care Program is actually a combination of three different groups: (1) The Permanente Medical Groups (providing professional services), (2) Kaiser Foundation Hospitals

(providing hospital care), and (3) Kaiser Foundation Health Plans (providing administrative and financial services). In the network model, the HMO contracts with two or more dependent group practices. Staff model HMOs (such as Group Health Cooperative of Puget Sound) employ most primary care physicians and major speciality physicians on a full-time, salaried basis. Hospital services and the rarer physician specialities are arranged through separate contracts. IPA-model HMOs forge the same types of hospital arrangements as staff-model HMOs, but physicians' services are established with a relatively large number of generally small or medium-sized group practices, with physicians receiving some type of discounted fee-for-service payment from the HMO, rather than the salaried reimbursement of staff-model HMO physicians.

As stated earlier, HMOs differ fundamentally from the true insurers (that is, commercials and Blue Cross/Blue Shield) because HMOs are not offering reimbursement for health care outlays; rather, HMOs actually guarantee the *provision* of covered health services. Like the historical record of Blue Cross and Blue Shield plans, HMOs generally have relied on community, not experience, ratings. (Indeed, the HMO Act of 1973 required federally qualified HMOs to price insurance in this manner.) Due to both competitive pressures and employers' increasing paranoia about perceived cream skimming by HMOs, however, HMOs are being pressured to engage in experience rating (which has been permitted since 1989 by subsequent amendments to the HMO Act of 1973). Another distinction between HMOs and their pure insurance colleagues is that HMOs often are regulated by an entirely different set of statutes and organizations than either commercial insurers or the Blues. In California, for example, there are state Insurance Department regulations for commercial

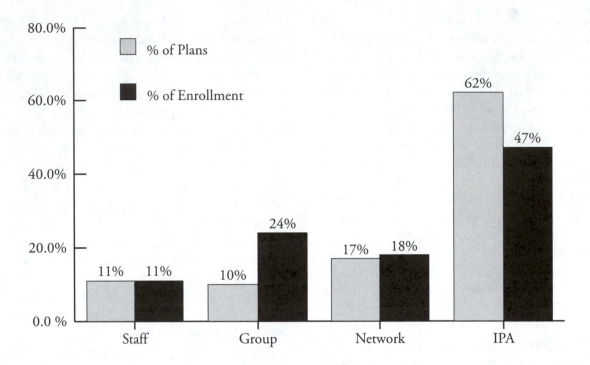

SOURCE: *Managed Care Outlook,* March 22, 1996, p. 7.

FIGURE 7–2 Distribution of plans and enrollment by predominant model type, year-end 1993

insurers, while HMOs are overseen by the Department of Corporations.

Not only can HMOs be freestanding organizations, but the Blues and commercial insurers also own and operate HMOs (see Table 7–7). Although the earliest large HMOs (such as Kaiser, Health Insurance Plan of New York, and Group Health Cooperative of Puget Sound), as well as some of the newer, well-respected HMOs (such as the Harvard Community Health Plan in Boston), were organized as not-for-profit entities, many of the newer, rapidly expanding HMOs (such as United HealthCare) and most of the commercial insurance company–sponsored HMOs are for-profit organizations.

PRIVATE HEALTH INSURANCE AS A FINANCING MECHANISM

Private health insurance is made up of the three principal entities just described (commercial carriers, the Blues, and HMOs), plus self-funded plans. As indicated in Figure 7–3, the importance of private health insurance as a source of financing for personal health care expenditures has increased slowly but steadily. In 1960, private health insurance funded more than one-fifth of these expenses; by 1995, nearly one in every three dollars spent for personal health care was reimbursed by private health insurance (Levit, et al., 1996).

As noted earlier, private health insurance began with coverage principally for hospital and

TABLE 7–7 Top ten general service HMOs, June 1996

Health Maintenance Organization	Members (Millions)	Tax Status
Kaiser Permanente Medical Care Program	7.0	Not for profit
United HealthCare Corporation	5.0	For profit
CIGNA Health Care	4.5	For profit
Prudential Health Care Group	4.5	For profit
Aetna/U.S. Healthcare	3.7	For profit
Pacificare Health Systems	1.9	For profit
FHP Healthcare	1.9	For profit
Health Systems International	1.8	For profit
Humana Inc.	1.8	For profit
Oxford Health Plans	1.3	For profit

Note: In 1997, FHP Healthcare and Pacificare merged.

SOURCE: *Business Insurance,* December 27, 1996, p. 1.

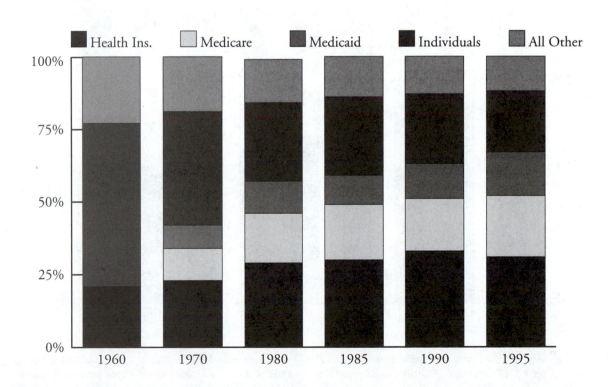

SOURCE: Adapted from "National Health Expenditures, 1995," by K. R. Levit, et al., 1996, *Health Care Financing Review, 18*(1), Table II, p. 205.

FIGURE 7–3 Private health insurance as a payor of personal health care expenditures

physicians' services. In 1960, virtually all of total net private health insurance payments were devoted to these two types of health care (see Figure 7–4). As Figure 7–5 depicts, private health insurance has funded a steady one-third of personal health care expenditures for hospital services since 1960. Between 1960 and 1990, however, private health insurance grew in importance as a source of financing for physicians' services, providing 30% of the funding in 1960 and 46% by 1990. The largest percentage impacts of health insurance financing have occurred in the areas of dental ser-

vices, nonphysician professional services, and pharmaceuticals. Private health insurance for these expenses was negligible until about 1970, and even at that time, reimbursements from private health insurance were less than 7% of total payments in each of the three categories. But by 1990, private health insurance was responsible for 43%, 38%, and 15% of personal expenses for dental services, nonphysician professional services, and pharmaceuticals and durable medical equipment expenses, respectively (Figure 7–5). Although in 1990 hospital and physicians' services still commanded about

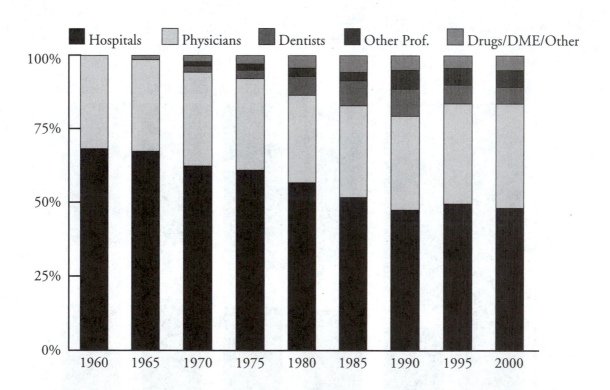

SOURCES: Adapted from "National Health Expenditures, 1985," by R. M. Gibson & D. R. Waldo, 1981, *Health Care Financing Review, 3*(1), pp. 45, 47; "National Health Expenditures, 1985," by D. R. Waldo, et al., 1986, *Health Care Financing Review, 8*(1), p. 20; "National Health Expenditures, 1990," by K. R. Levit et al., 1991, *Health Care Financing Review, 13*(1), p. 51; "Projections of National Health Expenditures Through the Year 2000," by S. T. Sonnefeld, 1991, *Health Care Financing Review, 13*(1), pp. 18–24.

FIGURE 7–4 Recipients of private health insurance payments

80% of private health insurance payments, almost $39 billion in private health insurance reimbursement was available for other types of medical care services (Levit, et al., 1991).

Projections of health care expenditures by the Health Care Financing Administration (HCFA) forecast total national health care expenditures of $1.6 trillion by the year 2000, of which $1.46 trillion will represent personal health care (Sonnefeld, 1991). Between 1990 and 2000, HCFA estimates that private health insurance expenditures will more than double, from $223 billion to nearly $508 billion. The proportion of personal health care expenditures funded by private health insurance, however, is expected to decline slightly during this period, from 32.5% to 30.5% (see Table 7–2), as publicly funded health care programs grow more rapidly than private financing.

As political debates in the United States continue regarding forms of national health insurance, there has been considerable argument and criticism about the "overhead" generated by the private health insurance mechanism ("Letters to the Editor," 1991; Woolhandler & Himmelstein, 1991). In 1995, the total administrative costs of public medical programs, philanthropic organizations, and the net cost of private health insurance amounted to nearly $48 billion, 4.8% of total national health expenditures (see Figure 7–6). (This estimate excludes the nontrivial administrative costs to providers regarding the filing of claims.) In 1990, Americans paid $217 billion in health insurance premiums and received $186 billion in benefit payments, resulting in a net cost of private health insurance equaling $31 billion (Levit, et al., 1991). This $31 billion includes

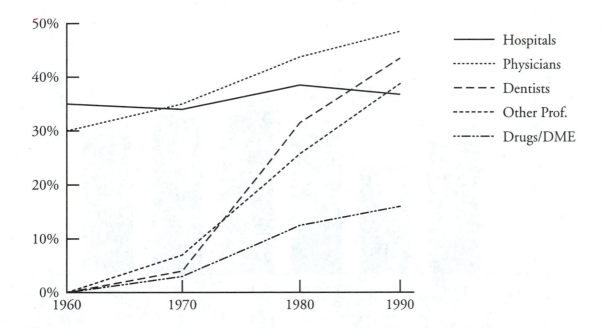

SOURCES: "National Health Expenditures, 1985," by D. R. Waldo, et al., 1986, *Health Care Financing Review, 8*(1), p. 20; "National Health Expenditures, 1990," by K. R. Levit, et al., 1991, *Health Care Financing Review, 13*(1), pp. 51–52.

FIGURE 7–5 Private health insurance as a percent of total payments for selected services

insurers' administrative costs, net additions to reserves, rate credits and policyholder dividends, premium taxes, and carriers' profits or losses.

Although there is no denying that some government health insurance programs such as Medicare deliver benefits at far less administrative cost per dollar of reimbursement than the private health insurance industry, health insurance *by itself* is not a significantly profitable business for most insurers. This is particularly true at the high end of the market, where self-funded "administrative services only" customers generate relatively narrow profit margins for most group insurers. Indeed, the health insurance industry has suffered a net underwriting loss (the difference between premiums and claims paid) in most of the years since 1976 ("Accident and Health Premiums," 1995). Health insurance is beneficial for many insurers primarily because it serves as a vehicle for selling other, more profitable products (such as life insurance) and because health insurance premiums generate revenues via investment income.

HEALTH-RELATED INSURANCE PROGRAMS

Individual Coverage

Although a number of insurance entities (mostly commercial carriers and the Blues) offer insurance

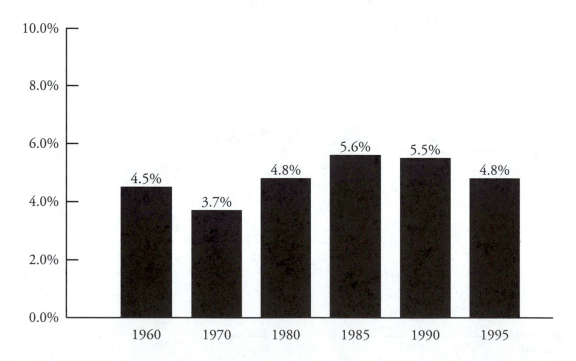

SOURCE: Adapted from "National Health Expenditures, 1995," by K. R. Levit, et al., 1996, *Health Care Financing Review, 18*(1), Table 9, p. 201.

FIGURE 7–6   Program administration and net cost of private health insurance as a percent of total national health expenditures

coverage for individuals, fewer insurers every year are interested in this line of business. Many of the nation's largest commercial accident and health insurers sell few or no individual policies. The number of people covered by commercial insurers' individual policies has decreased steadily since the late 1970s (Figure 7–7).

Much of the current individual insurance sold today is "supplementary" in nature—for example, to pick up coverage for the many expenses that Medicare does not cover, or covers only with significant cost sharing. Ordinary individual policies for basic medical (hospital and physician) coverage are extraordinarily expensive, as policy premiums can easily reach several thousand dollars, even for plans with extensive cost-sharing provisions.

Underwriting guidelines for individual policies have become increasingly stringent, so many people who might wish to purchase coverage are not able to do so. In some states, the only recourse for such individuals is through high-risk state insurance pools. Many states have enacted broad-based pools for uninsurable individuals to provide some protection.

Demand for individual medical policies has diminished with enactment of PL 99-272, the Consolidated Omnibus Budget Reconciliation Act of 1985 (COBRA). Under this statute, employers with twenty or more employees are required to extend group health care coverage to former employees for up to eighteen months after they leave their jobs (voluntarily or not) and for up to

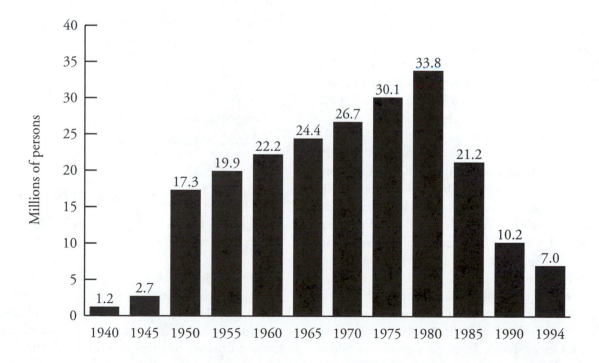

SOURCE: Reprinted with permission from *Source Book of Health Insurance Data, 1996* (Table 2.5, p. 41), Health Insurance Association of America, 1997, Washington, DC: Author.

FIGURE 7–7   Persons covered by commercial insurers' individual health policies

thirty-six months for dependents of employees following events such as death or divorce. Employers can charge a premium not to exceed 102% of the average cost of group health insurance for that employer.

Group Coverage

In the United States, employment not only provides the financial means of support for families, but it is the principal source of insurance protection against medical expenses and income loss associated with both on- and off-the-job illness and injury. Through sponsorship by a number of different groups (principally employers, but also unions, employer/union Taft-Hartley plans, multiple-employer trusts [METs], and multiple-employer welfare arrangements [MEWAs]), Americans receive the preponderance of their health insurance protection. Indeed, according to a study by the Employee Benefit Research Institute, the United States is the only major industrialized country in which voluntary, employment-based health plans are the primary source of health insurance for its citizens (Schachner, 1990).

In 1990, and likely currently as well, 70% of the population under age sixty-five obtained its health insurance through some employment-based group (Congressional Budget Office, Congress of the United States, 1991). The rapidly accelerating costs associated with medical care, and the tax-exempt nature of employee medical benefits, have stimulated the expansion of group health coverage. The importance of this latter factor is evidenced by calculations of the Congressional Budget Office that, in 1991, employers and employees were able to exclude $56–$58 billion in taxation from employer-paid employee benefits (Congressional Budget Office, Congress of the United States, 1991).

As noted earlier, small employers often provide meager health insurance benefits, if they provide them at all. But for workers of medium-size and large employers, medical insurance protection is nearly a universal benefit. For example, in a survey by the United States Chamber of Commerce of 957 firms (including 100 firms with fewer than 100 employees), various types of health insurance were provided as follows (U.S. Chamber Research Center, 1990):

Medical: 99%

Long-term disability: 65%

Dental: 56%

Short-term disability: 41%

Retiree medical: 33%

A more scientific survey of 1,647 medium-size and large business establishments by the Bureau of Labor Statistics produced these results (U.S. Department of Labor, Bureau of Labor Statistics, 1990):

Medical: 92%

Dental: 66%

Long-term disability: 45%

Sickness and accident: 43%

FUNDING ALTERNATIVE FOR GROUP HEALTH-RELATED INSURANCE

As mentioned earlier in this chapter, there are three principal options to funding health-related insurance: (1) fully insured, (2) partially insured, and (3) self-funding. At least for "conventional" health insurance (defined as non-HMO and non-PPO health plans), substantial differences exist in the use of funding alternatives among the Blues, commercial insurers, and self-administered/third-party administrator plans (Figure 7–8). For certain

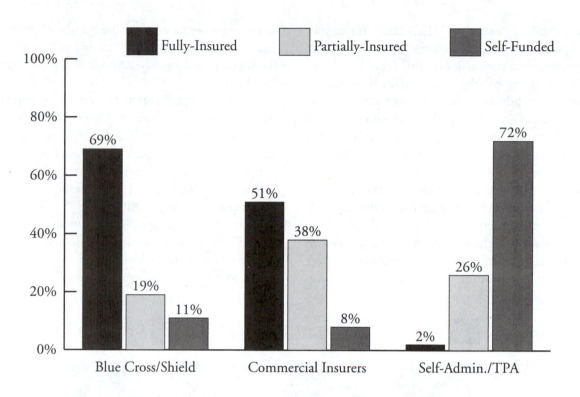

SOURCE: "Conventional Health Insurance: A Decade Later," by S. DiCarlo & J. Gabel, 1989, *Health Care Financing Review, 10*(3), p. 83.

FIGURE 7–8 Type of funding for conventional health insurance, by type of intermediary, 1987

health-related benefits, such as accidental death and dismemberment (AD&D), travel accident, long-term care, and long-term disability, funding (even within large corporations) is usually on a fully insured basis. This funding mechanism is employed because premiums are relatively small and stable, and the frequency of loss is so small that the only sound actuarial basis for establishing a premium is to combine exposures from many different employers.

For medical and dental employee benefits, however, all three of the aforementioned funding alternatives are used. Which one makes most sense to an employer is primarily a function of the size of its employee population and the employer's degree of

risk-aversion. Clearly for employers with more than several thousand employees, pure self-funding is actuarially viable, because medical expenses are relatively predictable. With one hundred percent self-funding, employers basically choose some organization (an insurer or third-party administrator) to administer their medical benefits program and perform claim adjudication. Depending on the self-funding contract, additional services (for example, actuarial, employee communications, and so on) also may be performed for the employer. Thus, the employer basically pays two types of employee benefits expenses: (1) medical service claim expenses submitted to the administrator for reimbursement by employees, and (2) an administrative fee, usually called "retention." This latter fee can be computed as a per capita charge, a percent of claim payments, or a transaction-related fee.

Self-funding of employee benefits is one of the principal trends in health insurance since the late 1970s (see Figure 7–9). There are four principal advantages to self-funding. First, the employer avoids the risk charges paid to the insurer that are inherent whenever any entity purchases insurance. Second, employers may be able to avoid administrative fees for services that are bundled with a normal insurance premium, but which the employer may wish to purchase through alternate channels (for example, actuarial or loss-prevention services). Third, since self-funding is technically not insur-ance, employers can avoid the nontrivial premium taxes (usually amounting to several percentage points) assessed by states on insured group health products.

Finally, and perhaps the biggest enhancement of self-funding, the Supreme Court ruled in June 1985 that the 1974 federal Employee Retirement Income and Security Act (ERISA) statute preempt-ed states from regulating self-funded group medical programs (*Metropolitan Life Insurance Co. v. Massachusetts,* 1985; Rublee, 1985). The most important advantage of this preemption is the abil-ity of employers to avoid the mandated benefit provisions of states, which require insured benefit plans to cover specific types of benefits. One tally

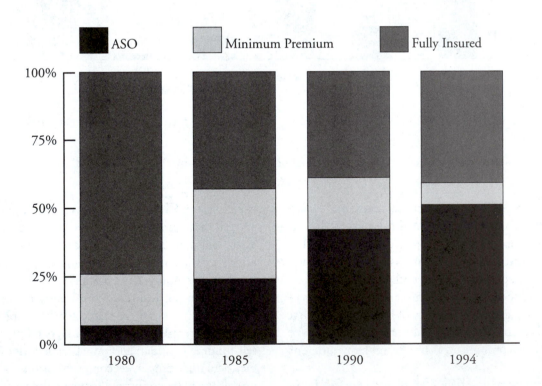

SOURCE: Adapted from *Source Book of Health Insurance Data, 1996* (Table 2.8, p. 44), Health Insurance Association of America, 1997, Washington, DC: Author.

FIGURE 7–9 Insurance company group hospital/medical claim payments, by type of funding

places the number of state-mandated health insurance benefits at nearly one thousand ("Tally of Mandated Benefits Nears 1000," 1991). These state mandates originally served as a useful stimulus to encourage appropriate coverage for types of care or for conditions not previously covered by typical group health plans (alcoholism is a notable example). In recent years, however, state legislatures have greatly expanded the scope and specificity of coverage to include personal preferences of powerful state legislators, and for care where cost-effectiveness is unproven.

Some observers blame mandated benefits for increasing the costs of medical benefits, especially for small employers, thereby exacerbating the uninsured problem (Goodman, 1991; Stipp, 1988). In effect, large employers began to see that their multimillion-dollar employee benefits programs were being crafted by politicians who bore no responsibility for the financial impact of their decisions. Thus, self-funding not only provides financial savings for large employers but also permits the employers significantly greater flexibility in designing benefit plans and establishing employee cost-sharing responsibilities. Some states, such as Texas, have become so concerned about the loss of tax revenues that they have attempted (so far without success) to seek legal rulings that would permit taxation of self-funded employee benefit expenses, which would reverse ERISA preemption ("Judge Strikes Down Texas Tax," 1989).

Many employers, particularly those with five hundred to five thousand employees, are reluctant to assume the financial risk of a fully self-funded arrangement. For these employers, there are several forms of "partial" self-funding (the most common of which is usually referred to as a "minimum premium plan"). Generally, these financial options permit the employer to self-fund claim expenses up to a certain predefined maximum amount, after which an "insured" policy assumes financial liability. Another variant of self-funding involves the purchase of "stop-loss" (or "specific and aggregate") insurance. Again, the employer pays directly for all medical claims, except for those that, either in the aggregate or individually, exceed a predetermined threshold.

Finally, there is the standard fully insured program, which remains the principal funding mechanism for the millions of small and medium-size businesses that form the foundation of employment for most Americans. For the small employer, premiums for this coverage are set prospectively (akin to auto insurance premiums, for example). For larger employers, a form of retrospective experience rating often is used, so that this year's premium is affected (either positively or negatively) by the previous year's claim expense history for each individual employer.

All three of these standard funding mechanisms are employed by both commercial carriers and the Blues. In contrast, most HMOs price their services prospectively, on a *per capita* basis. HMOs then are financially responsible for providing all necessary, covered medical services for this capitated premium. Historically, these capitation amounts were community-determined, unrelated to the claim experience of individual employers. As stated earlier, however, competitive pressures and amendments to the 1973 HMO Act are now stimulating funding approaches for HMO services that are more similar to the approaches used by the Blues and commercial insurers, particularly in the area of experience rating.

"CORE" MEDICAL EMPLOYEE BENEFITS

Today's core medical employee benefits consist primarily of medical and dental coverage. In addition, larger employers may offer separate plans for coverage of prescription drug and vision services (although coverage for these expenses can be combined under the general medical plan).

Medical Plans

This coverage is the oldest and most vital form of health insurance, since it protects against those financial expenses that can be truly catastrophic. For most major types of providers (for example, hospitals, physicians, nonphysician providers, laboratory and radiology, and so on), there is somewhat uniform coverage under indemnity group policies, but with different cost-sharing responsibilities for employees. The most generous plans (but also the type of plan rapidly losing favor with employers) are called "base/major medical" plans. Under these arrangements, there is first-dollar coverage for a few key providers (for example, hospitals and sometimes physicians), then more limited coverage (for example, with 20% employee coinsurance required) for all other services. Except for so-called "corridor" deductibles that may exist between the "base" and "major medical" expenses, these plans generally contain no up-front employee cost sharing. Perhaps the biggest disadvantage of base/major medical plans is that many do not place any upper limit on the expenses borne by the patient in a calendar year.

In contrast, the most prominent type of medical benefit plan today, the "comprehensive" design, retains little (if any) first-dollar coverage. A comprehensive plan design usually has a relatively small annual deductible (for example, $200) that pertains to all medical expenses, then it reimburses the patient a fixed percentage (most commonly 80%) of all medical claims that exceed the deductible, up to a maximum out-of-pocket patient expense (typically $1,000 to $2,000 per insured person). When the patient reaches this out-of-pocket maximum, 100% of all subsequent expenses are borne by the medical plan. Both base/major medical and comprehensive plans usually place lifetime maximums

on the total amount of benefits that will be paid to any individual. A 1989 Bureau of Labor Statistics survey found that while 78% of plan participants were so restricted, about half of these limits were set at $1 million or more (U.S. Department of Labor, Bureau of Labor Statistics, 1990).

In a 1989 Bureau of Labor Statistics survey of medium and large firms, 74% of medical insurance participants were covered by a fee-for-service medical plan, with the remainder of participants covered by an HMO (17%) or PPO (10%) (U.S. Department of Labor, Bureau of Labor Statistics, 1990). This survey also found that 53% of workers had their own coverage wholly financed by the employer, but this percentage was much smaller (34%) for dependent coverage (U.S. Department of Labor, Bureau of Labor Statistics, 1990). Forty-two percent of employees with a medical plan became eligible for coverage on the date of hire, while another 37% became eligible within three months of employment (U.S. Department of Labor, Bureau of Labor Statistics, 1990). Most medical plans today impose at least some managed care requirements on plan participants, the most common programs being utilization review and case management.

The benefit structure of medical plans offered by HMOs is somewhat different from fee-for-service "indemnity" coverages. First, the scope of coverage often is broader in HMO plans than in indemnity programs (although there are notable exceptions, particularly regarding the coverage of psychiatric and substance abuse illnesses). Second, the more generous HMO plans usually have no deductibles. Third, instead of coinsurance, HMOs feature fixed-dollar copayments for selected services, most commonly physician office visits ($5 to $15 per visit) and medications ($5 to $10 per prescription). Finally, HMOs traditionally have displayed greater attentiveness to fostering health promotion than have indemnity insurers.

Therefore, covered expenses in HMO benefit plans often include medical care not covered in indemnity plans, such as immunizations, well-child care, and physical examinations.

Dental Plans

Although Continental Casualty Company, in 1959, was the first commercial insurer to issue a comprehensive group dental insurance plan, insurance for dental expenses was not generally available until the 1970s. Plan designs for dental insurance generally follow more of a "comprehensive" than a "base/major medical" structure. Usually there are three tiers of benefits. For preventive services (for example, semiannual prophylaxis and routine dental X-rays), coverage often is 100%, without a deductible. For the two remaining benefit tiers, there is a small annual deductible ($50 to $100 per insured person) the patient must satisfy before any benefits are paid. Restorative services (for example, amalgams), oral surgery, endodontics (for example, root canal), and periodontics then are paid with relatively standard coinsurance (usually 80%). Services such as crowns, inlays, and prosthetics are reimbursed only 50% by the dental plan. Cosmetic dentistry (for example, bonding) usually is covered at this lower level, or it may be excluded from coverage entirely. Orthodontic services usually receive a relatively limited lifetime benefit (for example, $1,000), unless special orthodontic coverage is elected. Plans of dental HMOs (DMOs) and Delta Dental plans are analogous to medical HMO coverages, with slightly broader coverage and fewer cost-sharing requirements for the employee, when compared to indemnity dental plans.

By 1989, a survey by the Bureau of Labor Statistics of medium-size and large firms demonstrated that 91% of dental insurance participants were covered by a fee-for-service plan, with the remainder covered about equally by dental HMOs and PPOs (U.S. Department of Labor, Bureau of Labor Statistics, 1990). This survey revealed that individual coverage required no employee contribution for 52% of participants, while dependent coverage was free to only 37% of participants (U.S. Department of Labor, Bureau of Labor Statistics, 1990). Unlike medical benefits, dental plans are more restrictive in terms of annual limits on reimbursement. The Bureau of Labor Statistics survey found that 82% of dental plan participants were subject to an annual maximum, and for 62% of participants this threshold was $1,000 or less (U.S. Department of Labor, Bureau of Labor Statistics, 1990).

Vision Plans

Expense benefits for vision care were first introduced by private insurers in 1957. Many health care observers believe that vision care is a prime example of what should not be covered by an insurance program, since vision care is relatively inexpensive for most Americans. According to a 1989 Bureau of Labor Statistics survey, approximately 35% of medical care plan participants in medium-size and large organizations retained insurance coverage for vision services (U.S. Department of Labor, Bureau of Labor Statistics, 1990). For those individuals covered for vision services, nearly all received coverage for examinations, while two-thirds were covered for eyeglasses and contact lenses. Usually there are limits regarding the frequency with which examinations and lenses are reimbursable. With the advent of managed care, vision care may be available as a "carve-out" benefit, sometimes with a separate deductible. These vision care programs usually are offered in conjunction with large, national chains of vision care products, offering employees substantial discounts on these products if they are purchased through the preferred providers.

Prescription Drug Plans

This benefit is another example of a specialized employee benefit that increasingly is carved out of the regular medical benefit program, in order to take advantage of managed care features. Generally, coverage assumes one of two forms. In the traditional fashion, prescription drugs simply are a covered expense under the medical benefit plan. There may be individual copayments per prescription, and sometimes these copayments are higher for branded drugs than for generics. (Traditional coinsurance, typically 80%, may be substituted for the copayment type of cost sharing.) Nearly all types of prescription drugs are eligible for reimbursement, with common exceptions being certain injectibles (except insulin), contraceptives, and experimental drugs. Prescription drugs for acute conditions (for example, antibiotics) may be covered in part by the regular medical plan, while "maintenance" drugs are available through mail order. Mail-order plans permit employers and employees to take advantage of steep discounts and some drug use review, while offering the convenience of home delivery. Mail-order programs have been particularly well received by older employees and retirees. The latest trend in pharmacy programs, however, is a full "carve-out" program for all prescription drugs, a feature that may or may not include a mail-order companion product.

Long-Term Care Coverage

The most recent option for a number of corporate employee benefits programs is long-term care insurance, which first became available for groups during the last half of the 1980s. In 1995, private health insurance paid only $2.5 billion of the nation's nearly $78 billion in nursing home expenditures (Levit, et al., 1996). Many of these benefits were paid by individual long-term care policies and group medical plans (although nursing home coverage usually is quite limited for the latter programs). By December 1989, 118 United States insurers had sold about 1.5 million policies (mostly individual) covering long-term care (Health Insurance Association of America, 1991). The group policies now available are largely one hundred percent employee-funded, as employers are fearful of assuming any additional fiscal liability for insurance protection, even though the long-term actuarial value of this type of insurance is highly uncertain. (Unlike the service benefits of most group medical and dental plans, long-term care insurance is largely an indemnity product, offering a fixed daily reimbursement payment for nursing home care and related services. Coverage generally is not allowed for custodial care, nor for chronic organic illnesses such as Alzheimer's disease.)

The purchase of long-term care insurance received a significant stimulus with the passage of the Health Insurance Portability and Accountability Act of 1996 (commonly known as "Kennedy-Kassebaum"), which modified the tax treatment of long-term care insurance. If a long-term care plan is provided by an employer, premiums are deductible by the employer, and the benefits received by the beneficiary are tax-free to specified limits.

Retiree Medical Coverage

The foregoing description of the principal forms of group health insurance applies to active employees. (Of course, a very small percentage of active employees or their family members may receive primary insurance coverage through Medicare, such as individuals with chronic renal failure who require dialysis.) For active employees between the ages of sixty-five and seventy, the Tax Equity and Fiscal Responsibility Act (TEFRA) of 1982 required employers' group health insurance plans to remain the primary payers, with Medicare retaining only secondary coverage. In 1984, the Omnibus Deficit Reduction Act (PL 98-369) extended Medicare as the secondary payer for aged spouses of workers under age sixty-five. (These statutes are just two examples of how the federal government has shifted fiscal responsibility for the financing of some medical care from government to the private sector.)

According to a 1989 Bureau of Labor Statistics survey of medium-size and small firms, 42% of plan participants were enrolled in plans that continued health insurance coverage after retirement (U.S. Department of Labor, Bureau of Labor Statistics, 1990). For 79% of retirees less than age sixty-five and 72% of retirees older than age sixty-five, there was no change in health insurance coverage from their active coverages (U.S. Department of Labor, Bureau of Labor Statistics, 1990). For those retirees with health insurance coverage, however, 29% under age sixty-five and 26% older than age sixty-five were subject to a minimum company service requirement. Another 26% of retirees under age sixty-five and 30% of retirees older than age sixty-five were required to qualify for the company pension program in order to be eligible for health insurance coverage.

For retirees, there has been a profound reexamination by employers of providing continuing medical expense protection, particularly for early retirees who have not yet reached age sixty-five (and therefore are ineligible for Medicare) (Solomon, 1990). This rethinking of retiree medical coverage has occurred for several reasons. First, the unrelenting growth in employers' medical benefit expenses acceleration, which is two or three times as rapid as the increase in other costs of doing business, has forced most employers to reassess whether they can afford to finance retiree medical expenses as generously as in the past.

Second, as one would expect, early retirees' average annual medical expenses easily can be double or triple those of the active population. For employers with significant numbers of retirees

(such as long-standing manufacturing companies like auto and steel producers), early retiree medical costs can significantly raise an employer's overall average financial liability for medical benefits. Third, all employers (even relatively young firms) are faced with the undeniable "aging" of America, so the pressures on employers' total medical benefit expenditures will become more severe over the next several decades.

Finally, regulations promulgated by the Financial Accounting Standards Board (referred to as "FASB 106") became effective at the beginning of 1993 ("Now That Wasn't So Bad," 1991). Before 1990, virtually all employers used the pay-as-you-go approach to value the cost of retiree medical benefits on their financial statements. Now employers must accrue retiree health care liabilities as an expense against earnings, from the date an employee is hired until that employee becomes eligible for benefits. In addition, retiree health liabilities that have accumulated as of the date that employers adopt FASB 106 accounting rules must be recognized at once or be amortized (generally over twenty years). In 1990 and 1991, a number of prominent corporations decided to take their FASB 106 medicine, with a number of these companies assuming multibillion-dollar write-offs. For example, General Motors estimates the value of its FASB 106 obligations at a whopping $16 to $24 billion (Templin, 1991).

Since incorporation of these amounts on corporate balance sheets results in only a minimal diminution of actual cash flow (since FASB 106 is merely an accounting acknowledgment of future liabilities), its direct effect on employers' day-to-day operations is minor. However, the enormous financial impact of FASB 106 has jolted senior corporate executives into explicitly acknowledging the increasingly onerous burden of all medical benefits (not just retiree obligations) on employers' overhead expenses, perhaps more than any other single legislative or regulatory rule enacted to date.

As a result of these combined forces, most employers are reexamining how (and even if) they want to provide medical coverage for retirees. Some employers have even attempted to rescind retiree health insurance coverage ("Now That Wasn't So Bad," 1991). The courts generally have ruled that employers retain the right to rescind or amend retiree medical benefit programs, as long as this option is clearly stated in employers' benefit documentation (Geisel, 1989). For retirees under age sixty-five, benefit protection often is the same as that for active employees. For retirees over age sixty-five, employers' liability is diminished significantly, since the group health insurance plan becomes secondary to Medicare coverage. For both groups, however, employers are reconsidering their funding options.

One approach is to eliminate retiree medical coverage entirely for all new hires, or to link coverage with length-of-service requirements, much as pension plans are linked with "vesting" periods. Another option is to require retirees to contribute much more generously than in the past to their medical coverage. Unfortunately, current tax laws impede the ability of employers to establish tax-exempt trusts to fund retiree medical benefits. There have been some proposals in Congress to make it easier to fund retiree medical expenses by both employers and employees, for example, via an analog of 401(k) pension plans.

But the most fundamental choice most employers must make these days is whether they will continue to offer medical benefits to retirees under a "defined-benefit" concept or whether (like pensions) retiree medical benefits should be switched to a "defined-contribution" program. This latter option generally limits employers' future liabilities by making them much more predictable (like pension benefits) and clearly places most of the concern over the ultimate magnitude of medical care cost escalation squarely on retirees. If defined-contribution programs for retiree medical benefits become the norm, retirees will need to be much more concerned about issues of plan design and cost containment than they have in the past. Active employees also will be required to assume significantly more responsibility for funding their retiree medical benefits far ahead of when they will be incurred, just as workers must plan now to ensure that they will retain enough retirement income via pension benefits and 401(k) plans.

Disability Insurance

Serious illness or injury not only creates economic hardship due to the high costs of medical care but also inhibits the ability of workers to maintain a wage stream to support the everyday costs of living. Thus, loss-of-income policies are one of the oldest forms of health-related insurance. In contrast to the disability programs available through Social Security for chronic loss of income via disability, private insurance vehicles have focused on the short to medium term. Unlike most health insurance, disability insurance pays indemnity benefits, not medical service benefits. Except for the compulsory temporary disability insurance programs mandated by five states (Rhode Island, 1942; California, 1946; New Jersey, 1948; New York, 1949; and Hawaii, 1969), which combine wage replacement with medical expense reimbursement for nonoccupational disabling illness or injury, short- and long-term disability programs do not reimburse for expenses associated with medical services.

Short-Term Programs

Coverage for loss of income due to illness can be available to workers through two avenues: (1) sick leave or salary continuation benefits, or (2) short-term disability insurance. A 1989 Bureau of Labor

Statistics survey of medium-size and large firms observed that 89% of the working population was covered by one or both of these programs (U.S. Department of Labor, Bureau of Labor Statistics, 1990). While sick leave benefits usually replace all or most of an ill employee's wages, reimbursement often is limited to no more than a few weeks, at best. Eligibility for sick leave and the length of sick leave benefits are usually related to an employee's length of service.

According to the Bureau of Labor Statistics survey, in 1989 approximately 43% of workers were eligible for short-term disability insurance (U.S. Department of Labor, Bureau of Labor Statistics, 1990). Of those workers eligible, 84% of their programs were employer-financed. Short-term disability insurance retains several important features, many of which differentiate disability insurance from health insurance. First, there is a short "elimination period" (usually one to seven days) between the onset of disability or illness and the date when benefits begin to be paid. In the most generous short-term income protection employee benefits, sick leave benefits dovetail with short-term disability insurance so that the ailing worker has no front-end gaps in coverage.

Second, as their name implies, short-term disability programs protect workers only for relatively brief periods. In the Bureau of Labor Statistics survey, 96% of long-term disability plan participants had coverage of six months or less (U.S. Department of Labor, Bureau of Labor Statistics, 1990). Finally, three-quarters of short-term disability insurance plan participants had a length-of-service requirement before they were eligible for coverage, usually three months or less (U.S. Department of Labor, Bureau of Labor Statistics, 1990). This period of time to become eligible for coverage is called a "waiting period."

Long-Term Programs

Long-term disability insurance can be perceived in two different lights. In its most generous version, this coverage dovetails with an employer's short-term income maintenance program to create a seamless layer of wage protection for periods of several years. In its more primal role, long-term disability insurance is the disability equivalent to a catastrophic medical benefit plan, because benefits are paid only after the insured has retained a significant amount of loss.

According to the Bureau of Labor Statistics survey, in 1989 45% of American workers were protected by long-term disability (LTD) insurance (U.S. Department of Labor, Bureau of Labor Statistics, 1990). For 78% of the workers eligible for coverage, premiums were entirely employer-financed. Like short-term coverage, long-term disability insurance maintains a waiting period before employees are eligible for coverage. Nearly two-thirds of the LTD participants surveyed by the Bureau of Labor Statistics were subject to a length-of-service requirement of generally less than one year (U.S. Department of Labor, Bureau of Labor Statistics, 1990). In addition, the Bureau of Labor Statistics survey found that nearly half of plan participants had an elimination period (no coverage) of six months (U.S. Department of Labor, Bureau of Labor Statistics, 1990).

In order to induce workers to return to the job and because long-term disability payments can be exempt from both state and federal taxation, benefits are paid at rates usually in the range of 50–67% of a worker's wages (U.S. Department of Labor, Bureau of Labor Statistics, 1990), although there are often maximums to these payments. Due to the existence of Social Security disability programs, most long-term disability policies include provisions that permit benefits to be reduced commensurate with the amount of Social Security disability benefits paid. This provision is analogous to the "coordination of benefits" feature common in near-ly all medical and dental insurance policies.

Workers' Compensation Insurance

Like Medicare, workers' compensation insur-ance is a "social insurance" program. Usually, employee benefits professionals do not consider workers' compensation a health insurance pro-gram. But changes in the nature of workers' com-pensation benefits over the years, as well as the way in which these programs are now being affected by new managed care techniques, argue that workers' compensation should be discussed as a vehicle pro-viding nontrivial medical benefits.

Workers' compensation programs really were the first types of broad-coverage, health-related insur-ance in the United States. Beginning with a federal statute in 1908, workers' compensation–type insurance programs were enacted by nine states in 1911, and by 1920, all but six states had inaugurat-ed such a program ("Workers' Compensation," 1991). Today, there are fifty-five workers' compen-sation programs in operation—one in each of the fifty states as well as in Puerto Rico, the District of Columbia, and the Virgin Islands. There are also two special federal workers' compensation programs covering government employees and longshoremen and harbor workers. In addition, there are unique occupational illness and injury programs for coal miners suffering from pneumoconiosis ("black lung" disease) and railroad workers.

Covering nearly 96 million employees in 1993, workers' compensation insurance is compulsory for most private employment, except in a very few states. This protection provides workers and their families with three types of benefits: (1) indemnity cash benefits to help replace lost wages, (2) medical expense reimbursement, and (3) survivors' death benefits. Despite generally broad-based coverage, many state workers' compensation programs do not cover domestics, agricultural workers, and

casual laborers. Also, many programs cover public employees, as well as workers in nonprofit and charitable institutions, with varying degrees of comprehensiveness. Initially focusing on workplace injuries, workers' compensation programs increas-ingly are being pressured financially by the long-term effects of occupational illness (even though nationwide, occupational disease accounts for only about 2% of all workers' compensation claims).

In 1993, employers paid $57 billion for workers' compensation insurance, and workers' compensa-tion benefits exceeded $43 billion (Schmulowitz, 1995). The large difference between premiums and benefit payments reflects the long payout time frame on workers' compensation claims, so premi-ums collected in one year must anticipate claims filed for many subsequent years. Employers pro-vide funding for virtually all workers' compensa-tion premiums. About 20% of premiums are contributed to state high-risk pools, which provide coverage for high-risk employers that cannot obtain workers' compensation insurance through commercial carriers. Each state establishes its own regulatory mechanisms, eligibility rules, benefit schedule, and funding alternatives.

In forty-four states, employers may purchase workers' compensation insurance through private insurers, either property/casualty single-line carri-ers or multiline carriers. In six states, however, commercial insurance is not permitted. Two of these states (North Dakota and Wyoming) have an exclusive state workers' compensation insurance fund. In the other four states (Nevada, Ohio, Washington, and West Virginia), employers can purchase workers' compensation coverage through the state program or they can self-fund. In 1993, commercial insurers were responsible for 55% of benefits, state funds for 20% of benefits, and self-insurers for 25% of benefits (Schmulowitz, 1995).

One important development in workers' com-pensation programs over time has been the degree to which they provide reimbursement for medical benefits. In 1993, 41% of all workers' compensation benefits (totaling $17.5 billion) were for medical care, the highest percentage since 1940 (Figure 7–10). As Figure 7–11 depicts, this percentage has been increasing slowly but steadily since 1980. This trend is due both to states' restrictions on cash compensation benefit levels, as well as to the higher growth rate for medical care when compared to wages. Clearly all standard employee benefit medical programs contain provisions that exclude coverage for medical care for work-related accidents, in order to avoid duplicate payments by both the medical plan and workers' compensation.

Between 1978 and 1988, workers' compensation benefits accelerated at an annual average rate of 12.4%, with self-funded programs rising even more

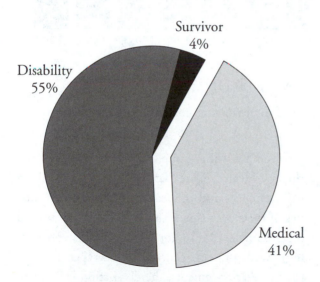

Benefits ($43 Billion)

SOURCE: "Workers' Compensation: Coverage, Benefits, and Costs 1992–93," by J. Schmulowitz, 1995, *Social Security Bulletin, 58*(2), pp. 51–57.

FIGURE 7–10 Workers' compensation benefit payments, by type of benefit, 1993

rapidly at 14.6% (Nelson, 1991). For this reason, many employers are beginning to observe their increasing workers' compensation expenses as closely as the accelerating costs of medical benefit programs. Thus, it is no surprise that many of the cost-management techniques (particularly managed care) that have been successful in moderating medical benefit plan expenditures are now being modified for workers' compensation programs. These strategies are more workable in some states than in others, however, as states differ in the degree of provider freedom-of-choice that is afforded to the injured worker. In most states, the employee may seek treatment from any physician, although in some cases this choice is restricted to lists of physicians established by state funds or insurers. In these states, therefore, it may be difficult or impossible to encourage workers to use a preferred provider network. Even utilization review may be only marginally effective in such circumstances. It is not surprising that some of the most aggressive transference of managed care techniques from the employee benefits arena to workers' compensation is occurring in those states that provide employers with unilateral physician selection powers.

CHANGES FACING THE HEALTH INSURANCE INDUSTRY

Profound changes have been sweeping through the private health insurance sector during the 1990s. The following themes are likely to continue throughout the end of the decade.

1. *Increasing challenges to control employers' medical benefit costs.* The cost-control mania of corporate America during the 1990s, coupled with employers' successes in drastically reducing medical benefit trend rates to the low single digits by mid-decade, have created an atmosphere of very aggressive cost-management expectations by group health

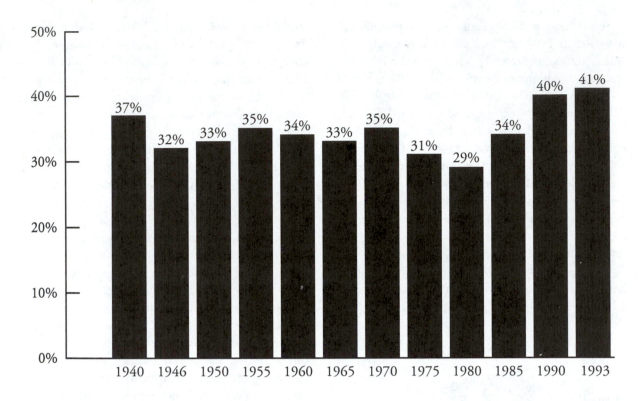

SOURCE: *Social Security Bulletin, Annual Statistical Supplement* (Table 9.B1, p. 347), 1995.

FIGURE 7–11 Medical care reimbursement as a percent of total workers' compensation payments

purchasers. Unfortunately, the very successes of private health insurers' managed care initiatives in reducing inpatient hospitalization utilization and garnering increasingly high levels of "discounts" from providers are likely to make continued low-growth trend rates more difficult to sustain. Successful health insurers will be required to either devise new cost-management programs or shift the interests of employers to other issues, such as quality improvement.

2. *Increasing competition from nontraditional health insurance models.* Health insurers face a growing array of competitive threats to their control of the medical benefits arena. First, providers are showing increased interest in direct contracting

involvement with group purchasers (witness the Buyers Health Care Action Group model in Minneapolis), and in creating managed care entities of their own (for example, provider-sponsored organizations [PSOs] for Medicare risk contracting). With the emergence of these types of managed care arrangements, the distinction is blurring between "providers" and "insurers." Second, private insurers are facing new competitors in the medical benefits administrative arena from human resources consultants and outsourcing firms. Third, the advent of technological developments such as the Internet permit many traditional health benefits activities (for example, enrollment) to be undertaken by firms that are primarily technology experts, not medical benefits experts.

3. *Continued consolidation of major health insurers.* Beginning with the purchase of Equicor's health insurance business by CIGNA in 1990, the private health insurance industry has undergone considerable and continued consolidation on two fronts. First, many smaller health insurers have elected to leave the health insurance arena entirely, and their business has been purchased by remaining large firms (for example, the purchase of John Hancock's group health insurance operations by WellPoint Health Networks). Second, there have been (and probably will continue to be) mergers among the largest of the health insurers. Examples are the 1995 merger of United HealthCare and MetraHealth (MetraHealth itself was the merger of the health insurance operations of Travelers Insurance Company and Metropolitan Insurance Company just a year earlier); the purchase in 1996 by Aetna of HMO powerhouse U.S. HealthCare; and two major mergers during 1997 of California-based HMOs (Foundation Health Corporation/Health Systems International and FHP/Pacificare).

4. *Movement away from "bricks-and-mortar" managed care structures.* Although staff model HMOs traditionally have been viewed as the "ultimate" form of managed care, the high fixed infrastructure costs are proving to be too onerous and inflexible in today's dynamic managed care competitive environment. In 1996, Caremark purchased CIGNA's large staff-model CIGNA medical group in Southern California (itself the successor of the venerable Ross-Loos medical group), and FHP Corporation sold its hospitals and essentially divested its long-standing staff-model medical practices. Even Kaiser Health Plans has been experimenting in different parts of the United States with operations that utilize nonowned hospitals and permit its HMO members to utilize non-Permanente physicians.

5. *Increasing growth of less restrictive forms of managed care.* The fastest-growing forms of managed care today are HMOs with opt-out provisions, and "open-access" HMO and POS plans (where members can seek care directly from any network physician, without gaining authorization from a primary care physician "gate-keeper"). Continued attacks by managed care critics are likely to force health insurers to decrease the "hassle factor" for both patients and providers. The strong growth and high consumer satisfaction levels for Oxford Health Plan in the Northeast is one example that members may be willing to pay more for managed care programs that focus on customer service.

6. *Escalating regulation and oversight of the managed care industry.* Critics of managed care, especially those groups whose vested self-interests are threatened by the increasing control of their activities by the managed care industry, are becoming much more sophisticated and successful in placing the health insurance industry on the defensive regarding its more aggressive cost-management practices. Mandated benefits at the state level (affecting primarily *insured* medical benefit programs) will be supplemented by attempts to also control the structure and process of managed care (for example, "any-willing-provider" statutes, "prudent layperson" restrictions on denial of emergency room usage, and so on). Of concern to large employers is the movement away from state-based legislative initiatives to federal ones, which remove the ERISA preemption and thus subject even self-funded medical benefit plans to their consequences (examples are the federal Mental Health Parity Law and the so-called "drive-though-delivery" restrictions that mandate minimum lengths of stay for pregnancies). Given the failure of broad-based health care restructuring initiatives such as the Clinton health plan in the early 1990s, more incremental legislative changes are being sought to

address more narrowly focused issues. The Health Insurance Portability and Accountability Act of 1996, which (among other impacts) dramatically limits the use of preexisting conditions in group health plans, is an example of legislation that was enacted relatively expeditiously and with considerable bipartisan support.

7. *Growing use of managed care in medical benefit programs, especially for retirees.* Given the level of provider "discounts" available from most major managed care insurers, very few employers any longer can afford to offer pure "indemnity" medical benefit offerings. And those employers with less aggressive forms of managed care (for example, PPOs) increasingly are attempting to move their employees toward more aggressive managed care alternatives (namely, POS and HMO plans). But, proportionately, the largest growth in managed care enrollment likely will come in the *retiree* population segment (both retirees younger than sixty-five and Medicare-eligible retirees) for three reasons. First, the FASB 106 accounting standards have significantly raised the visibility of retiree medical expenses, so there is increased pressure to manage these costs as aggressively as feasible. Second, corporate America's hard look at providing *any* retiree medical benefits will pressure employees to accept more stringent medical plan offerings. Finally, the enormous growth of interest by most major managed care insurers in Medicare risk programs will offer employers powerful financial incentives to migrate Medicare-eligible retirees to such plans as quickly as possible.

8. *Increasing focus on measuring and monitoring "quality."* As medical benefit trends have moderated, and as the stridency of managed care criticism has escalated, both employers and health insurers have faced mounting pressure to define, measure, and monitor medical care "quality." Three iterations of the Health Plan Employer Data and Information Set (HEDIS) standards, and growing demands for health plans to be formally accredited, are the most visible signs of slow progress in this arena. Particularly as other avenues of cost-management opportunities continue to dwindle, progressive insurers and employers finally are beginning to realize that quality improvement and health promotion strategies ultimately may be the biggest weapons of the future in continuing to moderate the cost escalation of employer-sponsored medical benefits programs.

REFERENCES

Accident and health premiums, 1989. (1990). *Best's Review (Life/Health Edition), 91*(8), 68–75.

Accident and health premiums, 1994. (1995). *Best's Review (Life/Health Edition), 96*(8), 16ff.

Blue Cross beset by financial problems. (1991, March 27). *Wall Street Journal,* p. A6.

Congressional Budget Office, Congress of the United States. (1980). *Tax subsidies care: Current policies and possible alternatives.* Washington, DC: U.S. Government Printing Office.

Congressional Budget Office, Congress of the United States. (1991). *Rising health care costs: Causes, implications, and strategies* (pp. x, 11–14, 67–80). Washington, DC: U.S. Government Printing Office.

Feldstein, M., & Friedman, B. (1977). Tax subsidies, the rational demand for insurance and the health care crisis. *Journal of Public Economics, 7*(2), 155–178.

Geisel, J. (1989, January 2). Court says firm can't alter retiree health plan benefits. *Business Insurance, 2,* 7.

Geisel, J. (1991, August 26). Relief for HMO costs. *Business Insurance, 27.*

Goodman, J. C. (1991, December 17). Health insurance: States can help. *Wall Street Journal.*

Greenspan, N. T., & Vogel, R. J. (1980). Taxation and its effects upon public and private health insurance and medical demand. *Health Care Financing Review, 1*(4), 39–46.

Health Insurance Association of America. (1991). *Source book of health insurance data, 1990* (pp. 1–2, 12, 103–109). Washington, DC: Author.

Health Insurance Association of America. (1997). *Source book of health insurance data, 1996* (pp. 21–22, 34, 49; Table 2.14). Washington, DC: Author.

HMOs: Employers shed casual attitudes, contracts. (1988). *Hospitals, 62*(12), 60–61.

In the future, employee health may tax employer. (1979). *Employer Benefit Plan Review, 34*(3), 38.

Journal of the American Medical Association. (1991, May 15). *265*(19).

Judge strikes down Texas tax on self-funded benefit plans. (1989, March 6). *Business Insurance* (pp. 1, 2).

Letters to the editor. (1991). *New England Journal of Medicine, 325*(18), 1316–1319.

Levit, K. R., et al. (1991). National health expenditures. *Health Care Financing Review, 13*(1), 38, 49.

Levit, K. R., et al. (1996). National health expenditures, 1995. *Health Care Financing Review, 18*(1) (Table 11, 205; Table 14, 208).

Metropolitan Life Insurance Co. v. Massachusetts, 84-325 (S. C. 1985).

National Center for Health Statistics. (1991, June 18). *Characteristics of persons with and without health care coverage: United States, 1989* (Advance Data #201, DHHS Pub. No. PHS 911250). Washington, DC: U.S. Government Printing Office.

National underwriter profiles, 1990, health insurers. (1991). Cincinnati, OH: National Underwriter.

Nelson, W.J. (1991). Workers' compensation: Coverage, benefits, and costs. *Social Security Bulletin, 54*(4), 17.

Now that wasn't so bad, was it? (1991, December 2). *Business Week, 3234,* 123–124.

Rublee, D. A. (1985). Self-funded health benefit plans. *Journal of the American Medical Association, 255*(6), 787–789.

Scanlon, J., & Austin, N. (1987). Bringing HMOs in line with cost management goals. *Business and Health, 5*(2), 12–17.

Schachner, M. (1990, October 22). United States has only health care system based on employer plans. *Business Insurance.*

Schmulowitz, J. (1995). Workers' compensation: Coverage, benefits, and costs, 1992–93. *Social Security Bulletin, 58*(2), 51–57 (Table 2, 53).

Shellenbarger, S. (1991, February 27). As HMO 1, 4 premiums soar, employers soar on the plans and check out alternatives. *Wall Street Journal.*

Solomon, J. (1990, May 17). Retirees, companies head for showdown over moves to reduce health coverage. *Wall Street Journal,* p. B1.

Sonnefeld, S. T. (1991). Projections of national health expenditures through the year 2000. *Health Care Financing Review, 13*(1), 1–27.

Stipp, D. (1988, December 28). Laws on health benefits raise firms' ire. *Wall Street Journal,* p. B1.

Tally of mandated benefits nears 1000. (1991). *Modern Healthcare, 21*(47), 8.

Templin, N. (1991, November 11). GM is facing a huge charge up to $24 billion. *Wall Street Journal,* p. A3.

Underwriting losses took a steep downturn. (1995). *Best's Review (Life/Health Edition), 96*(8), 16ff.

U.S. Chamber Research Center. (1990). *Employee benefits, 1989* (p. 35). Washington, DC: U.S. Chamber of Commerce.

U.S. Department of Labor, Bureau of Labor Statistics. (1990). *Employee benefits in medium and large firms, 1989* (pp. 4, 6, 22, 29, 33, 34, 37, 38, 50, 53, 62, 66, 67, 71, 124). Washington, DC: U.S. Government Printing Office.

Vaughn, E. J., & Elliott, C. M. (1978). *Fundamentals of risk and insurance* (p. 7). New York: Wiley.

Woolhandler, S., & Himmelstein, D. (1991). The deteriorating administrative efficiency of the U.S. health care system. *New England Journal of Medicine, 324*(18), 1253–1258.

Workers' compensation. (1991). *Social Security Bulletin, 54*(9), 28–36.

PART IV

PROVIDERS OF HEALTH SERVICES

CHAPTER

The Evolution of Public Health: A Joint Public-Private Responsibility

Paul R. Torrens

Lester Breslow

CHAPTER TOPICS

LEARNING OBJECTIVES

Upon completing this chapter, the reader should be able to:

- Understand the role of public health services in protecting the health of populations.
- Differentiate the various levels of prevention.
- Appreciate the history of public health in the United States
- Understand the roles and duties of each level of government in providing public health services.
- Appreciate the increasingly important role of the private sector in public health.
- View public health services as a collective requirement of all participants of the health care system.

In the past, if one were discussing the organization of health services in the United States, that discussion would most likely not include a great deal of detail with regard to health promotion or disease prevention. It would probably not cover in very great detail the organization of governmental public health services either. "Health services" in the past meant curative and treatment services for the most part, and health promotion or disease prevention services were considered only peripherally, if at all.

This is not to suggest that the providers of health care services in the past were uninterested in keeping their patients healthy over a long period of time. Rather, it is meant to suggest that the model of health care in the past was focused around acute treatment of short-term illnesses (with some notable exceptions). "Public health" was the job for governmental agencies and was seen as something quite distinct and very rarely overlapping with curative and treatment services.

In recent years, fortunately, a new paradigm for health promotion and disease prevention has emerged that is based on a public/private partner-

ship to protect and preserve the health of the American public. This chapter will examine this new paradigm of health promotion and disease prevention and will provide the modern health care practitioner with a better framework for understanding and dealing with the major health problems of the public.

LEVELS OF PREVENTION

In order to understand the new framework for health promotion and disease prevention, it is important first to provide background information about the levels of prevention, as included in the terms *primary, secondary,* and *tertiary prevention* (Commission on Chronic Illness, 1957; Leavell & Clark, 1958). Without a clear understanding of the levels of prevention, it would be difficult to understand the relative roles of the public and the private sectors with regard to the enhancement of the health of the public.

Primary prevention means averting the occurrence of disease. It includes those measures that are applied or brought into effect *before* disease is present. These may include general attempts to promote better health by efforts to educate the public, to establish standards of appropriate sanitation, and to apply specific methods of protection such as immunizations, removal of occupational hazards, and protection from known carcinogens. Primary prevention focuses on the promotion of healthy lifestyles and specific protections from known hazards.

Secondary prevention means halting the progression of disease from its early unrecognized stage to a more severe one and preventing the complication or sequelae of disease. It focuses on early diagnosis and/or prompt treatment of a health problem that would otherwise have serious impacts on the health of individuals. This means identifying the presence of a problem before it breaks the clinical horizon and before it becomes symptomatic in most cases, although it also includes attempts to discover disease early while it is still effectively treatable. In the case of coronary artery disease, for example, secondary prevention would focus on identifying individuals at high risk for disease—people, for example, who have a strong family history of heart disease, a history of heavy smoking, a lack of exercise, or a blood lipid profile that is abnormal. These early screening efforts can point the direction to more specific and focused tests and examinations that might further establish the early diagnosis of potential disease while it can still be constructively handled.

Tertiary prevention involves the prevention (or at least, the limitation) of the effects of disease once it has been identified. This level of prevention operates on the premise that simply because disease is present does not mean that its course should be allowed to run unhindered. In the case of coronary artery disease, for example, tertiary prevention would include efforts at cardiac rehabilitation and exercise programs, control of stress, maintenance of optimum weight and diet, and possibly adherence to a medical regimen that might reduce the future risk of further worsening of the disease.

In the new paradigm of public/private partnership in health promotion and disease prevention, there is a role for both the public and the private sectors at each level of prevention. Sometimes the roles are quite different and separate; other times the roles are similar, and perhaps overlapping, requiring some collaboration and coordination. The important message, however, is that there are several different levels on which health promotion and disease prevention can focus and a wide variety of interventions that can be sponsored by both public and private sectors.

HISTORICAL EVOLUTION OF HEALTH PROMOTION AND DISEASE PREVENTION IN THE UNITED STATES

In order to understand the present circumstances in the United States with regard to health promotion and disease prevention, it is important to review the history of public health activities in the United States. Much of our tradition and organizational framework for public health activities in the United States today is the product of the thinking and actions of previous generations. Therefore, it is important to know these developments and to understand how they affect our current thinking.

In the eighteenth century in the United States, public health activities were, for the most part, limited to individual cities and were focused on protection of the public in those cities from diseases introduced by travelers arriving from elsewhere. Early public health efforts in the United States in the eighteenth century focused on inspection of ships arriving in harbors along the eastern sea coast and included laws for the isolation and quarantine of persons suspected to be carrying diseases that might be spread to the general population. In some of these cases, local governments established institutions ("pest houses") to voluntarily (or involuntarily) contain suspected disease carriers until they either became noninfectious or, more likely, expired from their illness. During this period of time, the focus of public health activity in the United States was carried out by local governments and was quite limited to preventing the introduction of disease into the populations of port cities.

The nineteenth century marked a great advance in public health and was described by C.E.A. Winslow as "the great sanitary awakening" (Winslow, 1923). In this period, problems of sanitation were identified as a cause of disease, and public health efforts were focused on the improvement of social and environmental conditions. Housing, water supply, and sewage disposal were all the focus of organized public health activities, with the intent of reducing the disease burden on the public by improving the physical environment. As in the eighteenth century, these activities in the nineteenth century were generally carried out by cities and local governments, with the thrust of organized public health services being carried out on a local level, not necessarily on a state or national one.

In Massachusetts, Lemuel Shattuck published a landmark report in 1850 (Report of the Massachusetts Sanitary Commission) which for the first time collected vital statistics on the population of Massachusetts, pointing out the variable threats to health throughout the state as a result of variable sanitary conditions (Shattuck, 1850). His report recommended, among other things, new census schedules, regular surveys of local health conditions, supervision of water supplies and waste disposal, and special studies on specific diseases such as tuberculosis and alcoholism. Probably most important was the recommendation of the establishment of a State Board of Health to enforce sanitary regulations. Massachusetts did set up such a State Board of Health in 1869, becoming the first state in the United States to do so.

From the late nineteenth century to the early twentieth century, many of the sanitary threats to the public health were brought under control, and emphasis shifted to the prevention of acute illnesses by use of the increasingly available immunizations and vaccinations. This shift of emphasis from sanitary and environmental threats toward individual bacteriological threats to health signaled a major change in the role of health departments with regard to their focus of activity. In previous years, organized public health services focused more on problems that were sanitary and environmental in nature and did not necessarily involve individual people; the efforts were more engineer-

ing in nature than they were directly clinical. After the turn of the century, public health activities began to turn more directly toward prevention of disease in individual people, who were seen and treated as individuals. Organized public health activities moved away from structural protections of food, water, sewage, and housing and moved toward more personal and individual protection through immunization of children. Organized public health activities remained largely local government activities, but there now began to be increasing state government activity in public health as well.

As the twentieth century began to progress, federal government activities grew with regard to specific health problems related to children. The United States Children's Bureau was formed in 1912, and the first White House conference on child health was held in 1919. The Sheppard-Towner Act of 1922 established the federal Board of Maternity and Infant Hygiene; this act provided administrative funds to the Children's Bureau and also provided funds to the states to establish programs in maternal and child health. It also established a pattern of federal-state relationship that was to become standard in later years, with the federal government requiring individual states to develop a plan for providing services, to designate a state agency to administer the program, and to report on operations and expenditures of the program to the federal government. States that did not wish to comply with these regulations were deemed ineligible to receive federal funding, thereby setting the model of the federal practice for establishing guidelines for public health programs and providing funds to the state to implement programs meeting these guidelines.

The Social Security Act of 1935 further expanded the federal government's leadership role in setting national directions for public health; it also further solidified the federal/state partnership with regard to the delivery of public health services in the United States. Under the terms of the Social Security Act of 1935, grants were provided to the states for aiding state and local health departments to provide maternal and child health services as well as the expansion of the work of state and local governments. This marked the first major effort of the federal government to see that a nationwide system of state and local government public health organizations were put into place. By the time that Joseph Moutin issued his landmark report on local public health services in 1946, almost eighty percent of the total United States population had some access to organized local public health services; these services may not have always been of great depth, but at least a national framework of organized local public health services had been established (Moutin, et al., 1947).

The period of the New Deal in the 1930s also had a profound effect on the development of governmental public health services, but this effect was unfortunately somewhat negative with regard to the leadership of state and federal government activities. During these times, there was considerable pressure to expand the delivery of personal health services, both curative and preventive, more broadly to the public at large, and there was even some consideration by Franklin Roosevelt's administration of a mandatory, universal health insurance program that would cover the entire population. Since the role of the federal government in so many other areas was aggressively expanding, it was felt that perhaps there might be a similar expansion of governmental role with regard to the direct provision of health services.

Unfortunately, the political backlash against the expansion of the role of the federal government in the direct provision of health services, led primarily by the American Medical Association, was successful in forcing public health officials to assume a more cautious attitude toward the role of govern-

ment assistance. It became quite clear that there was no strong political support for the expansion of governmental health services, at least in the curative area, and many public health officials limited their activities to those programs and functions that were of a more traditional nature (that is, sanitation, immunization, early detection, and confinement of communicable diseases) rather than risk the wrath of organized medicine. This did not mean that the organized public health efforts of local, state, and federal government were reduced in volume, but it did mean that the governments were much more cautious in expanding the scope of their services, being careful to keep them within the confines of prevention and not venturing into treatment.

Indeed, it should be pointed out that the feeling in the United States was so conservative with regard to the federal government's role in health care that a cabinet-level department focusing on the health of the United States people was not established until 1953, almost one hundred and eighty years after the establishment of the republic! Various public health activities had been initiated by the federal government over the years, but it was not felt necessary, or possibly, politically possible, to have a federal "department of health," since health was seen as a personal matter involving private physicians and their patients. It should be pointed out that this same type of thinking governed our nation's thoughts with regard to education and social welfare: these also were seen as "local" matters in which federal government should not be involved, at least not directly. The creation in 1953 of a federal Department of Health, Education and Welfare (HEW) provided a national focus for developing and implementing federal government policy with regard to these three important areas.

In the period of 1953 to the present, there has been a great expansion of governmental activity focused on the public's health, much of it in the traditional public health areas, but much more in programs and functions related to the provision of personal health services. The passage of the Medicare and Medicaid programs in the mid-1960s is generally not seen as an expansion of the federal government's traditional public health role, but in retrospect, the passage of these financing mechanisms for the expansion of personal health services probably has had as major an impact as any of the previous, more traditional public health activities.

One further important development in public health thinking and theory was the passage of the federal Health Planning and Resource Development Act of 1974 (PL 93-641). Under this law, the federal government provided the funds to individual states for the establishment of a State Health Planning and Development Agency whose purpose was to plan and control the future development of health services, primarily hospitals, in the United States. The thinking behind the passage of this law was that there needed to be a coordinated planning effort to ensure that the proper type and volume of health services were available in equitable fashion throughout the United States, and that this could be carried out only by some type of publicly mandated planning effort to coordinate and regulate the development of these services. Although this national health planning effort was really a "public health" effort in the broadest sense, it was never fully connected to the already existing public health structures in the country and was never fully accepted as a legitimate public health activity by many formal public health professionals. The implementation of the Health Planning and Resource Development Act of 1974 was complicated and filled with significant controversy throughout the country; the law has since been allowed to lapse on both federal and state levels, and there is presently no direct attempt, by either federal or state governments, to "plan" the distribution of personal health services.

Lessons from History

What can be learned from this review of the evolution of organized public health efforts in the United States? What important political, social, and cultural trends can be identified that will tell us more about the current and future status of public health in the United States? There are several major points to emphasize.

First, it should be pointed out that organized public health activities in the United States began in local, seaport communities and only gradually expanded to state and federal government agencies. Indeed, the Constitution of the United States reserves to the states all functions (such as health) not specifically earmarked to the federal government. For most of our country's history, public health was an activity that was primarily carried out by a local or state governmental agency, and it was only after World War II that it was seen necessary or appropriate to have a federal cabinet-level Department of Health, Education and Welfare.

In many ways, this development would suggest that our country sees public health activities (and perhaps health activities in general) as a local and state matter; federal government involvement developed mostly after World War I, and mostly because of the abundance of federal tax revenues to be redistributed to states and local governments. The continuing efforts to reduce the size and scope of the federal government and to return basic functions (and funds) to local and state governments in recent years may be seen as a continuation of this general idea.

Organized public health activities in the United States began with quarantine and isolation of potential disease carriers, moved on to the improvement of sanitation in the environment, then went on to focus on immunization of children and control of individuals with contagious infectious disease. Almost all of these activities focused on acute infectious diseases, regardless of their origins. This has given rise to an unofficial and generally unspoken agreement that the primary mission of organized public health efforts in the United States should be toward the prevention and control of acute illness rather than chronic disease.

Organized public health efforts in the United States have focused on outbreaks of illnesses such as diphtheria and polio because of the suddenness and the severity of any outbreaks of these illnesses. In reality, however, the much more serious and major public health problems of the United States are no longer acute infectious diseases, but rather are chronic long-term degenerative conditions such as heart disease, cancer, and stroke. Organized public health efforts throughout the United States have a well-recognized role in protecting the public from "outbreaks" of infections, but they spend considerably less time and energy on problems of a much more serious and long-term nature, such as cancer, alcoholism, and mental illness. By default, organized public health agencies in the United States have accepted an acute illness prevention role as being appropriate, but they have not accepted a chronic disease prevention role to the same degree of intensity.

Because of the unfortunate political controversies of the 1930s around a possible national health insurance program, it would have to be admitted that there has been a relatively guarded relationship between the private medical sector and organized public health agencies throughout the country. As long as the organized public health agencies kept to the more traditional public health roles of sanitation, immunization, and infectious disease control, their activities were generally supported by the private sector. However, whenever the public health sector became more active in the provision of general health services or in the governance or planning of facilities and personnel in the private sector, considerable opposition arose. As a result of this opposition, organized public health agencies have been rather cautious about expanding their efforts beyond the boundaries of what was seen as "traditional" public health activities.

This is probably most marked and most obvious in reviewing organized public health's unwillingness or inability to assert any major role in the planning or regulation of the provision of health services in the United States. Although a broad definition of *public health* would certainly include the necessity of ensuring that the public has adequate access to personal health services, this planning or regulatory role has not been one that public health agencies have been willing to assume, or been allowed to assume by other forces in society. As a result, the health care system of the United States is a relatively unplanned and poorly coordinated system compared to most major industrialized countries throughout the world. In these countries, it is assumed that public health must protect the interest of the public in obtaining access to appropriate health services of high quality, but that has not been an accepted role for organized public health in the United States until now.

THE STRUCTURE OF ORGANIZED PUBLIC HEALTH EFFORTS IN THE UNITED STATES

The United States utilizes a very intricate combination of local, state, and federal government public health agencies to accomplish the public sector's responsibilities to the American public. Compared to other countries of the world, the United States has one of the most complex set of governmental relationships of any country in the world, a set of relationships that reflects the unique social and political values of the people of the United States. To understand how public sector activities in health promotion and disease prevention accomplish their objectives, it is important to understand each of the three elements in the public sector—the local, state, and federal government efforts—and then, after understanding how each segment works, understand the relationship between and among them.

In its important 1988 review of public health in the United States, "The Future of Public Health," the Institute of Medicine stated that the mission of public health was to assure conditions in which people can be healthy; it further stated that the governmental role in public health was made up of three functions: assessment, policy development, and assurance (Institute of Medicine, 1988). Looked at in another way, these functions could be described as identification of the major public health problems, mobilization of necessary effort and resources, and assurance that vital conditions are in place so that crucial services are received.

With regard to *assessment,* under this heading are included all of the activities involved in community diagnosis, such as surveillance, identifying needs, analyzing the causes of problems, collecting and interpreting data, case finding, monitoring and forecasting trends, research, and evaluation of outcomes. Assessment was seen by the Institute of Medicine committee as inherently a public function because policy formation, in order to be legitimate, is expected to take in all relevant information and to be based on neutral and objective factors. Moreover, public decisions take place in the context of limited resources so that a function of government is to provide a central mechanism by means of which competing proposals can be evaluated with only the best interest of society in mind. A fully developed assessment function is absolutely essential for an ideal public health system, since without it the society's real problems cannot be accurately measured, nor can alternative solutions be objectively evaluated.

Policy development is the process by which a society makes decisions about public health problems, chooses goals and the proper means to reach them, handles conflicting views about what should be done, and allocates resources. The Institute of Medicine felt that government provides overall guidance in this process, since it alone has the power to give answers that are binding on the entire society. In order to maintain its credibility in this policy development role, the governmental public health agency must pay attention to the quality of the policy development process itself and must raise the crucial questions that no one else can raise. To carry out this function effectively, the governmental public health agency must be equipped for its policy role with technical knowledge and professional expertise; this knowledge base of public health can therefore temper the excesses of partisan politics and make for fair social decisions.

The *assurance* function of governmental public health agencies makes sure that necessary services are provided to reach agreed-upon goals, either by encouraging private sector action, by requiring it, or by providing services directly. The assurance function in public health involves the implementation of legislative mandates as well as the maintenance of statutory responsibilities. It includes regulation of services and products provided in both the public and private sectors, as well as maintenance of accountability to the people by setting objectives and reporting on progress. Carrying out the assurance function requires the exercise of social authority; therefore, this is not a responsibility that can be delegated to the private sector. Members of society expect government to make certain that they enjoy at least adequate safety and security.

In reviewing the activities of the various governmental levels with regard to public health functions, it will be clear that some levels carry out more of one function than another. For example, the federal government level of public health in the United States has more of an assessment and policy development function than it does an assurance function, whereas state and local government public health activities have more of an assurance and assessment function than they do of policy development.

Federal Government Public Health Activities

The federal government's role in public health was relatively limited until the passage in 1913 of the Sixteenth Amendment to the United States Constitution which authorized a national income tax. Prior to that time, the federal government's role in much of public life in the United States was relatively limited, but particularly with regard to public health, since the government had neither statutory nor regulatory authority, nor did it have financial resources available to carry out its will. After the passage of a national income tax in 1913, the resources of the federal government in the United States became so overwhelming that federal government authority in all aspects of life, including public health, became the dominant aspect of governmental activity in the United States. Although the local and state governments actually have more formal and official responsibilities placed upon them to carry out public health functions than does the federal government, the federal government has by far the greater financial resources and power to make possible implementation of laws and regulations throughout the country. The federal government, therefore, has the predominant role in public health activities in the United States, not necessarily because of its explicitly assigned public health functions under the United States Constitution, but rather because it

has more financial power and authority available to it because of the national income tax.

The federal government's activities in public health in the United States are carried out through the Department of Health and Human Services, a cabinet-level department in the federal government. Although the exact internal organization of the Department of Health and Human Services varies somewhat from Congress to Congress and president to president, there is one descriptive characteristic that seems to remain: the Department of Health and Human Services is composed of a series of relatively separate superagencies that have comparatively little interaction with each other and that relate to quite different specialized constituencies, both public and professional. The Department of Health and Human Services is not a carefully designed and well-integrated organization that was intentionally put together to accomplish very specific functions of the whole organization; rather, it is an historical collection of powerful, individual, specialized agencies that at various times in their history were added into an already-existing federation of superagencies. As a result, the Department of Health and Human Services cannot be seen as functioning as a single, well-coordinated organization with a clear operating agenda that governs all of its parts; rather, the agendas of the individual separate superagencies, taken together, make up the policy of the department itself.

The federal Department of Health and Human Services can most easily be understood as having two major subdivisions, one related to health activities and the other related to human services activities. On the human services side of the department would be found organizations such as the Administration on Aging; the Administration for Children, Youth, and Families; and the Social Security Administration (the agency that administers the Social Security program). On the health services side of the department would be found health-related organizations such as the Centers for Disease Control and Prevention, the Food and Drug Administration, the Health Resources and Services Administration, the National Institutes of Health, the Alcohol/Drug Abuse/Mental Health Administration, and the Health Care Financing Administration (which manages the Medicare and Medicaid programs). Approximately two-thirds of the total budget of the entire Department of Health and Human Services is devoted to human services activities (and the vast bulk of that is specifically devoted to the Social Security Administration), while approximately one-third of the total Department of Health and Human Services budget goes to health-related activities (and the vast majority of that goes to the Health Care Financing Administration for the Medicare and Medicaid programs). Looked at in another way, more than eighty percent of the total budget of the federal Department of Health and Human Services is absorbed by two major programs, Social Security and Medicare/Medicaid (Institute of Medicine, 1988).

The major activities of the federal Department of Health and Human Services with regard to public health can be described through its eight primary functions: (1) documenting the health status and health situation in the United States through the gathering and analysis of statistical data (National Center for Health Statistics and Centers for Disease Control and Prevention); (2) sponsoring research in both basic and applied sciences (National Institutes of Health and the Alcohol/ Drug Abuse/Mental Health Administration); (3) formulating national objectives and policy (Office of the Assistant Secretary for Health); (4) setting standards for performance of services and protection of the public (various agencies within the department); (5) providing financial assistance to state and local governments to carry out predetermined programs

(Health Resources and Services Administration); (6) ensuring that the personnel, facilities, and other technical resources are available to carry out national policies and goals through support for training, construction, and program development (National Institutes of Health, Alcohol/Drug Abuse/Mental Health Administration, and Health Resources and Services Administration); (7) ensuring public access to health care services by the provision of special health insurance programs (Health Care Financing Administration); and (8) providing limited direct services to certain subgroups of the population (Indian Health Services and the former United States Public Health Services Hospitals for Merchant Seamen).

The major portion of the federal government's health activities is conducted through contracts and grants to states, localities, and private providers and organizations. The federal government acts through financing intergovernmental and interorganizational contracts to encourage various public health initiatives, convening participants around an issue, coordinating activities and developing state and local provider coalitions. In return for federal funds, states, localities, and private organizations must follow the federal standards and policies set in the contract. In most of its activities, the federal government takes an oversight, policy-setting, and technical assistance role, rather than a direct provider role. Most contracts to states and localities were initially offered as "categorical" grants, focusing on particular health issues or populations (such as research training grants for education, nutrition information programs, substance abuse and mental health programs, and family planning programs). In the early 1980s, the federal government grouped numerous categorical grants to states into four major "block" grants: one in preventive health, one in maternal and child health, one in primary care, and one in alcohol/drug abuse/mental health.

The more traditional "public health" functions of the Department of Health and Human Services are generally channeled through the Health Resources and Services Administration and the Centers for Disease Control and Prevention, but these are by no means the only channels by which federal public health finances and resources are channeled to state and local governments.

It should be noted that one of the federal government's major health activities, the provision of a large volume of direct patient care through the Veterans Administration, has no formal or organizational connection with the Department of Health and Human Services. The Veterans Administration, and its extensive network of hospitals and clinics throughout the United States, does not operate under the authority or jurisdiction of the Department of Health and Human Services at all.

State Government Public Health Activities

States are the principal governmental entity responsible for protecting the public's health in the United States. In the Tenth Amendment to the United States Constitution, states are designated as the repository of all government powers not specifically designated to the federal government. States carry out most of their responsibilities through their "police" power—the power to enact and enforce laws to protect and promote the health and safety of the people.

There are fifty-five state health agencies in the United States (the fifty states plus the District of Columbia, Guam, Puerto Rico, American Samoa, and the Virgin Islands). It is probably safe to say that each state agency is somewhat different from all the rest, since there is wide variation in the exact way in which state health agencies are organized. In general, each state agency is directed by a health commissioner or a secretary of health. Each agency

also has a state health officer (who is required to be a licensed physician) who is the top public health medical authority in the state; in many states, the state health officer is the director of the state agency, but in some states, the state health officer works for a nonphysician director who is the administrator of a larger agency or department. In approximately half of the states, there is also some type of state Board of Health or similar appointive body that is charged with responsibility for approving policy in the public health area and for reviewing the use of public funds; approximately half the states do not have Boards of Health and operate their public health agencies as administrative units of state government without any outside appointive oversight.

In discussing the federal Department of Health and Human Services, the department was described as a somewhat loose collection of superagencies, each of which operated in a semi-autonomous fashion from all the rest. State public health agencies, on the other hand, are relatively compact in the organization of their public health services and function as a single operational unit that is usually fairly well integrated within itself. The variation among state public health agencies, however, is that the public health function may be gathered together with a wide variety of other health-related agencies under some type of superagency or department. In some states, the traditional public health functions, usually gathered together in a single operational unit, are housed in a superagency that also contains organizations that deal with environmental issues, mental health services, services for retarded or disabled individuals, as well as the state Medicaid program. There is no uniform arrangement for these state-level superagencies, so that the public health unit may stand alone as an organizational unit or may be associated with up to four or five other health-related units in a superagency. In the state of California, for example, the Department of Health Services contains not only the traditional public health functions but also the state Medicaid program, which vastly overshadows the much smaller public health function; in California, the public health agency has responsibility for certain aspects of environmental issues as they relate to health, but a state environmental agency also has somewhat overlapping concerns in the same area.

Regardless of the organizational arrangement, there are certain functions and activities that seem to be common throughout the fifty-five state public health agencies in the United States. These include the following general functions: (1) collect and analyze health statistics to determine the health status and general health situation of the public, (2) provide general education to the public on matters of public health importance, (3) maintain state laboratories to conduct certain specialized tests that are required by state public health law, (4) establish and police public health standards for the state as a whole, (5) grant licenses to health care professionals and institutions throughout the state and monitor and inspect performance of personnel and institutions as appropriate, and (6) establish general policy for local government public health units and provide them with financial support as may be appropriate.

In general, state public health agencies nationwide receive half of their financial resources from state taxes, approximately one-third from federal government grants and contracts, and the remainder from special sources such as licensing fees and reimbursements (Institute of Medicine, 1988). In discussing federal public health agencies, it was pointed out that the financial resources of the federal public health activities draw on the very large national income tax for the financing of their operations, and at the same time, the federal government agencies have relatively few mandated responsibilities that must be carried out. By contrast, state governments must depend on a less robust state income tax for approximately half of their funding and, at the same time, have many more mandated services that they must provide. In general, state health departments are moderately well funded for the services that they are required to provide but considerably underfunded in terms of the potential health promotion and disease prevention services that they could provide.

If it can be said that the federal government public health agencies focus their energies on the identification of major health problems in the country and the establishment of national policies to attack these problems, state public health departments concentrate their energies on translating national health goals and objectives into state policy and spend a considerable bit of their time seeing that that policy is carried out. Many of these policies are carried out by the state public health agencies themselves, and many of them are carried out by local public health agencies under the direction and supervision of state health departments.

Local Government Public Health Activities

Local health departments are the "front line" of public health services in the United States. It is here in the local government agencies that the actual daily work of public health takes place, and it is here that the policies and strategies decided upon by federal and state public health agencies must be carried out. It is here where the stress of meeting public health challenges is greatest and where deficiencies or shortfalls are most visible and obvious.

Local health departments carry out their activities under the authority delegated by either their state or their local jurisdictions. Depending upon the interests and the resources of the local government, the local government public health function may either be very broad and energetic or very narrow and restricted. Some local health departments serve a single city or county, while others cover a group of counties. In about one-third of the states, the local health units are actually district offices of state health agencies, and in another one-third, the local health agencies are responsible to both local governments and the state public health agency.

The organization of the local public health agency is generally relatively simple, with the local public health agency responding directly to the local elected authority—either a mayor, county administrator, or board of supervisors. In its operations, however, the local public health authority must depend on state or federal funds for approximately half of its operating budget, so the leaders of the local public health agencies must continuously maintain a dual reporting function, one to their local government and the other to the state and/or federal government that provides them with the bulk of their operating revenues.

A special committee of the American Public Health Association, chaired by Haven Emerson in 1945, defined the six basic functions of a local health department as follows (Emerson, 1945):

1. Vital statistics—recording, tabulating, interpreting, and publishing of essential facts of births, deaths, and reportable diseases
2. Communicable disease control—tuberculosis, venereal disease, measles, hepatitis, and AIDS
3. Sanitation—supervision of milk, water, and eating places
4. Laboratory services
5. Maternal and child health services, including supervision of the health of children in schools
6. Health education of the public

For the most part, local public health departments continue to carry out the vital statistics, communicable disease control, environmental sanitation, and maternal and child health functions even up to the present time. They also, for the most part, maintain active public health education programs, although these efforts have become increasingly endangered by budgetary deficiencies. For the most part, laboratory services are no longer provided by local public health departments but are now provided by state health departments. And for the most part, the local public health department's functions are very immediate and in direct contact with the public: recording births and deaths, trying to maintain control or contact of individual people with serious communicable diseases, inspecting restaurants and other public gathering places to identify sanitary problems, and making sure that newborn infants receive their immunizations for infectious diseases and that children in school have some degree of health supervision. If the federal government's functions can be described as distant, nationwide, impersonal, and related to policy, the local government public health function can be described as immediate, individual, pragmatic, and personal. The basic operating unit of local government public health only serves to enhance this sense of immediate contact with the public, since it is usually represented by the local health center or local public health office; this is usually situated in areas of the greatest public health problems and at locations that provide easiest access to the most susceptible segments of the population.

Unfortunately, the disconnection between mandated required services and financial resources becomes most apparent at the local public health level. In the United States, local governments are usually the least well financed of the three levels of government, and it is no different for local public health agencies (Institute of Medicine, 1988). It is almost universally the case that local public health agencies are inadequately financed to perform even the minimum functions required by local or state law, let alone to provide an expanded and aggressive public health activity in keeping with the real needs of the public and potential for health improvement (Gordon, et al., 1997). It must be sadly admitted that local public health departments in the United States are probably the weakest link in the public health "chain," not because they are inadequately organized or poorly led, but rather because they seldom have the financial resources they need to meet their real potential.

Integrating Public Health Services

From this description, it can be seen that the public portion of our nation's health promotion and disease prevention activities depends upon an intricate collaboration and cooperation between three levels of governmental agencies: federal, state, and local. It involves elaborate transfer of financial resources from the federal government (where the resources are most abundant) to state governments (where resources are less abundant but still sufficient) and through to local public health agencies (where resources are scarcest and responsibilities most intense). The public portion of our nation's health promotion and disease prevention activities is, for the most part, focused first on the protection of the public from potential threats to health and only secondarily on the active promotion of healthier lifestyles.

Although the public health professionals in governmental health agencies know very well that the greatest long-term impact on the health of our nation's people probably depends upon changes in styles of living, those same public health professionals very often find themselves limited in their ability to engage in activities that are directly focused on lifestyle change. The federal, state, and local government public health agencies can create policies and goals to encourage individual personal lifestyle change, but for the most part, the actual implementation of those changes probably rests with the private sector, with the providers of medical care. The governmental public health agencies can go only so far with the resources available to

them in creating an atmosphere for major lifestyle change and improvement and, therefore, must depend upon their private-sector colleagues to carry the effort more directly into the homes of individual people. Nevertheless, governmental public health agencies have played a vital and essential role in the protection of the public, in setting strategies and goals for the improvement of the health status of the public, and in motivating the public to move to an even higher level of healthful living.

For that next level of health promotion and disease prevention, however, the full involvement and participation of the private sector is necessary. The importance of the private-sector clinical role was stressed in the United States Preventive Services Task Force Report in 1989 and was reinforced by the United States Public Health Service's major report, *Healthy People 2000,* which set national health promotion and disease prevention objectives for the country (U.S. Preventive Services Task Force, 1989; U.S. Public Health Service, 1990).

THE ROLE OF THE PRIVATE SECTOR IN HEALTH PROMOTION AND DISEASE PREVENTION

It is comparatively easy to discuss the role of governmental public health agencies, since usually they have been in existence for some time, have clearly defined roles, and have well-documented track records extending over many years. When one approaches the role of the private sector in health promotion and disease prevention, however, discussion becomes more difficult and more diffuse, if no less important. Indeed, in the minds of many individuals, the role of the private sector, particularly the physician in private practice, is increasingly central and important in creating the major lifestyle changes that are viewed as being so important to the prevention of disease over the long term.

McGinnis and Foege (1993) reviewed the actual causes of death in the United States for the year 1990 and determined that almost half of all of those deaths were attributable to lifestyle and personal actions on the part of individuals, such as tobacco use, improper diet and activity patterns, overuse of alcohol and firearms, unsafe sexual behavior, and vehicular accidents while under the influence of alcohol. They point out that most of these causes of death are only partially amenable to change by broad social or legislative actions and that only individual behavior change will really affect many of them. They also point out that the physician in medical practice is in a key position to influence behavior change, since research has shown that individuals are more likely to follow improved health habits if they are encouraged to do so by their usual medical practitioner. The central role of the practicing physician in encouraging and enhancing improved personal life habits has long been acknowledged and must be central to any future national plan of health promotion and disease prevention.

There are two major barriers to the individual physician's assuming the central role in health promotion and disease prevention: (1) the individual physician's willingness and ability to perform these health promotion and disease prevention activities, and (2) the ability of the population to access the services of a private physician.

With regard to the physician's interest in and ability to perform health promotion and disease prevention activities, it has long been noted that physicians are generally more interested and more competent in matters related to curative and treatment activities than they are in matters related to health promotion and disease prevention. This may be a reflection of their early medical training which

may have lacked emphasis on health promotion and disease prevention, or it may be related to the physician's natural human tendency to see curative treatment as "doing something" while seeing health promotion and disease prevention as "not doing something." Physicians are by nature activists and are more naturally drawn to the interventions where they are likely to see results in a relatively short period of time as opposed to events where the consequences of their actions will be known only, if at all, many years later.

It should also be pointed out that in the previous era of fee-for-service medicine, physicians were only reimbursed for treatment activities and were usually not reimbursed, either by insurance companies or by individuals paying their own bills, for prevention services. The former methods of payment for medical services encouraged increased active treatment of illness but did not encourage its active prevention. It is only natural, therefore, that physicians in the past should have responded to obvious incentives by spending more of their time and energies on treatment and less on prevention.

Probably a greater barrier to enhancing the role of the private physician in health promotion and disease prevention is the limited access that a significant portion of our population has to medical care. If a significant portion of the United States population is uninsured (estimates run between twelve and fifteen percent at any single point in time) or if a significant portion of the population has very limited insurance with relatively large financial burdens still resting with the individual patient, it is unlikely that individuals will visit a physician on a regular basis (Brown, et al., 1994). If individual people in the United States discover that their insurance plans do not cover health promotion and disease prevention and that they must pay for such tests themselves, they are less likely to use such tests and procedures and to visit a physician on a regular basis to obtain the counseling and encouragement that might be possible there.

It would seem natural to suggest, therefore, that if our nation wishes to involve the private sector in extensive health promotion and disease prevention activities that reach our entire population, it must be arranged in some fashion for the entire population to have health insurance coverage that ensures adequate access to medical care. Without universal health insurance coverage of some kind, it is an illusion to talk about a nationwide health promotion and disease prevention effort, since a significant percentage of the population (and, perhaps, those at highest risk) cannot access the one place where the most influential health promotion and disease prevention counseling might take place, the office of a private medical practitioner. Universal health insurance coverage, therefore, is central to any nationwide effort of health promotion and disease prevention.

Merely having universal health insurance coverage, however, is not enough if that health insurance coverage does not include financing for health promotion and disease prevention tests, procedures, and counseling. Many of the health insurance plans issued at the present time do not include reimbursement for health promotion and disease prevention, and as a result, individuals who may actually have health insurance coverage of a general nature are not covered for health promotion and disease prevention services. Therefore, it is essential that the design of future health insurance packages include financing for these services. Without such financing, individuals may be actively discouraged from seeking health promotion and disease prevention tests and procedures, as well as advice and counseling, from their primary physician.

The Role of Managed Care in Health Promotion and Disease Prevention

The advent of managed care health insurance coverage around the United States may present an opportunity to accomplish some of these health promotion and disease prevention objectives, particularly if the specific managed care plans are those of the health maintenance organization (HMO) type, which reimburse physician groups on a *per capita* basis. The advent of managed care of the HMO type presents opportunities for the expansion of health promotion and disease prevention in ways that have not been previously available (Breslow, 1996).

It is important to note two essential elements of the HMO type of managed care plan: (1) the official assignment of the long-term responsibility for supervising all aspects of an individual's care to a specific physician or medical group, and (2) the reimbursement of that physician or medical group on a *per capita* basis. Each of these specific aspects of HMO managed care are very supportive of the general long-term thrust in health promotion and disease prevention.

With regard to the first (that is, the assignment of long-term responsibility for an individual's care to a specific physician), HMO managed care plans require the identification of a specific primary care physician for each person covered by that type of insurance. This puts a particular physician on notice that this individual patient (or family unit) is his/her long-term responsibility. This identification of the individual physician as having an official long-term and continuing responsibility for an individual or a family changes the perspective of the individual physician away from the provision of specific individual services and toward the long-term health of the individual or the family. The designation of an individual physician as a patient's "primary care" doctor further solidifies the long-term role of that physician in managing the entire health-related set of activities in the minds of both the physician and the patient.

The use of *per capita* reimbursement to the primary care physician further reinforces the long-term nature of the relationship and particularly emphasizes the long-term role of attempting to reach maximum health outcomes, not just providing individual fee-for-service interactions. The HMO *per capita* reimbursement method serves as a reminder to the physician that his/her financial rewards are dependent upon keeping the individual patient as healthy as possible, rather than simply providing a series of individual services to a sick person. The dynamics in the HMO managed care plan thereby provide more incentives for keeping people healthy.

Managed care insurance coverage of the HMO type also has a great advantage over the previous fee-for-service type of coverage in that not only does it assign official responsibility to an individual physician or medical group, but it also holds that physician or medical group accountable for what happens to the patient. In the past, no physician or medical group was responsible for reporting to any insurance plan or purchaser of health care about the long-term pattern of services and their results. The individual physician merely provided one service after another on an individual and relatively unconnected basis, and no accountability was ever really required as to how the pattern of individual services eventually affected the overall health of an individual patient.

Under the new forms of HMO managed care, not only is it possible to assign individual long-term responsibility to a specific physician or medical group, but it is also possible, and, indeed,

increasingly the rule, to designate certain specific actions that the physician or group must take during the course of a particular year. It is increasingly common for HMO managed care plans to outline certain specific services or practices that a physician must follow and also to require documentation of the completion of those services (Schauffler & Rodriguez, 1996).

For example, many HMO managed care plans require that physicians provide certain health promotion and disease prevention services (such as immunizations for children, provision of mammograms for women over a certain age, blood cholesterol measurements, and the like). Not only are the HMO managed care plans able to require physicians to provide these services, but they are also able to require the physicians to report that these services have actually been completed. In this sense, not only are the services specified, but their accurate documentation is also included.

What this means for the encouragement of health promotion and disease prevention behaviors and activities on the part of the physician should be obvious. In the future, if it is judged that a certain pattern of health promotion and disease prevention services or activities should be provided to an individual patient during the course of a particular year, that requirement can be written into the contract with the individual physician before he/she is allowed to assume long-term responsibility for the patient. Unwillingness to perform these health promotion and disease prevention actions would bar the physician from being able to contract with the HMO managed care plan in the first place. The contract language also can ensure that the physician agrees to provide information that will allow the plan to determine whether the services have actually been delivered to the patient as agreed upon.

There are many aspects of managed care that are cause for concern among thoughtful observers of health care in the United States, but the enhancement of health promotion and disease prevention activities is not one of them. Indeed, one of the major positive aspects of managed care is its potential ability to install an organized, well-financed, and well-documented system of care that emphasizes health promotion and disease prevention. Despite whatever other concerns may exist about managed care, it is clear that the growth of managed care health insurance coverage offers an opportunity for an entirely new era with regard to the promotion of better health and the prevention of future disease in the United States (Schauffler, et al., 1993, 1994).

SUMMARY: THE FUTURE OF PUBLIC HEALTH

It should be clear from this discussion of health promotion and disease prevention in the United States that this is a shared responsibility between the public (governmental) and the private sectors of health care in this country. Neither sector can do what the other can do, and neither sector can do it alone. For the people of this country to reach their maximum health status, it will be necessary to forge an even stronger public/private partnership that allows both sectors to use their unique roles and advantages to advance the health of the public in ways that have never before been possible.

REFERENCES

Breslow, L. (1996). Public health and managed care: A California perspective. *Health Affairs, 15,* 92–99.

Brown, E. R., et al. (1994). *Who are California's uninsured?* Los Angeles: University of California, Center for Health Policy Research.

Commission on Chronic Illness. (1957). *Chronic illness in the United States:* Vol. I, *Prevention of chronic illness.* Cambridge, MA: Harvard University Press.

Emerson, H. (1945). *Local health units for the nation.* New York: Commonwealth Fund.

Gordon, R., Gerzoff, R., & Richards, T. (1997). Determinants of U.S. local health department expenditures, 1992 through 1993. *American Journal of Public Health, 87,* 91–95.

Institute of Medicine of the U.S. National Academy of Sciences. (1988). *The future of public health.* Washington, DC: National Academy Press.

Leavell, H. R. & Clark, E. G. (1958). *Preventive medicine for the doctor in his community.* New York: McGraw-Hill.

McGinnis, J., & Foege, W. (1993). Actual cases of death in the United States. *Journal of the American Medical Association, 270,* 2208.

Moutin, J., Hankela, E., & Druzin, G. (1947). *Ten years of federal grants-in-aid for public health, 1936–1946.* (Bull. No. 300). Washington, DC: Public Health Service.

Schauffler, H., et al. (1993). Managed care for preventive services: A review of policy options. *Medical Care Review, 50,* 153–198.

Schauffler, H., et al. (1994). Availability and Utilization of Health Promotion and Disease Prevention Programs and Satisfaction with Health Plan. *Medical Care, 32,* 1182–1196.

Schauffler, H., & Rodriguez, T. (1996). Exercising purchasing power for preventive care. *Health Affairs, 15.* 73–85.

Shattuck, L. (1850). *Report of the Sanitary Commission of Massachusetts.* Boston: Dutton & Wentworth. (Reprinted by Harvard University Press, Cambridge, MA, 1948).

U.S. Preventive Services Task Force. (1989). *Guide to clinical preventive services: An assessment of the effectiveness of 169 interventions.* Baltimore: Williams & Wilkins.

U.S. Public Health Service (1990). *Healthy people 2000: National health promotion and disease prevention objectives* (DHHS Pub. No. PHS 91-50212). Washington, DC: Department of Health and Human Services.

Winslow, C. E. A. (1923). The evolution and significance of the modern public health campaign. *Journal of Public Health Policy.*

CHAPTER

Ambulatory Health Care Services

Stephen J. Williams

CHAPTER TOPICS

LEARNING OBJECTIVES

Upon completing this chapter, the reader should be able to:

- Understand the role of ambulatory care services.
- Appreciate the evolution of ambulatory care as a delivery setting.
- Review the primary ambulatory care providers.
- Outline the organizational role and control mechanisms of ambulatory care services.
- Assess the allocation of responsibility for coordination, integration, appropriateness, and rationalization between ambulatory care and other sectors.

The evolution of our nation's health care system, particularly trends in the technology of medicine and surgery, and changes in financial arrangements have shifted the focus of the provision and control of health services to the ambulatory care arena. For many years, the hospital was the principal focus of the health care delivery system, but over the past decade, the role of the hospital has eroded while the advantages of shifting control and services to the ambulatory sector have been increasingly recognized by payers and providers alike. The ambulatory arena is likewise more tolerable for the patient, as well.

This chapter addresses the historical development and current and future roles of ambulatory care services, placing these services in a broader context that recognizes both the direct provision of care and mechanisms of controlling patients and providers within various payment arrangements. Descriptions of various ambulatory care provider settings, quantitative descriptions of the volume and nature of such services, and the increasingly important role of these services in the coordination and organization of the system are addressed.

The role of ambulatory care services in organizing and rationalizing the health care system has been greatly enhanced by the rapid growth of managed care, by the changing nature and role of hospitals and hospital systems, and by enhancement of the gate-keeper and coordinating function of front-line providers of care. The increasing shift of many services that have been traditionally performed on an inpatient basis such as many surgical services, maintenance-oriented care that is now provided in the home rather than in the hospital, and other practical and technological changes have also heightened interest in ambulatory care. Finally, the increasing consolidation and vertical integration of the health care system is greatly increasing the linkages between ambulatory care and other services.

Many of these changes and trends are discussed in other chapters of this book; their relevance to ambulatory care and ambulatory care's enhanced role in the system is discussed in detail in this chapter. Ambulatory care has long had a central role in health care, a role that is now increasing in scope and importance. An interesting history characterizes the evolution of these services.

Traditionally ambulatory care services have been viewed as the primary source of contact that most people have with the health care system. Although there are few concise definitions of ambulatory care, these services can be defined as care provided to noninstitutionalized patients. Sometimes ambulatory care is termed care for the "walking patient." Ambulatory care includes a wide range of services, from simple, routine treatment to surprisingly complex tests and therapies.

HISTORICAL PERSPECTIVE AND TYPES OF CARE

Ambulatory care originated with the healing arts themselves. In primitive societies and for many years thereafter, until the advent of institutional care, all care was provided on what might be referred to as an *ambulatory care basis*. Of course, the types of care given then bear little resemblance to today's health care, but the history of civilization demonstrates a consistent commitment to caring for the sick, using whatever knowledge has been available at the time. Remarkable forms of medical practice occurred in Greece, Rome, and other relatively sophisticated societies. In fact, many primitive societies had, and most, if not all, countries still have, their own indigenous practitioners such as religious healers and medicine men.

In more recent times, ambulatory care was provided in many new settings by a variety of more advanced practitioners. In Europe, and later in the United States, many of these services were given to wealthy patients in their homes, and poor people were cared for in dispensaries and public clinics. With improvements in hospital care, more patients of all social classes received both inpatient and outpatient care in hospital settings. In the United States, the poor have always been more likely than wealthier people to obtain care from the hospital than from private physicians.

In the United States, ambulatory care services were traditionally provided by individual medical practitioners working in their offices and in patients' homes and by public clinics operating primarily for poor and indigent patients. The limited technological armament that physicians required allowed them to travel easily, carrying with them their principal equipment and supplies. Thus home care was common, especially among wealthier patients. Physicians' offices were frequently located in their homes or in other small buildings, as opposed to today's medical office buildings or large medical centers. The general practitioner who made house calls, provided guidance, and offered available treatments was typical of the primary care provided before World War II.

Since World War II, however, an explosion of medical knowledge has led to increasing specialization, more complex technology, and rapid changes in the setting and nature of services. Fewer physicians are able or willing to travel to the patient's home, and many can no longer carry with them either the equipment and supplies or the specialized personnel available in an office. The growth of technical specialization, in particular, has led to the rapid expansion of new settings for providing care, such as group practices and, more recently, a profusion of specialized facilities. Increased knowledge has also led to the partial phasing out of the "traditional" general practitioner, although a new form of generalist is now taking hold, encouraged by managed care and concerns over comprehensivenes of care.

For the poor, in both Europe and the United States, care, when available, was often limited to public or philanthropic clinics or dispensaries. Private practitioners may have given their time to serve the poor, but their devotion to the patient was probably limited, as was the availability of care and the facilities in which services were provided.

Early efforts to link ambulatory care services and integrate them formally with inpatient care were promoted in this country and in Europe, in part, through the concept of regionalization. In Great Britain, the concept was presented in the Dawson Report, which eventually led to the National Health Service. In the United States, however, centralization of authority under government of the health care system has not been accepted as a politically viable alternative, a principle most recently affirmed by the rejection of the Clinton health care initiatives discussed later in this book.

The increasing sophistication of insurance mechanisms and the use of ambulatory care services as a control mechanism on the use of all services have led to an increase in the degree of structure of the health care system over the past few years. This increasing structure has primarily occurred in the private, nongovernmental sector. The concept of social and economic regulation of the system through governmental intervention, carried to a high level of sophistication in the Dawson Report, has largely been abandoned, at least for the foreseeable future. Integration of services will focus largely on multiple, independently organized systems of care that are competitive with one another.

The diversity of services, providers, and facilities involved in ambulatory care today is truly amazing and growing all the time. Many of these services and organizations are discussed in this chapter. Particular attention is directed toward rapidly expanding and innovative settings, such as group practice, and integration of settings and services through organized systems of care, especially in managed care. The role of ambulatory care is also discussed in other chapters of this book, especially those dealing with insurance and organizational arrangements.

Levels of Ambulatory Care Services

Ambulatory care services can be differentiated into a number of distinct levels or types of care. Primary prevention seeks to reduce the risks of illness or morbidity by removing or reducing disease-causing agents and opportunities from our society. These activities include efforts to eliminate environmental pollutants that are suspected to cause diseases such as cancer. Other examples of primary prevention include encouraging people to use automobile seat belts, treatment of water and sewage, and sanitation inspections in restaurants. Preventive health services are more direct personal interventions to detect and prevent disease. Examples of these services include hypertension, diabetes, and cancer screening clinics and immunization programs. The combination of primary prevention and preventive services is our first line of defense against disease.

Medical care that is oriented toward the daily, routine needs of patients, such as initial diagnosis and continuing treatment of common illness, is termed *primary care.* This care is not highly complex and generally does not require sophisticated technology and personnel. The vision of the general practitioner of bygone days, traveling from house to house ministering to the sick, represents the traditional role of primary care, which is replaced in today's society by considerably more skilled practitioners in relatively complex facilities.

In addition to providing services directly, the primary care professional should serve the role of patient advisor, advocate, and system "gatekeeper." In this coordinating role, the provider refers patients to sources of specialized care, gives advice regarding various diagnoses and therapies, and provides continuing care for chronic conditions. In many organized systems of care, such as managed care programs, this role is very important in controlling costs, utilization, and the rational allocation of resources.

The evolution of technology and medicine's increasing ability to intervene in illness have led to greater specialization of health care services. These more specialized services, termed *secondary* and *tertiary care,* are provided in both ambulatory and inpatient settings. The content of secondary and tertiary care practices is usually more narrowly defined than that of the primary care provider. Subspecialists, who provide the bulk of secondary and tertiary care, also often require more complex equipment and more highly trained support personnel than do primary care providers.

In recent years, the evolution of health care services has led to greatly expanded provision of secondary care on an outpatient, or ambulatory care, basis. Numerous surgical services of increasing complexity have been shifted to the ambulatory arena; recent advances in the use of fiber optic and other technologies suggest that this trend will continue. Diagnostic and therapeutic procedures that used to require hospitalization are also increasingly being performed in ambulatory settings.

There are no clear dividing lines for primary versus secondary and secondary versus tertiary care. Secondary services include "routine" hospitalization and specialized outpatient care. These services are more complex than those of primary care and include many diagnostic procedures as well as more complex therapies. Tertiary care includes the most complex services, such as open heart surgery, burn treatment, and transplantation, and is provided in inpatient hospital facilities. Most of the care discussed in this chapter involves primary care and those secondary services that can be provided in such settings as office-based practice, hospital outpatient departments, or community clinics.

SETTINGS FOR THE PROVISION OF AMBULATORY CARE

Use of Ambulatory Care Services

Historically, and at the present time, most ambulatory care services are provided in solo and group practice, office-based settings. Institutional settings for care, primarily the hospital, although an important component of the health care system, remain less prominent. Overlap between office-based practice and institutional settings is increasingly common, however, as the dividing lines between various components of the health care system continue to blur. Managed care programs especially tend to integrate these services.

An indication of the use and sites of ambulatory care visits is contained in Tables 9–1, 9–2, and 9–3, which present survey results on utilization patterns, based on national data that are representative of the entire United States population. These data are taken from the National Health Interview Survey (Adams & Marano, 1995), a national survey of

TABLE 9–1 Physician contacts, according to selected patient characteristics: United States, 1994

Characteristic	Physician Contacts Per Person
Total	6.0
Sex and age	
Male	5.2
Under 5 years	7.0
5–14 years	3.5
15–44 years	3.7
45–64 years	6.3
65–74 years	10.1
75 years and over	11.6
Female	6.7
Under 5 years	6.5
5–14 years	3.3
15–44 years	6.2
45–64 years	8.3
65–74 years	10.5
75 years and over	13.4
Family income	
Less than $14,000	7.6
$14,000–$24,999	5.9
$25,000–$34,999	5.8
$35,000–$49,999	6.2
$50,000 or more	6.0
Geographic region	
Northeast	5.9
Midwest	6.0
South	5.6
West	6.4

SOURCE: *Health, United States, 1996–97,* National Center for Health Statistics, 1997, Hyattsville, MD: Public Health Service.

Americans' use of health care services, and they complement the utilization data presented in previous chapters.

Table 9–1 describes the number of physician contacts experienced by Americans in various sex

TABLE 9–2 Physician contacts, according to place of contact and selected patient characteristics: United States, 1994

Characteristic	Place of Contact (Percentage)				
	Doctor's office	Hospital outpatient department[a]	Telephone	Home	Other[b]
Total	56.8	13.6	13.2	3.5	12.8
Age					
Under 15 years	60.6	13.1	14.3	0.8	11.1
Under 5 years	59.2	12.7	15.4	0.9	11.8
5–14 years	62.1	13.5	13.1	0.8	10.5
5–44 years	55.7	14.1	13.1	1.8	15.2
45–64 years	55.1	15.0	14.2	3.6	12.2
65 years and over	53.4	10.1	8.6	18.6	9.3
65–74 years	55.4	11.9	9.4	12.4	10.9
75 years and over	51.1	7.9	7.8	25.8	7.4
Sex					
Male	55.4	15.6	11.7	3.5	13.9
Female	57.7	12.2	14.3	3.5	12.2
Race					
White	58.4	12.5	14.1	3.3	11.8
Black	47.9	20.3	8.1	4.2	19.4
Family income					
Less than $14,000	43.9	19.0	11.2	5.7	19.5
$14,000–$24,999	53.8	16.0	13.0	3.9	12.7
$25,000–$34,999	61.5	13.8	12.7	2.0	11.6
$35,000–$49,999	56.9	11.5	16.3	3.9	11.2
$50,000 or more	63.8	9.4	15.5	1.6	9.8
Geographic region					
Northeast	59.0	13.0	12.8	4.0	11.2
Midwest	55.8	14.0	15.1	2.2	12.9
South	58.4	14.0	12.5	4.3	10.8
West	54.1	13.5	12.8	3.2	16.5

a   Includes hospital outpatient clinic, emergency room, and other hospital contacts
b   Includes clinics or other places outside a hospital

SOURCE: *Health, United States, 1996–97,* National Center for Health Statistics, 1997, Hyattsville, MD: Public Health Service.

and age categories as well as for family income and geographic regions. The very young and the very old report higher utilization of ambulatory services, and females generally experience higher utilization than males. The lowest-income groups in our population, not coincidentally those of lower health status as well, experience the highest utilization of ambulatory services when the data are examined by

TABLE 9–3 Interval since last physician contact, according to selected patient characteristics: United States, 1994

Characteristic	Percent Distribution		
	Less than 1 year	*One year to less than 2 years*	*Two years or more*
Sex and age			
Male	74.2	10.7	15.2
Under 15 years	84.8	9.5	5.7
15–44 years	63.8	13.7	22.6
45–64 years	73.5	9.3	17.2
65–74 years	85.9	5.2	8.9
75 years and over	90.5	3.5	6.0
Female	84.1	8.3	7.5
Under 15 years	84.7	9.7	5.6
15–44 years	82.2	9.2	8.5
45–64 years	83.8	6.8	9.3
65–74 years	89.5	4.3	6.2
75 years and over	92.0	3.3	4.7
Family income			
Less than $14,000	78.0	9.2	12.7
$14,000–$24,999	76.0	10.2	13.8
$25,000–$34,999	78.5	9.9	11.6
$35,000–$49,999	79.8	9.4	10.8
$50,000 or more	83.7	8.3	8.0
Geographic region			
Northeast	83.4	8.1	8.6
Midwest	79.5	9.4	11.1
South	77.3	10.5	12.2
West	78.4	9.2	12.4

SOURCE: *Health, United States, 1996–97,* National Center for Health Statistics, 1997, Hyattsville, MD: Public Health Service.

income groups. In examining the data by geographic regions, ambulatory services utilization is highest in those areas where managed care is most prevalent, particularly the West and Midwest regions of the country.

Examining these data by place of contact (Table 9–2) reflects higher utilization of hospital outpatient departments by minorities and by those individuals with lower incomes. Relatively little care,

except in the oldest age groups, is provided in patients' homes, quite a contrast from years gone by.

Table 9–3, also based on data from the National Health Interview Survey, indicates that most Americans have utilized physician resources in the prior year, with relatively few individuals reporting no utilization for two or more years. Again, females are more likely to report utilization for one- and two-year periods as compared to males, and the very young and the very old are also more likely to use services within the prior one or two years.

Use of Office Setting Services

Most utilization data are available from survey research results. To obtain more detailed information on health care use in physician office settings, the federal government has conducted periodic surveys of private, office-based physicians—the National Ambulatory Medical Care Survey (Woodwell, 1997). This survey involves a random sample of the nation's office-based, nonfederal physicians. Physicians are asked to complete a data collection form for each patient treated during a two-week interval.

Tables 9–4 and 9–5 list the most common reasons and the principal diagnoses for all office visits, respectively. The relative prominence of routine care, of follow-up or ongoing care, and of relatively simple primary care is rather striking and reflects the predominance of "routine," day-to-day needs of patients seeking ambulatory care services.

TABLE 9–4 Number and percent distribution of office visits by the twenty principal reasons most frequently mentioned by patients, according to patient's sex: United States, 1996

Principal Reason for Visit	Number of Visits in Thousands	Patient's Sex (Percent Distribution)	
		Female	Male
All visits	734,493	100.0	100.0
General medical examination	50,669	7.4	6.2
Progress visit, not otherwise specified	28,804	3.6	4.4
Routine prenatal examination	23,948	5.5	—
Cough	22,800	3.0	3.3
Postoperative visit	18,663	2.6	2.4
Symptoms referable to throat	17,967	2.2	2.8
Well-baby examination	15,236	1.8	2.4
Skin rash	11,997	1.6	1.6
Stomach pain, cramps, and spasms	11,721	1.7	1.4
Back symptoms	11,438	1.5	1.7
Earache or ear infection	11,321	1.5	1.7
Nasal congestion	11,245	1.4	1.7
Fever	10,719	1.1	2.0
Vision dysfunctions	10,410	1.5	1.4
Knee symptoms	9,822	1.2	1.5
Hypertension	9,719	1.2	1.5
Blood pressure test	8,554	1.0	1.3
Chest pain and related symptoms	8,190	1.0	1.3
Depression	8,169	1.2	1.0
Headache, pain in head	8,126	1.2	0.9
All other reasons	424,975	56.8	59.5

SOURCE: *National Ambulatory Medical Care Survey: 1996 Summary* (Advance data from vital and health statistics; No. 295), D. A. Woodwell, 1997, Hyattsville, MD: National Center for Health Statistics.

Further understanding of the nature of the visits is obtainable from additional data regarding the services provided to patients and the interactions shared between patients and physicians. Table 9–6 presents the source of payment for patients. The principal sources of payment for patient office visits are private and commercial insurance, Medicare, and HMOs and other managed care arrangements. The percentage of visits included in this last cate-gory likely will increase in future years while man-aged care grows in popularity. The drugs prescribed during the physician office visits included are clas-sified in Table 9–7. The most prevalent categories of drugs include cardiovascular and renal, anti-microbial, and pain-relief agents. As technology changes, the classification distribution of various drug categories will likely change in prevalence as well.

TABLE 9–5 Number and percent distribution of office visits by selected principal diagnosis groups, according to patient's sex: United States, 1996

Principal Diagnosis Group	Number of Visits in Thousands	Patient's Sex (Percent Distribution)	
		Female	Male
All visits	734,493	100.0	100.0
Essential hypertension	27,690	3.4	4.3
Acute upper respiratory infections, excluding pharyngitis	27,063	3.3	4.3
Routine infant or child health check	25,275	2.9	4.2
Normal pregnancy	24,530	5.6	—
Malignant neoplasms	21,431	2.4	3.7
General medical examination	19,708	3.0	2.3
Otitis media and Eustachian tube disorders	18,848	2.0	3.3
Arthropathies and related disorders	16,243	2.3	2.0
Diabetes mellitus	15,896	2.0	2.4
Dorsopathies	14,299	1.7	2.2
Chronic sinusitis	14,295	1.9	2.0
Rheumatism, excluding back	14,065	2.1	1.6
Chronic and unspecified bronchitis	10,253	1.2	1.7
Ischemic heart disease	10,216	1.0	2.0
Acute pharyngitis	10,065	1.2	1.7
Heart disease, excluding ischemic	9,861	1.3	1.4
Asthma	9,051	1.3	1.2
Sprains and strains of neck and back	8,663	1.2	1.2
Allergic rhinitis	8,376	1.0	1.3
Potential health hazards related to personal and family history	7,793	1.1	1.1
All other	420,872	58.1	56.1

SOURCE: *National Ambulatory Medical Care Survey: 1996 Summary* (Advance data from vital and health statistics; No. 295), D. A. Woodwell, 1997, Hyattsville, MD: National Center for Health Statistics.

TABLE 9–6 Number and percent of office visits by patient's source of payment: United States, 1996

Source of Payment[a]	Number of Visits in Thousands	Percent Distribution
All visits	734,493	100.0
Insurance	639,065	87.0
Insured, fee-for-service	263,878	35.9
Other	16,104	2.2
Unknown	7,336	1.0
HMO/other preiaid	190,804	26.0
Private insurance	100,513	13.7
Other	36,716	5.0
Unknown	24,647	3.4
Preferred Provider Option	98,318	13.4
Private insurance	69,730	9.5
Other	12,452	1.7
Unknown	6,014	0.8
Unspecified type of payment	86,065	11.7
Private insurance	23,634	3.2
Other	5,812	0.8
Unknown	2,662	0.4
Self-pay	64,016	8.7
No charge	8,142	1.1
Other	11,233	1.5
No answer	12,038	1.6

a   Only one type of payment (preferred provider option, insured fee-for-service, HMO/other prepaid, self-pay, no charge, or other) was coded for each visit. These figures may not always add to totals because of rounding. For payment types of preferred provider option, insured fee-for-service, and HMO/other prepaid, respondents were also asked to check all of the applicable expected sources of insurance. As a result, expected sources of insurance will not add to totals because more than one source could be reported per visit.

SOURCE: *National Ambulatory Medical Care Survey: 1996 Summary* (Advance data from vital and health statistics; No. 295), D. A. Woodwell, 1997, Hyattsville, MD: National Center for Health Statistics.

Table 9–8 presents the distribution of office visits by the duration of the visit. Relatively few visits require either very short or very long physician contacts. The typical physician office visit requires only about five to thirty minutes of time; nearly three-fourths of all visits require fifteen minutes or less. A high percentage of visits concluded with the recommendation that the patient return at a specified time interval for a follow-up visit.

The National Ambulatory Medical Care Survey thus provides some insight into the nature of office-based ambulatory care. Much more extensive documentation of the survey and results for various types of services, providers, and patient characteristics is available from the federal government. The survey data are an aid to planning health services in the ambulatory care setting and provide perspectives on national patterns of utilization. The applicability of the data to setting standards of

TABLE 9–7 Number and percent distribution of drug mentions by therapeutic classification: United States, 1996

Therapeutic Classification	Number of Drug Mentions in Thousands	Percent Distribution
All drug mentions	983,718	100.0
Cardiovascular-renal drugs	144,445	14.7
Antimicrobial agents	124,272	12.6
Drugs used for relief of pain	114,158	11.6
Respiratory tract drugs	101,571	10.3
Hormones and agents affecting hormonal mechanisms	92,440	9.4
Central nervous system	72,455	7.4
Skin/mucous membrane	62,995	6.4
Metabolic and nutrient agents	53,407	5.4
Gastrointestinal agents	44,196	4.5
Immunologic agents	39,729	4.0
Ophthalmic drugs	29,732	3.0
Neurologic drugs	23,433	2.4
Hematologic agents	17,677	1.8
Oncolytic agents	10,205	1.0
Other and unclassified	53,002	5.4

Note: Numbers may not add to totals because of rounding.

SOURCE: *National Ambulatory Medical Care Survey: 1996 Summary* (Advance data from vital and health statistics; No. 295), D. A. Woodwell, 1997, Hyattsville, MD: National Center for Health Statistics.

performance in managed care settings or under contracted agreements for service, however, is limited because of the many variables that could not be adequately measured.

AMBULATORY PRACTICE SETTINGS

Significant differences exist among physician practice settings, and these are discussed in the following sections of this chapter. The two primary noninstitutional settings for the provision of ambulatory care are solo and group practice. Each of these settings may be a component of larger systems of care through such integrating mechanisms as referral arrangements, insurance contracts, and direct ownership of practices. An organized system of care can, in turn, be comprised of various settings or types of ambulatory care providers.

Although the solo practice of medicine has traditionally attracted the greatest number of practitioners, group practice and institutionally based services are now expanding dramatically, continuing a trend that has been building over the past thirty years. Changing lifestyles, the cost of establishing a practice, personal financial pressures on practitioners, contracting and affiliation opportunities under managed care, and the burdens of running a business have enhanced the attractiveness of group practice for many physicians. With sharp increases in the number of physicians beginning practice, the growth of alternative settings, and especially of group practice, has been dramatic.

TABLE 9–8 Number and percent distribution of office visits by duration of visit: United States, 1996

Duration	Number of Visits in Thousands	Percent Distribution
All visits	734,493	100.0
0 minutes[a]	108,164	14.7
1–5 minutes	30,348	4.1
6–10 minutes	136,690	18.6
11–15 minutes	214,076	29.1
16–30 minutes	194,098	26.4
31–60 minutes	46,223	6.3
61 minutes and over	4,893	0.7

a Visits in which there was no face-to-face contact between patient and physician

Note: Numbers may not add to totals because of rounding.

SOURCE: *National Ambulatory Medical Care Survey: 1996 Summary* (Advance data from vital and health statistics; No. 295), D. A. Woodwell, 1997, Hyattsville, MD: National Center for Health Statistics.

Although solo practice remains an important avenue for providing ambulatory care services, these other settings have rapidly assumed a more prominent and visible role in the health care system, particularly as they provide a further mechanism for the integration, management, and control of health care services.

Solo Practice

Solo practitioners are difficult to uniformly characterize. Early sociological studies focused on specific questions, such as referral patterns or quality of care, and they did not provide a comprehensive picture of what the solo practitioner does. The studies that did contribute to a more complete understanding of the activities of solo practitioners were based on physicians in one geographic area or a particular specialty, and the results of these stud-

ies, although interesting and useful, may not be applicable to other practices or areas. In addition, solo practitioners are heterogeneous; they include many types of health care professionals who provide an immense array of services.

Many solo practitioners are subspecialists who provide secondary care primarily on referral from primary care practitioners. Under managed care, these subspecialists are being squeezed by reduced payment for specialty services, by capitation payment for population coverage, and by the increasing trend for gate-keepers to perform services that otherwise might have been referred to subspecialists. Some subspecialists provide both primary and secondary care, since they have insufficient work in their own specialties to achieve desired income levels.

Many solo practitioners, including those trained in general and family practice, internal medicine, pediatrics, and obstetrics and gynecology, provide primary care services. There is some controversy and competition among practitioners concerning which specialists should be providing primary care. The specialty of family practice, in particular, represents a challenge to general internal medicine in providing adult primary care and to pediatrics in providing child care, although the role of family practice is now firmly established, especially in managed care.

Most solo practitioners perform a number of functions in the office, including patient care, consultations, and administration and supervision of office staff. The requirements for administration and for supervision of personnel have been increasing in recent years. Solo practitioners are increasingly affiliating with managed care networks that help ensure a viable patient population.

Solo practice is often associated with an increased feeling that the provider cares about the welfare of the patient, possibly resulting in a stronger patient-provider relationship than occurs in other settings. There is some evidence that this situation, where it occurs, is a result of the lower level of bureaucracy or organizational complexity in solo practice. Since there is also some evidence that the relationship between patient and physician is related to patient compliance with medical regimens, patients who perceive that they are receiving more personalized care may respond to the care process more positively.

Solo practitioners may not be as restricted in referrals to specialists as are providers in some other settings, such as group practice, where organizational loyalties intervene. Managed care contracts, however, may severely limit referral options.

The solo practitioner may feel a greater identification with the community served, since there is a more direct relationship between patient and provider. Organizational forms, especially managed care, that incorporate solo practitioners into larger systems of care may be decreasing some of this physician-patient bond, especially as providers are forced to discount fees, increase productivity, and focus on the cost-effectiveness of their practices.

From the provider's perspective, solo practice offers an opportunity to avoid organizational dependence and to be self-employed; there is also no need to share resources or income with other providers. Philosophically, solo practice is most closely aligned with the traditional economic and political organizations that have characterized medicine; younger physicians faced with discounting, contracting, and networks for care, however, may no longer identify with the more traditional perspectives.

All of the increasingly complex problems of administering a practice must be dealt with in solo practice unless a professional manager is hired. Furthermore, competitive pressures in the health care industry are leading many practitioners to question the feasibility and desirability of going it alone. Many solo practitioners are now affiliated

with larger entities such as independent practice associations, practice management companies, and other organizations. Thus solo practice offers distinct opportunities and has philosophical and emotional appeal but is far from devoid of problems and constraints, especially in light of the realities of medical practice today.

Group Practice

Office-based practice includes, in addition to solo practice, group practice. This form of practice has been growing in popularity in recent years, especially as the increasing pressures of practice have led many providers to seek alternative settings in which to work.

Group practice is an affiliation of three or more providers, usually physicians, who share income, expenses, facilities, equipment, medical records, and support personnel in the provision of services through a formal, legally constituted organization. The formal definition of group practice, developed by the American Medical Association and the Medical Group Management Association, is three or more physicians formally organized to provide medical care, consultation, diagnosis, and/or treatment through the joint use of equipment and personnel, and with income from medical practice distributed in accordance with methods previously determined by members of the group. Although definitions of a group practice vary somewhat, the essential element is formal sharing of resources and income.

Traditionally, group practice has meant participation and ownership by physicians. Increasingly, however, as new and more diversified models for the provision of services are developed, other practitioners will participate in group practices. In some communities, for example, group practices of nurse practitioners may be the only sources of health services. Dentists, optometrists, podiatrists, and other specialized personnel are also increasingly developing group practices.

History of Group Practice. Some of the earliest group practices in the United States were started by companies that needed to provide care to employees in rural sites where medical care was unobtainable. For example, the Northern Pacific Railroad organized a practice in 1883 to provide care to employees building the transcontinental railroad. This industrial clinic was one of a number of such clinics founded in the nineteenth century.

Even more significant, however, was the establishment of the Mayo Clinic in Rochester, Minnesota—the first successful nonindustrial group practice. The Mayo Clinic, originally organized as a single-specialty group practice in 1887 and later broadened into a multispecialty group, demonstrated that group practice was feasible in the private sector. The Mayo Clinic also represented a reputable model for group practice in a national atmosphere of fierce independence where group practice was viewed with skepticism and distrust. By the early 1930s there were about one hundred and fifty medical groups throughout the country, many of which were located in the Midwest. Most included or were started by someone who had practiced or trained at the Mayo Clinic.

In 1932 a national committee, the Committee on the Costs of Medical Care, was established to assess health care needs for the nation. It issued a report that suggested a major role for group practice in the provision of medical care. The committee recommended that these groups be associated with hospitals to provide comprehensive care and that there be prepayment for all services. The report strongly supported the concept of regionalization that eventually gained wide recognition in the establishment of the British National Health Service, our own military health care systems, and other national models of organized health service systems.

Other constituencies, including some unions, also developed group practices. After World War II, a number of pioneering groups were established. In New York City, the Health Insurance Plan of New York was organized to provide prepaid medical care to the employees of the city—an idea promoted by Mayor Fiorello LaGuardia. On the West Coast, the Kaiser Foundation Health Plan was established to provide health care to employees of Kaiser Industries; Kaiser is an affiliation of plans and providers that is now serving millions of Americans across the nation. In Seattle, a revolutionary development included the establishment of Group Health Cooperative of Puget Sound, a consumer-owned cooperative prepaid group practice. It was founded by progressive individuals who were dissatisfied with the private medical care available to them in the late 1940s.

Developments in medical practice also spurred the group practice movement. Perhaps most notable was the increasing specialization of medicine and the rapid expansion of technology. This increasing sophistication meant that no individual practitioner could provide all the expertise that patients would require. It also meant that more complex and expensive facilities, equipment, and personnel were needed to care for patients. Group practice provided a formal structure for sharing these costs among providers. Many people believed that resources would be used more efficiently in groups. In addition, multispecialty groups, encompassing more than one specialty, could provide patients with more of their health care under one roof and, hence, reduce problems of physical access to care and coordination of services.

Group practice was also thought to promote higher-quality care, since most of the different specialists that a person required would be practicing together and would thus have the opportunity to discuss patient problems among themselves, share a common medical record, and be more able to ensure the quality and continuity of care. Therefore, group practice was viewed by many as being advantageous for the physician—offering opportunities such as easily developed referral arrangements, sharing of after-hours coverage, greater flexibility in working hours, and less financial risk—while also benefiting the patient.

Opposition to group practice occurred mostly for political and philosophical reasons. The American Medical Association and local medical societies have, at times, opposed group practice. Many early group practices had difficulties when physicians were denied admitting privileges in local hospitals. Community-based specialists sometimes refused to treat patients referred by group practice physicians. In more recent years, however, opposition to group practice has lessened dramatically, and restrictive laws have been challenged. The need to form affiliations for contracting under reimbursement programs and for achieving efficiencies in organizing health services more generally has resulted in little remaining formal opposition to group practice.

Survey of Group Practice. The American Medical Association has conducted surveys of physician-oriented medical group practices in the United States on a periodic basis since 1965. These surveys represent the most comprehensive data available concerning the growth and characteristics of group practice in this country. Group practices that qualified within the American Medical Association's definition were identified from a variety of data sources and were then surveyed through a mail data collection instrument. Numerous items of information were collected regarding the nature of the practice and its facilities and relationships to other entities.

The dramatic increase in popularity of practices is reflected in Table 9–9. The number of reporting

TABLE 9–9 Number of medical groups and number of physicians in group practice: United States, selected years

Year	Total Number of Groups	Number of Physician Positions in Group Practice
1969	6,371	40,093
1975	8,488	66,842
1980	10,762	88,290
1984	15,186	139,127
1988	16,495	155,628
1991	16,576	184,358
1995	19,787	210,811

SOURCE: Adapted from *Medical Groups in the U.S., 1996 Edition. A Survey of Practice Characteristics,* by P. L. Havlicek, 1996, Chicago: American Medical Association.

group practices has more than doubled since 1975. There are now over 16,000 group practices in the United States, the majority of which are single-specialty groups.

Even more dramatic is the growth in the number of physicians in a group-practice setting. Over 155,000 physicians in the United States are now working in group practices, which represents a marked increase from 67,000 in 1975 and 88,000 in 1980. A higher percentage of all physicians in group practice work in multispecialty-oriented groups as compared to the percentage of total groups that are multispecialty, largely because the average multispecialty group is substantially larger than the average single-specialty group. The average size of all group practices in the United States in 1988 was about nine physicians, an increase from 1980. These data reflect only physician "positions" and exclude other medically related professionals such as nurse practitioners.

Most group practices are professional corporations. The dramatic shift toward professional corporations since 1969 is primarily a result of changes in federal and state laws pertaining to taxation, the increasing size and complexity of the practices themselves, and interrelationships among physicians participating. Changes in federal tax law may result in further shifts in patterns of legal organizational forms.

Specialty distribution of physicians in group practice has not changed dramatically in recent years. The specialties that account for the largest percentage of physicians participating in group practice include family and general practice, internal medicine, anesthesiology, obstetrics and gynecology, pediatrics, and radiology; many groups are now involved in managed care contracting.

Relatively few groups account for a significant percentage of all physicians in group practice as presented in Table 9–10. There are relatively few groups that employ more than fifteen physicians. As would be expected, most of the larger groups are multispecialty, while the smaller groups are predominantly single specialty.

The geographic distribution of group practice in the United States is dominated by seven states, which account for forty percent of all groups. These states are California, Pennsylvania, New York, Texas, Illinois, Florida, and Ohio. The origin, growth, and current distribution of group practice and group practice physicians are not homogeneous throughout the various regions, which reflects a greater acceptance of group practice in some regions as well as a varied distribution of larger urban population centers in the country. As might be expected, physician groups and group-practice physicians are substantially more prominent in metropolitan areas than in nonmetropolitan areas of the country. The development of prepaid group practice also varies by region.

Interestingly, most group practices employed a business manager or administrator, although far fewer had an identifiable medical director. Multispecialty groups were more likely to employ a group administrator, and, as might be expected, larger groups were much more likely to employ administrators and have medical directors than were smaller groups. Nearly all the larger groups did employ an administrator. The market for trained group-practice administrators has grown substantially over the past few years, and its growth is likely to continue as the number of group practices increases.

TABLE 9–10   Total groups and group physician positions by size of group, 1995

Size of Group	Groups		Group Physician Positions	
	Percent	*Number*	*Percent*	*Number*
3–4	45.9	8,926	14.7	30,941
5–6	22.9	4,451	11.4	23,929
7–9	12.6	2,453	9.0	19,001
10–15	8.8	1,714	9.6	20,337
16–25	4.8	943	8.8	18,576
26–49	2.7	527	8.6	18,063
50–99	1.2	226	7.2	15,193
100 or more	1.2	238	30.7	64,770

SOURCE: Adapted from *Medical Groups in the U.S., 1996 Edition. A Survey of Practice Characteristics,* by P. L. Havlicek, 1996, Chicago: American Medical Association.

New Forms of Group Practice

Managed care has led to the development of new forms of group practice to allow physicians alternative settings in which to participate in contracting arrangements such as the independent practice associations (IPAs) discussed in Chapter 6. Most of this innovation is the result of the need to form contractual arrangements with health systems, managed care organizations, and insurers. These new organizational forms are continuing to evolve. Smaller practices, in particular, have needed to seek out alliances that facilitate contractual arrangements under managed care. Smaller practices face disadvantages with regard to availability of capital investment, professional management, and often overhead and other costs. Larger practices and new approaches to creating affiliations of groups facilitate potential economies of scale, efficiencies in management and operations, improved contracting potential and market involvement, and enhanced deployment of capital.

Group practices may be formed by or affiliated with larger organizations such as hospitals or health systems. The larger entity may provide capital, management services, patient flows, and contracting assistance to the smaller group. Groups may be affiliated with one another through various mechanisms which may provide management services and contracting potential for solo and smaller group practitioners while preserving a degree of independence for these practitioners. A group practice without walls is another avenue utilized to affiliate practitioners—in essence, practices are merged but are able to maintain their existing locations with administrative services carried out in a central office or through a contract with a management services organization. There are increasing numbers of for-profit management companies and some not-for-profit entities providing these services to physician groups and, in some instances, actually purchasing groups outright, as well.

From a pragmatic point of view, many of these new forms of group practice are designed to facilitate the participation of solo- and group-practice physicians in the rapidly changing world of managed care where practices must be managed efficiently and have easy access to contracting mechanisms. The specific legal and operational approaches to organizing these integrated forms of group practice vary considerably and are continuing to evolve. Key issues include physician autonomy and involvement in governance and management; sources and uses of capital investment; control over physician clinical practice patterns; extent of control by a larger entity over physician staff, facilities, and daily operation; and relationships with other entities such as hospitals, insurers, managed care organizations, and, of course, patients. Many physicians and physician practices as well as other provider organizations may elect to continue within the more traditional parameters of such managed care organizations as independent practice associations and preferred provider organizations. Other practices may determine that the assistance available through management-related contractual arrangements warrants the loss of autonomy. Finally, some practitioners may simply sell out to hospitals, health systems, physician management companies, and other organizations and elect to focus on their clinical practice itself.

An Assessment of Group Practice

A critical assessment of group practice yields distinct advantages and disadvantages for both patients and providers as compared to other modalities for providing ambulatory services. Some of these are summarized in Table 9–11. Specific advantages and disadvantages vary from group to group, and Table 9–11 also lists major considerations generally associated with group practice.

TABLE 9–11   Some advantages and disadvantages of group practice[a]

Advantages	Disadvantages
From perspective of the provider	
Availability of professional manager	Less individual freedom
Organizational responsibility for patient	Possible excessive use of specialists
Less physician administrative time	Fewer outside consultants
Shared capital expense	Possible reduced identity with patient and community
Shared financial risk	Group rather than individual decision making
Improved contracting and negotiating ability	Sharing of all problems
Better coverage and shared on-call shifts	Necessity of working with others
More flexible working hours	Less individual incentive and more orientation toward security
More peer interaction	
Increased access to specialists	Income limitations
Broader array of ancillary services	Income distribution arguments
Stable income for providers	
No direct financial concerns with patient	
Lower initial investment	
More time for continuing education	
More flexible vacation time	
Generally excellent benefits	
Possible efficiencies of scale	
Use of nonphysician practitioners	
From perspective of the patient	
Care under one roof	Possible lessening of provider-patient relationship
Availability of specialists, laboratories, and so on	Possible overuse of ancillary services
Improved coverage and emergency care	Possible high provider turnover
Central location of medical and administrative records	Heavy patient loads and possible increase in waiting time
Simplified referrals	Less provider incentive for care
Peer interaction among providers	More bureaucracy
Better administration of group	
Possible promotion of efficiency in patient care	

a   Some advantages and disadvantages could be included under both provider and patient categories.

Some of the topics listed under patient or provider perspectives could readily pertain to both.

The advantages of group practice from the perspective of the provider include shared operation of the practice; joint ownership of facilities and equipment; centralized administrative functions; and, in larger groups, a professional manager. The professional manager can provide expertise in areas often lacking among the providers such as billing; personnel management; patient scheduling; ordering of supplies; and, recently, of particular importance, negotiating, contracting, and related matters.

Financially, the group relieves the provider of the heavy initial investment often required to establish a practice. In most groups, however, coownership requires that new members buy into the group through purchase of a share of the group's capital over a period of time.

The burden of operating costs is also lessened for any individual member of a group. Rather than having to independently absorb the ups and downs of a practice, as do solo practitioners, those involved in a group practice share the income and expenses within the group, allowing for moderation of those fluctuations experienced in individual practices. For example, a solo practitioner who becomes ill may have no practice income aside from disability insurance, whereas a group member's income may continue during a short period of illness, since other providers are simultaneously generating revenue. However, the provisions of income distribution plans vary substantially among groups.

The participation of physicians in group practice also has a significant advantage in facilitating the development of definitive arrangements for contracting and negotiating. The group can support increased levels of participation, has a knowledgeable group practice administrator to manage the contracts, and can respond to the market with a wider range of services. Even single-specialty groups, with shared on-call services and subspecialization of group members, are able to offer more to the market on a contractual basis than the individual practitioner. Having a professional manager to negotiate on behalf of the group further enhances the relative attractiveness of group practice, particularly for physicians who lack experience in interpreting and negotiating contracts.

Patient care responsibilities are also shared in group practice. This sharing results in greater flexibility of working hours for the provider, as well as more time for vacation and continuing education, without sacrificing the quality of care for the patient. For example, providers cover for each other during vacations and after normal working hours. Although most practitioners in solo practice arrange for patient care coverage, the continuity of care and the extent of coverage are probably greater in group practice, since the patients' medical records and the full resources of the group are always available, even if specific providers are not working.

Sharing of patient care may have some other potential benefits. These include more peer interaction as a result of informal discussions and referral of patients among providers. The inclusion of more providers also results in the availability, by necessity, of a wider range of specialists and ancillary services, which represents a convenience for both providers and patients as well as a source of added revenue for the group.

Does the sharing of administrative and patient care activities within group practice produce better care at lower cost? Although many people believe that effective group management uses resources more efficiently than solo practice, the evidence is mixed. Some evidence tends to refute this belief, but more analytical research indicates some economies of scale, or efficiencies, attributable to the grouping of resources for smaller groups, but possibly less so for larger and more bureaucratic groups. The use of personnel may be more advantageous in group than solo practice. Receptionists, medical records specialists, laboratory and radiology technicians, nurses, and other types of personnel may be used more efficiently and in the specialized areas of their training in many medium- and larger-sized groups. In addition, there is some question about whether any savings that are achieved will be returned to consumers or simply represent higher income for providers. Further, the increasing supply of physicians may reduce the desirability of employing mid-level practitioners, except in certain prepaid settings.

The effect of groups on patient care, especially on the quality of care, is an important issue. Sharing of medical records, peer interaction, easy referrals and consultations with specialists, more sophisticated and accessible ancillary services, and more skilled and diversified support personnel are all arguments suggested in support of higher-quality care in group practice. Pressures from managed care contracts, however, may affect quality-related issues such as use, access, and appropriateness of care.

Group practice also offers advantages to patients and their communities. For the patient, the group offers a wide range of services under one roof so that travel between providers is reduced and access increased. A unified medical record can contribute to continuity of care and less duplication in diagnosis and treatment. Some groups also own or operate hospitals and thus further extend the integration and scope of the services that they provide, an especially important consideration in negotiating with employers and insurers.

Group practices usually offer more accessible care after normal working hours. Some groups also offer emergency services through their own emergency rooms or clinics. Groups with a broader community perspective may even be involved in programs such as school health services and community immunization efforts, and the use of a professional manager should benefit the patient through more efficient scheduling and patient flow and improved overall management of the practice.

On a communitywide basis, group practice may offer a means of attracting providers to areas with inadequate numbers of medical care personnel. By offering peer interaction, support services, and other advantages, groups may increase the appeal of practicing in rural or inadequately served urban centers.

There are also distinct disadvantages to group practice for providers, patients, and communities. From the perspective of the provider, practicing in a group implies less individual freedom, with a variety of restrictions imposed through the sharing of a practice. Ideologically, the limitations of a group in this regard may be difficult for some people to accept, since medicine has traditionally been an individualistic enterprise. In addition to reduced freedom, group practice entails sharing responsibilities and problems with others. The interpersonal requirements for working out these responsibilities may not appeal to all practitioners. Older individuals who have been working in solo practice may be especially unlikely to adapt readily to group practice.

The financial advantages for group practice are a trade-off against some restrictions on income generation and the necessity of complying with the group's income distribution and practice pattern requirements. Thus, there often is more security and less risk but also less incentive and reward for individual initiative and production.

The shift of some patient care responsibilities from the individual practitioner to the group may adversely affect the patient-provider relationship by introducing a degree of impersonalization. If a group has high physician turnover, which is rare, patients may have to change providers frequently. Groups that have too few providers for the number of patients they serve, a common occurrence when excess capacity is being avoided, especially under managed care financial pressures, also have waiting times for appointments in the office that patients may believe to be excessive. The group may impose greater restrictions on referral practices, consequently limiting the practitioner's willingness to use the expertise of other specialists in the community.

From a community perspective, groups may reduce the geographic dispersion of providers and thus increase difficulties of physical access to care. In addition, groups may reduce competition in the health care marketplace by consolidating what would otherwise be competing providers. Consolidation may eventually reduce the ability of insurers, employers, and other plan sponsors to negotiate favorable terms for contracted care.

The changing organizational structure of the health care system is also changing some aspects of the role of ambulatory care services from the perspectives of providers, consumers, and the community. Ambulatory care is assuming a much greater role in the rationing of care, especially for primary care, and in the control of referrals and use of specialty, laboratory, and other services. These changes are especially notable in managed care and for hospital-sponsored systems of care. Ambulatory care is substantially affecting other provider organizations, especially the hospital, as more and more care is provided on an ambulatory basis. There are important fiscal, organizational, and utilization implications for all components of the system as a result of these changes.

The implications of these structural changes in the provision of health care are profound. Consumers are affected in terms of where and how they receive services. Providers are affected by changes in their affiliations, referral patterns, incentives, and practice characteristics. And, finally, the community is obviously affected by the changing organization of services, by the formation of alliances, and by shifts in the economic and political clout of various providers.

INSTITUTIONALLY BASED AMBULATORY SERVICES

In addition to solo and group practice in the traditional private sector, many institutions have expanded their involvement in ambulatory care. These institutionally based settings, especially those associated with hospitals, are discussed next.

The hospital has evolved from an institution for poor people who could not be cared for at home to a provider of a full range of health services from primary to tertiary care. As technological advances have brought more services into the hospital and expanded the scope of care provided, the hospital has assumed an especially important role in the provision of highly complex health services. At the same time, an increasing number of people have sought primary care from hospitals, sometimes as a result of lack of access to other sources of care.

Outpatient and Ambulatory Care Clinics

The increased demands placed on hospitals for care taxed the ability of many facilities to respond with appropriate and adequate resources. The result was overcrowded facilities; the wrong mix of services, equipment, and personnel to respond to patient needs; and extremely dissatisfied consumers and providers. Most hospitals have now successfully responded to these demands by expanding outpatient services and hiring full-time providers to staff redesigned hospital ambulatory facilities.

Traditional hospital outpatient services have been provided in clinics and emergency rooms. In many hospitals, clinics have had second-class status as compared to complex and expensive inpatient services. However, as hospitals are increasingly recognizing the important role of primary care, especially in managed care contracting, and are seeking to expand the base of patients who are potential users of inpatient and ancillary services, more attention is being directed toward improving clinic operations and services.

Hospital clinics include both primary care and specialty clinics. Many hospitals differentiate between clinics for walk-in patients without appointments and those for scheduled visits. Specialty clinics are usually organized by department and provide services such as ophthalmology, neurology, and allergy care. In teaching hospitals, clinics serve as important settings in which house staff members provide ongoing care to patients and follow-up after hospitalization. Increasingly, clinics also provide an opportunity to expose medical students and house staff to ambulatory care services in order to complement the traditionally more extensive experience with inpatient care. With ambulatory care's increasing role in health services, this trend is significant.

Many hospital primary-care clinics evolved from an orientation of service to the poor and were staffed by physicians who served without reimbursement in exchange for staff privileges. The level of commitment to the patient under such circumstances was, not surprisingly, less than desirable. Many hospitals now employ physicians and other practitioners as full-time clinic staff. Some hospitals have established primary-care group practices to complement other outpatient services and to assume the burden of providing primary care to patients who seek most of their care from the hospital.

The development of a group practice has advantages for both consumers and the hospital by providing comprehensive and accessible care and by removing primary-care patients from facilities that are not designed to serve their needs, such as emergency rooms. Development of these group practices also has the potential of increasing use of the hospital's inpatient and ancillary services, an advantage if occupancy is low. Hospitals with ambulatory care resources can negotiate contracts for providing a wide range of both inpatient and outpatient services. They are subsequently also able to more effectively control the use of services and thus costs. Questions have been raised, however, concerning the ability of hospitals to compete effectively in an arena in which they have not been overly successful in the past. But the increasingly competitive nature of the hospital and the health care marketplace is forcing many hospitals to enter this area of practice even if they are uncertain about doing so.

Ambulatory Surgery Centers

A further innovation in hospital-based care has been the development of ambulatory surgery cen-

ters. Originating in hospitals in Washington, D.C., Los Angeles, and elsewhere, these organized hospital units provide one-day surgical care. Patients are usually screened for acceptability by their personal surgeons and then report at an assigned date and time for surgery. The surgeon is supported by the unit's facilities, equipment, and personnel, and the patient is discharged one to three hours after surgery when recovery from anesthesia is sufficiently complete.

In the early 1970s, freestanding ambulatory surgery centers were opened; one of the first was in Phoenix, Arizona. These facilities are independent of hospitals and usually provide a full range of services for the types of surgery that can be performed on an outpatient basis. Community surgeons are granted operating privileges and can perform surgery in these facilities when the patient agrees and when there are no medical contraindications.

Other facilities are also used for ambulatory or outpatient surgery. Many physicians traditionally performed surgery in their offices, although this practice has declined in some specialties as a result of malpractice concerns and the increasing availability of better-equipped and -staffed alternative facilities. Some specialties, such as oral surgery, plastic surgery, and ophthalmology, extensively use office-based facilities.

Freestanding emergency centers have also opened in many cities, paralleling the success of ambulatory surgery centers. These emergency centers sometimes provide a wide range of primary care in addition to responding to urgent problems. The future of specialized ambulatory centers, both in hospitals and as freestanding facilities, will probably include further expansion into other areas of health care, ranging from sports medicine to women's health care.

Even greater innovation has occurred in recent years. Freestanding postsurgical recovery centers for short nonhospital stays of one to three nights are under development to provide a less intensive recovery setting for less complex surgical cases. Mobile diagnostic facilities with sophisticated imaging equipment have been operational for a number of years. Even mobile physician vans are now in use to return the house call to more frequent clinical use by transporting the physician along with his/her office to the patient's home without sacrificing technological capabilities. The challenge for the future remains to identify economically feasible and innovative approaches to providing patient care that expedite the care process and are accepted by consumer, providers, and payers.

Emergency Medical Services

The emergency room, like other hospital departments, has undergone transformation in recent years. The emergency room has expanded in the range of services offered and in complexity. An especially important long-term trend has been the increasing use of the emergency room for primary care. Since the emergency room requires sophisticated facilities and highly trained personnel and must be accessible twenty-four hours a day, costs are high and services are not designed for nonurgent care. To reduce the burden on the emergency room and to meet patient need more effectively, many hospitals treat patients on a triage basis. In this process, often performed by a nurse, the patient's health care needs are determined and the patient is referred to a more appropriate source of care within the hospital. Misuse of the emergency room has received considerable attention over the past twenty years.

Emergency medical services have also been increasingly integrated with other community resources. Included are drug and alcohol treatment programs, mental health centers, and voluntary agencies. Most major urban centers have developed formal emergency medical systems that incorporate all hospital emergency rooms as well as transporta-

tion and communication systems. In these communities, people needing emergency care either transport themselves or call an emergency number (such as 911). An ambulance is dispatched by a central communications center that also identifies and alerts the most appropriately equipped and located hospital. In many communities, regional hospital-based trauma centers have been built with extremely sophisticated capabilities. Specialized ambulance services, including mobile coronary care units and shock-trauma vans, are also increasingly prevalent.

GOVERNMENT PROGRAMS

In addition to private sector and institutionally initiated efforts, government programs have been designed to increase the availability of health care resources in many communities. These programs have adapted some of the concepts of private institutional settings, especially those of group practice.

Neighborhood health centers were funded starting in 1965. Originally intended to serve approximately twenty-five million people, this federal program never reached its initial objectives. The program was designed to provide primary medical care with a family orientation. It was targeted for population groups in need of services, as reflected by such indicators as disease prevalence and income level. At the same time, the centers were intended to employ people from the communities they served in positions that would offer opportunities for training and advancement. Responsiveness to community needs was to be ensured by a community board or advisory panel. The centers were to recognize that the broad attributes of a community, such as housing and employment, contributed to health and illness.

Although these health centers were originally intended to serve the poor, changes in federal policy that encouraged them to collect fees from patients and from third-party insurers have broadened the socioeconomic mixture of patients obtaining care. However, the centers still predominantly serve the medically indigent. Sources of funding have been broadened to include local government as well. Pressures for achieving self-sufficiency have been very powerful in recent years.

A related category of provider, the "free clinic," evolved from a strong social commitment but has had to face similar financial realities. The combination of former free clinics, neighborhood health centers, public agency clinics, and some hospital clinics and groups now forms an informal "safety net" of providers for individuals who lack private insurance or access to other sources of care, or who simply need care from an available, sympathetic provider. Many of these providers now contract on their own or in coalitions with other providers to provide care to various individuals under government entitlement programs, sometimes in managed care arrangements, as well.

Other community health centers that have been funded by the federal government include migrant health centers serving transient farm workers in agricultural areas and rural health centers. The National Health Service Corps supported practitioners who were placed in urban and rural areas with shortages of medical resources. Other innovations, such as mobile health vans in rural areas, have also been used to expand the scope of services. The Community Mental Health Center program was established to provide ambulatory mental health services in underserved areas. Community mental health centers were intended to provide outpatient services and emergency care and to work with other community agencies to foster action and concern for mental health.

In recent years, community health centers have evolved into larger practices with multiple sources of support, including increasing reliance on patient fees and private donations. Many of these centers have become more businesslike in their operations. Yet most still face serious problems in attracting adequate financing, in attracting and retaining physicians, and in diversifying their patient mix, especially with regard to patients with insurance or the ability to pay for services on their own. The shift of funding for entitlement programs to prepaid contracts may provide more financial stability for some of these providers in the future. Conflicts exist in some centers over the historical mission of serving the medically indigent versus the need for enhanced fiscal diversity and adopting a more business-oriented approach to operations.

Other Federal Government Programs

The federal government, in addition to supporting a variety of community-based health services organizations, directly operates many health facilities. The Veterans Administration includes the largest health services system under a unified management structure in the United States with more than one hundred and seventy hospitals and clinics. This system provides needed care to millions of veterans throughout the nation. The military services also provide health care to millions of individuals in the armed forces and have developed extensive regionalized facilities throughout the world.

Government has a special responsibility for providing health care to a number of groups within the country. The Indian Health Service is charged with ensuring access to medical care on Indian reservations and in certain other locations. Although the difficulties of operating a largely rural system are immense, the Indian Health Service has succeeded in bringing modern medicine to many people.

NONINSTITUTIONAL AND PUBLIC HEALTH SERVICES

As noted in the introduction to this chapter, there are many ways in which ambulatory and community health services are provided. Although only the most prevalent types of provider and service are discussed here, each helps to meet the many health care needs of a community. The list is nearly endless, and a number of services warrant further discussion.

Home health services are provided by visiting nurse associations, proprietary companies, some hospitals, public health departments, and other agencies. These services allow people to remain in their homes and yet receive essential health services, thereby reducing costs and increasing the quality of life for many.

Rural health care has required unique and innovative solutions in many communities, especially in the absence of adequate supplies of physicians and facilities. In rural Alaska, many towns are served by physicians and other professionals who regularly fly in to treat patients. Satellites are used to facilitate communications with specialists in urban medical centers, since even ordinary communications in remote areas may be difficult. Rural health care in many areas remains a challenging test of the ingenuity and resourcefulness of the health services system and community residents.

Other community health services not discussed in detail here include, but are not limited to, school health services; prison health services; vision care; dental care provided by solo, group, and institutionally based practitioners; foot care from podiatrists; and drug dispensing from pharmacists, who often also extensively advise and educate consumers. Voluntary agencies also provide health care services such as cancer screening clinics and health education. Finally, many indigenous health practitioners offer their services in this country and abroad. These practitioners include chiropractors, "medicine men," naturopaths, and others. The supportive and sometimes curative role of these individuals is often underestimated.

Among the most important contributions to reductions in mortality and morbidity in the twentieth century have been such public health measures as the improvement of sanitation, ensurance of potable water supplies, and upgraded housing. In recent years, there has also been an increased awareness of the need to control air and water pollution, to reduce exposure to carcinogens, and to improve and ensure the quality of the environment. The contribution of these efforts to health far exceeds, dollar for dollar, efforts to treat illness once it occurs. Their importance to ambulatory care is mentioned here, however, because public health agencies have responsibility for a remarkable range of relevant services.

And in this context it is important to emphasize that health care and ambulatory care services also must successfully interact with other aspects of our society. These other areas include social and welfare services, accident prevention in industry and in transportation, protection of the environment, improvement of food and water supplies, and even the general economic well-being of society, since health is directly correlated with employment and income security.

ORGANIZATION OF AMBULATORY CARE SYSTEMS

The changing structure of the health services system has had tremendous implications for ambulatory care services. The increased movement toward integrated systems of care and managed care has led ambulatory care services to assume a central role in the design and operation of many insurance and delivery programs. In addition, those paying for health services, including employers and insurers, have increasingly focused attention on the role that ambulatory care services can provide in improving the coordination and control of care as well as in reducing costs through the reduction of duplication and the shifting of services to lower-cost settings.

Those organizations constructing large-scale, integrated systems of care are continuing to seek existing ambulatory care structures, or are building new ones, as a means to complete their systems. In particular, insurers, hospitals, and other organizational entities are developing or purchasing ambulatory care resources such as medical practices, clinics, and other existing networks. Government units, such as the military, have long recognized the key attributes of ambulatory care in coordinating and controlling the overall utilization of services and, then, the cost and quality of care. These trends are likely to continue.

There are many key design attributes of ambulatory care that are essential for both the effective operation of ambulatory services and for the full integration of these services into larger systems of care. Ambulatory care is important in providing access to care, particularly within larger integrated systems. Access considerations include scope of services provided and hours of operation as well as distribution of resources throughout a geographic region populated by the target group of consumers. Physical access to the facilities must also be assured, including such considerations as parking, access to public transportation where appropriate, and access to physician facilities for the handicapped.

The scope of services provided must respond to population needs. These needs differ depending on whether the population is enrolled through insurance or entitlement programs or fee-for-service. How the population is served differs substantially in each situation. For both situations, however, decisions must be made concerning the type of care to be provided on an ambulatory versus an inpatient basis.

Marketing advantages can be achieved in the ambulatory care setting by recognizing the special needs of consumers, such as having multilingual staff available where appropriate. The friendliness of the staff and the attractiveness of the physical facilities can have dramatic effects on patient attitudes and satisfaction, not only with the ambulatory care provider but in the larger system of care as well. Thus, ambulatory care provides an influential marketing function in any system of care. Ambulatory care services also generally provide an opportunity for educating the consumer in terms of both health behaviors and "appropriate" use of the system. This educational role can contribute to cost containment by having patients help in "managing" their use.

Ambulatory care can provide a key role in the overall provision of coordinated and continuous care. By accepting the gate-keeper role of the primary care physician, using medical records and other administrative tracking of patients, and avoiding duplication of services and unnecessary care, the ambulatory care setting can contribute handsomely to the overall effectiveness of all care provided to the patient. Physician payment incentives can facilitate an enhanced coordinating role for ambulatory care. Centralization of responsibility for patient care thus must be clearly assigned. Mechanisms for monitoring patient and provider behavior to ensure compliance with health system operating guidelines are essential. There is also evidence that more effective continuity of care is associated with higher levels of patient compliance regarding medical regimens, which, in turn, may lead to better health outcomes and eventually lower subsequent utilization rates. Patient satisfaction is generally greater when continuity and coordination of care are achieved—both effective marketing and cost-containment tools.

The quality of care should reflect not only adequate medical skills but also a caring attitude on the part of the provider. Consumers in ambulatory care are capable of detecting some aspects of the technical quality of care, but they are even more aware of provider and system attitudes and behavior. Responding to the consumer is increasingly important in the competitive environment.

AMBULATORY CARE AND THE CHALLENGE OF MANAGED CARE

Ambulatory care services have been and will continue to be dramatically affected by the evolution of managed care. Managed care serves to shift considerable risk to practitioners and forces greater efficiencies in the ambulatory care arena. Clinical responsibility in many ambulatory care practices not only for patient care but also for allocation of resources and broader aspects of clinical decision making have also been enhanced by the pressures of managed care. Since managed care is focused on controlling provider and patient behavior, most of that control is being exercised through the ambulatory care arena. These pressures have allowed ambulatory care providers to gain greater power within the health care system, but with enhanced power comes increased responsibility, risk, financial pressures, and frictions with providers, insurers, and patients. Increasingly, the shift of managed care toward organizational forms that are associated with greater controls over resources, providers, and patients is increasing the pressure on those involved in the provision of ambulatory care services. The move toward more integrated health care systems has decreased practitioner autonomy and imposed additional managerial controls and pressures on all participants.

The role of ambulatory care in controlling the patient, particularly through such mechanisms as gate-keepers and various forms of utilization control, places the provider in a more difficult position with regard to patient satisfaction and clinical decision making. Rationing, both directly and indirectly, may result from fiscal pressures and risk shifting under managed care and is exacerbating these pressures. Practitioners in ambulatory care increasingly must face new realities regarding incentives for income and the quality and quantity of the patient's care services. All of these changes are appreciably affecting the ambulatory care arena and its participants.

At the same time as the financial and clinical practice pressures build, competition in the health care marketplace is requiring ambulatory care practitioners to provide friendly but efficient care that is customer-oriented in a manner that attracts the patient but also controls the resources.

Clinical and managerial information systems have gained increasing importance in ambulatory care. Fiscal reports that reflect costs, expenditures, and other financial indicators are important in light of risk shifting under managed care contracts. Clinical measures of performance are increasingly utilized to assess physician practice patterns and relative performance among physicians in multispecialty groups. Managed care organizations and insurers are also utilizing such data for economic credentialing and other assessments of not only clinical but also financial performance on the part of practitioners. These trends concern many observers, since access, utilization, quality, and rationing are all affected by use of resources and allocation of services.

The future of health services, particularly with the pressures inherent in managed care and technological advances, will be characterized by further shifts in services from inpatient to ambulatory care settings. Ambulatory care practices will need to respond with appropriate and innovative service delivery options including new equipment, technology, specialized personnel, and facilities. Competition will be driven in managed care contracting in part by the ability to provide cost-effective care in more innovative and appropriate settings.

Affiliations of provider organizations ranging from direct ownership in integrated systems to loose confederations and affiliations developed through contractual arrangements will enhance integration, coordination, managerial efficiency, and provision of clinical services. All group practice, and even solo, practitioners must be prepared to participate in various forms of networks, integrated systems, coordinated service provider organizations, and other innovative approaches to organizing the health care delivery system.

SUMMARY

The challenge in ambulatory care is to effectively shift from a traditionally reactive set of providers, attitudes, and operational approaches to the proactive leadership role needed in today's competitive environment. Ambulatory care once meant a large-ly unaffiliated and unstructured set of small providers responding as business walked in the door. Now ambulatory care is a key vital element in the structuring of large-scale systems. These systems require financial and contractual arrangements with providers, and these ties are critical to all parties concerned.

The system's structure itself vitally affects the role of ambulatory care services; ambulatory care can, in turn, be vital to the success of the system. In managed care systems, the ability to control providers and consumers, and hence costs, depends on structuring the system based on the controlling role of ambulatory care and performing needed services through ambulatory delivery vehicles where feasible, while also maintaining quality. Ideally, quality and access will attain acceptable minimum levels under any delivery system, and controls will be built in to monitor both.

From a health care delivery perspective, as opposed to the financial focus of other chapters, the demands on ambulatory care to provide a marketing, integrating, controlling, and organizing function are great. At the same time, services must retain the attributes of high quality, meeting specific patient needs, and offering a stimulating and rewarding environment for the providers as well. This is no small challenge.

REFERENCES

Adams, P. F., & Marano, M. (1995). Current estimates from the National Health Interview Survey, 1994. National Center for Health Statistics. *Vital Health Statistics, 10,* 193.

Albrecht, K. G., & Bradford, L. J. (1990). *The service advantage: How to identify and fulfill customer needs.* Homewood, IL: Dow Jones-Irwin.

Benson, D. S., Townes, M. D., & Townes, P. G., Jr. (1990). *A practical guide to developing effective quality assurance programs.* San Francisco: Jossey-Bass.

Cunningham, L. (1991). *The quality connection in health care: Integrating patient satisfaction and risk management.* San Francisco: Jossey-Bass.

Havlicek, P. L. (1990). *Medical groups in the U.S., 1990 ed. A survey of practice characteristics.* Chicago: American Medical Association.

Hsiao, W. C., Braun, P., et al. (1988). Results, potential effects and implementation issues of the resource-based relative value scale. *Journal of the American Medical Association, 260*(28), 2429–2438.

Peterson, O. L., Andrews, L. P., Spain, R. S., et al. (1956). An analytical study of North Carolina general practice 1953–1954. *Journal of Medical Education, 31*(Pt. 2), 1–165.

Rorem, R. (1931). *Private group clinics.* Chicago: University of Chicago Press.

Ross, A., Williams, S. J., & Schafer, E. L. (1997). *Ambulatory care management* (3rd ed.). Albany, NY: Delmar.

United Kingdom Ministry of Health. (1920). *Dawson report, interim report on the future provision of medical and allied services.* London: His Majesty's Stationery Office.

Woodwell, D. A. (1997). National ambulatory medical care survey: 1996 summary. Advance data from vital and health statistics (No. 295). Hyattsville, MD: National Center for Health Statistics.

CHAPTER

Hospitals and Health Systems

William L. Dowling

CHAPTER TOPICS

LEARNING OBJECTIVES

Upon completing this chapter, the reader should be able to:

- Understand the role of the hospital in today's health care system.
- Appreciate the historical trends that have shaped the hospital industry.
- Understand the types of hospitals, ownership patterns, and differentiating characteristics of various hospitals.
- Comprehend the development of health systems and the role of hospitals in such systems.
- Follow the impact of competitive pressures and other developments on the structure and operation of hospitals and health systems.
- Understand the internal organizational structure of hospitals.

The dramatic advances in medicine around the turn of the century transformed the hospital into the key resource and organizational hub of the American health care system. Hospitals became central to the delivery of patient care, the training of health personnel, and the conduct and dissemination of health care research. They were built by communities as a collective investment in the sophisticated technology and specialized personnel required to provide modern medical care—a community resource available for the benefit of all. As the repository for the equipment and personnel needed by physicians to support them in providing care, hospitals became the physician's "workshop," ever more the economic and professional heart of medical practice as the pace of advances in medical knowledge and technology accelerated. In recent years, hospitals have expanded beyond their inpatient role to become comprehensive community health centers, often formally linked with physicians, offering a broad range of outpatient, community-based, and home-based, as well as institution-based, services. As highly advanced, scientific institutions, hospitals manifest the complexity and detached efficiency of a clinical laboratory. As human service organizations, they deal with the emotions of life and death, and triumphs and tragedies. Hospitals are frequently the caregivers of last resort for many of the nation's poor who have nowhere else to turn for health care.

Current forces in health care are once again transforming the role of hospitals. Many predict that efforts to contain spending for hospital services, declining inpatient volumes, competition from other providers, and outpatient technology will erode the central role of hospitals. Over the years, however, hospitals have proved to be remarkably resilient to even the most powerful changes in health care.

Hospitals are big business. Collectively, they are among the largest industries in the United States measured by the dollars they consume or the size of the workforce they employ. By far the largest single component of the nation's health care system, hospitals employ about half of all health care personnel and consume 40% of the nation's health expenditures. Fifty-three percent of all federal health expenditures and 30% of all state and local government health expenditures go for hospital care (Levit et al., 1996).

The magnitude of the hospital industry and the central role hospitals play in the delivery of health services place hospitals at the root of many of the health care system's most pressing problems—rising costs, duplication of services, bed surpluses, overemphasis of specialized services versus primary care, depersonalization of care, and so forth. Furthermore, because the public sees hospitals as community or quasi-public institutions, and because hospitals are heavily dependent on public dollars, hospitals are often targeted by community groups, business coalitions, insurance companies, government agencies, and others as instruments of social change and health system reform (Shortell, 1977).

The hospital industry is a mix of public and private for-profit and not-for-profit institutions. Hospitals range from small institutions in rural areas providing limited basic medical care, to large regional referral centers providing a comprehensive range of sophisticated, highly specialized services. Many hospitals have expanded their roles to include primary care clinics, home care, health promotion, and long-term care services. Other hospitals have reorganized to develop for-profit entities or to sponsor managed care plans.

While hospitals are traditionally thought of as inpatient institutions, they now play an increasingly important role in the provision of outpatient care. Hospitals are evolving toward a new role as providers of a comprehensive and integrated continuum of health services (Shortell et al., 1995). To illustrate, outpatient services, virtually nonexistent until the 1960s, today generate 30% of total hospital revenue (American Hospital Association, 1966), and if the present trend continues, outpatient revenue will exceed inpatient revenue by the year 2003 (Philip, 1990). In 1986, for the first time the number of outpatient visits seen in the nation's hospitals exceeded the number of inpatient days. Today, 89% of the nation's community hospitals have organized outpatient departments, 92% have emergency departments, 94% have ambulatory surgery units, 90% have health promotion programs, and 42% offer home health services (American Hospital Association, 1966). Many hospitals are also now actively engaged in long-term care and geriatric services. In 1995, 28% of community hospitals had long-term care units.

In recent years, the structure of the hospital industry has changed dramatically in response to the changing health care marketplace and the growth of managed care. Up to the mid-1980s, most hospitals were independent and locally owned. Their focus was mainly on inpatient care. Rarely did they employ or have formal "business" relationships with physicians to share responsibility for patient care. Consolidation of hospitals into local, regional, and even national systems began in earnest with Medicare's switch from cost reimbursement to diagnosis-related group (DRG) payment of hospitals in 1983, because this put great pressure on hospitals to control costs and make up for declining inpatient volumes. Consolidation picked up momentum through the 1990s as a result of the increasing competition among hospitals for the patient volumes controlled by health plans and other purchasers. Consolidation first took the form of horizontal integration—the coming together of independent hospitals into hospital systems—to gain administrative cost savings and economies of scale. More recently, consolidation has increasingly taken the form of vertical integration—the coming together of physicians, hospitals, and other providers into organized delivery systems—in order to contract with health plans and assume financial risk for the care of defined populations.

Changes in the health care environment continue to motivate providers to come together into organized delivery systems, both to increase their negotiating power with health plans and to be able to assume risk for managing care under capitation or other risk-sharing arrangements. Today, 50% of all community hospitals are members of systems, up from 30% in 1980. Individual providers cannot very well assume risk; this takes an organization of some size. Size also brings economies of scale and the ability to invent information systems and other care management technology. Delivery systems can also bring all health care resources—physicians, hospitals, long-term care, home care, and so on—into a single organization so as to facilitate coordination of care across the entire range of health services.

It is unclear how many health plans will try to create their own provider networks by contracting directly with individual physicians and hospitals, and how many will contract with already-organized, provider-based delivery systems. Nor is it clear whether physician- or hospital-based systems will predominate. What is clear, however, is that health plans and providers are well on the way to fundamentally restructuring the way health care is delivered. Competition and managed care are driving the transformation of the fragmented "nonsystem" of the past into formally organized, vertically integrated systems capable of assuming the risk for managing the care of defined populations.

The purpose of this chapter is to characterize the hospital system in the United States, emphasizing major issues and trends. Because the character of the modern hospital reflects its past, the chapter begins with a discussion of the historical development of hospitals. The second section describes the hospital system as it exists today. The third section describes the internal organization of hospitals.

HISTORICAL DEVELOPMENT OF HOSPITALS

The history of hospitals in this country (Figure 10–1) can be traced back to the almshouses and pest houses that existed in some form in most cities of any size by the mid-1700s (MacEachern, 1957). Almshouses, also called poorhouses or workhouses, were established by city governments to provide

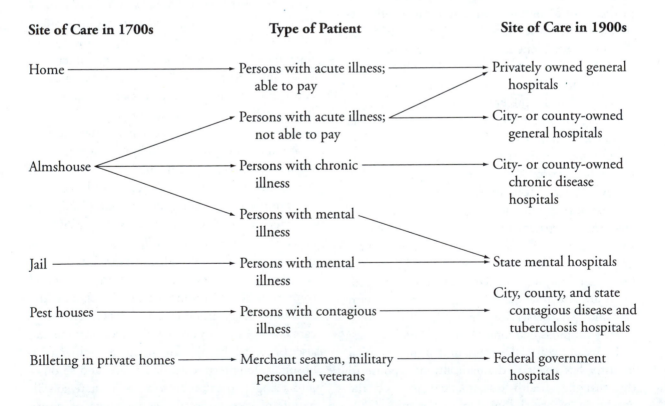

FIGURE 10–1 Evolution of institutional care sites

food and shelter for the homeless poor, including many aged, chronically ill, disabled, mentally ill, and orphans. Medical care was a secondary function of the poorhouse. In some facilities, however, those who became sick were isolated in infirmaries where care, such as it was before the advent of modern medicine, was provided, typically by other residents. Not until the late 1800s did the infirmaries or hospital departments of city poorhouses break away to become medical care institutions on their own—the first public hospitals.

Pest houses were operated by local governments in seaport towns where it was necessary to quarantine people exposed to contagious diseases aboard ship. During epidemics, these institutions were also used to isolate victims of cholera, smallpox, typhus, and yellow fever. Their primary purpose was to control the spread of contagious diseases by removing infected persons from the community. As with almshouses, medical care was a secondary function—in this case, secondary to protecting the community from disease. Pest houses were often established during epidemics and discontinued or closed down when the threat of disease subsided. These institutions were the predecessors of the contagious disease and tuberculosis hospitals that later emerged.

Almshouses and pest houses were maintained for the poor and the homeless and were avoided by everyone else. These institutions were dismal places: crowded, unsanitary, and poorly heated and ventilated. Nutrition was often inadequate, nursing care incompetent, and separation of different types of patients minimal. The contagious, the disabled, the dying, and the mentally ill were often crowded together. Cross-infection was rampant and mortality high. All those who could afford to, were cared for at home or in the homes of neighbors.

The first community-owned or voluntary hospitals in this country were established in the late 1700s and early 1800s, often at the urging of influential physicians who had been trained in Europe and needed facilities to practice obstetrics and surgery in the manner in which they had been taught. These physicians also sought a setting where they could provide preceptor-type instruction for medical students. These early hospitals depended on philanthropy, and contributions were solicited from both private citizens and the local government. Voluntary hospitals generally preceded both religious and public hospitals in the United States, representing a departure from patterns in England and Europe. Voluntary hospitals admitted both indigent and paying patients. For example, in its first year of operation in 1751, Pennsylvania Hospital in Philadelphia admitted twenty-four paying patients and forty poor patients. Except in the largest cities where the concentration of poor was too great, the early voluntary hospitals cared on a charitable basis for the sick who were unable to pay. These hospitals relied upon philanthropy and donations of time by the physicians who comprised their medical staffs (MacEachern, 1957; Rosen, 1963).

The first hospitals of this type were the Pennsylvania Hospital, Philadelphia, 1751; New York Hospital, New York City, 1773; Massachusetts General Hospital, Boston, 1816; and New Haven Hospital, New Haven, Connecticut, 1826. Voluntary hospitals were established in Savannah, Georgia, in 1830; Lowell, Massachusetts, in 1836; and Raleigh, North Carolina, in 1839. Voluntary hospitals cared for patients with acute illnesses and injuries but did not admit persons with contagious diseases or mental illnesses. Isolation of these unfortunates from the rest of the community was seen as a government responsibility. Therefore, during the same period, a number of city, county, and state mental hospitals were established. These included hospitals in Williamsburg, Virginia, 1773; Lexington, Kentucky, 1817; Columbia, South Carolina, 1829; Worcester, Massachusetts,

1832; Augusta, Maine, 1834; Brooklyn, New York, 1838; and Boston, Massachusetts, 1839.

Although voluntary hospitals provided better accommodations and care than had the poorhouses that preceded them, the efficacy of care improved little, and it was not until the late 1800s that hospitals became accepted by persons of all economic strata as the best setting for the care of serious illness and injury. Then, their growth was dramatic. In 1873, there were only 178 hospitals with 35,604 beds in the United States. By 1909, the number of hospitals had increased to 4,359 with 421,065 beds, and by 1929, to 6,665 hospitals with 907,133 beds. This rapid growth was brought about by advances in medical science that rapidly transformed the hospital's role from a custodial institution in which to isolate or shelter the poor to a curative institution in which communities concentrated their health care resources in support of the local physicians for the benefit of all (Corwin, 1946; Rosen, 1963). Starr (1982) has characterized this redefinition of the hospital as a transformation from a social welfare facility to an institution of medical science, from a charitable organization to a business, and from an orientation toward patrons and the poor to a focus on professionals and patients.

FORCES AFFECTING THE DEVELOPMENT OF HOSPITALS

Beginning in the late 1800s and early 1900s, six major developments were particularly significant in transforming hospitals into the institutions of today: (1) advances in medical science increased the efficacy and safety of hospitals, (2) the proliferation of technology and specialization within medicine necessitated the institutionalization of medical care, (3) the development of professional nursing brought about more humane patient care,

(4) advances in medical education added teaching and research to the hospital's role, (5) the growth of health insurance provided adequate and certain funding, and (6) government began to exert greater influence over the activities of hospitals (Commission of Hospital Care, 1947; Rosen, 1963; Starr, 1982).

Advances in Medical Science

Most notable in terms of their impact on hospitals were the discovery of anesthesia, followed by rapid advances in surgery, and the development of the germ theory of disease with the subsequent discovery of antiseptic and sterilization techniques. By the early 1800s, enough was known about anatomy and physiology that surgeons were able to perform a variety of fairly complex surgical procedures; however, the inability to deaden pain meant that surgery was extremely traumatic and had to be carried out at great speed. In addition, infection from surgery was common. Ether was first used as an anesthetic in surgery by Long in 1842 and Morton in 1846, and its use then spread rapidly. Great advances in the efficacy of surgery followed.

Before formulation of the germ theory of disease, a few scientists, most notably Holmes in the United States and Semmelweis in Vienna, had observed and reported that fever, infection, and mortality could be reduced through cleanliness. Both concluded that childbed fever, which was the cause of high maternal mortality, was an infection transmitted by physicians, midwives, and medical students to women in labor. In 1861, Pasteur proved that bacteria were living, reproducing microorganisms that could be carried by air or on clothing and hands. It became clear that germs were the cause rather than the result of infection and that germs could be destroyed by chemicals and heat. Lister built on Pasteur's work and, in 1867, introduced carbolic acid spray in operating rooms as an antiseptic to keep air and incisions clean. In 1886, steam sterilization was introduced, providing a means of freeing medical equipment from microorganisms. Surgical infection rates fell. Advances in surgery led to the need for skilled preoperative and postoperative care and well-equipped operating rooms, which could be provided only in an institutional setting. By 1900, 40% of all hospitalizations were for surgery.

The discovery of sulfa drugs in the mid-1930s and antibiotics in the mid-1940s changed the prevalent causes of death in the United States from infectious diseases to the diseases of old age, particularly heart disease, cancer, and stroke. Hospitals responded slowly to the health care needs of an aging population. Even today most of the nation's medical resources are still concentrated on curable illnesses that respond quickly to medical treatment, rather than on chronic conditions that must be managed over long periods of time. By the mid-1990s, however, hospitals began to broaden their role, adding skilled nursing units, inpatient and outpatient rehabilitation programs, day care, home care, and other services aimed at the elderly and chronically ill.

Advances in medical science today are generating a growing debate about the right balance between cost and improvements in medical diagnosis and treatment. Cost-effectiveness and outcomes research are producing a body of knowledge about the relative value of alternative approaches to care and of new technology. Because hospital care is so costly, much of this research focuses on the effects of shorter stays and of substituting alternative care settings for the hospital. Outcomes research now complements traditional medical research and underpins the development of clinical treatment protocols and utilization parameters that increasingly guide medical practice today.

Development of Specialized Technology

In the late 1800s, medical technology began to proliferate. The first hospital laboratory opened in 1889, and X-ray films were first used in 1896. These developments greatly increased the diagnostic effectiveness of hospitals. The discovery of blood types in 1901 made blood transfusions safe; the electrocardiogram (EKG) was first used in 1903 and the electroencephalogram (EEG) in 1929. In addition to increasing the efficacy of medical care, these advances in technology affected the site and organization of care. As the tools of medicine could no longer be carried in the physician's bag, hospitals became the place where the equipment, facilities, and personnel required by modern medicine were housed. In addition, since physicians could no longer be competent in all areas of medical practice, specialization began to occur within medicine, and new professional and technical occupations began to emerge. Again, the hospital became the place where physicians and support personnel came together to provide patient care.

Developments in specialized technology in recent years have proceeded at such a rapid pace as to prompt one observer to describe the United States system as a "medical-industrial complex" (Relman, 1980). Advances in diagnostic imaging and minimally invasive surgery are two hallmarks of late-twentieth century technology breakthroughs. Advances have occurred in administrative as well as clinical technology. Hospital managers now use sophisticated management information systems to analyze costs, utilization patterns, quality, and other dimensions of performance, and employ continuous quality improvement (CQI) techniques to measure and monitor workflow processes. These developments pose economic and political challenges as expenditures for the expensive equipment and highly trained personnel they require drive up hospital costs.

As physicians and the public came to expect that a wide range of advanced technologies would be available in their local hospitals, new discoveries were quickly diffused from large medical centers to smaller institutions. Duplication became commonplace, giving rise to calls to regulate capital expenditures by hospitals. Most states established certificate of need (CON) programs to control capital spending. Comparisons with other countries are striking. In the late 1980s, for example, there were more magnetic resonance imaging (MRI) units in Pennsylvania than in all of Canada.

Many types of clinical technology—surgical lasers and laparoscopes for ophthalmologic and thoracic procedures, lithotripsy machines for kidney stones, computerized tomography (CT) and MRI units for imaging, and pharmacology agents for behavioral illness—either were developed for use in outpatient settings or reduced the need for all but a few days in the hospital. The emergence of such technology has prompted the shift of many procedures to outpatient settings. In recent years, many states have eliminated or weakened their CON programs, relying on market forces rather than regulation to contain spending on new technology (Katz & Thompson, 1996). Today, hospitals increasingly face competition from physician clinics and other freestanding entities that offer high-tech health care services once provided only by hospitals. Thus, recent trends affecting specialized technology have created significant economic and strategic challenges for hospitals.

Development of Professional Nursing

Humane treatment of hospital patients awaited the development of professional nursing. Before the late 1800s, nursing care was provided primarily by Catholic sisters and Protestant deaconesses, who were dedicated but minimally trained. Some religious orders established hospitals, and occasionally were called on by city officials to provide nursing care in public institutions. Almshouses used untrained female residents, and hospitals relied on poorly paid, unskilled labor.

The transformation of nursing into a profession is credited to Florence Nightingale, who completed four months of nurses' training in a deaconess school in Germany. In 1854, Nightingale and thirty-eight nurses were sent by the British government to the Crimea to take charge of nursing care for wounded soldiers. The nurses found conditions deplorable and instituted cleanliness and sanitation, dietary reforms, simple but humane care, discipline, and organization. As a result, mortality dropped dramatically. On her return to England, Nightingale wrote of her experiences in the Crimea and about the contributions of sanitation to the recovery of wounded and ill patients. In 1860, she founded the Nightingale School for Nursing in England.

In the United States, President Abraham Lincoln called on religious orders to provide nursing care for the wounded during the Civil War, but more nurses were needed. Dorothea Dix was appointed Superintendent of Nursing for the Union Army. She began a recruitment program and encouraged a one-month hospital training program for new nurses. By the end of the war, there were two thousand lay nurses in the United States. The first permanent schools of nursing were established at Bellevue Hospital, New Haven Hospital, and Massachusetts General Hospital in 1873. There was some initial reluctance on the part of hospital administrators and trustees to establish nursing schools, but the benefits of good nursing soon became apparent. In addition, student nurses provided better care and were less expensive than the untrained women previously employed to do this work. By 1883, there were 22 nursing schools and 600 graduates; by 1898, these totals had grown to 400 schools with 10,000 graduates.

Advances in nursing contributed to the growth of hospitals in two ways: (1) increased efficacy of treatment, cleanliness, nutritious diets, and formal treatment routines all contributed to patient recovery; and (2) considerate, skilled patient care made hospitals acceptable to all people, not just the poor. The public's fear of hospitals began to give way to an attitude of confidence and respect.

As of 1995 there were over two million registered nurses in the United States. About two-thirds of working nurses are employed by hospitals. Developments in nursing today are being shaped in no small measure by the economic pressures on hospitals and by declining inpatient volumes. Following highly publicized shortages in the 1980s, nurses now find their professional autonomy and even their jobs in jeopardy (Lumsdon, 1995). In many hospitals, pressures to contain costs have led to layoffs and to the replacement of professional nurses with less-skilled personnel. In addition, in some hospitals the use of CQI techniques to "re-engineer" patient care and achieve process improvements has reduced the demand for professional nurses.

Contemporary trends in the employment of nurses by hospitals reflect two counteracting forces. On the one hand, the increasingly complex case mix of hospital patients as a result of earlier discharge of patients and substitution of outpatient for inpatient care for less complex conditions, combined with the ever more sophisticated technology found in hospitals, has created a demand for more and more highly trained nurses. Acting to reduce the demand for nurses are declines in patient volumes and pressures to cut costs. The net effect of these forces has been a steady rise in the total number of registered nurses employed by community hospitals from about 750,000 in 1985 to 890,000 in 1995. Registered nurse (RN) employment grew from 95 per adjusted 100 census in 1985 to 100 in 1995. In contrast, the substitution of more highly trained for less trained nurses plus cost cutting resulted in a significant drop in employment of licensed practical nurses (LPNs) from 24 per adjusted 100 census in 1985 to 18 in 1995 (American Hospital Association, 1996).

Advances in Medical Education

Changes in medical education brought about by the Flexner report in 1910 had a major impact on the development of hospitals. Before 1900, great variation characterized the nature and quality of medical education. There were no uniform standards for the academic training of physicians. Most medical schools were proprietary and were not connected with universities. They were dominated by influential practitioners, and most instruction was through didactic (often unscientific) lectures. Apprenticeship practices varied greatly. Clinical and laboratory instruction was minimal, and there was little research.

The Flexner report led to changes in the content and methods of instruction to emphasize the scientific basis of medicine. The standards of education established by the report were widely accepted by both the profession and the public; as a result, medical schools that did not meet the standards were forced to close. State laws were established requiring graduation from a medical school accredited by the American Medical Association as the basis for a license to practice medicine. A four-year course of study at a medical school based in a university became standard, as did clinical training on the wards of a hospital.

These changes expanded the role of the hospital to include education and research as well as patient care. The hospital's role in education became even more prominent as medical specialization led to a proliferation of internships and residencies in the 1920s and 1930s. The requirements of medical education necessitated the expansion of hospital facilities and services and the addition of equipment and personnel. Hospitals were called on to assume a greater role in acquiring and organizing these resources. Quality of care improved through advances in medical education, especially for patients with complex and serious illnesses. On the other hand, specialization led to a fragmentation of care among different physician specialists and ancillary personnel, and decreased interest in chronic, routine, and other "uninteresting" medical conditions.

Medical education in the United States continues to favor the training of specialists. The growing influence of managed care and the recognition of the oversupply of specialists, however, have gradually led educators, industry representatives, and legislators to shift more training to ambulatory care settings and to increase the number of training slots in the primary care disciplines of family practice, pediatrics, internal medicine, and obstetrics/gynecology. As medical students and residents experience additional community-based education, the traditional focus on the diagnosis and treatment of the individual patient will be balanced by more of an orientation toward population-based care, health promotion, managed care, physician participation on patient care "teams," and with patterns of practice consistent with high-volume outpatient settings.

Growth of Health Insurance

The growth of health insurance contributed significantly to the development of hospitals. Private insurance for hospital care expanded rapidly from the end of World War II through the 1960s, increasing both the portion of the population with insurance and the adequacy and scope of coverage. Today, the out-of-pocket cost of hospital care at time of use is relatively modest for most of the population, because most hospital bills are covered by either government or private health insurance.

A variety of factors led to the growth of hospital insurance. From the public's perspective, of course, a hospital stay is sufficiently expensive to warrant the purchase of insurance protection. The hospital industry's interest in insurance began with the Great Depression of the 1930s, when the number of patients who could not pay increased markedly and hospital use declined. The financial solvency of many hospitals was threatened, and the number of hospitals dropped from 6,852 in 1928 to 6,189 in 1937. A study of not-for-profit hospitals in 1935 revealed that on average, total income was three percent less than total expenses. In response, acting through the American Hospital Association, hospitals took the initiative to encourage the development of hospital insurance plans, primarily Blue Cross (Commission of Hospital Care, 1947; Starr, 1982).

The growth of health insurance provided the dollars to finance the great expansion of facilities and services and the prompt implementation of new technology that have characterized the hospital industry since the end of World War II. Insurance also contributed to the increased demand by the public for health services. Because hospital care has been better covered by insurance than care provided in other settings, patients have been reluctant to substitute less-well-insured out-of-hospital services even though they are less costly. This resulted in a bias toward hospital care relative to ambulatory, home, or nursing care settings and a general overuse of hospitals. In recent years, however, concern over the rising costs of hospital care and hospital overuse has given rise to actions to reverse this trend. Insurance plans now actively promote nonhospital alternatives and exercise stringent control over inpatient admissions and lengths of stay. The belief that hospital admissions were often unwarranted was underscored by an influential Rand Corporation study that examined a sample of hospital records from 1974 to 1982.

The study concluded that 23% of the admissions studied were inappropriate and another 17% could have been avoided through the use of ambulatory surgery (Siu, et al., 1986).

The rapid rise in hospital costs through the late 1960s and 1970s was caused in part by cost-based reimbursement, the method of payment adopted by Medicare and Medicaid when these programs were enacted in 1965 following the practice of most Blue Cross plans at the time. Cost reimbursement did not provide hospitals with an incentive to contain costs. The result was inefficiency, duplication of services, and overbuilding. To stem rising hospital costs, public and private payers tried both regulatory and competitive approaches (Luft, 1985). Regulatory approaches—most notably certificate-of-need (CON) review of new hospital beds and equipment, and hospital rate regulation—were initiated by a large number of states in the 1970s. As hospital costs continued to rise, however, economists, businesses, and policy makers began suggesting that market competition would provide greater incentives for controlling health care costs (Havighurst, 1986). The 1980s witnessed a weakening of regulatory approaches to controlling costs and a growing emphasis on market forces. One hallmark of the marketplace model is the buying power of major purchasers of health care such as employer coalitions, managed care plans, Blue Cross, Medicare, and Medicaid. These purchasers have replaced payment systems based on retrospective costs with payment based on negotiated prices or prospectively set rates.

A major step toward the introduction of economic forces to contain costs occurred with the Tax Equity and Fiscal Responsibility Act (TEFRA) of 1982 (PL 97-248) which converted Medicare reimbursement to a prospective, per-case system based on diagnosis-related groups (DRGs). In turn, many states revised their Medicaid payment methods to pay prospective rates. Additionally, cost-containment pressure has come from health maintenance organizations (HMOs) and other types of managed care plans that employ financial incentives and utilization controls, as they have rapidly grown to dominate the private insurance market.

National expenditures on hospital care exceeded $350 billion in 1995—up 36% from 1990. The sources of these funds were private insurance (32%), out-of-pocket payments (3%), federal programs including Medicare and veterans benefits (50%), and state and local government programs including Medicaid (11%) (Levit, et al., 1996). This breakdown illustrates the pluralistic public/private financing system that exists today. Critics suggest that a substantial portion of hospital overhead is caused by the administrative costs of interacting with the multiplicity of private insurance companies, health plans, Medicare, and Medicaid.

While cost-based reimbursement is widely blamed as the root cause of runaway hospital costs, it allowed hospitals to remain current with advances in medical technology, and with demands from communities and physicians for ready access to the latest services. In sharp contrast, hospitals now find themselves competing for the growing enrollment of managed care plans on the basis of price and quality. In 1995, 65% of community hospitals had formal contracts with health maintenance organizations (HMOs), 78% had contracts with preferred provider organizations (PPOs), and 12% contracted directly with employers (American Hospital Association, 1996). Quality measures are increasingly used as a tool to assist purchasers and consumers in choosing among health plans and providers, although there is currently little consensus on uniform measures of quality. A fundamental public policy issue yet unresolved is how to assure the poor and disadvantaged access to needed care in a system driven by competitive forces.

Role of Government

Patterns of hospital financing and ownership differ from country to country. Most advanced nations recognize health care as an essential service to which all should have access, and government plays a major role. In Great Britain and many other industrialized nations, government owns and operates most hospitals and employs the physicians who work in them. In other countries, the government limits its role to financing care that is provided by privately owned hospitals and private practitioners. In countries like Canada, where universal health insurance is in effect, hospitals operate primarily on public funds and hence are essentially controlled by the government even though they are not government-owned. In the United States, by contrast, government's role has been generally limited to financing care for needy groups such as the aged, the poor, and the disabled. This role has grown, however, to the point where community hospitals now receive almost half of their income from government sources (primarily Medicare and Medicaid). The rest comes mainly from private health insurance, supplemented by direct payments by patients. In short, the United States has a pluralistic public-private financing system with largely privately owned hospitals. However, as the portion of hospital income financed by government has increased (from about 25% in 1960 to 47% today), so has government's influence.

Government's role in the hospital industry has changed over time. During colonial times, government involvement was mainly at the local level through cities and towns establishing almshouses and pest houses and making grants to help construct and support voluntary hospitals. The initial thrust of federal involvement began in 1935, with federal categorical grants-in-aid to state and local governments to assist in the establishment of public health programs: public health departments; communicable disease programs; maternal and child health programs; and public assistance for specific groups such as crippled children, the aged, the blind, the disabled, and poor families with dependent children. These programs were part of the general social reform movement initiated during the Depression with the recognition that state and local government and voluntary efforts alone were not sufficient to meet the needs of out-of-work and vulnerable populations.

Direct federal involvement in the hospital industry began in 1946 with the Hill-Burton (Hospital Survey and Construction) Act. Few hospitals had been constructed during the Depression and World War II, and by the end of the war, a severe shortage of hospitals existed. The Hill-Burton program was enacted to help states and communities plan for and construct hospitals and other health facilities by providing federal grants on a matching basis to supplement funds raised at the community level.

The Hill-Burton program assisted in the construction of nearly forty percent of the beds existing in the nation's short-term general hospitals by 1960 and was the greatest single factor in the increase in the nation's bed supply during the 1950s and 1960s. Another positive impact of the program was that hospital facilities became more evenly distributed across rural and urban areas and high- and low-income states. In retrospect, however, Hill-Burton also contributed to the overbuilding of hospitals and to the preponderance of small rural hospitals that continues to exist today.

From assisting with the financing of hospital construction and promulgating basic life-safety codes for hospitals, government's role expanded to the financing of care with the introduction of Medicare and Medicaid in 1965. In the mid-1980s, the federal government implemented a major policy shift that set the stage for the managed care era by shifting Medicare payment from cost reimbursement to the payment of prospective

DRG rates. Resource-based, relative-value rates (RBRVs) were introduced in the early 1990s as the basis for physician payment. By lowering Medicare and Medicaid hospital payments (relative to payments by private insurers), government programs accelerated the introduction of managed care in the 1990s by large private-sector purchasers to counter the practice of cost-shifting by hospitals. The concept of payment based on prospectively set rates, first introduced by the Medicare program, has now been adopted by most state Medicaid programs, private insurance companies, and managed care plans.

Patterns of Ownership

In the United States, government ownership of hospitals is limited. This is due to several historic factors. First, government was relatively weak in the nineteenth century when hospitals were first established in response to advances in medical science; initiative generally came from private citizens. At that time, the perception prevailed that the needs of the poor could be addressed through charity care financed by philanthropy in private hospitals. In major cities with large concentrations of the poor, however, public hospitals were established to care for the needy.

Second, government responsibility for the health of the public was viewed narrowly before the Depression of the 1930s. Government's job was seen as protecting healthy citizens from persons with contagious diseases and mental illnesses and providing care for special groups such as merchant seamen, military personnel, and the poor. State governments operated hospitals for the mentally ill, and city and county governments in urban areas operated hospitals for the poor and persons with tuberculosis and other contagious diseases. Third, in the United States, government traditionally becomes involved in a sector of activity only when the private sector clearly fails to provide important services. Chronic,

psychiatric, and tuberculosis hospital care would have been difficult to finance privately, given the lengthy stays that prevailed and the fact that the incidence of these conditions was greatest among the poor. As a result, care for people with these conditions became a public sector function. The private sector proved better able to finance short-stay hospital care through philanthropy, direct payments, and private health insurance, and government's role here was supplementary.

Current trends in hospital ownership reflect a significant interest on the part of investor-owned companies in the profit potential of efficiently run hospitals. Although for-profits comprised only 14% of all short-stay community hospitals in 1995, the slight growth in total hospital beds and admissions in the for-profit sector in the 1990–1995 period was in contrast to the decline in facilities and patient volumes in public or community-owned hospitals (Tables 10–1 and 10–2). As competition increases among hospitals to reduce costs, the emphasis of for-profit hospitals on efficient management and reduced labor costs is being imitated widely in the not-for-profit sector. In an industry that remains over capacity in the 1990s, facilities that do not do well become vulnerable to closure or acquisition by stronger for-profit and not-for-profit systems.

CHARACTERISTICS OF THE HOSPITAL INDUSTRY

Hospitals today comprise a complex and diverse industry that is experiencing significant change. As hospitals evolve from the central role in the delivery of health care they occupied in the past to a role as one component of organized networks of providers, they are diversifying services, forming systems, competing for contracts with managed care plans as an important source of patients, seeking new sources of capital to finance their transformation to

TABLE 10–1 Community and other hospital activity by ownership: United States, 1995

	Hospitals		Beds		Admissions		Outpatient Visits	
	Number	*Percent*	*Number*	*Percent*	*Number*	*Percent*	*Number*	*Percent*
Community								
Private/nonprofit	3,092	60%	609,729	70%	22,556,693	73%	303,850,987	73%
Investor-owned	752	14%	105,737	12%	3,427,850	11%	31,939,860	8%
State/local government	1,350	26%	157,270	18%	4,960,814	16%	78,553,990	19%
Subtotal	5,194	100%	872,736	100%	30,945,357	100%	414,344,837	100%
Federal	299		77,079		1,559,089		59,933,639	
Other	798		130,786		777,678		8,916,444	
Total U.S.	**6,291**		**1,080,601**		**33,282,124**		**483,194,920**	

SOURCE: *Hospital Statistics,* 1996/97, Chicago: American Hospital Association.

TABLE 10–2 Trends in hospital activity by ownership: United States, 1990–1995

	Private/Nonprofit	*Investor-Owned*	*State/Local Government*	*Federal*	*Other*	*Total U.S.*
Hospitals						
1990	3,191	749	1,444	337	874	6,595
1995	3,092	752	1,350	299	798	6,291
% change	–3%	0%	–7%	–11%	–9%	–5%
Beds						
1990	656,755	101,377	169,228	98,255	174,441	1,200,056
1995	609,729	105,737	157,270	77,079	130,786	1,080,601
% change	–7%	4%	–7%	–22%	–25%	–10%
Admissions						
1990	22,878,443	3,066,198	5,236,405	1,759,058	810,068	33,750,172
1995	22,556,693	3,427,850	4,960,814	1,559,089	777,678	33,282,124
% change	–1%	12%	–5%	–11%	–4%	–1%
Outpatient visits						
1990	221,073,380	20,109,508	60,145,874	58,527,091	6,947,280	366,803,133
1995	303,850,987	31,939,860	78,553,990	59,933,639	8,916,444	483,194,920
% change	37%	59%	31%	2%	28%	32%

SOURCE: *Hospital Statistics,* 1996/97, Chicago: American Hospital Association.

new roles, and expanding linkages with other providers and community-based partners.

Traditionally, hospitals have been classified in three ways: according to length of stay, type of service provided, and ownership. The most common type of hospital is the short-stay, community hospital, in which the average length of stay is now under seven days. In long-term institutions, including chronic disease, psychiatric, and tuberculosis hospitals, the average length of stay can range from two to four months.

A second method of classification is by type of service. General hospitals offer a wide range of medical, surgical, obstetric, and pediatric services, whereas specialty hospitals provide care for a specific disease or population group. Examples of specialty hospitals are children's hospitals and psychiatric hospitals. During the first part of the twentieth century, many specialty hospitals were established by philanthropic support of prestigious physicians who wanted to develop a hospital in their own area of practice. Financial difficulties and advances in medical science eventually made general hospitals more appropriate and efficient, and most specialty hospitals either closed or converted to general hospitals.

A third method of classification is according to form of ownership, including private, not-for-profit ownership; government or public ownership; and for-profit ownership. Regardless of ownership, hospitals today face many common challenges, including accessing capital for new ventures, cutting costs to lower prices, and measuring quality and outcomes of care using advanced information systems. And as a result of hospital industry consolidation in the 1980s and 1990s, many not-for-profit and for-profit hospitals, and even academic medical centers, are now part of large, multihospital systems (Etheredge, et al., 1996).

Community Hospitals

Short-stay, general hospitals—whether for-profit, not-for-profit, or public in ownership—are often referred to as community hospitals because they are available to the entire community and meet most community needs for hospital care. In 1995, community hospitals represented 83% of the total number of hospitals in the United States. They provided 81% of all hospital beds and 93% of all hospital admissions that year, in addition to

86% of all hospital-based outpatient care (Table 10–1).

The average length of stay in community hospitals was 6.5 days in 1995, a decrease of 9% from 7.1 days in 1985. The steady decline in length of stay is due to several factors, including an increased emphasis on outpatient care; the utilization management practices carried out by health insurance plans, Medicare, and Medicaid to reduce unnecessary hospital stays; and the shift to prospective payment by Medicare and other payers. Taken together, community hospitals admitted just under 31 million inpatients in 1995, an 8% decrease from 1985. This downward trend in admissions, combined with the shrinking average length of stay, led to a 16% decrease in total acute care "volume" from 1985 to 1995 as measured by inpatient days of care (American Hospital Association, 1996). Traditionally, the major role of community hospitals has been to provide short-term, inpatient care for patients with acute illnesses and injuries; however, the outpatient role of hospitals has been growing in importance and accounted for 30% of gross hospital revenues in 1995. Between 1985 and 1995, total community hospital outpatient visits (including emergency room visits) jumped 89% from approximately 219 million to 414 million. Where there were about 6.5 outpatient hospital visits for every community hospital admission in 1985, this ratio increased to 13.4 hospital visits per admission by 1995 (American Hospital Association, 1996).

Community hospitals fall into three ownership categories: private/not-for-profit (owned and operated by community or religious organizations), for-profit (investor-owned), and public (owned by state or local government).

Private/Not-for-Profit Hospitals. Private/not-for-profit hospitals comprised three-fifths of all community hospitals in 1995 and provided 70% of the nation's hospital beds and 73% of both admissions and outpatient visits (Table 10–1). In past years, these hospitals have been pressed to expand their roles to become true community health systems (Goldsmith, 1981). The rationale is that they represent their community's collective investment in health resources financed by a population's insurance premiums. In this view, access to these resources should not be limited to patients who happen to need inpatient hospitalization. Initially, because of limited physician interest, poor reimbursement for nonhospital services, and resistance by nursing homes and other providers, hospitals were slow to expand their roles beyond inpatient care.

More recently, diversification of services has been undertaken by community hospitals to offset declining inpatient revenues, to contain costs by substituting less expensive care settings for expensive inpatient stays, and to respond to community needs. Over the last five years, for example, outpatient visits at private/not-for-profits grew by 37%, a higher rate of increase than for all hospitals nationally in this period (Table 10–2). Hospitals are now adding a wide variety of ambulatory care and health promotion services, and a significant proportion have expanded mental health and rehabilitation services as well (Table 10–3). Community hospitals are seeking to play a central role in planning and coordinating the entire range of community health services. For example, in the American Hospital Association's 1995 Annual Survey, 75% of community hospitals reported working with other providers, public agencies, or community representatives to conduct health assessments in their communities; 70% reported using population-based health status indicators to design or modify services; and 74% reported having a long-term plan for improving the health of the community (American Hospital Association, 1996).

A major trend during the 1980s and 1990s has been that of industrywide consolidation, whereby many community hospitals have affiliated or

merged with other hospitals or joined larger hospital systems (Table 10–4). In 1995, half of all community hospitals were in systems, with beds in private/not-for-profit systems comprising 41% of all beds in systems nationally.

Public Hospitals. Public hospitals are owned by agencies of federal, state, or local government. Federally owned hospitals are maintained primarily for special groups of federal beneficiaries: Native Americans, military personnel, and veterans. State governments have generally limited themselves to the operation of mental and tuberculosis hospitals, reflecting government's early approach to protecting the public by isolating the mentally ill and persons with contagious diseases. Nonfederal public hospitals comprised 26% of all community hospitals in 1995 and provided 18% of beds, 16% of admissions, and 19% of outpatient visits (Table 10–1).

Most local government hospitals are short-stay general hospitals, and most fall into two general types. The first category includes city, county, or hospital district institutions of small or moderate size, with medical staffs consisting of private physicians. Many of these hospitals are located in small cities and towns. They serve both indigent and paying patients. Their costs are met primarily through patient care revenues, and they generally function the same as private, not-for-profit hospitals.

The second category of public hospitals consists of large city or county hospitals in major urban areas. The National Association of Public Hospitals recently identified sixteen different categories of vulnerable populations among their patients (Andrulis, et al., 1996). These hospitals serve a wide range of primarily local residents, but concentrate on the poor. The typical large, urban public hospital is staffed mainly by salaried physicians and residents in training. Most are affiliated with medical schools; their operating costs often exceed patient revenues, and deficits are often made up through

TABLE 10–3 Selected facilities and services, U.S. community hospitals, 1990–1993

Facility or Service	1990	1993	Change 1990–1993
Emergency department	94%	92%	–2%
Trauma center	13%	17%	4%
Ambulatory care			
Medical clinics	85%	89%	4%
Surgery	95%	94%	–1%
Hemodialysis	27%	28%	1%
Acute care			
AIDS/HIV program	NA	74%	NA
Open heart surgery	17%	19%	2%
Geriatric care unit	10%	11%	1%
Behavioral health services			
Acute care psychiatry	28%	33%	5%
Partial hospitalization	13%	18%	5%
Emergency psychiatry	34%	35%	1%
Ambulatory care psychiatry	20%	23%	3%
Ambulatory care substance abuse	21%	21%	0%
Education	22%	24%	2%
Rehabilitation services			
Ambulatory care rehabilitation	52%	58%	6%
Physical therapy	85%	86%	1%
Speech therapy	46%	50%	4%
Occupational therapy	40%	55%	15%
Other services			
Women's health center	21%	28%	7%
Reproductive health	21%	28%	7%
Home care	36%	42%	6%
Health promotion program	77%	90%	13%
CT scanner	70%	77%	7%
MRI unit	18%	31%	13%
Hospice	16%	20%	4%

SOURCE: *Hospital Statistics,* 1994, Chicago: American Hospital Association.

tax subsidies and Medicare and Medicaid disproportionate share payments. Large, urban public hospitals play an important "safety net" role in the health care system. They provide care for all patients regardless of ability to pay, and offer services that many private hospitals cannot or will not provide, including burn and trauma care, alcohol and drug abuse treatment, psychiatric services, care for persons with communicable diseases, and treatment of persons with AIDS. They are located in inner-city

TABLE 10–4   Hospitals and beds in nonfederal multihospital systems by ownership, 1980–1995

	Private/Nonprofit	Catholic Church	Other Church Related	Investor-Owned	All Nonfederal Systems
Total systems					
1980	88	124	20	35	267
1990	165	72	15	54	306
1995	162	57	14	45	278
% change, 1980–1990	88%	–42%	–25%	54%	15%
% change, 1990–1995	–2%	–21%	–7%	–17%	–9%
Hospitals in systems					
1980	426	533	137	701	1,797
1990	806	531	99	1135	2,571
1995	866	488	97	1156	2,607
% change, 1980–1990	89%	0%	–28%	62%	43%
% change, 1990–1995	7%	–8%	–2%	2%	1%
Beds in systems					
1980	91,356	139,767	20,590	89,635	341,348
1990	180,097	123,959	19,248	137,318	460,622
1995	187,320	109,622	19,009	143,183	459,134
% change, 1980–1990	97%	–11%	–7%	53%	35%
% change, 1990–1995	4%	–12%	–1%	4%	0%

SOURCE: *Hospital Statistics,* 1996/97, Chicago: American Hospital Association.

areas where private physicians are often in short supply, and their outpatient departments are often the chief source of ambulatory care for the poor. In addition, public hospitals play a major role in medical education; most are affiliated with a medical school and offer residency training programs. More than half of all practicing physicians receive at least some of their training in public hospitals.

The introduction of the Medicare and Medicaid programs had the potential to reduce the demands on public hospitals by giving the elderly and the poor access to "mainstream" providers. The anticipated shift did not occur, however, in part because private practitioners were in short supply in many inner-city areas; those who were there often limited the number of Medicaid patients they would

accept because of low Medicaid payment rates. In addition, cultural and social barriers often discourage the poor from approaching private physicians and hospitals, and as a result, a large proportion of charity care continues to be provided by public hospitals. Given the increasing demands on and limited financial support for large, urban public hospitals, their futures are uncertain. Characteristically, these hospitals are old and outmoded, and tend to be underequipped, underfinanced, and understaffed. Administration is often constrained by the bureaucratic red tape of city or county government. Ironically, amid this change, the public hospital has become the darling of several American television dramas over the last ten years.

Many public hospitals offer highly specialized tertiary services such as regional trauma services, burn care, neonatal intensive care, and kidney dialysis for all segments of the population, including privately insured patients. Future strategies recommended for public hospitals include continuing as the regional provider of the most costly, high-technology services for the entire population, shifting nonurgent services to lower-cost community sites, partnering with other public and private agencies to provide health care and social services for the chronically ill, and working with medical schools to adapt clinical training programs to the ambulatory environment (Andrulis, et al., 1996).

For-Profit Hospitals. For-profit, investor-owned hospitals are operated to provide a financial return to their owners or shareholders, although spokespersons for the investor-owned hospital companies are quick to point out that profits come from providing good patient care, and satisfying the demands of physicians, patients, and purchasers. In 1995, for-profits represented 14% of community hospitals and provided 12% of beds, 11% of admissions, and 8% of outpatient visits (Table 10–1). At the turn of the century, more than half of the nation's hospitals were proprietary. As late as 1950, there were still over 1,200 proprietary hospitals, but their number declined to under 800 before beginning to rise in recent years. An important underlying shift took place during this period: large, national, investor-owned corporations acquired proprietary hospitals formerly owned by single individuals or partnerships. In recent years, the growth of these companies has been mainly through the purchase of not-for-profit and public hospitals—often those in financial difficulties because of declining inpatient volumes, high debt, and an inability to compete successfully for contracts with managed care plans.

The investor-owned hospital companies assert that their institutions are able to earn profits while maintaining quality by operating more efficiently than not-for-profit hospitals. In addition, investor-owned systems often respond first to strategic opportunities such as population shifts because of their ability to raise capital quickly. They point to the availability of management specialists, the application of modern management techniques, cost savings in construction, economies of scale, and group purchasing as key factors enabling them to control costs without compromising quality.

For-profits have expanded outpatient volumes by almost 60% over the last five years, compared to 32% for the industry as a whole—and the for-profit sector is the only part of the hospital industry in which the total inpatient capacity (that is, number of beds) has grown during this period (Table 10–2). For-profit hospitals report lower average lengths of stay, fewer personnel, and lower expenses per inpatient stay than their not-for-profit counterparts. Critics claim, however, that these apparent efficiencies and the profits they generate are actually attributable to admitting patients with less serious medical conditions, not offering expensive services that do not pay for themselves, and concentrating on those patients able to pay the full costs of hospitalization. Critics also note that the profits derived from these cost savings are passed on to shareholders rather than to the community in the form of lower prices. By not admitting uninsured patients, for-profit hospitals can avoid charity care and bad debts, which may run as high as 10% of total expenses in not-for-profit and public hospitals in certain locations. By not admitting seriously ill patients, for-profit hospitals can avoid providing expensive or unprofitable services. The for-profits reply that they provide community benefits through the taxes they pay, and that these taxes often exceed the amount of charity care provided by tax-exempt not-for-profits.

Do for-profit hospitals really act any differently than not-for-profits? The literature comparing the two supports a number of inferences. Not-for-profits do provide more charity care than for-profits, although the differences are often small. Not-for-profits generally treat a higher portion of Medicaid patients. Not-for-profits are more involved in education and research, and more frequently offer high-cost, unprofitable services such as neonatal intensive care units (NICUs), transplant surgery, burn care, and trauma centers. They are more likely to be located in lower-income areas and to provide community services such as free clinics, HIV/AIDs care, and outreach workers. Few hospital studies have looked carefully at quality of care in relation to ownership, although for-profit hospitals have equal or higher rates of accreditation than not-for-profit hospitals. Studies of nursing homes, however, consistently find more quality problems in for-profit homes. And for-profit nursing homes and home care agencies are more likely to select patients based on ability to pay.

Perhaps most surprising, given the constant claim of the for-profits that they are more efficient than not-for-profits, is a growing body of evidence suggesting that the opposite is true. Several recent studies have compared costs, productivity, revenues, and profits in not-for-profit and for-profit hospitals, adjusting these measures for case-mix complexity and outpatient activity. For-profits were found to have higher profit margins and higher gross and net revenues per case-mix adjusted patient stay. Not-for-profits, however, had lower costs per adjusted stay, even after crediting for-profits for the taxes they pay. Efficiency and productivity were not found to differ significantly between the two types of hospitals. In short, the higher profits earned by the for-profits were due to higher prices and "revenue management" rather than better management of costs or productivity (Shukla & Clement, 1997).

A very important current issue, given the health care industry's shift toward market-oriented reform, is whether health care purchasers place enough value on the availability of charity care, needed but unprofitable services, and other community benefits to contract preferentially with hospitals or systems that provide these services. It does not appear that this is the case. This could be due to the current preoccupation with price. It could also be due to the lack of unequivocal measures of community service. Some purchasers are even wary of providers that give substantial community service, fearing that the costs of these services will be shifted to them in higher prices. Purchasers do weigh the overall reputation of hospitals, and they are beginning to look at Health Plan Employee Data Information Set (HEDIS) and patient satisfaction measures, but these measures focus mainly on a plan's "members," not on benefits provided to the community as a whole. To date, there is little to suggest that purchasers place much value on a comprehensive range of services, on health promotion, on serving all segments of the population, or on actions aimed at optimizing the community's overall health. Perhaps, as economists suggest, not until competition has forced down the prices of all providers and narrowed the price differences among them, will other factors be given more weight (Dowling, 1996).

Small and Rural Hospitals

Small and rural hospitals constitute a large part of the United States hospital industry. In 1995, 45% of all community hospitals had fewer than one hundred beds, and despite some regional variation, this figure has not changed in the last ten years. Most small hospitals are located in rural communities. The preponderance of small hospitals is a legacy of the Hill-Burton program which channeled funds to thinly populated rural areas least able to finance hospital construction without outside help.

In general, small hospitals care for less seriously ill patients than do larger hospitals; their average length of stay is shorter and their care less specialized. The national average daily census for community hospitals with fewer than one hundred beds declined rapidly in the 1980–1990 period, although the rate of loss in census has abated in the last five years (Table 10–5). Due perhaps to hospital closures in many small communities, the average occupancy rate among the very smallest hospitals (37%) increased slightly in recent years (Table 10–6).

Small and rural hospitals face a number of problems that threaten their future viability. Several hundred hospitals have closed since the early 1970s, and many have become part of for-profit or not-for-profit multihospital systems. In general, small hospitals cannot afford as broad a range of services as their larger urban counterparts and find it difficult to keep abreast with developments in medical technology. In addition, labor requirements are high in small hospitals for the services

TABLE 10–5 Trends in U.S. community hospital average daily census (ADC) by bed size, 1980–1995

Hospital Bed Size	ADC, 1980	ADC, 1990	ADC, 1995	% Change 1980–1990	% Change 1990–1995
6–24 beds	2,308	1,431	1,878	–38%	31%
25–49 beds	19,806	14,645	14,650	–26%	0%
50–99 beds	67,630	48,617	44,359	–28%	–9%
Subtotal >100 beds	89,744	64,693	60,887	–28%	–6%
100–199 beds	137,774	112,987	110,117	–18%	–3%
200–299 beds	133,931	120,469	110,562	–10%	–8%
300–399 beds	111,144	97,212	78,509	–13%	–19%
400–499 beds	95,559	72,642	58,881	–24%	–19%
500+ beds	179,254	151,272	129,345	–16%	–14%
Grand total	747,406	619,275	548,301	–17%	–11%

SOURCE: *Hospital Statistics*, 1996/97, Chicago: American Hospital Association.

TABLE 10–6 Trends in U.S. community hospital occupancy rates by bed size, 1990–1995

Hospital Bed Size	Occupancy Rate, 1990	Occupancy Rate, 1995	Change 1990–1995
6–24 beds	32.30%	36.84%	4.54%
25–49 beds	41.30%	42.52%	1.22%
50–99 beds	53.80%	53.67%	–0.13%
100–199 beds	61.50%	58.74%	–2.76%
200–299 beds	67.10%	63.03%	–4.07%
300–399 beds	70.00%	64.73%	–5.27%
400–499 beds	73.50%	68.10%	–5.40%
500+ beds	77.30%	71.40%	–5.90%

SOURCE: *Hospital Statistics*, 1996/97, Chicago: American Hospital Association.

offered, and small hospitals tend to operate at far less efficient occupancy levels than larger hospitals. On the other hand, the few studies that have examined quality in relation to size suggest that small hospitals that treat only conditions they are equipped to handle can achieve equally good outcomes as larger hospitals.

Small and rural hospitals have historically been strongly affected by Medicare and Medicaid funding (due in part to less adequate private health insurance coverage in rural areas and a higher elderly population). In the 1980s, the Medicare Prospective Payment System effectively penalized rural hospitals because the low-wage scales in rural areas resulted in low DRG payment rates. Coupled with the depressed economies of some of these communities, these pressures caused a number of small hospitals to incur operating losses and threatened the survival of many.

Strategies employed by rural hospitals focus on linking with other local and regional hospitals, joining managed care contracting networks, and seeking additional resources by broadening their role in the communities they serve. The key to the future of small and rural hospitals would appear to lie in regional networking, especially since managed care organizations favor wide geographic availability of health care services for their enrolled populations (Brown, 1996). These arrangements should encourage referral of patients to the institutional setting most appropriate to their needs. Rural communities are also seeking to strengthen their hospitals by entering into contractual relationships with their physicians that unify the interests of the two.

Strategic relationships between urban and rural providers today range from informal agreements to formal affiliations, joint programs, and the merger of institutions into multihospital systems. The objectives of such relationships include: a two-way flow of patients, with patients referred to larger hospitals for specialized services and returned to smaller communities for long-term, follow-up, and home care; participation in the continuing educational programs of the larger hospital; management assistance from the larger hospital; consolidation of services; and group purchasing. Many rural hospitals have begun to collaborate with urban health care systems in "telemedicine" programs that provide clinical support and educational programming across great distances. The success of regional networks depends on community support, collaboration between management and physicians, and synchronized financial incentives. The number of examples of effective regional relationships involving hospitals, public health departments, physician groups, and even school districts, is growing. In the long run, community and regional networking may preserve rather than threaten the independence and viability of smaller hospitals.

Academic Medical Centers

Academic medical centers (AMCs) are university-owned hospitals. They are typically large, urban institutions. AMCs' patient care activities are included in the overall statistics for community hospitals. Despite significant strategic challenges facing AMCs today in the form of increased competition and reduced financial support, these institutions are largely responsible for the major advances in twentieth-century American medical treatment, technology, and training.

Historically, AMCs have performed several distinct functions simultaneously: they operate as tertiary-care referral centers offering state-of-the-art technology for the diagnosis and treatment of the most complex medical problems; they function as the primary clinical teaching site for their medical schools; they house much of the nation's medical research; and they care for a large portion of the poor in the areas in which they are located. Care in AMCs is provided primarily by faculty and residents whose patient care activities are administered by faculty practice plans. Many patients are enrolled in clinical trials run by faculty researchers.

The expansion of AMCs in number and degree of sophistication roughly parallels a fifty-year period of substantial investment in medical research by the federal National Institutes of Health. AMCs were given an additional boost by Medicare and Medicaid reimbursement. In the early 1980s, however, with Medicare's introduction of the DRG prospective payment system to contain Medicare spending, the fortunes of many AMCs began to change. AMCs in general have been slow to respond to the cost-cutting incentives implicit in prospective payment and managed care.

Historically, teaching hospitals relied heavily on public subsidies in the form of Medicare and Medicaid payments for direct and indirect medical education costs, and "disproportionate share" payments in recognition of the high portion of poor patients they serve. These subsidies are seriously threatened by the current cutbacks in public health care spending and by market pressures to contain private spending. Teaching hospitals have also been able to "cost-shift" some of their higher costs to private insurers in the form of higher rates. In addition, like all hospitals, many teaching hospitals are experiencing declines in admissions and lengths of stay (Carey & Engelhard, 1996).

Congressional debate today centers on slowing the growth of Medicare spending. Because AMCs have depended on Medicare payment supplements to help cover the costs associated with teaching, they are especially vulnerable to payment cuts. In addition, AMCs must compete with community hospitals to be included in the provider networks of managed care health plans. Hence, they are under great pressure to reduce costs, but given their salaried physician staffs and relatively high operating costs, this transition will be difficult. In fact, a major national commission appointed to study the future of AMCs recommended in 1995 that a substantial number of medical schools and their hospitals close by the year 2005, and that training resources be redirected to primary care (Bolognia & Wintroub, 1996).

The societal pressures that led AMCs to expand expensive teaching and research programs and acquire advanced technology have reversed course, and now challenge AMCs to compete for contracts with managed care plans and other purchasers based on competitive prices. As a result, many AMCs that in the last two generations built national and international reputations through the growth of state-of-the-art technology are now trying to adapt by developing primary care delivery networks, revising teaching programs, downsizing, and aligning with not-for-profit or for-profit systems in order to be better positioned in the new medical marketplace.

HOSPITALS AND HEALTH SYSTEMS

Consolidation of hospitals and other providers into networks and systems—first in the form of hospitals coming together into multihospital systems, and more recently, in the form of hospitals, physicians, and other providers consolidating into integrated health care systems—has been a dominant trend in the health care industry since the early 1970s. Consolidation is fundamentally changing the landscape of the nation's health system and, even more significantly, is reshaping the relationships among purchasers, health plans, providers, and the people they serve. Consolidation can take many organizational forms: acquisition of one entity by another, the merger of two or more entities to create a new organization, or the formation of more loosely structured alliances and networks.

Consolidation in the health care industry is of two basic types: horizontal integration and vertical integration. Horizontal integration refers to the coordination or consolidation of facilities or services that are at the same stage of the patient care "production process." Examples include the coming together of hospitals into multihospital systems, which is the focus of this chapter; the joining of individual physician practices into medical groups; and the merger of a number of home care agencies into a single, larger home care organization. The primary goals of horizontal integration are economies of scale, elimination of redundant or underutilized facilities, group purchasing, streamlining operations, and, in recent years, strengthening the resulting system's hand in competing for and negotiating contracts with health plans.

Vertical integration refers to organizing the "production" of patient care so that the sequential stages in the process are carried out or coordinated by a single organization (Gillies, et al., 1993; Mick & Conrad, 1988). Comprehensive integration would entail coordinating the entire range of services for protecting, maintaining, and restoring peoples' health, from disease prevention and health promotion at one end of the spectrum to treatment and rehabilitation at the other. Coordinated provision of a full continuum of services, in turn, would require coordination of the work of physicians, one or more hospitals, long-term care facilities, home care agencies, and a variety of other providers. The goals of vertical integration are cost-effectiveness, continuity and quality of care, and better positioning of the providers comprising the integrated health care system to compete, assume risk, and manage the care of the population served.

Two fundamental motives propelled the multihospital system movement of the 1970s and 1980s that so dramatically changed the character of the hospital industry: organizational survival and organizational growth. For many freestanding hospitals, the increasingly complex, fast-changing, demanding, even hostile health care environment made survival problematic. Competition, financial pressures, regulation, and other external forces were so threatening that hundreds of hospitals turned to systems for the strength to survive, albeit under different ownership. For the systems, acquisition of additional hospitals provided a means to grow—to add new services, enter new markets, establish new referral patterns, or build more financial and political power.

In 1995, 278 nonfederal multihospital systems, defined as corporations that own, lease, or manage two or more acute care hospitals, accounted for 2,607 (50%) of the nation's community hospitals (Table 10–4). These systems operated 52% of the nation's community hospital beds. Of the 278 multihospital systems, 57 (21%) were Catholic; 14 (5%) had other religious affiliations; 162 (58%) were secular not-for-profit; and 45 (16%) were investor-owned. Although representing only 16% of the nation's multihospital systems, the investor-owned systems tend to be large, averaging 26 hospitals and 3,200 beds per system, compared to 6 hospitals and 1,350 beds per not-for-profit system. As a result, investor-owned systems contain 44% of all system hospitals and represent 31% of all system beds.

The growth of horizontally integrated hospital systems began in earnest in the late 1960s, spurred by the entry and expansion of investor-owned systems in response to the improved financial climate for hospitals following the enactment of Medicare and Medicaid. Not-for-profit system growth picked up in the mid-1970s. Today, hospital acquisitions, mergers, and affiliations are aimed at better positioning the participants to compete for market share. Since health care markets are local in nature, local or metropolitan groupings of hospitals have gained in importance, and large multistate systems have tended to plan their strategies and investments on a market-by-market basis, even divesting hospitals in markets where they have a limited presence. Luke and Olden (1996) have explored the "local hospital system" phenomenon and report that over 1,000 (25%) of the nation's hospitals belong to one of 400 urban-centered local groupings. Over half of all urban hospitals are in some type of local alliance, network, or system.

How well have multihospital systems actually performed? Shortell's (1988) seminal review of the evidence on system performance, based on the handful of then-available studies and on comparative data from nearly one thousand system and freestanding hospitals, concluded that "there is little support for any of the alleged advantages of system hospitals relative to their nonsystem counterparts. . . . Little if any economic or service 'value added' appears to be present." Areas of performance examined by Shortell included:

- Costs, economies of scale, efficiency, productivity
- Prices
- Financial performance, profitability
- Access to capital
- Charity care provided
- Services offered
- Managed care involvement
- Quality, patient care outcomes

Shortell hypothesized that the unimpressive performance of systems was due largely to the fact that many systems had formed mainly as a defensive reaction to the increasingly hostile health care environment. Systems were seeking security rather than lower costs or greater community health benefits. Nor did most systems really behave like systems in the sense of "operating as an organic whole with a strategic intent." Shortell's findings undoubtedly also reflected the fact that in the mid-1980s, many systems were in the formative stages, and most saw

themselves as horizontally integrated hospital systems, not as vertically integrated delivery systems.

Vertical Integration

The pressures to transform today's fragmented financing and delivery structures into rationally designed, integrated health care systems come from the growth of managed care and the movement toward health care reform. These forces are giving rise to two new realities: (1) Medicare, Medicaid, and private purchasers are curtailing their spending to the point that the flow of dollars into health care will not sustain the delivery system as it exists today, and (2) capitation-based payment is ending the separate flow of payments to each category of provider and putting providers at financial risk. But today's fragmented "nonsystem" of still largely independent physicians, hospitals, and health plans is not structured to manage care within fixed dollar limits or to deploy resources more rationally.

There is growing recognition that the changing financial and market pressures call for a restructuring of the way health care is delivered. Providers are responding by coming together into organized delivery systems able to accept responsibility for the health of enrolled populations, manage care across the full spectrum of services, reduce fragmentation and redundancy, and do so within fixed financial resources determined increasingly by purchasers. This model is generally referred to as a "vertically integrated delivery system." An extreme form of vertical integration intended to capture patients at the source (that is, when they choose a health insurance plan) entails integration of the delivery and financing functions. A number of delivery organizations are starting health plans or contracting with a health plan to be the plan's exclusive or preferred provider resource. At the same time, a number of health plans are approaching this from the other direction and assembling their own provider networks through selective contracting. The integrated delivery system is clearly "an idea whose time has come," although most providers are just beginning to assemble all the elements (Dowling, 1995).

The generic elements or properties that characterize a vertically integrated delivery system include (Dowling, 1995; Shortell, et al., 1995):

1. *A broad range of facilities and services*— prevention, promotion, primary care, specialty care, acute care, long-term care, home care— under a single organizational umbrella. This facilitates coordination and continuity of care and the use of the sites of care most appropriate to each patient's needs.
2. *A group or network of primary care physicians* formally linked with the delivery system through arrangements that align the interests of both parties. The primary care physicians should be organized to manage care and promote health within available resources. They should be geographically located to provide access to the system throughout the area served. Economic incentives and organizational loyalties should be structured so that the primary care physicians share responsibility with the system for costs, outcomes, and system performance.
3. *Specialists* and other providers formally linked with the delivery system through arrangements and incentives that align the interests of both parties and encourage the delivery of cost-effective, quality care.
4. *Mechanisms for coordinating/integrating care* across the entire spectrum of services that facilitate cost-effective, quality care and reduce fragmentation, duplication, and redundancy. Examples include primary care physicians as care managers, clinical nurse specialists in care coordination roles, coordination by interdisciplinary teams, case management, treatment guidelines, an integrated information system, a single medical record, and discharge coordinators/ social workers in both inpatient and outpatient settings.
5. *Health promotion services* that prevent or reduce the risks of illness and injury. Examples include immunizations and other prevention services, health education, lifestyle change programs, fitness programs, self-care education, and occupational health and safety programs. Mechanisms for identifying high-risk people and bringing them into specially tailored health maintenance programs are especially important.
6. *Information systems* that enable planning, monitoring, evaluating, and publicly reporting on cost-effectiveness, quality, and outcomes. Information systems should be able to track populations/patients over time and across providers/sites, integrate data from all settings, and relate outcomes to treatment. Information systems should be able to support the management of patient care as well as the management of financial risk. Information should enable the profiling of both providers and treatment patterns.
7. *Integrated strategic planning, resource allocation, and assessment of system performance* facilitated by cross-functional management and organizational structures. Systematic assessment and deployment of new technologies.
8. *Unified marketing and contracting* such that the delivery system approaches the market as a single entity.
9. *Integration of financing and delivery* through common ownership and/or exclusive or preferred relationships with health plans.

The growth of managed care has made integration of financing and delivery especially important. Previously, insurers paid for the services rendered by whatever providers individuals chose to go to. Few providers were excluded. With the advent of

HMOs, PPOs, and selective contracting, insurers and health plans began to contract only with selected providers and to employ financial disincentives to discourage their enrollees from using other providers. Hence, health plans became the providers' source of patients. Integration of finance and delivery gives providers a direct link to the source of patients. It also enables the delivery system to (1) align incentives, (2) rationally deploy resources internally (which is almost impossible if insurers pay each provider independently and often in a contradictory manner), and (3) benefit financially from being efficient. A few major integrated health care systems like Kaiser and Group Health Cooperative of Puget Sound own their own health plan; most systems contract to assume the financial risk for the care of the enrollees of health plans they do not own. The delivery system's goal, however, is to be in the position to control the methods and levels of payment to its providers, that is, to "manage the capitation dollar."

System leaders believe vertical integration can cut costs substantially through improved cost-effectiveness of care, lower admissions, lower service utilization, shorter lengths of stay, economies of scale, greater volumes, and increased productivity. Reductions in length of stay and service utilization are widely reported to result from the use of clinical treatment guidelines, case management, discharge planning, coordination of posthospital services, and filling gaps in the availability of services. Where systems are at financial risk as a result of capitated contracts for the health of a defined population, greater emphasis is placed on health education, health promotion, and prevention. Vertical integration, driven by capitation and guided by population-based planning, also tends to lead to efforts to achieve a better fit between a system's resources and the needs of the populations it serves. Attention focuses, for example, on the balance between primary care physicians and specialists.

Hospital beds are eliminated in favor of outpatient facilities and long-term care beds. The matching of system resources to the needs of the population served has come to be called "rightsizing" (Coddington, et al., 1996).

Consolidating a substantial portion of an area's providers into a single system can greatly strengthen the system's bargaining power with purchasers. In some cases, this has gone so far as to raise antitrust questions. It may be that many systems first pursue integration mainly to cut costs and/or to gain market power. But once the elements of integrated service delivery are assembled, systems faced with increasing pressures from purchasers to cut costs may then turn their attention to the efficiencies achievable through better coordination of care. Coddington, Moore, and Fischer (1996) concluded from a study of ten integrated health care systems that the strategies pursued by these organizations were primarily aimed at gaining competitive advantage. "However, when properly implemented . . . these strategies also enable organizations to increase the value added they bring to their customers and communities" (p. 181).

Many observers see the hospital- or hospital system–sponsored integrated delivery system as the ideal organizational form and inevitable end point toward which health care delivery is transitioning. Hospitals have capital, community ties, and management leadership, and most have already diversified vertically into a broad range of services. Some enjoy dominant market positions. Hurley (1993), however, has challenged this "conventional wisdom" by highlighting a number of obstacles to provider leadership of delivery reform, many of which are rooted in the reality that "provider-sponsored integration proposals are inherently self-serving." Hurley notes that neither communities nor purchasers seem inclined to trust providers to redeploy the resources they have historically controlled to convert from hospital-centered to continuum of care–centered systems. In addition, a basic conflict exists between the desire of purchasers to spend less and providers' appetite for the latest technology. Medical staff politics which often stymie change is another major impediment.

Competition for the central role in reorganizing delivery is coming from increasingly aggressive purchasers. As meaningful information on costs, efficacy, and customer satisfaction becomes more readily available, and as the oversupply of hospital beds and physicians in many markets gives purchasers alternative providers from which to choose, purchasers will be in a position to selectively contract with whatever providers they believe give them the most value. In short, purchasers will be able to put together their own provider networks.

Between the provider-sponsored and purchaser-sponsored models, Hurley defines a third model—a long-term, bilateral contract between a provider network or system and an intermediary who plays the role of exclusive distributor of the providers' health benefits product to one or more purchasers. A group model HMO marketed by a single insurer or health plan approaches this model. Typically, the intermediary is in the driver's seat in this model. A fourth candidate for the central role in integrating the delivery of care and controlling the flow of dollars is the conglomerate of medical groups. Such "supergroups" can pursue contracts with health plans on behalf of their participating physicians and accept financial risk, often for hospital as well as physician services.

Hospital Responses to Competition and Cost-Containment Pressures

In addition to the trend toward consolidation, hospitals are actively adapting to the new competitive environment in other ways. Prospective payment and price competition create a strong incentive for hospitals to achieve more efficient staffing levels, since labor represents approximately 54% of the average hospital's costs. Hospitals are looking at ways to utilize nurses more efficiently by "re-engineering" how patient care is provided, and many hospitals are substituting less highly trained support personnel for professional nurses. Total Quality Management and Continuous Quality Improvement (TQM/CQI) techniques are being applied to streamline work processes and restructure the way ancillary departments support nursing and other direct patient care departments. Hospitals are also attempting to increase the productivity of their workforce by cross-training employees to fill multiple positions. Unfortunately, this emphasis on cost containment and productivity is likely to create new conflicts between hospitals, nurses, and labor unions.

Hospitals are investigating other methods of increasing their efficiency and competitiveness, including product- or service-line management. The practice of analyzing hospital programs and services as strategic business units (SBUs) in order to identify and enhance profitable services and turn around or eliminate unprofitable services is being advocated by many as a more businesslike approach to hospital management (Ruffner, 1986). The concern is that some hospitals may discontinue services that are unprofitable but needed by the community. Still, a positive aspect of product-line management is the development and organization of services to meet the special needs of specific subgroups in the population. Examples include diabetes programs, women's programs, and sports medicine clinics. It can be argued that competition is forcing hospitals to be much more sensitive to the needs and desires of people for convenient, specially tailored services.

Under Medicare's DRG payment system, there is a strong incentive for hospitals to discharge patients as soon as medically warranted, and this has done a great deal to foster the effectiveness of discharge planning. The role of the discharge planner is critical in ensuring that patients receive proper care after leaving the hospital. For elderly patients in particular, rehospitalizations may result unless proper discharge instructions and support services are provided. In many instances, the elderly patient cannot be discharged from the hospital until placement in a nursing home is secured or arrangements are made for home care. This has heightened the interest of many hospitals in operating their own skilled nursing units and home care programs. A major concern of the Medicare program is that hospitals not discharge patients too soon. Hospitals are under great pressure to deliver exactly the right amount of care to Medicare patients, since too much care may result in reimbursement denials and too little care can result in penalty assessments or lawsuits. As a result, hospitals are placing more emphasis on complete documentation of patient care in medical records.

INTERNAL ORGANIZATION OF COMMUNITY HOSPITALS

From the outside, hospitals appear as cohesive organizations with a united sense of purpose and a clear goal of providing high-quality patient care. From the inside, however, hospitals are comprised of several different components, each of which has distinct goals and roles: the management team, which is responsible for the efficient operation of the institution as a whole; the medical staff, which is responsible for the quality of patient care provided by physicians; and the governing board, which sets institutional policy and goals and has responsibility for the fiscal health of the organization (see Figure 10–2).

Each party has distinct responsibilities. The governing board is ultimately responsible for everything that goes on in the hospital, both administratively and clinically. The board's role is often described as one of stewardship for the insti-

tution. It carries out this responsibility by adopting policies and plans to guide the hospital's operation; selecting and delegating management responsibilities to a chief executive and supervising the chief executive's performance; and appointing physicians to the medical staff, approving the medical staff's organization for governing itself and for supervising the professional activities of its members, and delegating responsibility to the medical staff for the provision of patient care.

In reality, boundaries between areas of authority among triad members are not always clear. For example, while it might seem there is a clear distinction between governance and the medical staff's responsibility for patient care, courts have concluded that hospitals have a corporate responsibility or legal liability for ensuring that patients receive high-quality patient care. Thus, the governing board must make sure that only qualified physicians practice in the hospital and that quality assurance mechanisms are established and working, yet only the medical staff has the expertise to assess qualifications and judge the care provided by individual physicians.

Although the medical staff is legally subordinate to the governing board's authority over the affairs of the institution, physicians are partially autonomous from the board through the structures set forth in the medical staff bylaws. And from an economic perspective, physician independence from the hospital exists because most are in private practice and are not employed by the institution. On the other hand, physicians in most specialty fields need access to the hospital to practice modern medicine, and only the governing board has the power to grant the privilege of practicing in a hospital. The unique relationship between physicians and hospitals is not without stresses and strains, and it makes the governance and management of hospitals a challenging responsibility.

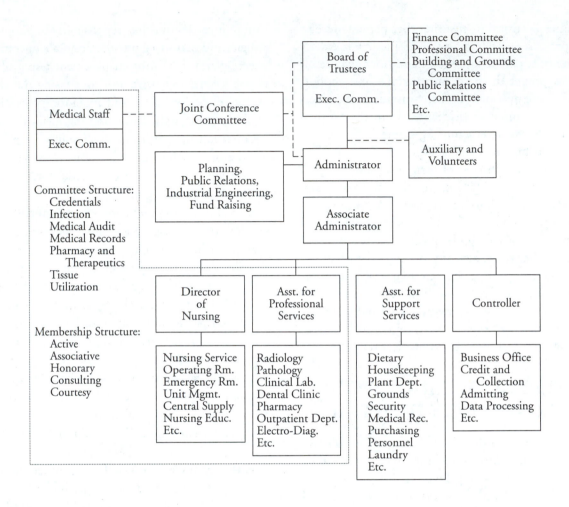

SOURCE: Reprinted with permisson from *A Primer for Hospital Trustees,* Chamber of Commerce of the United States, 1974, Washington, DC: Author.

FIGURE 10–2 Prototypical hospital organization chart

Delineating the roles of the board and management, distinctions are not always clear between the board's responsibility for adopting policies to guide the hospital and management's responsibility for implementing these policies and managing the hospital's activities on a day-to-day basis. Problems can arise when the governing board becomes involved in administrative matters. On the other hand, management may make decisions that overreach specific (or implied) board policies. Teamwork and communication are necessary to avoid conflict or misunderstandings.

Hospital executives have developed significant expertise in recent years in dealing with the increasingly complex operational, market, and regulatory issues confronting hospitals. But since the internal triad does not always agree on directions and priorities, hospitals often experience internal tensions and find it difficult to respond in a systematic way to environmental conditions and changing community needs. Given the challenges within today's health care industry, it is more imperative than ever that hospital leadership work as a team.

The Governing Board

The governing board of the community hospital has evolved in function and structure as the hospital itself has developed new roles. During the late 1800s and early 1900s, when advances in medical science were transforming hospitals from custodial institutions for the sick poor to sources of effective and safe care for the entire community, board members were often wealthy benefactors who gave money to establish and equip the hospital and meet its deficits. The primary function of the board at that time was trusteeship, that is, preserving the assets that they and others like them donated. The trustees' job was seen as providing the facilities and equipment the medical staff needed to care for patients with little direct involvement in medical matters. Administrative duties were divided among board members; the hospital manager often functioned as a clerk.

After World War I, the complexity and size of hospitals exceeded the ability of board members to personally handle day-to-day administration. Business managers were employed to handle administrative and financial matters; the business manager and superintendent of nurses reported to the board, and the board coordinated their work. As operational complexity and the competence of hospital managers increased, they gradually assumed administrative responsibility for nursing and all of the hospital's departments, so that only one person reported directly to the board. The business manager's title evolved to "superintendent."

The governing board's role changed further as hospitals became ever more complex and as philanthropy yielded to patient revenue as the primary source of financial support. The board's role became one of overall policy making and planning, and board membership was used to augment and supplement the skills of the administrative staff. Hospital boards included fewer philanthropists and more individuals with specific management skills including business executives, attorneys, bankers, architects, and contractors. Reflecting these areas of expertise, board decision making tended to focus on finance, personnel, and physical plant matters. Boards typically deferred to the medical staff regarding physician qualifications and patient care.

Since the 1960s, several major trends have brought further change in the governing board's role. Continuing advances in medical science, the proliferation of medical technology, and the rapid growth in hospital sophistication have given hospitals a central role in the United States health care system, while also creating public concern about the cost of hospital care. Public expectations regarding hospitals' responsibility to the community have also changed, so that hospitals are now viewed as community resources with obligations to address community needs. In addition, the regulation of hospital construction, costs, quality, and use, as well as labor relations, have become more stringent, particularly following the establishment of Medicare and Medicaid. Finally, court decisions have clearly established the concept of corporate or institutional responsibility for ensuring the quality of patient care. As a result of these forces, the governing board's role has broadened and become more demanding.

Boards have become quite active in monitoring the changing environment, becoming knowledgeable about community concerns and external trends, and interpreting the significance of these trends for the hospital. External competitive pressures have forced hospitals to reexamine their priorities and programs, and boards have found it necessary to provide clearer direction and stronger leadership in strategic planning. Boards have expanded community representation within their membership and assumed the role of mediating between the demands on the hospital from the community, the medical staff, employees, and interest groups. Board members often take the lead in discussions with other hospitals about an alliance and merger, and boards assume the central role in exploring system opportunities. Finally, boards have been forced to take a more active role in quality control, rather than abdicating this responsibility to the medical staff. Although the function of quality monitoring is still delegated to the medical staff, boards are more actively involved in scrutinizing how well this function is carried out.

Research on the topic of effective hospital governance has suggested five success factors for effective performance: (1) a common definition of governance, (2) a clearly defined mission for the organization, (3) a decision-making process based upon continuing education, (4) an efficient board structure with clear priorities, and (5) a communication and reporting system for clear information (Umdenstock, et al., 1990).

The board is responsible for ensuring that the mechanisms for evaluating the credentials of physicians and monitoring the care they provide are established and working. Courts have held the board and the hospital responsible in malpractice cases in which reasonable precautions were not taken to ensure the careful selection of the medical staff; establishment of high standards of care; and enforcement of policies, rules, and regulations. In practice, direct board control over medical staff performance is limited and depends more on the medical staff's commitment to quality than on formal sanctions such as suspending or terminating a physician's hospital privileges. As governing boards have become more actively involved in medical and patient care matters, an increasing number have added physicians to their membership. More than half of all community hospital boards now include physicians.

Governance functions and structures in multihospital systems are an important issue for the hospital field. Several models for structuring governance in multihospital systems have been developed. In the parent holding company model, governing bodies exist at both the system and institutional levels. Some systems have adopted a variation of the parent holding company model in which there is a system-level governing board and boards at the institutional level that serve in an advisory rather than governing capacity. The corporate model exists when a single system-level governing board carries out all governance activities for both the system and the individual institutions that make it up. In all three models, the corporate-level board is likely to retain responsibility for decisions regarding the transfer or sale of assets, formation of new companies, purchase of major assets, changes in hospital bylaws, and appointment of local board members. The corporate model has the advantage of structural simplicity and clear lines of authority, while the holding company model provides for greater input and involvement at the community level. In general, the more decentralized the governance model, the more likely it is that activities such as service development, strategic planning, capital and operating budget, medical staff privileges, and appointment and evaluation of the hospital chief executive officer will be under "local" board control.

Today, governing boards are being challenged as never before. They are called on to oversee system and institutional costs and effectiveness in meeting community, patient, and purchaser demands in an environment of constant change. They seek to balance the institution's overall mission, quality, and community benefit, while also seeking to compete effectively. Hospital boards are increasingly required to understand the long-term implications of significant business decisions, such as physician practice acquisitions or the signing of managed care contracts. The boards of investor-owned systems are also concerned about profits and the financial return to the company's shareholders. This shift in trustees' roles is a significant adjustment from traditionally passive asset management and short-term financial oversight. Some boards are clearly rising to the new challenges. They are being more selective in choosing members, they are educating themselves more fully, and they are streamlining board structures to expedite decision making.

Management

Hospital, and more recently, health system, management has grown in importance as hospitals have grown in size and sophistication and combined into multihospital systems. The job of implementing board policy and the responsibility for day-to-day operations are delegated by the board to the chief executive officer. The chief executive officer has direct responsibility for the management team, the institution's finances, acquiring and maintaining equipment and facilities, planning and implementing new services, and hiring and supervising personnel. A key aspect of the job is to coordinate and serve as the "channel of communication" among the governing board, medical staff, and hospital departments. Even more critical today is strategic planning to position the hospital to compete effectively in the managed care marketplace.

In addition to financial, personnel, and physical plant matters, the management team plays an important role in patient care. It is responsible for coordinating the work of the patient care and support departments, ensuring that departments are adequately equipped and staffed and functioning smoothly. Under the chief executive, the management team is actively involved in planning for new patient care services and in ensuring that the hospital meets accreditation, licensure, and regulatory standards. Because the medical staff is normally not employed by the hospital, the chief executive must establish a cooperative working relationship with physicians to accomplish tasks that involve both administrative and clinical considerations. The management team acts as the liaison with the community and with external agencies, both bringing information from these sources into hospital decision making and planning processes, and representing the hospital to outside parties. Because of the increasing impact of external and regulatory pressures on hospitals, this latter role has become one of the most important aspects of hospital managers' jobs.

Medical staff relations have, in the last decade, become a critical area of concern for management. Although the nature of physicians' hospital practice has historically been voluntary, today numerous alliances and joint ventures between hospitals and physicians are being formed, including physician-hospital organizations (PHOs) for joint contracting with health plans. Many hospitals and integrated delivery systems are actively pursuing the acquisition of physician practices and entering into contractual relationships with medical groups to be better positioned to compete for contracts with health plans, assume risk, and manage care for contracted populations. In these scenarios, the arrangements between the hospital and physicians resemble a business partnership more than the traditional hospital–medical staff relationship.

Historically, hospital administration has advanced rapidly as a profession, moving from "business manager" in the 1920s, to management "coordinator" in the 1950s, to the modern-day corporate chief executive with authority for directing all aspects of the hospital's strategy and operations. As professional management has broadened from hospitals to ambulatory care, long-term care, home care, health plans, medical groups, and other organizations, the title "hospital administration" has given way to "health care administration," and the chief executive's title is commonly "president" or "chief executive officer" rather than "administrator." To survive the challenges encountered in today's competitive environment, the successful chief executive and management team must continuously develop new skills, including the ability to articulate a clear and compelling vision for the organization, formulate and execute strategies, empower the organization's people, innovate, practice value-based management, satisfy consumers and purchasers, and accept increasing levels of entrepreneurial risk.

Hospital Medical Staff

The governing board delegates responsibility for assuring high-quality patient care to the medical staff, which is formally organized to carry out this responsibility and is accountable for it to the board. Unlike in many advanced countries, where hospital medical staffs are composed of salaried physicians, the medical staffs of most hospitals in the United States are composed of private practitioners who are not employees of the hospital. The relationship between the hospital and its medical staff is a mutually dependent and sometimes stressful one. The hospital is dependent on the medical staff to admit and care for patients and monitor the quality of patient care. In a sense, physicians are the clients of the hospital, since it is they who admit patients, decide how long they will stay, order tests and procedures, and direct the care provided by the hospital's staff. On the other hand, physicians are dependent on the hospital because, in order to practice modern medicine, they must have access to its diagnostic and therapeutic services. Thus, a

quid pro quo relationship exists—physicians agree to abide by hospital policies and medical staff rules and to devote time to the medical staff's quality assurance functions (in the past, they also contributed time to care for indigent patients), in return for the privilege of using the hospital to care for their patients. This traditional relationship is under intense pressure today, however, as the competitive, managed care marketplace has created an alphabet soup of physician-hospital arrangements for contracting with health plans and has intensified competition between physicians.

In carrying out its responsibility for ensuring the quality of patient care, the medical staff organizes and governs itself, establishes qualifications for appointment to the staff and for clinical privileges, establishes standards of care and rules and regulations to guide the provision of care, and supervises the professional performance of its members. These duties are accomplished in accordance with the medical staff bylaws, which set forth the form, functions, and responsibilities of the medical staff. Bylaws must be approved by both the medical staff and the governing board.

Different categories of appointment to the medical staff carry different privileges and responsibilities. *Active medical staff* members have full hospital privileges and provide most of the medical care in the hospital. They are responsible for the governance and administrative activities of the organized medical staff. The *associate medical staff* consists of physicians and dentists who are being considered for advancement to the active medical staff; *courtesy medical staff* members meet the qualifications for active membership but admit patients to the hospital only occasionally (usually because they are on the active staff of another hospital); and the *consulting medical staff* includes physicians and dentists who are recognized for their professional expertise and who act as consultants to the hospital medical staff physicians, although they practice primarily in other hospitals. Finally, the *honorary staff* consists of physicians recognized for their past service to the hospital; and *residents* are employed as the house staff of hospitals with formal teaching programs, functioning under the supervision of attending physicians.

The administrative head of the typical community hospital's medical staff organization is the president or chief of staff. The chief of staff acts as liaison among the governing board, the chief executive, and the medical staff; chairs the executive committee of the medical staff and serves as an ex officio member of all medical staff committees; enforces governing board policies and medical staff bylaws; maintains standards of medical care in the hospital; and provides for continuing education for the medical staff. Although the chief of staff is usually elected by the medical staff, this position is also in a sense part of the hospital's administrative structure, directly accountable to the hospital's governing board. Larger hospitals often employ a full-time salaried medical director to augment the chief of staff in linking administrative and medical staff activities, to direct the administrative infrastructure that supports quality assurance and utilization review, and to participate with the governing board and management team in strategic planning and program development. This trend is growing rapidly in light of the challenges inherent in integrating physicians and hospitals to assume quality care and be better positioned for managed care.

Most of the organizational responsibilities of the medical staff are carried out by committees. The *executive committee* is the key administrative and policy-making body of the medical staff. It governs the activities of the medical staff, and all other committees are advisory to it. It is typically composed of the chief of staff, the chiefs of the clinical departments, and a number of at-large members elected by the active medical staff. The

joint conference committee is the formal liaison between the governing board and medical staff and includes members from both groups plus the chief executive. This committee is a forum for discussing medical administrative matters of mutual concern. The *credentials committee* reviews the qualifications of applicants to the medical staff and makes recommendations regarding appointments, annual reappointments, and clinical privileges. Recommendations are transmitted through the medical staff executive committee to the hospital's governing board, which has final authority over medical staff membership and privileges. Other medical staff committees oversee specific functional areas or departments (for example, emergency room, nursing, pharmacy, special care, and surgery) and manage important quality assurance and monitoring activities, including medical audit, utilization review, and tissue review.

Under pressure from managed care organizations and other purchasers of health care services, hospitals have moved rapidly in the 1990s to gain greater control over the appropriateness and cost-effectiveness, as well as quality, of the care provided within their walls. Recent shifts in reimbursement toward prospective payment have significantly changed the financial incentives for hospitals. To a greater extent than ever before, hospitals now must ensure that hospital admissions are justifiable, that lengths of stay do not exceed accepted norms, and that treatment regimens are medically appropriate. As an extension of their traditional responsibility for quality, it is critical that medical staff now share in the process of evaluating utilization, particularly under health plan contracts in which there is fixed reimbursement. Evidence-based practice guidelines, continuous quality improvement (CQI) techniques, and other quality/cost-management tools have become commonplace with hospital medical staffs. More recently, hospitals have been faced with health plans' and purchasers' interest in quality report cards and outcomes measurement (Hanchak, 1996).

The growing pressure on hospitals to exercise greater influence over physician behavior to control costs and utilization and improve outcomes represents a significant threat to physician autonomy and can result in increased conflict between hospital management and the medical staff. Methods used by hospitals to influence physician behavior include direct appeals, adding physicians to the governing board, establishing medical director positions, joint ventures between medical services and technology, "economic credentialing," and the employment of physicians (Glandon & Morrisey, 1986). Additional approaches include education, peer review and feedback, administrative rules, participation in developing treatment guidelines, and incentives (Grieco & Eisenberg, 1993).

In heavily managed care–driven markets, hospitals and physicians are pursuing a variety of strategies depending on the leverage that managed care organizations have in the selection of providers and pricing of managed care contracts. In some markets, integrated physician/hospital arrangements have been formed as a vehicle for sharing the benefits and risks of health plan contracting, while in other markets intense competition for ambulatory care services and health plan contracts has left hospitals struggling to utilize excess capacity while their physicians migrate to other facilities, or consider selling their assets to practice management companies.

The responsibilities of the hospital medical staff (credentialing, appointing, privileging, reviewing, and reappointing) and its formal structure (officers, committees, departments, and links to the governing board and management), as commonly defined and practiced, are often referred to as the "Joint Commission Model" (White, 1997). This is because of the great influence the standards and accreditation process of the Joint Commission on the Accreditation of Healthcare Organizations (JCAHO) has had over the years on the quality assurance activities of medical staffs. Even hospitals that do not seek accreditation tend to adhere to the JCAHO's prescriptions as the best "conventional wisdom" about how medical staffs should work. The influence of the JCAHO goes beyond what might be expected of a voluntary accreditation process because accreditation is accepted by the federal Medicare program as meeting its standards for participation (and payment), and by most states as meeting their hospital licensure requirements. Over the years, the standards spelled out in successive versions of the JCAHO's *Accreditation Manual for Hospitals* have essentially defined, some would say dictated, what is considered good practice with regard to the design, roles, and functions of the organized hospital medical staff.

The Joint Commission Model, however, evolved during the years before competition, managed care, and the resulting consolidation of providers into networks and systems. Today, physicians and hospitals are joining together to form physician-hospital organizations (PHOs) or even larger vertically integrated delivery systems to better position themselves to compete for contracts with health plans and public purchasers, and to be able to assume risk and manage the care of the populations for which they contract. Many believe the realities of the new medical care marketplace make the Joint Commission Model an anachronism.

Without question, many of the characteristics of the competitive marketplace differ from the assumptions that underlie the Joint Commission Model. In contrast to the tradition of an "open" hospital medical staff, with privileges dependent only on clinical qualifications, health plans, networks, and systems typically select only a subset of the community's physicians, with selections based on economic as well as quality criteria. Too, managed care organizations have a strong preference for primary care physicians versus specialists. Some hospitals are actively "downsizing" their medical staffs to fit more closely the size of the population for which they contract to care. Health plans and provider organizations often do their own credentialing, no longer relying on the hospital. Further, as hospital utilization is closely scrutinized and admissions discouraged, care is shifted to the clinic or physician's office, away from the reach of hospital credentialing and peer review. In addition, purchasers are demanding "report cards" that call for outcome measures of quality quite different from the structural measures traditionally emphasized by the JCAHO. And perhaps most important, as physicians increasingly compete with each other as participants in rival provider organizations, is it reasonable to expect them to dispassionately judge each others' credentials and patient care as members of the same hospital medical staff? In short, as medical groups and provider organizations position themselves for a more competitive marketplace, these organizations are taking over functions historically performed by hospital medical staffs. In addition, adherence to treatment guidelines and utilization parameters may subsume chart-by-chart peer review. Despite all of these trends, as of today, many hospital medical staffs continue to take their traditional quality assurance responsibilities seriously. It would seem, however, that new structures, more suited to the changing marketplace, will emerge as hospitals face the future.

REFERENCES

American Hospital Association. (1996). *AHA hospital statistics* (1996–97 ed., pp. xix–xxix).

Andrulis, D. P., Acuff, K. L., Weiss, K. B., & Anderson, R. J. (1996). Public hospitals and health care reform: Choices and challenges. *American Journal of Public Health, 2,* 162–165.

Bolognia, J. L., & Wintroub, B. U. (1996, September). The impact of managed care on graduate medical education and academic medical centers. *Archives of Dermatology,* 1078–1084.

Brown, M. (1996). Mergers, networking, and vertical integration: Managed care and investor-owned hospitals. *Health Care Management Review, 1,* 29–37.

Carey, R. M., & Englehard, C. L. (1996). Academic medicine meets managed care: A high impact collision. *Academic Medicine, 8,* 839–845.

Coddington, D., Moore, K., & Fischer, E. (1996). *Making integrated health care work.* Colorado: Center for Research in Ambulatory Health Care Administration.

Commission of Hospital Care. (1947). Expansion of hospitals, 1840–1900. In *Hospital care in the United States* (pp. 454–526). Cambridge, MA: Harvard University Press.

Corwin, E. H. (1946). *The American hospital* (pp. 193–213). New York: Commonwealth Fund.

Dowling, W. L. (1995). Strategic alliances as a structure for integrated delivery systems. In A. Kaluzny, H. Zuckerman, T. Ricketts, III (Eds.), *Partners for the dance, forming strategic alliances in health care* (pp. 139–175). Ann Arbor, MI: Health Administration Press.

Dowling, W. L. (1996, Summer). The community-oriented integrated health care organization: How viable? *Frontiers of Health Services Management, 12*(4), 58.

Etheredge, L., Jones, B. J., & Lewin, L. (1996). What is driving health system change? *Health Affairs, 4,* 93–104.

Gillies, R. R., Shortell, S., Anderson, D., Mitchell, J. B., & Morgan, K. L. (1993, Winter). Conceptualizing and measuring integration: Findings from the Health Systems Integration Study. *Hospital and Health Services Administration, 38*(4), 467–489.

Glandon, G. L., & Morrisey, M. A. (1986). Redefining the hospital-physician relationship under prospective payment. *Inquiry, 23,* 166–175.

Goldsmith, J. C. (1981). *Can hospitals survive?* Homewood, IL: Dow Jones-Irwin.

Grieco, P. J., & Eisenberg, J. M. (1993, October 1). Changing physician practices. *New England Journal of Medicine, 329*(17), 1271–1273.

Hanchak, N. A. (1996). Managed care, accountability, and the physician. *Medical Clinics of North America, 2,* 245–261.

Havighurst, C. C. (1986). Changing the locus of decision making in the healthcare sector. *Journal of Health Politics, Policy and Law, 11,* 697–735.

Hurley, R. (1993, Summer). The purchaser-driven reformation in health care: Alternative approaches to leveling our cathedrals. *Frontiers of Health Services Management, 9,* 5–35.

Katz, A., & Thompson, J. (1996). The role of public policy in health care market change. *Health Affairs, 2,* 77–91.

Levit, K. R., et al. (1996, Fall). National health expenditures, 1995. *Health Care Financing Review, 18*(1), 175–214.

Luft, H. S. (1985). Competition and regulation. *Medical Care, 23,* 383–400.

Luke, R. D., & Olden, P. (1996). Foundations of market restructuring: Local hospital clusters and HMO infiltration. *Medical Interface, 8*(9), 71–75.

Lumsdon, K. (1995). Faded glory: Will nursing ever be the same? *Hospitals and Health Networks, 23,* 31–35.

MacEachern, M. T. (1957). *Hospital organization and management* (3rd ed.). Chicago: Physicians Record Company.

Mick, S., & Conrad, D. (1988). The decision to integrate vertically in health care organizations. *Hospital and Health Services Administration, 33*(3).

Philip, J. (1990, Fourth Quarter). Standard indicators of hospital activity have failed to keep pace with changes of hospitals and in the practice of medicine. *HMO,* 14–17.

Relman, A. S. (1980). The new medical-industrial complex. *New England Journal of Medicine, 17,* 963–970.

Rosen, G. (1963). The hospital—historical sociology of a community institution. In E. Freidson (Ed.), *The hospital in modern society* (pp. 1–36). New York: The Free Press.

Ruffner, J. K. (1986). Product line management: How six healthcare institutions make it work. *Healthcare Forum, 29,* 11–14.

Shortell, S. (1988, Fall). The evolution of hospital systems: Unfulfilled promises and self-fulfilling prophesies. *Medical Care Review, 45,* 177–214.

Shortell, S. M. (1977). Organization of hospital resources. In *Hospitals in the 1980s.* Chicago: American Hospital Association.

Shortell, S., Gilles, R., Anderson, D., Erickson, K., & Mitchell, J. (1996). *Remaking health care in America.* San Francisco: Jossey-Bass.

Shortell, S. M., Gillies, R. R., & Devers, K. J. (1995, Summer). Reinventing the American hospital. *The Milbank Quarterly, 73*(2), 131–160.

Shukla, R. K., & Clement, J. (1997, Spring). A comparative analysis of revenue and cost-management strategies of not-for-profit and for-profit hospitals. *Hospital and Health Services Administration, 42*(1), 117–134.

Siu, A. L., Sonnenberg, F. A., Manning, W. G., et al. (1986). Inappropriate use of hospitals in a randomized trial of health insurance plans. *New England Journal of Medicine, 315,* 1259–1266.

Starr, P. (1982). *The social transformation of American medicine* (pp. 145–179). New York: Basic Books.

Umbdenstock, R. J., Hageman, W. M., & Amundson, B. (1990). The five critical areas for effective governance of not-for-profit hospitals. *Hospital and Health Services Administration, 4,* 481–492.

White. (1997). *The hospital medical staff.* Albany, NY: Delmar.

CHAPTER

The Continuum of Long-Term Care

Connie J. Evashwick

CHAPTER TOPICS

LEARNING OBJECTIVES

Upon completing this chapter, the reader should be able to:

- Understand the role and scope of services included in long-term care.
- Appreciate who uses long-term care and under what circumstances.
- Assess how long-term care services are organized, integrated, evaluated, and paid for.
- Be introduced to forward-looking delivery systems and approaches for long-term care for the future.
- Understand national policy issues pertinent to long-term care and our aging population.

Long-term care is one of the greatest challenges facing the health care delivery system. In terms of population need, consumer demand, resource consumption, financing, and system organization, long-term care will be a dominant issue during the twenty-first century. The components of long-term care have grown during the past decade. Integration is beginning to occur. In order for the limited available resources to meet increasing demand, the system that currently exists—an unevenly financed array of fragmented services—must evolve into a well-organized, efficient, client-oriented, cost-effective continuum of care.

A case study illustrates an extreme of the issues and current challenges of long-term care.

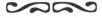

Mrs. Jackson is a sixty-six-year old widow, a successful librarian, still working, who lives alone in a third-story suburban apartment in a relatively small Midwestern town. She is generally healthy but has mild hypertension and is diabetic. One night during the winter, she slips on the ice while carrying groceries up the front steps of her building and breaks her hip. A neighbor calls the 911 emergency number, and eventually an ambulance arrives. The ambulance takes Mrs. Jackson to the emergency room of the nearest hospital. Mrs. Jackson cannot be admitted because she does not have proof of insurance, her Medicare card, credit cards, or even her checkbook on hand, and her condition is determined not to be life-threatening. She is thus transferred to another hospital. Mrs. Jackson's only physician is an internist who cannot handle a fracture, so Mrs. Jackson is operated on by the surgeon on call.

After the surgery, Mrs. Jackson spends two weeks in the hospital, one on the surgical floor and one on a step-down unit. Her physician stops by to visit, but her care is the responsibility of the surgical residents who change on an undetermined schedule. Her employer has recently reduced the health benefits that the group policy covers. Her insurance covers only the first thirty days of hospital care, and Medicare, as a secondary payer, picks up some of the uncovered expenses. Nonetheless, she has a daily copay, so she is anxious to be discharged as quickly as possible. The physician recommends that Mrs. Jackson go to a rehabilitation hospital. The nearest one, however, is in the next town. Instead, Mrs. Jackson agrees to spend a week or two at a nursing home until she is able to move about more easily. Mrs. Jackson knows that she will be responsible for all payments, since she has no insurance for nursing home care, and neither her primary insurance nor Medicare will cover her convalescence in the nursing home because she does not meet the rather stringent criteria for requiring twenty-four-hour nursing care. Despite the cost, she does not feel strong enough to go home alone.

Mrs. Jackson finds that the majority of patients in the nursing home are quite elderly, with most in their late eighties, and most suffering from Alzheimer's or some other form of dementia. There is little independence. Mrs. Jackson is glad when she feels strong enough to go home. The nursing home orders a walker for her before she leaves so that she can get around her apartment on her own.

At home, Mrs. Jackson must recuperate before she is able to ambulate easily. She has no way to get down the stairs, let alone to the grocery store, post office, or pharmacy. A neighbor who is a nurse arranges for a homemaker from a local agency to come in three days a week for two hours to help her. She is not quite ill enough to qualify for home health care as defined by the regulations of her health insurance or Medicare, that is, "homebound," thus she pays the homemaker directly. A colleague from work offers to stop by the pharmacy to pick up prescriptions for her. As a widow, Mrs. Jackson never cooked much for herself. A friend arranges for Meals on Wheels to deliver a hot meal at lunch and a cold snack for dinner. However, no food comes on the weekends. Meanwhile, bills begin to flood in from the emergency room, the hospital, the nursing home, several different physicians, and the home health agency. She is not sure what her private insurance will pay, what Medicare will pay, and what she must pay herself.

Mrs. Jackson returns to the hospital outpatient department for rehabilitation therapy, but she must depend on one of her neighbors being at home to help her get up and down the stairs. She cannot drive, so she calls a cab, which does not always come to the suburbs on time and is expensive. The therapists at the outpatient department are different than those in the hospital or at the nursing home, and Mrs. Jackson feels as though no one quite knows her clinical history or recent condition. Her insurance does not cover outpatient rehabilitation, but the office clerks tell her that Medicare Part B may cover the services.

Mrs. Jackson struggles along for several weeks and eventually is able to return to work. She believes that the medical care and therapy she received have been good quality. She comes out of the experience, however, with huge bills and negative feelings about the impersonality of the health care system, the high costs and low insurance coverage for long-term care, the fragmentation of services and payment, and the frustrating helplessness of even the professionals in mobilizing resources to facilitate the simple functions of daily living. She realizes that if she were twenty years older, were no longer covered by her employer's insurance or a Medicare supplemental, had spent much of her savings, and lived in an isolated two-story house in a rural area rather than in an apartment complex filled with friends and neighbors, her experience would have been far worse.

❧❧❧

The implications? The existing formal system of providing care to persons with long-term, complex problems is both complicated and fragmented. With some notable exceptions, the long-term care system functions because of individual expertise and informal relationships. On a broad scheme, it is highly regulated, costly, and occasionally arbitrary, with access to services limited by place, patient characteristics, and knowledge. Most of all, it does not consistently meet the needs of consumers, providers, or payers.

As described in the following text, the demand for long-term care will grow exponentially during the early part of the twenty-first century. The Baby Boom generation, also known as the "Me Generation," will begin to swell the population of older adults with chronic illnesses and those caring for family members with chronic illnesses, and thus consumer interest in arranging long-term care services will likely soar. The size of the younger disabled population will also grow. The combined consumer-based demand for well-organized long-term care will exacerbate the forces of managed care and integrated health care delivery systems that are already prompting change in the organization and financing of the health care delivery system.

This chapter describes the various facets of long-term care as they exist in the late 1990s and presents a conceptual framework for understanding how the many pieces of long-term care can be molded into a rational system for the future.

WHAT IS LONG-TERM CARE?

Long-term care refers to health, mental health, and social and residential services provided to temporarily or chronically disabled persons over an extended period of time with a goal of enabling them to function as independently as possible. There is no single regulatory or academic definition of long-term care. Long-term care has been defined as:

> A wide range of services which address the social, custodial and medical needs of individuals who lack some capacity for self-care and whose continuing incapacity will necessitate the provision of care for a relatively long and indefinite period of time (Young, 1985).

> Those services designed to provide diagnostic, preventive, therapeutic, rehabilitative, supportive and maintenance services for individuals of all age groups who have chronic physical and/or mental impairments, in a variety of institutional and non-institutional settings, including the home, with the goal of promoting optimum levels of physical, social and psychological functioning (Weissert, 1978).

> A range of services that addresses the health, personal care, and social needs of individuals who lack some capacity for self care. Services may be continuous or intermittent but are delivered for a sustained period to individuals who have a demonstrated need, usually measured by some index of functional dependence (Kane & Kane, 1982).

Throughout these differing definitions, several themes are consistent:

- Long-term care may be needed because of conditions that are physical or mental, temporary or permanent.
- Long-term care is targeted at those with functional disabilities.
- The goal is to promote or maintain health and independence in functional abilities and quality of life. For those who are terminally ill, the goal is to enable them to die peacefully and with dignity.
- The multiple services required, the professions involved, and the settings of care span broad spectrums.
- Care is multifaceted, recognizing all sphere's of a person's life: physical, mental, social, and financial.
- Care is orchestrated around the unique needs of each individual and family, and thus the patterns are many.
- Service delivery can be expected to change over time as the patient's and family's needs change.

WHO NEEDS LONG-TERM CARE?

The primary consumers of long-term care are persons who have chronic and/or complex health problems accompanied by functional disabilities. Clients may require care for a relatively short period of time, such as several months, or for an extended or indefinite period of time.

The first group includes those who have relatively short-term problems but ones that require orchestration of a complex set of community-based services. This group includes those with acute injury or illness who ultimately will achieve complete recovery or independence but who require an extended period of convalescence or treatment, such as persons suffering from cancer, head trauma, hip fracture, or stroke.

The second group comprises those who have ongoing ("chronic") and multiple health and/or mental health problems and who are unable to care for themselves ("functionally disabled") and thus require nursing or supportive health care for a prolonged or indefinite period of time.

Definitions

Chronic connotes permanent, or at least indefinite. For technical data collection purposes, chronic is defined by the National Health Interview Survey as any condition that lasts three months (or ninety days) or more (Adams & Marano, 1995). Chronic conditions may be derived from physical or mental conditions; over the progression of a disease, both may occur. Chronic conditions may be as life-threatening as coronary artery disease or as harmless as mild arthritis. Figure 11–1 shows the variety of courses chronic illness can take. In 1995, an estimated 99 million people had some type of chronic condition (Hoffman & Rice, 1996). By 2020, a projected 134 million people will have a chronic condition, and this number will grow to

167 million by 2050 (Hoffman & Rice, 1996). Figure 11–1 shows the projected growth in the prevalence of chronic illness.

Chronic illnesses vary by age and other patient characteristics. For example, asthma is most common among children; arthritis is most common among seniors. Table 11–1 shows the prevalence of the top twelve physiological chronic conditions and shows the difference in prevalence between the total adult population and those age sixty-five and older. Chronic conditions vary in the extent to which they are stable and the extent to which they require formal care. Some conditions, such as stroke, may have a progressive improvement over time; some conditions have episodic flare-ups; yet others are stable but require daily attention indefinitely.

An *impairment* is defined as "a chronic or permanent defect, usually static in nature, that results from disease, injury, or congenital malformation. It represents a decrease in or loss of ability to perform various functions" (Adams & Marano, 1995). Permanent impairments, such as limb amputation or blindness, may require an initial adjustment and are then more or less stable.

Disability is a general term that refers to any long- or short-term reduction of a person's activity as a result of an acute or chronic condition (Adams & Marano, 1995). The National Health Interview Survey compiles data on "ability to perform major activity." Major activity is defined according to age: playing for young children up to age 5, attending school for school-age children 5–17, working or keeping house for adults age 18–69, and self-care and independence for people age 70 or older (Adams & Marano, 1995). In 1994, approximately 15% of the United States population had some degree of activity limitation due to a chronic condition (Adams & Marano, 1995). Table 11–2 shows the percentage of the population, by age,

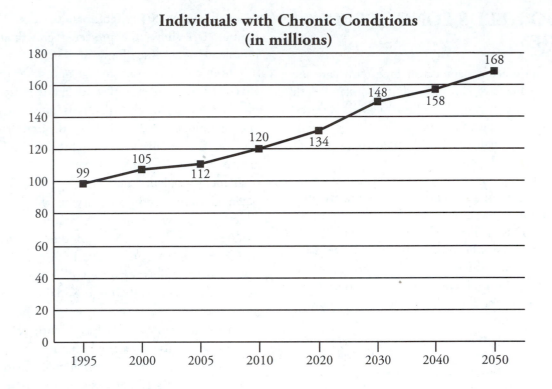

Individuals with Chronic Conditions (in millions)

SOURCE: Reprinted with permission from *Chronic Care in America: A 21st Century Challenge* (p. 9), by D. Rice & C. Hoffman, 1996, Robert Wood Johnson Foundation.

FIGURE 11–1 Projected growth in the number of persons with chronic conditions: United States, 1995–2050

who experience activity limitations due to chronic conditions.

In addition to the measure used by the federal government of ability to perform major activity, a much more common indicator of disability is functional ability. *Functional ability* has been described as a person's ability to perform the basic activities of daily living. Initially defined by Katz and colleagues, years of research have produced commonly accepted measures and scales of functioning. These are referred to as activities of daily living (ADL) (Katz, et al., 1985) and instrumental activities of daily living (IADL) (Lawton & Brody,

1969). Activities of daily living include the ability to eat, dress, perform personal care and grooming, transfer from bed to chair, bathe, walk, and maintain bowel and bladder continence. The instrumental activities of daily living include handling monetary affairs, telephoning, grocery shopping, housekeeping, doing chores, and arranging for transportation. Functional ability declines with age. Table 11–3 shows the level of functional ability among the older population. However, estimates are that as many as 50 million people need help with the basic activities of daily living, and 42% of these are under age sixty-five (McNeil, 1992).

TABLE 11–1 The twelve most prevalent physical chronic conditions, for total adult population and adults age 65+, 1994

	Total Adult Population*		Adults Aged 65+	
	Per 1000	*Number in millions*	*Per 1000*	*Number in millions*
Sinusitis	134	34.9	151	4.7
Arthritis	129	33.4	502	15.6
Orthopedic impairment	120	31.1	166	5.1
Hypertension	109	28.2	364	11.3
Allergies without asthma	101	26.1	80	2.5
Hearing impairment	86	22.4	286	8.9
Heart conditions	86	22.3	325	10.1
Bronchitis	54	14.0	61	1.9
Asthma	56	14.5	51	1.6
Migraine headache	43.4	11.3	48.1	0.7
Diabetes	29.9	7.8	48.1	3.1
Visual impairment	33.1	8.6	82.2	2.6

* Total U.S. population, 1994: 259,634,000; total aged 65+: 31,026

SOURCE: "Current Estimates from the National Health Interview Survey, United States, 1994," National Center for Health Statistics, 1995, *Vital and Health Statistics* (Series 10, No. 193), Tables 57, 62, 78.

TABLE 11–2 Percent distribution of persons by degree of activity limitation due to chronic condition, by age, 1994

	Percent Distribution			
Age	*No activity limitation*	*Some limitation*	*Limited in major activity*	*Unable to do major activity*
All people	85.0	15.0	10.3	4.6
Under 18 years	93.3	6.7	4.9	0.7
18–44 years	89.7	10.3	7.1	3.2
45–64 years	77.4	22.6	17.1	9.2
65+ years	61.8	38.2	22.6	10.7

SOURCE: "Current Estimates from the National Health Interview Survey, United States, 1994," National Center for Health Statistics, 1995, *Vital and Health Statistics* (Series 10, No. 193), Table 67.

Functional disabilities may be due to physical or mental problems, and over time, both may occur. Alzheimer's disease is one example. Estimates are that 25% of those age eighty-five and older have Alzheimer's or a related dementia (Alzheimer's Association, n.d.). Alzheimer's begins by affecting mental functioning and behavior. Ultimately, it affects a person's physiological systems as well. In

TABLE 11–3 Functional disability among older adults

Age	Needs Help with One or More Activities of Daily Living* (Percent)	Needs Help with One or More Instrumental Activities of Daily Living** (Percent)
65–69 years	14.7	19.9
70–74 years	21.1	24.7
75–79 years	24.1	29.2
80–85 years	34.4	40.0
85+	49.8	55.2

* Activities of daily living include bathing, dressing, eating, getting in and out of bed and chairs, walking, going outside, and toileting.

** Instrumental activities of daily living include preparing meals, shopping for personal items, managing money, using the telephone, doing heavy housework, and doing light housework.

SOURCE: Adapted from "Aging in the Eighties: Functional Limitations of Individuals 65 and Over," by D. Dawson, G. Hendershot, & J. Fulton, June 10, 1987, *Advance Data* (No. 133), National Center for Health Statistics.

1996, approximately 4 million people suffered from Alzheimer's disease. The number of persons with Alzheimer's disease will increase as the population ages, to as many as 14 million by 2050 (Alzheimer's Association, n.d.).

Chronic illness, impairments, and functional disabilities are interrelated. Of those with chronic conditions and/or impairments, some portion will be limited in activity. Of those who are limited, some will nonetheless be independent, and some will be limited in functional activities of daily living (ADLs and IADLs). All of those who are unable to perform the basic activities of daily living need help—from devices, from informal sources, or from formal sources. Regardless of their physical or mental limitations, those most likely to need assistance from formal sources are people who are very old, have multiple chronic conditions, live alone, and have minimal or no support system of family and/or friends. Figure 11–2 shows the multiple paths to needing assistance. Those requiring the assistance of formal long-term care services are the users of the system described in this chapter.

Understanding Demand

In brief, the users of long-term care represent a mosaic of subsegments of the population. Projecting the demand for long-term care requires an understanding of the definitions and subsets of the population with chronic illnesses, impairments, functional disabilities, and the portending growth of each, tempered by projections of advances in biomedical technology, changes in the workforce, other demographic and clinical factors, and social policies. Projections on the older population alone estimate that by 2020, of those age sixty-five and older, about 10–12 million people will have major disabilities (Manton, 1989; Rivlin, et al., 1988; Zedlewski, et al., 1990). The total number of people of all ages who will be unable to go to school, to work, or to live independently due to a chronic condition is projected to reach 17 million by the year 2020 (Hoffman & Rice, 1996). Many of these people will need long-term care from informal and/or formal sources at some point during their lives, if not indefinitely.

Because there is no single identifier or uniform pattern of long-term care users, long-term care services can be organized on numerous dimensions: demographic characteristics (for example, age, gender, economics), affinity (for example, veterans), disease category/diagnosis (for example, mental status, AIDS/ARC), or impairment (for example, blind). Examples of these subsets of potential users of long-term care provide concrete examples of the array of conditions leading to long-term care. They also warrant particular attention because of the

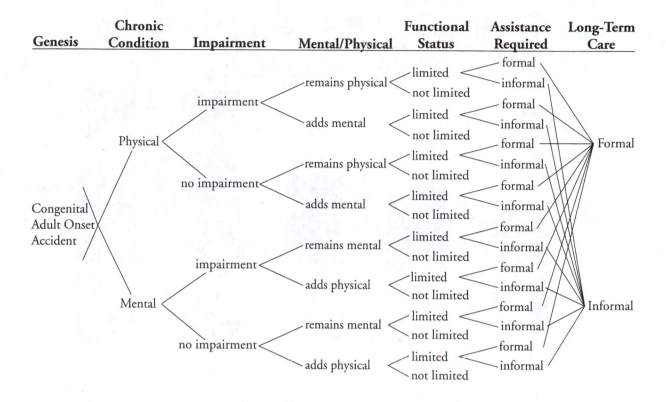

FIGURE 11–2 Progression of chronic illness

magnitude of their demand and because of the policy and financing vehicles likely to address their concerns.

The Aged. As shown in Tables 11–1 and 11–2, chronic illness and functional disabilities increase with age. Of persons age 65 and older, 80% have at least one chronic health problem, and the majority have multiple problems. As shown in Table 11–3, of those age 65–69, less than one in six, or 15%, experience functional ADL disabilities, while half of those age 85 and older suffer functional disabilities.

The changing demographic composition of the United States will make long-term care an increasingly significant aspect of the health care system. As

shown in Figure 11–3, the number of people over the age of sixty-five will increase from 33.5 million in 1995 to 70 million in 2030 (American Association of Retired Persons, 1996). Older adults will increase from under 13% of the United States population in 1995 to 20% of the total population by the year 2030 (American Association of Retired Persons, 1996). The very old, or those over age eighty-five, are increasing the most rapidly in terms of percentage. As stated previously, the very old suffer the most functional disabilities and thus are those who most need long-term care. As the number of old and very old people increases, the need for long-term care will rise.

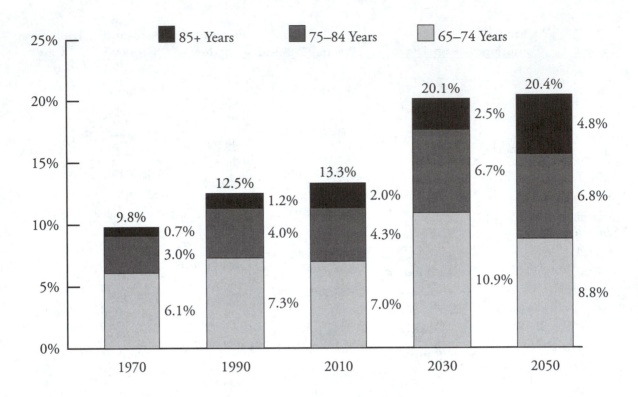

Note: Details may not sum to totals because of rounding.

SOURCE: Georgetown University IHCRP based on Hobbs and Damon, 1996; data from the U.S. Bureau of the Census.

FIGURE 11–3 Projected growth in the older population as a percentage of U.S. total population, 1970 to 2050

The Young Disabled. The total demand for long-term care includes younger people who have disabilities. Rice estimates that of the 99 million with chronic conditions in 1996, 75% were younger than age sixty-five (Hoffman & Rice, 1996). And, as noted earlier, 42% of those with functional disabilities are under age sixty-five. Younger population groups requiring long-term care include those with mental conditions, neurological diseases or degenerative neurological conditions, accidents resulting in paralysis, children with chronic congenital abnormalities, paralyzing strokes, end-stage cancer, blindness, early Alzheimer's disease, and AIDS/ARC.

Veterans. Because women outnumber men among the very old, long-term care is often associated with women. However, men, too, need long-term care. The Department of Veterans Affairs is facing the challenge of caring for aged veterans, the vast majority of whom are men (American Association of Retired Persons, 1989; General Accounting Office, 1987; Levenstein, 1995; U.S. Department of Veterans Affairs, 1989). In 1988, of the 27.3 million total veterans, 5.7 million, or 24%, were age sixty-five or older. By 2000, 8.9 million, or 37% of veterans, will be seniors, and by 2020, 7.7 million, or 45% of living veterans, will be age sixty-five or above (assuming no new major wars) (Keenan, 1989). The Department of Veterans Affairs, which has its own health care services, faces the same challenge as the public and private sectors in trying to construct an efficient, integrated system to care for those with multifaceted, chronic illnesses and functional dependencies.

AIDS/ARC. The AIDS epidemic began in the 1980s. By the mid-1990s, considerable progress had been made in preventing and treating the disease. However, the sudden and rampant expansion and the initial deadliness of the disease brought national attention to the care needed by those suffering from this disease. Special programs with special funding have been established throughout the nation to meet the extended care needs of those with AIDS/ARC. In 1995, the number of living people reported to have AIDS totaled approximately 205,000 (AIDS Hotline, 1997). However, thousands more are estimated to be HIV-positive, the precursor of AIDS/ARC.

Mentally Ill. Estimates are that about 51 million people, or more than one-quarter of those living in the community or in institutions, experience a mental disorder in any given one-year period (Kraus, et al., 1996). Between 3 and 5 million people have a severe mental disorder, and about three-fourths of these are limited by their mental condition (Kraus, et al., 1996). In addition, about 1%, or 2.5 million people, not residing in institutions, and approximately 700,000 residing in various types of institutions, are mentally retarded (Kraus, et al., 1996). Many of these people are limited in major activities and/or require assistance with functional tasks.

The Blind and Visually Impaired. Among those age sixty-five and above, more than 8%, or 2.7 million people, have some form of vision impairment, even when wearing glasses (Adams & Marano, 1995). Of adults under age forty-five, more than

2%, or 3.9 million people, are visually impaired, meaning they are blind in one or both eyes or have trouble seeing, even with glasses. Even among children under age eighteen, nearly 1% are blind in one or both eyes or have difficulty seeing, even with glasses. Many adaptive technologies have been developed to help those who have difficulty seeing, ranging from the widespread use of Braille on elevator buttons, to books in large print or on tape, to computers with large fonts and special color-contrast screens. Nonetheless, the blind and visually disabled may require assistance with the functions of daily living on a regular basis or at some point in time, and when ill, require all the more help.

The demand for long-term care extends beyond those suffering directly from some type of disability. Caregivers, family members, and employers are also affected—and have the potential to impact the system for providing long-term care.

Caregivers. People with functional disabilities need help to perform the ADLs and the IADLs. The majority of care is provided by family and friends on an informal basis (Doty, et al., 1996). Thus, the consumer demand for long-term care must include caregivers and employers, as well as the disabled themselves. Caregiving, which has always existed, became recognized as a health care issue during the 1980s. For the first time in history, the average American family has more parents than children. It has been estimated that women spend an average of seventeen years of their lives caring for children and eighteen years caring for their parents ("The Daughter Track," 1990). Nearly one in four households in the United States is involved in family caregiving to elderly relatives or friends.

A recent survey by the National Alliance for Caregiving revealed the following (National Alliance for Caregiving, 1997). Nearly three-fourths of caregivers are women (72%). About half are spouses, and one-third are children of the disabled person. More than one-third are caring for two or more elderly relatives or friends at the same time. Forty percent are caring for children under eighteen at the same time as elderly relatives or friends. The average caregiver provides eighteen hours of care per week, but in 4.1 million households the caregiver provides forty or more hours of care per week.

Caregivers are susceptible to health problems. The physical and emotional demands of caregiving can be extensive. Caregivers who can no longer meet the needs of functionally disabled persons often turn to nursing homes. The health care system has begun to accommodate by organizing services for caregivers, such as respite, educational programs, counseling, and support groups. Trends for an increasing number of women working and smaller families mean that in the future, the United States will face a significant decline in available family caregivers at the same time that the population in need of help increases dramatically. The formal health care system must do whatever it can to support those who are willing and able to be informal caregivers in order to maximize their involvement with the functionally disabled.

Employers. Employers have recognized that caregiving adds to their costs both in the health consequences for caregivers and the days of work lost due to caregiving responsibilities. Travelers Company was one of the first to study the prevalence of caregiving. In a 1985 survey, they found that 28% of their employees age thirty or older cared for an aged parent an average of ten hours per week ("The Daughter Track," 1990). The productive time lost by employees in caring for elderly relatives is estimated to cost American businesses billions of dollars each year.

As a result of the attention given during the 1980s to the effect of caregiving on work productivity, employers have set up programs to facilitate

caregiving. These range from education to access to national networks of case managers. These reduce stress and time lost while enabling employees to fulfill their responsibilities to their family members. A well-organized system of long-term care is thus sought not only by those suffering from complex chronic illnesses but also by family, friends, employers, providers, and payers.

Terminology

Users of long-term care are referred to variously as *patients, clients, participants,* and *residents,* depending upon the perspective of the service provider. This chapter uses the terms *patients* and *clients* as general terms and uses specific terms as appropriate for individual services.

HOW IS LONG-TERM CARE ORGANIZED?

Most long-term care is provided by friends and family. The formal system of providing long-term care has no single structure or financing. Just as each person requires care for a unique set of conditions, each community has its own combination of available resources, funding sources, and organization. A distinct arrangement is made for each individual and is usually more informal than formal. A major dilemma in long-term care is the incongruence between the way long-term care services should be ideally and how they operate currently.

As described previously, long-term care is designed for people who require multiple and ongoing health, mental health, and social support services over an extended period of time and whose needs are likely to change. The ideal system is one that provides comprehensive, integrated care on an ongoing basis and offers various levels of intensity that change as a client's needs change. The goal is to provide the health and related support services that enable a person to maximize functional independence. This contrasts with the goal of acute care, which is to "cure" the patient of an illness. Many clients may use only select components of the system and may remain involved with the organized system of care for a relatively short period of time; others may use only a limited and stable set of services over a prolonged period of time.

This ideal system of long-term care is referred to throughout the remainder of this chapter as the *continuum of care*. A continuum of care is defined as:

> a client-oriented system composed of both services and integrating mechanisms that guides and tracks patients over time through a comprehensive array of health, mental health and social services spanning all levels of intensity of care (Evashwick, 1987).

The continuum of care concept extends beyond the definitions of long-term care. A continuum of care is a comprehensive, coordinated system of care designed to meet the needs of patients with complex and/or ongoing problems efficiently and effectively. A continuum is more than a collection of fragmented services. It includes mechanisms for organizing those services and operating them as an integrated system.

The goal is to facilitate the client's access to the appropriate services at the appropriate time, quickly and efficiently. Ideally, a continuum of care:

• Matches resources to the patient's condition
• Monitors the client's condition and changes services as the needs change
• Coordinates the care of many professionals and disciplines
• Integrates care provided in a range of settings
• Enhances efficiency, reduces duplication, and streamlines patient flow
• Maintains a comprehensive record incorporating clinical, financial, and utilization data

By doing these things, a true continuum of care should: (1) achieve cost-effectiveness by maximizing the use of resources, and (2) enhance quality through appropriateness and continuity of care.

Services

Over sixty distinct services could be identified in the complete continuum of care. For simplicity, the services are grouped into seven categories: (1) extended care, (2) acute inpatient care, (3) ambulatory care, (4) home care, (5) outreach, (6) wellness, and (7) housing. Table 11–4 lists the major services within these categories. This chapter approaches the continuum of care from the perspective of health care. In theory and in practice, even more services that affect health status or health care use could be included, such as retirement planning, social activities, and guardianship. In brief, the seven categories represent the basic types of health care assistance that a person would need over time, through periods of both wellness and illness.

Extended inpatient care is for people who are so sick or functionally disabled that they require ongoing nursing and support services provided in a formal health care institution but who are not so acutely ill that they require the technological and professional intensity of a hospital. The majority of extended care facilities are referred to as nursing facilities, although this is a broad term that includes may levels and types of programs. Subacute units and rehabilitation units also offer extended inpatient care.

Acute inpatient care is hospital care for those who have a major and acute health care problem. For the majority of people, a typical hospital stay of four to eight days is the intensive aspect of a longer spell of illness, preceded by diagnostic testing and succeeded by follow-up care.

Ambulatory care services are provided in a formal health care facility, whether a physician's office

TABLE 11–4 Services and service settings of the continuum of care

EXTENDED CARE	Durable medical equipment
Skilled nursing facilities	Home visitors
Step-down units	Home-delivered meals
Swing beds	Homemaker and personal care
Nursing home follow-up	OUTREACH AND LINKAGE
ACUTE CARE	Screening
Medical/surgical inpatient unit	Information and referral
Psychiatric inpatient unit	Telephone contact
Rehabilitation inpatient unit	Emergency response system
Interdisciplinary assessment team	Transportation
Consultation service	Senior membership program
AMBULATORY CARE	WELLNESS AND HEALTH PROMOTION
Physicians' offices	Educational programs
Outpatient clinics	Exercise programs
Interdisciplinary assessment clinics	Recreational and social groups
Day hospital	Senior volunteers
Adult day care	Congregate meals
Mental health clinic	Support groups
Satellite clinics	HOUSING
Psychosocial counseling	Continuing care retirement communities
Alcohol and substance abuse	Independent senior housing
HOME CARE	Congregate care facilities
Home health—Medicare	Adult family homes
Home health—private	Assisted living
Hospice	Short-term housing for families and/or patients
High technology	

SOURCE: Adapted from "Definition of the Continuum of Care," by C. Evashwick, in *Managing the Continuum of Care,* edited by C. Evashwick & L. Weiss, 1987, Gaithersburg, MD: Aspen.

or the outpatient clinic of a hospital or an adult day care program. They include a wide spectrum of preventive, maintenance, diagnostic, and recuperative services for people who manifest a variety of conditions, from those who are entirely healthy and simply want an annual checkup to those with major health problems who are recuperating from hospitalization to those with chronic conditions who need ongoing monitoring.

Home care represents a variety of nursing, therapy, and support services provided to people who are homebound and have some degree of illness or functional disability but who are able to satisfy their needs by bringing services into the home setting. Home health programs range from formal programs of high-technology drug therapy or high-touch skilled nursing care to relatively informal networks that arrange housekeeping for friends.

Outreach programs make health and social services readily available in the community rather than within the formidable walls of a large institution. Health fairs in shopping centers, senior membership programs, and emergency response systems are all forms of outreach. They are targeted at the relatively healthy who are living in the community for the purpose of keeping them connected with the health care system.

Wellness programs are provided for those who are basically healthy and want to stay that way by actively engaging in health promotion. Wellness programs include health education classes, exercise programs, and health screenings.

Housing for frail populations increasingly includes access to health and support services and, conversely, recognizes that the home setting affects health. Housing incorporating health care ranges from independent apartments affiliated with a health care system that sends a nurse to do weekly blood pressure checks to assisted living with nursing and social services provided around the clock on site.

The categories are for heuristic purposes only. The order of the categories and the services comprising them can vary. The categories can be appropriately reordered on the basis of the dimension being considered: duration of stay, intensity of care, stage of illness, disciplines of professionals, type of facility, availability of informal support, and primary payer. Within each category are health, mental health, and social services, potentially provided by professional clinicians, provider organizations, families, and/or patients themselves. A more accurate diagram would be a multidimensional matrix showing the interrelationship of all of these factors in caring for a single individual and family. Such a matrix would be dynamic, not static, for the relationships would be different for each individual client and would change over time as the client's needs changed.

Within the categories as well as between them, the services of the continuum are distinct. Each has different regulatory, financing, target population, staffing, and physical requirements. Each has its own admission policies, patient treatment protocols, and billing system. Each organization has its own referral and discharge networks. A primary reason for organizing services into a continuum is to achieve integration, yet the differences among services make unified planning and operations quite difficult. One challenge faced by administrators in the initial creation of a continuum of care is that each service must be dealt with separately and brought into a cohesive whole.

The continuum of care is so extensive that it is unlikely that any single organization can offer a complete continuum for all of its clients. The goal of the provider should be to facilitate access for clients to the services they need. In brief, an organization need not have all services under its direct ownership or control; rather, it may have a variety of formal and informal relationships with other providers in the community.

The trend in the 1980s was for organizations to broaden the scope of the services provided and lay the groundwork for the continuum of care to be created during the 1990s. Some organizations bought others; some started new entities; some simply added new staff and new divisions. The 1990s saw the further expansion of long-term care services and the recognition that fragmented services do not meet the needs of those with multifaceted, chronic conditions nor the needs of providers or payers to achieve cost-effective, efficient care, particularly under managed care and at-risk arrangements. This groundwork of service availability, consumer demand, and provider and payer financial attention is a prerequisite for a continuum of care.

Integrating Mechanisms

By definition, a continuum of care is more than a collection of fragmented services; it is an integrated system of care. To gain the system benefits of efficiencies of operation, smooth patient flow, and quality of service, integrating mechanisms are essential. Four integrating management systems are required: interentity structure, care coordination, information systems, and financing.

Inter-entity structures means that management arrangements and operating policies are in place to enable services to coordinate care, facilitate smooth patient flow, and maximize use of professional staff and other resources. Examples include product line management organization, joint planning and operating committees, transfer arrangements, and joint budgeting.

Care coordination refers to the coordination of the clinical components of care, usually by a combination of a dedicated person and established processes that facilitate communication among

professionals of various disciplines at multiple sites. Case management, extended care pathways, interdisciplinary teams, and single-access referral are all techniques for achieving care coordination.

Integrated information systems refers to one patient record that combines financial, clinical, and utilization information being used by multiple providers and payers across multiple sites, with automatic updating of information.

Integrated financing removes barriers to continuity and appropriateness of care by having adequate financing for long-term care as well as acute care, preferably paid by a capitated system to allow maximum flexibility of service arrangement.

Figure 11–4 presents a schematic diagram of the services and integrating mechanisms of the

Services and Integrating Mechanisms of the Continuum of Care

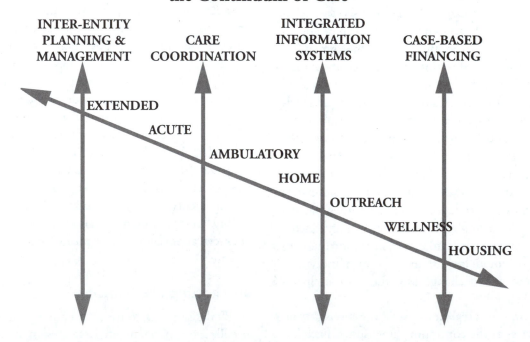

FIGURE 11–4   Services and integrating mechanisms of the continuum of care

continuum of care. The following sections describe in detail select services and the four basic integrating mechanisms.

SERVICES

Hospitals

The common vision of the acute hospital is one of complicated machines, bustling staff, and patients arriving and departing quickly, cured of their ailments. In reality, the hospital plays a significant role in providing the continuum of long-term care.

Of the 6,291 hospitals in the United States in 1995, many served patients with long-term needs (American Hospital Association, 1997a). Table 11–5 shows the breakdown of hospital by type. Tuberculosis, rehabilitation, orthopedic, chronic disease, and psychiatric hospitals all serve patients with long inpatient lengths of stay. Of the 258 million inpatient days in 1995, more than 43 million were in hospitals serving long-term patients (American Hospital Association, 1997b).

Medicare recognizes a specific category of "long-term hospitals," which by definition are hospitals that have an average length of patient stay greater than twenty-five days. In 1995, the nation had 112 general long-term hospitals with nearly 19,000 beds.

A high proportion of long-stay hospitals are psychiatric and are integral parts of the continuum of care for the mentally ill. Psychiatric hospitals numbered 657 in 1995, with over 100,000 beds and more than 707,000 admissions.

In addition to long-term hospitals, community hospitals provide many of the services of the continuum of care. Nationwide surveys conducted in 1981 (Evashwick, et al., 1985) and 1985 (Hospital Research and Educational Trust, 1986) to ascertain the activities of hospitals in long-term care and geriatrics demonstrated that hospitals provide a wide array of programs and services that reach patients and families before and after a stay in the inpatient unit. Table 11–6 shows some of the geriatric and chronic care services offered by hospitals as of 1995.

Many hospitals also own, contract with, or operate freestanding nursing homes and hospital-based step-down units. These enable the hospital to continue to care for patients who are not yet ready to be discharged into the community but whose needs can be met in an institutional setting less intense

TABLE 11–5 Hospitals in the United States, by type, 1995

	Hospitals	*Beds*	*Admissions*	*Average Daily Census*
All U.S.	6,291	1,080,601	33,282,124	708,746
General	5,249	911,302	31,826,926	576,592
Psychiatric	662	113,168	754,273	90,416
Mental retardation	13	7,195	1,456	5,873
Tuberculosis/respiratory	3	214	1,067	166
Rehabilitation	171	15,328	185,292	11,246
Orthopedic	25	1,681	35,600	705
Chronic disease	22	9,076	27,970	7,903
All other	119	20,127	296,783	15,563

SOURCE: Adapted from *AHA Hospital Statistics, 1996–7 Edition* (Table 3A), 1996, Chicago: American Hospital Association.

TABLE 11–6 Number and percent of hospitals reporting long-term care services, 1995

	Long-Term Care Related Services Provided by Hospitals, 1995	
	Number	Percent
Adult day care	840	15.6
Arthritis treatment center	559	10.4
Assisted living	433	8.0
Burn care unit	441	8.2
Case management	2,500	46.4
Geriatric services	2,205	40.9
Health screenings	3,475	64.5
HIV-AIDS services	2,403	44.6
Home health services	3,454	64.1
Hospice	2,551	47.4
Meals on wheels	1,106	20.5
Physical rehabilitation outpatient services	4,022	74.7
Physical rehabilitation inpatient unit	1,679	31.2
Psychiatric care	1,723	32.0
Psychiatric geriatric services	2,062	38.3
Retirement housing	381	7.1
Skilled nursing care unit	2,213	41.1
Social work services	4,707	87.4
Support groups	2,897	53.8

SOURCE: American Hospital Association, Data & Information Business Group, special run from the 1995 AHA Annual Survey, produced February 1997.

than that of the acute hospital. In 1995, 1,467 hospitals, or about one-fourth of short-term non-federal community hospitals, had a hospital-based skilled nursing unit, and a total of 40% offered skilled nursing through off- or on-campus sites (see Table 11–6). Nearly two-thirds of hospitals also operate their own home health services.

Rehabilitation is yet another long-term service offered by hospitals. Patients who are discharged quickly from a short-term inpatient stay often continue to receive therapy for months. They may transfer to a rehabilitation hospital or unit for intense therapy; transfer to skilled nursing to regain their strength, then to a rehabilitation unit; or go home and return as outpatients to the hospital or a freestanding outpatient rehabilitation center. In 1995, the United States had 171 rehabilitation hospitals with a total of 15,328 beds and over 185,000 annual admissions.

Federal hospitals, short-stay as well as long-stay, include Department of Veterans Affairs (DVA) facilities. The DVA operates its own continuum of care for veterans, which is "the largest coordinated system of health and long-term care services in the world" (U.S. Department of Veterans Affairs, 1986). DVA complexes often include short-stay hospitals, long-stay hospitals or units within the acute hospital, geriatric evaluation units (GEUs), skilled nursing facilities or units, adult day care, hospice, home health, residential care homes, and respite. The DVA has also been on the forefront of developing geriatric research, education, and clinical centers (GRECCs). Since 1975, the DVA has established fifteen GRECCs, which are based in DVA hospitals throughout the nation. In previous times, the largest proportion of the DVA health care budget was for hospital care. As noted earlier, by 2020, 45% of veterans will be age sixty-five or older. Thus, in the future, the proportion of the DVA health care budget spent on long-term care will increase dramatically.

The rationale for hospitals to be involved in long-term care is clear. Nationally, 35% of hospital admissions and 47% of all inpatient days are for persons age sixty-five and older (American Association of Retired Persons, 1996; National Center for Health Statistics, 1996). One in four older adults is admitted to the hospital each year, and of those admitted, more than 50% are readmitted at least once ("Health Data on Older

Americans," 1993). As noted earlier, the health problems of seniors are characterized as chronic and multifaceted. For hospitals to provide high-quality care to seniors, they must address the needs of these patients beyond the few days spent in the hospital. As the older population grows in number and proportion, the hospital will be faced with an increasing demand for comprehensive, coordinated, continuing care by senior consumers and their families.

The trend toward outpatient care also contributes to the hospital's role in providing long-term care. Futurists project that by the year 2000 more than half of a hospital's income will derive from outpatient services (Coile, 1991); this is already the case for many institutions. The more that can be done on an outpatient basis, the more the patients who are admitted are those with multiple and/or long-term conditions who need multifaceted, continuing care.

A third trend prompting hospitals' involvement in the continuum of care is financial. In 1995, nearly 41% of community hospitals' revenues came from Medicare (American Hospital Association, 1997b). As comprehensive, capitated, and managed care payment systems grow, the acute hospital finds it advantageous from a financial standpoint and essential from a marketing standpoint to provide a spectrum of services. To ensure viable financial performance, the hospital must manage access to services beyond those of acute inpatient care. Diversification of owning and operating multiple levels of service may also contribute to the hospital's revenues.

Today's hospital cannot realistically expect to remain in business by providing only short-term, curative care. The 1980s saw the beginning of hospital diversification into a wide array of services, including long-term care. The early 1990s saw hospitals developing comprehensive continuums of care that combined not only services but the integrating mechanisms as well. Hospitals with vision will concentrate during the beginning of the twenty-first century on refinement and expansion of the integrating mechanisms to give their patients access to comprehensive care over time and across settings. Hospitals are evolving from a focus on inpatient activity to becoming comprehensive health care systems, with the hospitals as only one of many services offered.

Nursing Homes

Nursing home is a broad term that encompasses a wide spectrum of facilities ranging from three-bed privately owned adult residential care homes to twenty-bed units of acute community hospitals to twelve-hundred-bed government-operated institutions. *Convalescent home, retirement center, long-term care facility, care center, nursing facility,* and other similar terms have no specific meaning. Nursing homes may be freestanding, units of hospitals, or integral parts of campus of care retirement centers. Many facilities have a combination of skilled nursing care and personal care beds. The common feature is that a person who is not able to remain at home alone due to physical health problems, mental health problems, or. functional disabilities resides at the facility. These persons are thus called *residents* rather than *patients*. Residents may stay for a short period of days or an indefinite period of time.

Each state licenses long-term care facilities, and each has its own licensing requirements, reimbursement policies, governing regulations, classification systems, and terminology. As part of the regulatory process, each state establishes its own definitions of nursing homes and related long-term care institutions.

For data collection purposes, the National Center for Health Statistics defined nursing homes in 1995 as "facilities with three or more beds staffed for use by residents, and routinely provided nursing and personal care services." The 1995 nationwide survey reported 16,700 nursing homes with 1,770,900 beds (Strahan, 1997). Table 11–7 gives key characteristics. The data do not include some step-down units of hospitals, intermediate care facilities for the mentally retarded, or supportive-living residences licensed by some states.

Two-thirds of nursing homes are proprietary. One-fourth are nonprofit, and the remaining 8% are owned and operated by federal, state, or local governments. Slightly more than half of nursing

TABLE 11–7 Characteristics of nursing homes, 1995

	Nursing Homes		Nursing Home Beds		Beds Per Home
	Number	Percent	Number	Percent	
Ownership					
Proprietary	11,000	66.1	1,151,700	69.0	104.7
Voluntary nonprofit	4,300	25.7	486,100	22.8	108.9
Government	1,400	8.2	151,000	8.1	107.9
Certification					
Certified, Medicare and Medicaid	11,600	69.7	1,378,400		118.1
Certified, Medicare only	1,000*	6.1	59,600		59.6
Certified, Medicaid only	3,400	20.1	280,300		82.4
Not certified	700*	4.2	52,600		75.1
Bed size					
Less than 50 beds	2,800	16.8	87,300		31.2
50–99 beds	5,900	35.6	430,400		72.9
100–199 beds	6,700	40.1	902,500		134.7
200 beds or more	1,300	7.5	350,800		269.8
Census region					
Northeast	2,900	17.1	378,800		130.6
Midwest	5,600	33.4	564,400		100.8
South	5,500	32.8	572,700		104.1
West	2,800	16.6	254,900		91.0
*Affiliation***					
Chain	9,100	54.3	978,000		107.5
Independent	7,600	45.5	788,200		90.7
Total	16,700	100	1,770,900		106.0

* Figure should not be assumed reliable because the sample size is between 30 and 59 or the sample is greater than 60 but has a relative standard error over 30%

** Excluded a small number of homes, beds, and residents with unknown affiliation

SOURCE: "An Overview of Nursing Homes and Their Current Residents: Data from the 1995 National Nursing Home Survey," by G. Strahan, *Advance Data from Vital and Health Statistics* (No. 280, DHHS Pub. No. PHS 97-1250; 7-0122, Table 3), January 1997, Hyattsville, MD: National Center for Health Statistics.

homes belong to a multifacility chain; just less than half are independent. Like hospitals, nursing homes range in size: 40% have 100–199 beds; 36% have 50–99 beds; only 8% have 200 beds or more. The average bed size ranges from 91 beds for independent homes to 108 beds for homes that are part of a chain. Occupancy averages 87%.

Nursing homes may be certified by Medicare (federal) and Medicaid (state) to accept patients whose care is paid for by these respective programs. To be certified by Medicare, a nursing home must qualify under Medicare's regulations for a skilled nursing facility (SNF). Certification categories formerly used by Medicaid of skilled nursing facility (SNF) and intermediate care facility (ICF) have been combined; Medicaid now recognizes only one category of nursing facility. By 1995, 96% of nursing facilities were certified for Medicare (6%), Medicaid (20%), or both (70%).

Table 11–8 shows how the nursing home field has evolved during the past two decades. From the 1973–1974 survey to the 1985 survey, the number of nursing homes increased by 22% and the number of beds increased 38% (Strahan, 1997). The number of residents increased, as did average occupancy. Between 1985 and 1995, the number of homes decreased, but the total number of beds and the average number of beds per facility increased. The average size of a home has grown over time; small homes have gone out of business. Nursing home membership in a multifacility system has grown; bed size and full-time equivalent staff (FTE/resident) have increased. Admissions also increased, but occupancy decreased, indicating shorter lengths of stay. Staffing ratios (the number of full-time staff per bed) also increased, reflecting a patient population who is sicker or needs more intense care. Whereas in the 1970s, relatively few facilities were certified for Medicare and many private facilities were not certified for Medicaid, by 1995, almost all facilities have recognized the

TABLE 11–8 Characteristics of nursing homes, 1973–1974, 1985, 1995

	1973–1974	1985	1995
Number of homes	15,700	19,100	16,700
Beds	1,177,300	1,624,200	1,770,900
Full-time equivalent (FTE) employees	485,400	793,600	933,600
FTEs per 100 beds	41.2	48.9	52.7
Current residents	1,075,800	1,491,400	1,548,600
Annual admissions	1,110,800	1,299,200	1,706,400
Occupancy	91.4	91.8	87.4

Note: FTE (full-time equivalent) employee includes only those providing direct patient care: administrative, medical, and therapeutic staff; registered nurses; licensed practical nurses; nurses' aides; and orderlies. Occupancy rate is calculated by dividing current residents by beds. Admissions are for the calendar year prior to the survey year.

SOURCE: "An Overview of Nursing Homes and Their Current Residents: Data from the 1995 National Nursing Home Survey," by G. Strahan, *Advance Data from Vital and Health Statistics* (No. 280, DHHS Pub. No. PHS 97-1250; 7-0122, Table 2), January 1997, Hyattsville, MD: National Center for Health Statistics.

imperative to be certified to care for Medicare and Medicaid patients.

Several factors have affected the nursing home market. Subacute units based in hospitals mushroomed during the early 1990s and took patients with short-term, high-intensity needs. Competition prompted more nursing homes to increase their ability to care for the high-intensity patient, thus improving the nursing facilities' staffing ratio and staff competence levels. Home care expanded in availability and in types of patients who can now be taken care of at home. Assisted living facilities increased in number and financial accessibility. Thus, the result is that those who enter nursing facilities are people with heavy care and intense nursing care needs.

The average cost of nursing home care ranged from $2,000 to $4,000 per month in 1993, varying by state and type of facility (American Health Care Association, 1996). Payment for nursing home care is made primarily by Medicaid (47%) and private individuals and families (42%) (National Center for Health Statistics, 1996). Medicare pays only about 8% of the annual costs of nursing home care. The Department of Veterans Affairs, private insurance, and other payers account for the remainder. The heavy dependence on state Medicaid payment poses a financial challenge for nursing homes. In some states, the expenditure for the nursing home component of Medicaid is the largest single expense in the budget. As states look for ways to control their budgets, funding for nursing home care is heavily scrutinized. States have used "certificate of need" authorities to limit the number of nursing home beds allowed in the state and thereby limit state spending.

Payment methods for nursing homes vary by state. A variety of payment systems have been tried. Most states have some form of cost-based per diem rates. Rates may be adjusted for case mix, and ancillary costs, such as physical therapy, may be included in the per diem rate or paid separately. Efforts to implement prospective case-mix payment systems are underway at both state and federal levels.

Nursing homes are highly regulated. Concern about quality is juxtaposed with the limited budgets of state Medicaid agencies and private families. The 1987 Nursing Home Reform Act, incorporated into the Omnibus Budget Reconciliation Act of 1987 (OBRA 1987), made significant changes in how nursing homes operate and how they are evaluated (Coleman, 1991). The survey process was changed from one focusing on physical and task criteria to one focusing on the caring process, resident feelings, and patient care outcomes. The minimum data set (MDS) was required to be completed for all residents, initiating standardization in record keeping and providing a basis for comparison of patient status. OBRA 1987 was implemented in phases throughout the 1990s.

The majority of employees of nursing homes are unskilled or low-skilled: nurses aides, housekeeping and maintenance and food service workers. Even in skilled nursing facilities that meet Medicare requirements, a registered nurse must be on duty only eight hours per day. On evening and night shifts, the highest professional staff may be a licensed vocational nurse. Other health care professionals who work with nursing homes include physicians; pharmacists; nutritionists; occupational, physical, speech, and respiratory therapists; and medical social workers. Except in very large homes, these professionals will work at the home on a part-time basis and are likely to associate by contract rather than be paid as employees. The number of full-time equivalents (FTEs) per 100 beds has increased over time from 41.2 in 1973 to 48.9 in 1985 to 52.7 in 1995 (Strahan, 1997).

Table 11–9 characterizes nursing home residents. Nursing homes serve primarily the very old, frail elderly. In 1995, 89% of the 1.5 million nursing home residents were age sixty-five and older; 36% were age eighty-five and over. Three out of four residents (72%) were women, and nearly nine out of ten (88%) were white.

The primary diagnoses of nursing home residents age sixty-five and older are circulatory system disorders (27%), mental disorders (17%), and diseases of the nervous system (11%) (Dey, 1997). Functional dependence is high among nursing home residents. Eight-six percent of those age sixty-five and older require assistance with at least one ADL (Dey, 1997). Many have suffered debilitating strokes and have not fully recovered mentally or physically. As many as one of three to two in five nursing home residents have some type of mental disorder, most often organic brain

TABLE 11–9   Nursing home and personal care home residents age 65 and older, by age, sex and race, 1995

Total Residents: 1,548,600	Percent
Age	100.0
Under 65 years	10.9
65–74 years	15.9
75–84 years	37.6
85 years and older	35.8
Sex	
Male	27.7
Female	72.3
Race	
White	88.0
Black	9.7
Other	1.4
Unknown	0.5

SOURCE: "An Overview of Nursing Homes and Their Current Residents: Data from the 1995 National Nursing Home Survey," by G. Strahan, *Advance Data from Vital and Health Statistics* (No. 280, DHHS Pub. No. PHS 97-1250; 7-0122), January 1997, Hyattsville, MD: National Center for Health Statistics.

syndrome or senile dementia. As the population ages, the number of people with Alzheimer's disease will increase, and many of these people ultimately go into a nursing home. Table 11–10 delineates the dependency status of nursing home residents and also shows how the level of dependency has increased over time.

The reasons people are admitted to nursing homes tend to be functional dependency rather than diagnosis alone. Research has shown that for every person in a nursing home, two equally ill people reside at home, cared for by family and friends. Admission to a home usually occurs because friends and family can no longer provide the level of support required. Night wandering and incontinence are two problems that frequently stress a family beyond its caregiving capacity and result in the frail person being admitted to a nursing home. People who are single and do not have strong social support systems are also more likely to be in nursing homes.

The lifetime chance of ever being in a nursing home is nearly one in two: 49% probability for women and 47% probability for men (Kemper & Murtaugh, 1991). The likelihood, however, increases with age. Of people age 65–74, only one in ten is in a nursing home. Of those age 85 and above, 20% reside in a nursing home. Contrary to popular belief, most people do not spend many years in a nursing home. Nearly one-third of those admitted to a nursing home are discharged within ninety days; an additional 20% are discharged within one year. Nineteen percent of women and 12% of men stay in a nursing home more than five years.

The use of nursing homes will continue to grow in the future. As the population grows older, there simply will be more people with the characteristics of those who enter nursing homes. The rate of use of nursing homes may decline as more community-based housing and service options are available and as the technological ability to provide care at home expands. The increase in numbers, however, is likely to outweigh any decrease in the use rate.

Home Health

Home health care is one of the oldest components of the continuum of care. A number of home health agencies across the nation have celebrated their centennial. Home health is also one of the most rapidly growing areas of health care. The expansion began in the early 1980s and has continued during the 1990s. It reflects the convergence of several major factors:

TABLE 11–10 Dependency status of nursing home residents, 1977, 1985, 1995

	1977*	1985*	1995**
	Percent	*Percent*	*Percent*
Type of dependency (requires assistance with:)			
Bathing	86.3	88.7	96.05
Dressing	69.4	75.4	88.70
Using bathroom	52.6	60.9	77.65
Mobility or transferring	66.1	70.7	73.88
Difficulty with bowel/bladder control	45.3	51.9	N/A
Eating	32.6	39.3	60.95
Number of Dependencies	*Number*	*Number*	*Number*
None	9.6	8.2	3.95***
One	12.4	9.3	7.35
Two	12.9	10.4	11.05
Three	10.7	9.2	3.77
Four	13.5	14.3	12.93
Five	17.6	19.5	60.95
Six	23.3	29.1	
Average	3.5	3.9	N/A

* SOURCE: "Nursing Home Utilization by Current Residents; United States, 1985," by E. Hing, National Center for Health Statistics, October 1989, *Vital Health Statistics, 13*(102), Table F.
** SOURCE: *Nursing Home Statistical Yearbook 1995* (Table II-1, p. 48), by C. C. McKeen, 1996, Tacoma WA: Cowles Research Group, Inc.
*** SOURCE: *Nursing Home Statistical Yearbook 1995* (Table II-7, p. 60), by C. C. McKeen, 1996, Tacoma WA: Cowles Research Group, Inc.

- Desire by both consumers and payers to minimize health care costs by substituting less intense alternatives to institutional care
- Financial pressures of hospitals and medical groups to diversify and to control patient flow under capitated and prospective payment systems
- An increase in demand due to the growing number of older people
- Preference of patients and families for care in their own home

- A lawsuit against the federal government in the 1987 that removed constraints on home care use by Medicare recipients
- Advances in technology that enable therapies that formerly would have been provided only in hospitals or doctors' offices by health care professionals to be provided safely and effectively in the home by home care professionals or patients and family members

Home care consists of several types of services: skilled nursing care and therapies, homemaker/ home health aide care, high-technology home therapy, durable medical equipment (DME), and hospice. The services may all be provided by one agency, or an agency may specialize in only one aspect of home care. However, high-technology home therapy and DME companies are likely to be distinct organizations, and hospice may be provided by organizations from a variety of venues, so these are discussed separately.

Skilled home health services include:

- Nursing care, provided by a registered nurse or licensed vocational nurse, ranging from patient education and basic nursing procedures to highly complex care
- Physical, occupational, and speech therapy
- Respiratory therapy
- Medical social service
- Nutrition counseling

Often several services are provided to a single patient by a multidisciplinary team. Each provider, however, may visit the patient at a different time. Patients are those who are recovering from an acute episode of illness, require rehabilitation, suffer from chronic illnesses that need ongoing monitoring or intense attention, are undergoing special short-term therapies, and/or are in the last stages of life.

Homemaker/home health aide care includes:

- Personal care
- Bathing and grooming
- Meal preparation
- Shopping
- Transportation
- Select household chores
- Other tasks that do not require trained health care professionals

Patients are typically those who are functionally impaired on a short-term or permanent basis and require assistance with the activities of daily living.

The agencies providing home health and homemaker care take an array of organizational forms. The Health Care Financing Administration has developed a classification system that involves ownership, control, and tax status. The categories are:

Freestanding

Visiting nurse associations—voluntary, nonprofit organizations governed by a board of directors and usually financed by tax deductible contributions as well as by earnings. (The term earlier had a more specific meaning and referred to home care agencies that were named Visiting Nurse Associations and shared a common history.)

Public agencies—government agencies operated by a state, county, city, or other unit of local government, such as public health departments, having a major responsibility for prevention of disease and for community health education.

Proprietary agencies—freestanding, for-profit home care agencies. These range from single agencies owned by individuals to large nationwide chains.

Private nonprofit—not-for-profit freestanding agencies that are privately developed, governed, and owned.

Other—freestanding agencies that do not fit one of the other categories for freestanding agencies.

Facility-based

Hospital-based—operated as an integral part of a hospital, such as a department or unit. Agencies that have working arrangements with a hospital or are owned by a hospital but operated as separate entities are classified under one of the freestanding categories.

SNF—agencies based in skilled nursing facilities.

Home health agencies are licensed in most states, and a few states require a certificate of need. The Joint Commission for the Accreditation of Health Care Organizations and the Community Health Accreditation Program of the National League of Nursing accredit home health agencies, and the National Home Caring Council accredits home care aide organizations.

Medicare-Certified Home Health Agencies. Home health agencies that meet stringent federal standards can be certified by Medicare to care for clients enrolled in Medicare Part A or Part B. The agency is shaped by federal requirements and serves a heavy proportion of patients whose payers are Medicare, Medicaid, workers' compensation, or private insurance. Medicare limits participation to home care agencies that are primarily engaged in providing skilled nursing services and other therapeutic services, as well as home health aide care. Organizations that provide primarily homemaker or nonclinical support services are not certifiable.

The number of Medicare-certified home health agencies doubled during the 1980s, from 2,924 in 1980 to 5,695 in 1990 (National Association for Home Care, 1996). Growth of another 50% occurred by 1995, when Medicare-certified agencies totaled 9,120. The field changed from primarily Visiting Nurses Associations and public agencies to hospital-based and private for-profit or nonprofit agencies. Table 11–11 shows this transition from 1967, when Medicare first certified home health agencies, to 1995. Although a home health agency may be part of a larger health care organization, it is typically structured as a distinct department or organization in order to maximize the financial benefits under Medicare. Home health agency productivity and size are generally measured by number of visits.

To be eligible for home health coverage by Medicare, a client must be homebound, be capable of improvement, and require short-term, intermit-

Table 11–11 Number of Medicare-certified home health care agencies, by auspice, 1967, 1985, 1995

Auspice	Number of Agencies		
	1967	*1985*	*1995*
VNA	642	573	617
Government	939	1,205	1,161
Proprietary	0	1,943	3,730
Nonprofit	0	832	667
Hospital	133	1,297	2,360
SNF	0	129	153
Other	39	4	59
Total	1,753	5,983	8,747

SOURCE: *Basic Statistics About Home Care,* National Association for Home Care, 1995, Washington, DC: Author.

tent nursing care, physical therapy, or speech therapy. Home health agencies may also provide occupational therapy, medical social work, and home health aide services. Medicare will pay for these, but only if the client first meets the preceding criteria and receives one or more of the primary services. All services must be prescribed by a physician.

Like the number of agencies, the number of persons who receive home health care from Medicare-certified agencies has increased, as has the average number of visits per person. The number of Medicare enrollees served suggests the magnitude of total growth (National Association for Home Care, 1996). In 1980, approximately 957,000 Medicare recipients received 22.4 million home health visits. The number of clients doubled by 1990, when 1.94 million clients received 69.5 million visits. In 1996, of the 37 million persons enrolled in Medicare, 3.9 million Medicare clients received 279 million home health visits. Similarly, the number of Medicaid clients increased from 392,000 in 1980 to 719,000 in 1990 to 1,376,000 in 1994 (National Association for Home Care, 1996).

The characteristics of home health users are shown in Table 11–12. The majority of clients served by Medicare-certified agencies are age sixty-five and older. The single largest group consists of patients being discharged from hospitals who require short-term follow-up to complete their recovery. Hospitals are the predominant referral source. The most frequent diagnosis is diseases of the circulatory system.

Despite its recent growth, the total amount of funds spent on home health is relatively small compared to the dollars spent on hospital and physician

TABLE 11–12 Characteristics of home health and hospice users, by age, sex, race, and marital status, 1994

	Home Health		Hospice	
	Number	*Percent*	*Number*	*Percent*
Total	5,272,200	100	328,000	100
Age *				
Under 45 years	668,700	12.7	18,600	5.7
45–64 years	677,100	14.8	69,800	21.3
65 years and older	3,778,300	71.7	239,100	72.9
65–74 years	1,251,300	23.7	91,200	27.8
75+ years	2,527,000	48.0	147,900	45.1
Unknown	151,300	2.9	—	—
Sex *				
Male	2,124,700	40.3	171,500	52.3
Female	3,147,500	59.7	156,500	47.7
Race *				
White	3,478,600	66.0	260,400	79.4
Black	455,300	8.6	24,000	7.3
Other or unknown	1,338,300	25.4	43,700	13.3
Marital status *				
Married	1,986,100	37.7	160,300	48.9
Widowed	1,616,200	30.7	97,300	29.7
Single or divorced	1,045,900	19.8	48,300	14.7
Unknown	624,000	11.8	22,200	6.8
Primary diagnoses (top 2 diagnoses only) **				
Malignant neoplasms	115,100	6.1	35,800	58.7
Circulatory system	502,900	26.6	7,800	12.8
Nutritional disorder	178,100	9.4	—	—

SOURCE: *An Overview of Home Health and Hospice Care Patients: 1994 National Home and Hospice Care Survey* (DHHS Pub. No. HS 96-1250 6-0294 (4.96), Vital and Health Statistics Advance Data, No. 274), Tables 5(*) and 6(**), by G. W. Strahan, April 24, 1996. Washington, DC: National Center for Health Statistics.

care. In 1996, approximately $36 billion was spent on home care, representing 3.7% of the national health care expenditures (National Association for Home Care, 1996). Medicare is the largest single payer of formal home care services, paying about 60% of all home care. Medicaid paid approximately 14.4%, private insurance 8.4%, and individuals and families paid approximately 3.1% of all home care costs (National Association for Home Care, 1996). In 1994, Medicare and Medicaid spent, respectively, 12.2% and 6.5% of their total annual budgets on home care (National Center for Health Statistics, 1996). The Older Americans Act, Title XX social services block grants, the Department of Veterans Affairs, CHAMPUS, and private insurance companies all also funded limited amounts of home care.

The average charge for a visit from a Medicare-certified agency was estimated at $78 in 1996, ranging from $99 for a registered nurse visit to $52 for a homemaker visit (National Association for Home Care, 1996). The charge varies according to the type of professional service rendered and the geographic area. Medicare currently pays on a cost-reimbursement basis and thereby limits the amount of profit an agency can make. The Health Care Financing Administration is exploring a prospective payment system based on severity of illness.

Private Home Health Agencies. "Private" home health agencies serve primarily private pay and contract patients. These agencies are not certified for payment by Medicare and, concomitantly, are not bound by Medicare regulations. Although in some states they must be licensed as health care providers, in many states these agencies operate under the auspices of only a business license. Noncertified agencies emerged during the 1970s and grew during the 1980s and 1990s to fill the demand for home care by patients who do not qualify for Medicare or Medicaid. In the mid-1990s, private home care agencies found a new market as contractors for managed care companies.

Private home care agencies offer the same professional services as Medicare-certified agencies, plus numerous others. Services include skilled nursing, physical therapy, occupational therapy, speech therapy, medical social work, home health aides, homemakers, high-technology home infusion therapy, ventilator care, and high-risk pregnancy monitoring and neonatal care, among others. In contrast to Medicare-certified agencies, which Medicare authorizes to provide only intermittent and skilled visits, noncertified agencies provide twenty-four-hour care, daily care, care for an indefinite period of time, and specialty services. Private agencies also offer homemaker/home health aide care such as personal grooming, bathing and shaving, housekeeping, transportation, shopping, meal preparation, and home repair.

Private home health agencies tend to be staffed differently than Medicare-certified agencies. Private agencies tend to draw from a large pool of home health aides and homemakers. Staff often work on an on-call basis and may work for several agencies. Professional staff are also likely to work on an as-needed basis rather than as full-time employees. The challenge for many private home care providers is to keep a minimum number of staff on full-time payroll and a large enough cadre of staff available on-call to meet demand. The loose association with staff makes quality control particularly important.

Clients comprise a broader group than those served by Medicare-certified agencies. While the latter receive the majority of their referrals directly from hospitals of patients who are being discharged, private home care agencies engage in active marketing to secure clients of many types. Clients range from young accident victims who require twenty-four-hour nursing care to ill children to workers' compensation clients who need rehabilitation before returning to work to seniors living alone who have no severe health problems but do have functional disabilities. Depending upon the payment source, private home care does not necessarily require a physician's prescription, and clients thus come from many sources. Social service agencies, Medicare-certified home health agencies, relatives, friends, and the yellow pages all refer to private home care. Some private agencies pursue contracts with various government agencies to be the preferred provider for particular types of patients.

Because private home care agencies are not reimbursed or certified by any federal agencies, precise statistics are difficult to obtain. The National Association for Home Care identified 7,897 home health agencies, home care aide organizations, and hospices in 1996 that did not participate in Medicare (National Association for Home Care, 1996). Thus, the total number of private agencies almost equals the 8,747 Medicare-certified agencies. The great majority of private home health agencies are proprietary; the few operated by churches or social service agencies are nonprofit. Several large nationwide chains characterize the private home care field.

Private home care agencies charge by the hour or by the visit. Often a minimum number of hours is required. Charges tend to be less than Medicare-certified agencies, even for the same service, because private agencies are not required to have comparable staffing by permanent employees, which adds to overhead.

Private home care agencies have many private pay patients. Other payers include private insurance and government contracts. Workers' compensation, Title XX of the Social Security Act, the Older Americans Act, state and local mental health departments, child welfare department programs, and local block grants may contract with a home care agency to care for the clients eligible for their particular program. As noted earlier, managed care has emerged during the 1990s as a major contractor for home health care.

Through the 1980s, private and Medicare-certified agencies tended to be separate and, hence, to compete with each other for some types of cases. The current trend is for companies to offer both services. Because of Medicare regulations, however, even if two such agencies are housed in the same office, the two programs must operate as separate businesses. Private agencies may choose to be accredited by JACHO. State licensing requirements vary, in some states, only a business license is required, while other states require the same licensing as Medicare-certified agencies if skilled care is offered.

High-Technology Home Therapy. High-technology home therapy appeared in the early 1980s as new technologies emerged. Cost-containment initiatives squeezing hospitals and advances in drug and equipment technology made it possible to deliver services in the home that had formerly been available to patients only in hospitals. A major advantage of providing high-technology therapy in the home is that it is much less expensive than providing the same care in a hospital or nursing home. The expansion of ambulatory care, especially ambulatory surgery, beginning in the late 1980s and continuing into the 1990s has further abetted the trend to move services out of the hospital and into home settings. High-technology services now provided in the home include:

- Intravenous antibiotics
- Oncology therapy
- Pain management
- Parenteral and enteral nutrition
- Ventilator care
- High-risk pregnancy monitoring
- Infant monitoring

High-technology home therapy typically involves pharmaceuticals and equipment that are expensive, require special staff expertise to use and monitor, and are available only from select sources. The total volume of patients requiring high-technology care is small, and the protocols can vary on an individual basis much more than for basic home care.

High-technology home therapy is provided by many Medicare-certified and private home health agencies. In addition, some agencies specialize only in providing high-technology home care. The cost for each patient can be quite high, and reimbursement is often negotiated on an individual basis. Companies with the requisite expertise have found that they can thrive just by specializing in this one component of home care. Continued growth in the high-technology arena is likely in the future.

Durable Medical Equipment. Durable medical equipment (DME), ranging from walkers to electric beds, is frequently provided in conjunction with home health care. The home health agency often assumes responsibility for arranging for equipment, and may have a formal or informal affiliation with a local durable medical equipment company to provide the needed equipment. If the equipment is to be paid for by Medicare, it must be prescribed by the patient's physician.

During the 1980s, the durable medical equipment business boomed as a fast-growing area of home health care less regulated and more lucrative than other areas of health care delivery. Many joint ventures were initiated; multi–health care systems acquired or started DME businesses; and home health conglomerates were tried, bringing all aspects of home health care together into one parent company. In the mid- and late-1980s, Medicare tightened its regulatory and payment policies. The DME field has since stabilized. In the 1990s, DME remains an essential but distinct component of home health care.

Home health care continues to be an area of growth. Because of the changes in technology, the increase in use of home care for younger persons, and the growth in the number of older persons, the use of home care is projected to be the most rapidly growing health care service (National Association for Home Care, 1996). The number of agencies, which leveled off during the late 1980s and early 1990s, has experienced significant growth again during the mid-1990s. The distinct split between Medicare-certified and uncertified agencies is blurring. Medicare is examining a prospective payment system for home care, but implementation is not likely until the late-1990s. The expansion of private managed care and the emergence of Medicaid-managed care during the 1990s have provided new impetus for home health care. The field is likely to continue to change and expand.

Hospice

Hospice is a concept of providing care for the terminally ill. It began as a formal program in Great Britain and spread to the United States during the 1970s. The philosophy of hospice is that terminally ill persons should be allowed to maintain life during their final days in as natural and comfortable a setting as possible. Every attempt is made to enable the person to remain at home; other services are brought in as needed. All aspects of hospice emphasize quality, rather than length, of life.

Elements common to all hospices include (Lack, 1978; U.S. Department of Health and Human Services, 1991):

• Service availability, including medical and nursing care, to home care patients and institutional inpatients on a twenty-four-hour-per-day, seven-day-per-week, on-call basis

- A full complement of skilled and homemaker home care services
- Inpatient care as needed
- Respite care for the family provided in the home, hospital, or nursing home
- Control of physical symptoms, including use of palliative drugs
- Psychological, social, and spiritual counseling for patient and family
- Physician direction of services
- Central administration and coordination of services, and collaboration among provider organizations (home health agencies, hospitals, nursing homes)
- Multidisciplinary team of care providers
- Use of volunteers as an integral part of the health care team
- Treatment of the patient and family together as a unit
- Bereavement follow-up for family and friends

The concept of hospice and its implementation received considerable national attention during the late 1970s and 1980s. Federally funded demonstration projects tested the impact of hospice on patient and family quality of life and cost-effective use of resources. Ultimately, service criteria and payment authorization by Medicare were included in the Tax Equity and Fiscal Responsibility Act of 1982 and extended in 1986. Payment benefits were revised in 1989 and 1991.

Under Medicare Hospital Insurance (Part A), defined hospice benefits are covered when provided by a Medicare-certified agency. In 1995, 1,857 hospices were accredited by Medicare (Hospice Association of America, 1996). Blue Cross, Blue Shield, Medicaid, and many private insurance companies recognize and pay for hospice care. Hospice services not organized as a special program may nonetheless be paid for as separate home health, hospital, or nursing home care.

Hospice is an approach to care and as such can be offered through a variety of organizational settings. As shown in Table 11–13, hospice programs vary in their organizational auspices. In 1996, the United States had approximately 2,000 formal hospices (Hospice Association of America, 1996). This is a 25% increase from 1,500 in 1986, indicating that hospice is still growing. The Joint Commission for the Accreditation of Healthcare Organizations accredits hospices.

To participate in a hospice program, a person must generally have a diagnosis of terminal illness fatal within six months or less. (Medicare requires

TABLE 11–13 Number of Medicare-certified hospices, by auspice, 1986, 1990, 1995, 1996

Auspice	1986 (number)	1990 (number)	1995 (number)	1996 (number)	1996 (percentage)
Home health agency	113	313	699	802	38
Hospital	54	221	460	506	24
SNF	10	12	19	20	1
FSTG	68	260	679	762	37
Total	245	806	1,857	2,090	

SOURCE: *Hospice Facts & Statistics,* Hospice Association of America, Washington, DC, 1996, and Hospice Data FY 93–95 by date of service, prepared by HCFA October 1996.

certification by a physician of impending death to participate in Medicare-sponsored hospice care.) However, the average length of stay in a hospice (for Medicare patients) was 59 days in 1994 (Hospice Association of America, 1996). The patient and the family must be willing to acknowledge the imminence of death and desire palliative care. Some hospice programs require the clients to have a caregiver; others care for patients who live alone and have no designated caregiver. The number of persons cared for annually by hospice was estimated in 1990 to be 200,000 (National Hospice Organization, 1995). By 1994, an estimated 328,000 people had received hospice care (Strahan, 1996).

Table 11–12 shows the characteristics of hospice users. More women than men use hospice, and almost half of the users are married. More than two-thirds of the users are age sixty-five or older (71.5%). Malignant neoplasms are the most common diagnosis of hospice patients, accounting for 71% in 1993 (Hospice Association of America, 1996). Cancer of the lungs, breast, colon, and prostate represented 60% of the neoplasms. Other frequent diagnoses include diseases of the circulatory system, diseases of the respiratory system, diseases of the nervous system, and infectious and parasitic diseases, including human immunodeficiency virus (HIV) (Strahan, 1996).

As noted earlier, all types of third-party payers cover hospice, but not all hospice care is billed as a discrete service. Thus, data on total expenditures are accurate for Medicare-certified and Medicaid-certified hospice care but underrepresent the total amount spent nationally on hospice. Total expenditures for Medicare hospice climbed from $118.4 million in 1988 to $1.3 billion in 1994 (Hospice Association of America, 1996). Medicaid expenditures for hospice in 1994 totaled approximately $198 million (Hospice Association of America, 1996). A special study by Catholic University esti-

mated that Medicare pays for about two-thirds of hospice care (67%), private insurance accounts for 15%, and Medicaid accounts for 9% (National Catholic School of Social Services, 1995). The cost of hospice varies by how long a person stays in the program and what type of services are rendered. Medicare caps what it will pay a hospice for a Medicare recipient; in 1995, the cap was at $13,469. The FY 1996 rates paid by Medicare for the four types of services it recognizes were $92 for routine home care, $539 for continuous home care, $96 per day for inpatient respite care; and $411 per day for inpatient care in a hospital, skilled nursing facility, or inpatient units of a freestanding hospice.

Adult Day Care

Adult day care is a daytime program of nursing care, rehabilitation therapies, supervision, and socialization that enables frail, often elderly, people to remain in the community. By attending adult day care, people who are functionally disabled and/or moderately ill but not in need of twenty-four-hour nursing care can remain in their homes at night with their families and friends while receiving the care that they need during the day. The goal is to foster the maximum possible health and independence in functioning for each client as well as the optimum combination of caregiving and respite for each family. For many, if a supportive home environment and adult day care are not available, the only alternative is to enter a nursing home.

Adult day care proliferated during the 1980s. Before 1975, fewer than 100 centers were identified (Von Behren, 1986). The number had grown to 1,200 in 1985 (Von Behren, 1986). By 1989, over 2,100 adult day care centers existed, providing care to nearly 42,000 people each weekday (Zawadski & Von Behren, 1990). By the mid-1990s, an estimated 3,000 day care centers existed, and adult day care had become an accepted and integral component of the continuum of care (Cox & Reifler, 1994).

No comprehensive reporting mechanism captures adult day care programs for the entire United States. The National Institute on Adult Daycare (NIAD) of the National Council on Aging (NCOA) has periodically surveyed adult day care programs in conjunction with the Health Care Financing Administration. Nationwide surveys were conducted in 1980 (Health Care Financing Administration, 1980), 1985 (Von Behren, 1986), and 1989 (Zawadski & Von Behren, 1990). A new survey of the universe of individual centers was conducted in late 1997, but no current data are available at the time of this writing. The characteristics described in the following text are believed to represent the field, but exact numbers and precise documentation are not available.

The services adult day care programs provide include: nursing, activities of daily living assistance, personal care, meals, recreation, nutrition counseling, social services, physical therapy, occupational therapy, medical assessment and treatment, family counseling, and transportation. Some adult day care centers provide all of these services; the remainder provide select services. Furthermore, some adult day care centers focus on a particular target population, such as those with Alzheimer's disease or mental retardation/developmental disabilities, and tailor their services accordingly. Most adult day care programs operate on Monday through Friday from 8 A.M. to 4 P.M.

Adult day care centers may be freestanding (about one-third) or sponsored by a parent organization (about two-thirds)—a hospital, nursing home, multipurpose senior center, community social services agency, government agency, or church. The majority are not-for-profit. Most adult day care centers cannot cover their costs, and about half operate at a loss. Adult day care centers depend heavily on philanthropy, volunteers, and in-kind contributions. The rationale for their existence is clearly to meet a service need, not to generate excessive revenues.

The average cost to attend an adult day care center is $50 per day (National Institute on Adult Daycare, 1994–1995). Charges vary depending upon the range of services offered, number of days attended per week, and various other factors. Many centers use a sliding fee scale for private pay patients to accommodate family incomes.

Despite the fact that most of the clients are over age sixty-five, Medicare does not pay for adult day care. The largest single payer is Medicaid. Fees paid directly by clients and families are the second largest source. Most adult day care centers patch together funds from several sources, including Title III of the Older Americans Act, Title XX social service block grants, Veterans Administration, state and local mental health and development disability programs, United Way, managed care, long-term care insurance, private foundation grants, and fundraising activities (National Adult Day Services Association, 1996).

Reflecting the growth and evolution of adult day care, many states now license and/or certify adult day care centers (National Institute on Adult Daycare, 1994–1995). There is, however, no federal certification or national accreditation. Each state sets its own licensing and accreditation criteria and payment policies.

Those who attend adult day care centers are typically in fragile mental or physical condition. According to the 1989 survey, about half suffer from cognitive impairment; an additional one-third have Alzheimer's disease or related disorders. Nearly 60% require assistance in two or more activities of daily living. One-fourth rely on a cane or walker; many are wheelchair-bound. The majority of participants come for an indefinite period of time; however, some come during the recuperative spell of an acute episode of illness until they have regained independence in physical or mental functioning. Clients may attend every day of the week or just select days, depending upon the caregiver's needs.

As of 1989, the average age of participants was seventy-six years. Two-thirds of all participants were women. Two-thirds of participants lived with a spouse, adult children, other family, or friends; one-fourth lived alone.

The functional and personal client characteristics suggest that adult day care centers do indeed offer an alternative to nursing home care for people who would be unable to function alone but who are able to live with family or friends, provided that respite and daily supervision are available.

Assisted Living

Assisted living is another service of the continuum that has burgeoned in the late 1990s. Assisted living facilities typically provide residents with one- or two-room apartments, meals, housekeeping, social services, limited transportation, and personal assistance. Residents are those who need assistance with the ADLs and IADLs, as well as perhaps with medication administration, but who are not so ill that they must be in a nursing home with twenty-four-hour supervision.

Assisted living facilities have emerged to fill a role previously played by the nursing home. As federal and state regulations for Medicare and Medicaid reimbursement have limited those who are eligible for admission to a nursing facility, assisted living facilities have evolved as a lower-cost, lower-intensity alternative that nonetheless offers a highly supportive environment. Assisted living facilities are not regulated by the federal government because Medicare does not recognize them as a provider of acute services. Some states license assisted living facilities, and a few, like forerunner Oregon, pay for the services provided through the state Medicaid program.

Because of the lack of comprehensive licensing and/or certification, the exact number of assisted living facilities and their characteristics are not known. One recent study identified 30,000 facilities serving approximately 1.5 million people (Assisted Living Federation of America, 1996).

INTEGRATING MECHANISMS

For a continuum of care to function as a system of care rather than as a collection of fragmented services, integrating mechanisms are essential. As described earlier, these include (1) an internal organization that coordinates the operations of various services; (2) a management information system that integrates clinical, utilization, and financial data and follows clients across settings; (3) a case management/care coordination program that works with clients to arrange services; and (4) a financing mechanism that enables pooling of funds across services. These integrating mechanisms are in various stages of development; few comprehensive systems that include all of these components exist. Considerable advancement was made, however, during the decade of the 1990s.

Inter-entity Structure

Inter-entity planning and administration must be structured both within an organization and across organizations. Patient services are not likely to be coordinated unless the units that are providing the services are coordinated administratively, particularly when budgeting and financial issues arise. A patient with a hip fracture may be cared for by the emergency room, acute care inpatient unit, skilled nursing facility, rehabilitation hospital or unit, home health, and durable medical equipment company. Even when all of these services are within the same parent organization, the patient fills out admissions papers six different times, deals with six different sets of clinicians and administrators, and receives bills from six distinct provider entities.

Administrative structures are necessary for a continuum of care to (1) ensure channels of communication and cooperation; (2) establish clear lines of authority, accountability, and responsibility for patient care services; (3) negotiate budgets and financial trade-offs; (4) address issues of risk management and liability; and (5) present a cohesive, consistent message in interactions with external agencies and the community.

During the 1990s, a variety of formal legal entities grew with the means of bringing together physicians, hospitals, and managed care entities. Physician-hospital organizations (PHOs) were formed to align the financial and market interests of physicians and hospitals. Foundations were established as a model way of combining the assets of hospitals, physicians, and managed care entities within a single organization yet allowing the relative autonomy of the components. Informal networks were incorporated as formal entities with the capability to contract on behalf of all members. Informal affiliations were changed to formal affiliations detailing respective performance expectations. Purchases and mergers continued among providers and payers. The number of independent hospitals, nursing homes, and home health agencies declined, and participation in multi–health care systems grew. But even though corporate relationships began to bring service providers together and to bring providers and payers together, the management mechanisms to ensure day-to-day collaboration are not necessarily universally in place.

Practicing in a continuum of care creates changes in the traditional roles of professionals. New roles and responsibilities develop in relation to patients and families, providers and payers, and other professionals (Evashwick & Weiss, 1987).

The human component is an essential dimension of the continuum of care for the patient and practitioner. The staff interactions and attitudes must be reoriented to have a systems approach, and thus the administrative mechanisms must be put in place to facilitate human resource management as well as all other aspects of management.

Administrative mechanisms within an organization essential for the seamless functioning of a continuum of care include:

- Committees that cut across service areas
- A multilevel structure and designated senior administrator responsible for decisions that affect several different departments or units
- An integrated budget that recognizes the contribution of each unit to the performance of the whole, including losses in one unit that produce larger gains in another unit
- Multidepartment/multientity planning teams
- Multidisciplinary and multidepartmental task forces focusing on specific short-term issues
- Product line management organized for a continuum of care

The organizational issues inherent in operating an efficient continuum of care began to be articulated during the late 1980s and 1990s (Evashwick, 1997; Evashwick & Weiss, 1987). Experts studied health care systems and physician groups (Coddington, et al., 1994; Gillies, et al., 1993). National associations delineated criteria for integration. The Joint Commission for the Accreditation of Healthcare Organizations added a segment on integration to its organizational analysis. The National Chronic Care Consortium (NCCC) arose. The NCCC is a cooperative of thirty-two members, each comprising a hospital and nursing home, that spearheads initiatives to tackle the issues of integrating financing and organization between acute and long-term care. The

NCCC has developed the SASI (Self-Assessment for Systems Integration) tool for measuring an organization's structural and process readiness for integration (National Chronic Care Consortium, 1996).

Organizations that exemplify continuum structure in the late 1990s are ones that have evolved over time with gradual modifications. Only as research and evaluation entities have articulated requisite administration structures and as the other three integrating mechanisms have evolved to the stage of being practical realities have organizations realized that they must consciously implement internal management structures in order to maximize the benefits of comprehensiveness, continuity, and integration offered by a continuum of care.

Integrated Information Systems

Integrated information systems are necessary for efficient management of the continuum. Many health and social service organizations still maintain separate clinical, financial, and utilization data systems. During the late 1990s, hospitals began to develop data systems to integrate the multiple components of inpatient and outpatient records. Nursing homes were forced to computerize patient records due to reporting requirements specified in the Omnibus Budget Reconciliation Act of 1987 (OBRA 1987). Many small organizations, however, particularly social service agencies, small community-based agencies, and housing facilities, do not have computerized clinical records, even in the late 1990s. Overall, very few health care organizations maintain data on patients as they move from one service to another, such as from acute hospital care to home care. Yet, financing of health care and social services is increasingly dependent on prepaid and/or capitated systems encompassing a comprehensive service package. In order to implement quality assurance and utilization review programs, assess efficiency of operations, and track

and aggregate patient experiences, comprehensive and integrated data systems and accompanying management reporting systems are imperative.

The ideal information system for a continuum of care was conceptualized in the mid-1980s (Zawadski, 1987). However, the computer technology to make such a system feasible and affordable depended on the development of new computer chips with expanded capacity and networking technology, both of which occurred during the latter part of the 1980s, and on the establishment of the Internet, which became widely available in the latter half of the 1990s. Figure 11–5 schematically shows an ideal integrated patient record.

In the 1990s, the individual services of the continuum have been upgrading their information systems to combine clinical, financial, and utilization data. Information systems that combine the financial, clinical, or utilization aspects of a patient's care across settings have been designed and slowly implemented. Payers and utilization review companies have enhanced their databases and tracking programs to evaluate the cost of caring for a patient through an episode of illness. And evaluators have specified criteria for quality that depend upon tracking patient data over time and data on a communitywide basis. Once these component information systems have been developed, they can be combined to the degree required for the ideal continuum.

Care Coordination

The clinical care for a person in the continuum must be coordinated over time, across settings, and among various professionals. Several techniques have evolved for doing so; case management, interdisciplinary teams, clinical liaisons, single-entry access points, and extended care pathways are among the most common.

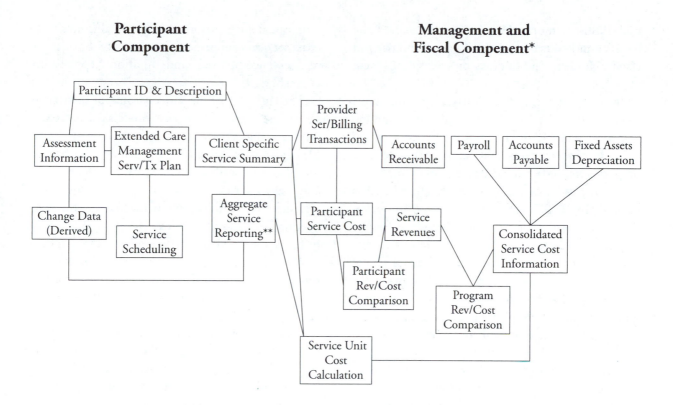

Participant Component

Management and Fiscal Compenent*

* These elements are repeated for each individual service
** Data from each individual service aggregated here

SOURCE: Adapted from *The Continuum of Long-Term Care: An Integrated Systems Approach,* edited by C. Evashwick, 1996, courtesy of Delmar Publishers: Albany, NY.

FIGURE 11–5 Model integrated information system for a chronic care organization

Case management is also referred to as service coordination or care management, and occasionally by other terms. The purpose of case management is to work directly with clients and families over time to assist them in arranging and managing the complex set of resources that the client requires to maintain health and independent functioning. Case management seeks to achieve the maximum cost-effective use of scarce resources by helping clients get the health, social, and support services most appropriate for their needs at a given time. It guides the client and family through the maze of services, matches service need with funding authorization, and coordinates with clinicians and provider organizations.

Case management began through public programs, often with social workers in the public welfare department, case workers in mental health, or nurses in public health departments. For years, it struggled for identity. The most frequent locus in the private sector was in social service agencies. During the late 1970s and continuing through the mid-1980s, demonstration projects examined the benefits and costs of care coordination and tried to classify models. The findings on cost savings were mixed.

In the latter part of the 1980s, care coordination began to be recognized as necessary to streamline care and negotiate the maze of long-term care services. Private insurance companies, managed care programs, employers, and private family members began to pay for case management. The result has been a proliferation of models and the confusion that accompanies growth. The 1990s saw further evolution and clarification of the role of the case manager. Table 11–14 shows the characteristics of different types of case managers and illuminates the dimensions that categorize case management programs: funding/reimbursement, targeting, gatekeeping, and organizational auspices.

Case management is defined as a process. The components are assessment, care planning, arrangement of services, monitoring, and reassessment (White & Gundrum, 1996). Assessment is usually done by a multidisciplinary team that includes a nurse, a social worker, a physician, and other professionals as indicated by the conditions of the particular client. When possible, assessment includes evaluation of the home environment and family situation. Based on the results of the assessment, the team concurs on a specific plan of action and recommends an array of appropriate services.

The ongoing care coordinator may be a nurse, social worker, or health care professional trained specifically as a case manager. The care coordinator is responsible for arranging the services ordered by the team and maintaining contact with the client and the service providers to confirm that services are being delivered and are meeting the client's needs. Reassessment of the client's status occurs either according to a regularly scheduled checkup with the clinicians or when the care coordinator detects a change that warrants reevaluation. Long-

term case management is distinguished from short-term service arrangement by intensity, breadth of services encompassed, and duration (Applebaum & Austin, 1990).

The authority of the care coordinator to arrange service use varies. Three basic models exist: broker, service management, and managed care (Applebaum & Austin, 1990). Under the broker model, care coordinators identify needed services and make referrals but have no authority over service delivery. With service management, the care coordinator has authority over payment but usually has a capitated or predetermined cap limiting how much can be spent. Managed care places the provider at risk, and thus the care coordinator has no set cap but clear financial incentives to use resources carefully and wisely.

A care coordinator can handle twenty to eighty active clients, depending on the breadth and intensity of the program, the dependence level of the clients, and the organizational resources supporting the care coordination operations.

The fee for case management is $50 to $150 for an initial assessment, and then a lesser fee for ongoing monthly service or follow-up consultation. Medicare does not pay for care coordination except under home health. A case management program may be paid for entirely or partially by certain state government programs, such as Medicaid, Title XX, mental health, or Older Americans Act funds; demonstration grants; private moneys, such as grants, foundations, or donations; select insurance companies who now cover this as a benefit; or directly by clients or families.

The role of the care coordinator is still evolving. Only during the 1990s has it received recognition as a separate and distinct role. New variations include care coordinators based in hospitals, HMOs, private insurance companies, employers, and managed care companies. Private pay case management is now sufficiently common that an

TABLE 11–14   Summary of case management types and key characteristics

Type	Population	Setting	Focus	Financing
Medical				
Primary care	Patients	Doctor's office; clinics	Prevent, diagnose, treat, monitor	Private pay; insurance; Medicare
Acute care	Patients	Hospital; acute, subacute facilities	Facilitate flow of care and discharge; prevent readmission	Private pay; insurance; Medicare; Medicaid
Other medical	Medically dependent	Skilled nursing facility; home	Treat, monitor, supervise, prevent, rehabilitate	Private pay; insurance; Medicare; Medicaid
Insurance/managed care	Enrollees; high risk, high cost	Primary/acute settings	Authorize, verify services and utilization; manage costs	Private pay; insurance; Medicare; Medicaid
Nonmedical				
Community/ in-home	Community functional/ cognitive disability	Noninstitutional	Coordinate wide range of nonmedical care	Private pay; waiver funds; grants/ contracts
Long-term care insurance	Ongoing need for care, supervision; chronic problems	In-home, community or facility	Monitor, prevent decline; link to needed resources	Private pay; some waiver funds; grants/contracts
Other	Usually well; need advice, counseling	Community	Resource/service information, referrals	Private pay; grants/ contracts

SOURCE: "Care Coordination," by M. White & G. Gundrum, in *The Continuum of Long-Term Care: An Integrated Systems Approach,* edited by C. Evashwick, 1996, Albany, NY: Delmar.

entire association has grown up of private geriatric case managers. Meanwhile, the traditional case manager brokers continue in social services agencies and government programs. Four dimensions characterize care coordination and provide a framework for classifying the myriad of models.

During the past decade, the providers and payers of health care have recognized the need to develop a cost-effective means of dealing with the complexity of patient's ongoing needs for comprehensive, continuing care. Case management has the potential to coordinate an array of resources, both within a given organization and externally in other community agencies, and to make astute use of a variety of financial resources to maximize the care affordable by the client. The trend to recognize the distinct role of a case manager/care coordinator is further enhanced by the expansion of health care organizations into continuums of care, with more than a single type of service available within the same organization and with a pool of funds for health and social support services that can be spent at the discretion of the provider.

Case management is likely to become even more prevalent in the future as part of the expansion of integrated health care delivery systems and capitated managed care arrangements. Its cost-effectiveness will likely continue to be examined, and refinement and streamlining of the models will likely continue to occur.

Other methods of care coordination include:

- Single-entry access
- Interdisciplinary team and team conferences for clinicians
- Clinical liaisons assigned to service programs that have frequent patient referrals
- Clinical pathways
- Extended care clinical pathways

The latter is perhaps the newest technique for coordinating clinical care across settings. The extended care pathways specifies what should happen to a patient in different settings as their episode of illness extends beyond the acute hospital into home and community-based venues of care.

Integrated Financing

Comprehensive, flexible, and adequate financing is a goal of the ideal continuum. This is the single component of the continuum of care most critical and most challenging in the 1990s. As with many other areas of health care, delivery system changes will be driven by financial incentives. The problems of fragmented financing and underfunded financing are discussed later in the chapter under the heading Policy Issues. For a continuum

to achieve the desired access to the full spectrum of long-term care services, financial barriers must not dominate placement and resource allocation decisions. Several trends and demonstrations offer hope that the financing of long-term care is moving in the direction required for the continuum.

The number of seniors enrolled in HMOs continues to increase. In 1990, 2,138,000 people, or approximately 6.7% of seniors, were enrolled in HMOs (Office of Prepaid Health Care Operations and Oversight, 1991). By January of 1997, 4.9 million seniors were enrolled in 336 Medicare-certified health plans, for a total of 13% (Health Care Financing Administration, 1997). Many people under age sixty-five with chronic illnesses are also enrolled in HMOs, and the enrollment of younger adults also continues to increase.

Several variations of Medicare HMOs have been formulated by the Health Care Financing Administration (HCFA). All offer a package of services that includes acute care with some preventive and long-term services. By having consumers pay for care on a capitated basis, HMOs overcome the access barriers of fragmented funding from the consumer's perspective for at least those services that comprise the service package. Providers may or may not be paid on a capitated basis. Risk sharing, which is now the predominant Medicare HMO model, has financial incentives for providers to be efficient in getting patients the services they need. The models also have the incentives and the flexibility to match services to a patient's needs rather than according to constrained payment policies.

As currently structured, HMOs are not required specifically to offer a comprehensive continuum of care nor to provide ongoing services for chronic problems. Nor do they coordinate care and monitor use as ideally as they might. However, many offer a fairly broad array of services. And, as evidenced by the experience of the S/HMOs described later, they do have a structure that can be expanded into an integrated continuum when the market and financial incentives are right.

Long-term care insurance emerged during the late 1980s as another way to fund long-term care. By 1994, 121 companies offered some type of long-term care product (Health Insurance Association of America, 1995). The number of people who had purchased policies grew from 815,000 in 1987 to over 1.65 million in June 1990 and to 3.8 million by 1994. A major trend during the 1990s has been to market long-term care insurance to younger adults as part of employer-sponsored benefit packages. Long-term care insurance aids the development of comprehensive financing for a continuum of services. For those who have Medicare Part A and Part B or indemnity insurance to cover acute services, long-term care insurance offers complementary coverage for the long-term, ongoing services.

When long-term care insurance policies began to be sold in the early 1980s, they reflected acute care health insurance by paying based on diagnosis and use of limited services, specifically either nursing homes or home health. By the early 1990s, the policies had changed to be based on functional disability and to pay on a per diem basis. Payout of such policies is based on being functionally disabled, not having a specific disease. The recipient can then spend the daily allotment to pay for whatever services they choose to use, including skilled nursing facilities, home health, homemakers, assisted living, or other formal or informal home support services.

Social HMOs, or S/HMOs, were begun in 1985 by the HCFA as a demonstration project. The purpose of the S/HMO was to examine the utilization and relative cost-effectiveness of a capitated payment system that includes chronic and extended benefits as well as medical services. The HCFA described the model as follows (Health Care Financing Administration, 1991a):

The S/HMO model includes four basic organizational and financing features. First, a single organizational structure provides a full range of acute and long term care services to voluntarily enrolled Medicare beneficiaries. Beneficiaries pay a monthly premium for services. In addition to the basic Medicare benefits, services include nursing home, home health, homemaker, transportation, drugs and others. Second, a coordinated case management system is used to authorize long term care services for those members who meet specific disability criteria, within a fixed limit of about $6,000–$12,000 per year. Third, the S/HMOs are designed to serve a cross-section of the elderly population, including both the functionally impaired and unimpaired elderly. Fourth, financing is accomplished through prepaid capitation by pooling funds from Medicare, Medicaid and member premiums. The initial financial risk was shared by the S/HMOs and HCFA. After 30 months of the demonstration, the S/HMO sites assume full financial risk for service costs.

Three of the four original S/HMOs have endured through the late 1990s: Kaiser Permanente in Portland, Oregon; Metropolitan Jewish Geriatric Center in Brooklyn, New York; and Senior Health Action Network (SCAN) in Long Beach, California. In the mid-1990s, the demonstration was extended and authorized to add new sites, with revised formulas for calculating payments. As of this writing, the six newly authorized sites have not yet opened, and the payment structure continues to be highly complex.

The original S/HMOs were slower to get started than had originally been expected (Harrington & Newcomer, 1990; Newcomer, et al., 1991). In 1990, after five years of operation, the four S/HMOs had 17,869 enrollees and had refined their benefit packages and operations to reflect financing realities and market competition. By the mid-1990s, one had ceased to operate. Rigorous evaluation of the S/HMOs has been minimal. In brief, the experiment by the federal government of funding both acute and long-term care through a single health plan remains more demonstration than norm as of the end of the 1990s.

The Program of All-Inclusive Care for the Elderly (PACE) is another program funded by HCFA. It began as a demonstration during the early 1990s to test a variation of a capitated payment program linked with a service system for the chronically ill. PACE attempts to replicate On-Lok, a program serving the Chinese community of San Francisco that centers around adult day care. On-Lok and its replicated sites organize a continuum of care for an extremely frail elderly population at considerably less than the cost of care for a comparably ill population not part of an organized system of care. The HCFA described the original model as follows (Health Care Financing Administration, 1991b):

> [It] includes as core services the provision of adult day health care and multi-disciplinary team case management through which access to and allocation of all health and long term care services are arranged. Physician, therapeutic, ancillary and social support services are provided on site at the adult day health center whenever possible. Hospital, nursing home, home health and other specialized services are provided extramurally. Transportation is also provided to all enrolled members who require it. Financing is accomplished through prospective capitation of both Medicare and Medicaid payments to the provider.

The PACE project differs from the S/HMO in that it focuses only on frail elderly people who are eligible for nursing home placement, while the S/HMO attempts to get a representative population over which to spread the risk of service use. The PACE projects serve 120–325 people, compared to the 5,000–10,000 served by each S/HMO. The provider network of PACE is smaller, more tightly controlled, and focuses around

adult day care. Finally, the financial arrangements are different. PACE receives a capitated amount from Medicare and Medicaid for a frail, high-use population and may also charge private pay clients on a sliding scale basis. The S/HMO functions more like an HMO, charging enrollees premiums and negotiating with Medicare and Medicaid for capitated payments based on a healthy population. As of 1997, eleven sites had waivers to operate as PACE sites from both Medicare and Medicaid; nineteen had Medicaid-only waivers; and more than thirty other sites were exploring the feasibility of developing a PACE program. The federal budget reconciliation of 1997 authorized PACE as a reimburseable service under Medicare, thereby moving the program from demonstration to permanent status.

Both S/HMOs and PACE are efforts to combine acute care and long-term care funding into an integrated system that enables a care manager to allocate resources according to need, rather than be stymied by the constraints of fragmented financing.

Although reaching only a very small number of people, the demonstrations and trends in private insurance and HMOs portend positively for future financial flexibility that will enable a continuum of care to integrate services according to client need rather than categorical funding.

POLICY ISSUES

The public policy issues pertaining to long-term care are complex, reflecting the diversity and breadth of the field. A comprehensive description would cover the policy issues pertaining to each service and integrating mechanism at federal, state, local, institutional, and society levels. This section highlights the major policy issues that should be considered by those involved in creating or managing a continuum of care.

The resolution of the issues identified in the following text is likely to take place gradually. Great impetus for major change may await the explosion of demand that will accompany the graying of the Baby Boom generation. In either case, managers must be aware that legislation and regulations may appear in any or all of the following areas, pertaining to any subset of the target population, and directed at any individual type of service provider or payer.

Financing

Financing is one of the primary problems inhibiting the provision and organization of long-term care on a coordinated, continuing basis. The definition of a continuum of care assumes: (1) adequate financing available to provide clients with an array of needed health, mental health, and social services; (2) access to such financing; and (3) the flexibility to apply funds in a variety of ways as needed by a given individual. At national and local levels, the current mechanisms of financing inhibit the operation of a continuum of care. Under existing financing:

- The federal government does not have a national policy or program that funds long-term care.
- The financing streams for long-term care are highly fragmented.
- The various payers have different eligibility criteria, service coverage, reporting and operating requirements, and payment policies.
- Most providers do not have control over all the pertinent financing streams, thus limiting their ability to pool funds and allocate resources from an internal process to match a client's needs with appropriate care.
- Much of long-term care is paid for by individuals. In effect, the national policy on long-term care is to leave care to the responsibility of individuals and families with states, through Medicaid, as a backup.
- The total amount of money expended by the nation may not be sufficient to meet the total need, thus resulting in rationing.
- The cost of a universal long-term care program paid for by government funds may prohibit a national policy from being developed in the foreseeable future.

To understand the challenges of changing long-term care financing from the existing situation to the financing required for the ideal continuum, knowledge of current and projected financing is useful. In 1994, the United States spent $949.9 billion on personal health care expenditures (National Center for Health Statistics, 1996). This includes expenditures for administration, research, construction, and public health. As shown in Table 11–15, of the total, more than one-third, or 36%, was spent on hospital care. An additional 20% was spent on physician services. The amounts spent on nursing home care and home health care were, respectively, 7.6% and 2.8%. Thus, the proportion of funds spent on acute care dwarfs the amount spent on long-term care. Political attention to revamping the health care delivery system focuses on hospitals and physicians; less attention is given to long-term care.

As noted earlier, the majority of those requiring long-term care are age sixty-five or older. Medicare is the federal insurance program for people age sixty-five and older. Medicare, however, pays primarily for acute care services. Medicare has two parts: Part A pays for hospital care, and Part B pays primarily for physicians and other outpatient care. In 1994, Medicare Part A and Part B accounted for $165 billion of the $949 billion of health care expenditures. More than one-sixth of the nation's health care funds were used by one-eighth of its population. Seventy-eight percent of Medicare

TABLE 11–15 National Health Care Expenditures, 1994

Category	Dollars	Percent
All expenditures	$949.4	100.0
Health services and supplies	919.02	96.8
Personal health care	831.67	87.6
Hospital care	338.94	35.7
Physician services	188.93	19.9
Dentist	41.77	4.4
Nursing home care	72.15	7.6
Other professional services	49.37	5.2
Home health care	26.58	2.8
Drugs and other medical nondurables	78.80	8.3
Vision products	13.29	1.4
Other personal health care	21.84	2.3
Program administration and net cost of health insurance	58.86	6.2
Government public health activities	28.48	3.0
Research and construction	30.38	3.2
Noncommercial research	16.14	1.7
Construction	14.24	1.5

SOURCE: *Health, United States 1995* (DHHS Pub. No. PHS 96-1232 6-0240, Table 119), National Center for Health Statistics, June 1996, Hyattsville, MD: Public Health Service.

Part A benefits and 22% of Part B benefits were for hospital care. Sixty-two percent of Part B benefits was for physician services. Medicare spent only 7.3% of its funds, or $7.6 billion, on nursing home care in 1994, and less than 13% of its funds, or $12.7 billion, for home health care in 1994.

Medicaid is a major payer of long-term care services (Table 11–16). Of the 35 million people eligible for Medicaid in 1994, 11.5%, or more than 4 million, were age sixty-five and over. Nearly 31% of Medicaid funds, however, were spent for enrollees age sixty-five and older. Total expenditures for Medicaid in 1994 were $108 billion, or about two-thirds as much as Medicare and just less than one-ninth of the total United States health care expenditures. Nearly 25% of Medicaid funds were spent on nursing home care. Over $27 billion was spent on 1.6 million people. Six-and-one-half percent (6.5%) of Medicaid funds, or approximately $7 billion, were spent on home health care for approximately 1.4 million people. Medicaid spent approximately 10%, or $10 billion, on care for Medicaid enrollees in inpatient mental hospitals and facilities for the mentally retarded and about 24% of its funds, or $26 billion, on acute hospital care.

Of the $26.6 billion spent on home health care in 1994, Medicaid paid approximately $7 billion, and Medicare paid $12.7 billion. The nearly $7 million remaining was paid by private individuals and an array of other private and public insurers.

Of the $72 billion spent on nursing home care in 1994, Medicaid paid $47 billion, and Medicare spent $8.2 billion. The amount paid by Medicaid for nursing home care is three times the amount paid for acute hospital care, and in many states, nursing home care is the largest single expenditure in the state Medicaid budget. All government programs combined paid for almost 58% of nursing home care; individuals paid for more than 37%; and the remaining 5% of expenditures were paid for by private health insurance and other private funds.

During the latter part of the 1980s and the early 1990s, state budgets began to tighten, and as a result, Medicaid programs were constrained. Since Medicaid is a major payer for long-term care, these budget cuts affected long-term care. States began to consider how to afford long-term care for their residents. The state of Oregon implemented a rationing program to limit Medicaid services to the ones proven to be most cost-effective. Should reduced budgets at state levels and rationing at

TABLE 11–16 Expenditures on hospital care, nursing home care, physician services, and all other personal health care expenditures, 1994

	Percent Distribution of Expenditures			
	Hospital	*Nursing home care*	*Physician services*	*Other personal health care*
Out-of-pocket payments	2.9	37.2	18.9	44.2
Private health insurance	34.2	3.0	47.3	25.6
Other private funds	4.0	1.9	1.6	4.5
Government				
Total	59.0	57.9	32.1	25.7
Medicaid	14.6	47.4	7.1	13.5
Medicare	30.0	8.2	20.1	8.8

SOURCE: *Health, United States, 1995,* (DHHS Pub. No. PHS 96-1232 6-0240, Table 124), National Center for Health Statistics, June 1996, Hyattsville, MD: Public Health Service.

state and federal levels expand, long-term care services are likely to suffer. Their availability will not keep up with the projected growth in demand.

Payment for long-term care is further complicated in that each state has its own payment system. Nursing homes are the largest single expenditure and thus have received the most attention. A variety of payment systems for nursing homes has been tried over the years to minimize cost, maximize quality, and provide desired incentives to providers. The most progressive systems base payment on acuity level of patients or intensity of care provided. Similarly, adult day care, other social support services, and much home care are paid for primarily by multiple state and local programs. Within a given state, payment may vary from one locality to another.

The private sector recognizes that a large share of long-term care funding falls on individual and families. The long-term care insurance market has grown, as described earlier. Further expansion of private coverage for long-term care may be enhanced by tax incentives. The Kennedy-Kastelbaum legislation passed in 1996 allows the cost of long-term care insurance to be deducted

from federal tax liability provided the policy is one of those qualified under federal standards and that the individual meets the income level specifications.

Expenditures for long-term care will rise dramatically in the near future. Because much of long-term care supports activities of daily living rather than acute illness, payers are hesitant to authorize funding for fear of unlimited demand. The public policy question, then, is how all this care will be funded.

Medicare is in the process of implementing systems to pay nursing homes and home health agencies on other than a fee-for-service basis. Demonstrations such as the PACE and S/HMO are being tried, and bundling of specific services is being considered. The Balanced Budget Act of 1997 attempted to increase the number of providers assuming capitated responsibility for Medicare beneficiaries by loosening the stringent requirements health plans must meet to be Medicare-certified health maintenance organizations. Further incremental changes in Medicare funding arrangements are likely to occur during the coming years. States may or may not adopt the federal system; hence, federal/state/private pay variations may continue for some time.

In outlining the considerations for a national health policy that would cover long-term care, the Pepper Commission of 1989 estimated the cost at $43 billion (U.S. Bipartisan Commission on Comprehensive Health Care, 1991). This represented about half of the total amount spent by Medicare in 1990 and ten times the amount Medicare spent on nursing home and home care. The amount was viewed as prohibitively expensive for a nationwide program. The Medicare Catastrophic Care Act of 1988 approached the long-term care arena by incrementally expanding select Medicare benefits. Funding relied on taxing the older population. The opposition by seniors was so great that the law was quickly repealed. In the early 1990s, the costs of long-term care were dealt a further blow by being excluded from President Clinton's proposal for national health reform. Although the total reform initiative failed, the fact that long-term care had been dropped before the program got to its final stages further indicates the high cost, the uncertainty, and the general preference of the nation that long-term care remain the responsibility of states and individuals.

Fragmentation

As is evident from the discussion of services, the continuum of care consists of a myriad of different services provided by many organizations, each governed by several different public and/or private sources. To provide any type of comprehensive, continuous care requires achieving cohesion. At the same time, flexibility must be maintained in order to tailor the program to the unique needs of each individual. Individual service providers and agencies must cooperate and share common goals. Although this is readily acknowledged, establishing the mechanisms to achieve such cooperation and sharing requires overcoming history and learned

preference; state, local, and federal regulations; as well as operational barriers.

Funding for long-term care services comes from health, mental health, social service, public welfare, social security, and housing programs, to mention only the main public funding sources. Individuals, families, employers, and a variety of insurers and managed care companies represent the private side. Each payer, whether private or public, has distinct requirements. Administration of long-term care services, particularly those that are paid for by public sources, reflects the financing fragmentation. For example, four or five different state agencies may be involved in paying for home health services. Fragmentation of delivery is likely to continue as long as the funding streams remain separate.

The intent of the continuum of care is to be able to pool funding streams in order to provide the services required by an individual. Putting in place the mechanisms to do this is the leading challenge of the twenty-first century. Several states have initiated programs to combine funds at the state agency level. Wisconsin and Minnesota are among those that have pooled dollars and authorities at the state level. As states move their Medicaid recipients into managed care, additional opportunities may arise to pool funding streams for long-term and acute care. Trends toward capitated financing for both Medicaid and Medicare are encouraging as eventual platforms for achieving integrated financing of long-term care services.

Availability and Accessibility

For years the cry in the community-based, long-term care arena was that services were simply not available. During the 1980s, the nation made great progress in this area. As can be noted from the earlier section on individual services, the number of providers grew during the 1980s and 1990s: home health agencies doubled, adult day care centers grew in profusion, hospice became a common and integral component of the system, and hospitals added services specifically for the elderly and chronically ill. In general, most urban areas now have a wide array of community-based services for those requiring long-term care.

Nonetheless, not all services are available to everyone when needed. Affordable homemaker and unskilled home support remains one of the services for which demand exceeds supply. Nursing home beds are in short supply in some areas because the state, in an attempt to limit Medicaid spending, has not allowed the construction of new beds. State Medicaid waivers may eliminate financial barriers to community-based services for those who qualify as low-income, but do nothing to minimize costs for those who are just above poverty-level income. Rural areas continue to suffer a lack of many services, not just health care. The operation of a continuum of care assumes the availability and accessibility of key services. To the extent that public policy and funding limit service access or availability, the continuum of care will be abbreviated and patient flow inhibited accordingly.

Quality

Quality has always been a hallmark of the American health care system. In previous years, the lack of quality in nursing homes was infamous (Vladeck, 1980). Many of the most egregious problems have been corrected. The growth during the 1980s in the number of organizations providing care for the elderly or chronically disabled has been accompanied both by more visible problems and a large enough nucleus of providers to warrant and fund the development of standards. As the population ages and the general public becomes more aware of long-term care, cries for high standards are prevalent.

During the 1980s, major initiatives were begun in both private and public sectors to measure the process and outcomes of acute and long-term care.

Perhaps because of early grievances, long-term care providers tend to be scrutinized for quality every bit as much as acute care providers. Chronic care per se and subsegments of the population suffering chronic illnesses have received increased attention during the late 1990s (Schroeder, 1996).

Public programs measuring quality are done under the auspices of payers, regulator, and funder of research. Stringent regulations are imposed by Medicare and Medicaid, as well as by state licensing and certification programs, to ensure a minimum level of quality.

In the past few years, considerable attention has been given to improving Medicare. The Omnibus Budget Reconciliation Act of 1986 (OBRA 1986) called for a study to "design a strategy for quality review and assurance in Medicare." The recommendations from this study, conducted by the Institute of Medicine (Lohr, 1986), had a major impact on subsequent legislation and regulations.

The single most significant event affecting the quality of long-term care during the late 1980s and 1990s was the passage of the Nursing Home Reform Act of 1987, which was incorporated in the Omnibus Budget Reconciliation Act of 1987, referred to as "OBRA 1987." This legislation, a series of amendments to the federal budget, created a series of changes affecting nursing homes, home health agencies, and hospitals, as well as other aspects of health care. The thrust of regulations was changed from process evaluation to outcomes. Increased training was required of aides, who are essential staff in nursing homes and home care. Decreased use of restraints was required in hospitals as well as nursing homes. Medicare eliminated the distinction between skilled nursing facilities and intermediate care, requiring instead that all facilities meet the requirements for skilled-level nursing care. OBRA 1987 required more structured patient assessments and care plans, and thus prompted computerization of clinical records of nursing homes. The implementation of OBRA 1987 was phased in over a period of years, and health care organizations spent much of the 1990s adapting to the changes.

The Agency for Health Care Policy and Research launched a major initiative during the 1980s to establish clinical pathways with outcome measures for select conditions. This policy helped publicize and promote projects by individual institutions to develop clinical pathways as a way of standardizing, streamlining, and, ultimately, improving quality of care. Although initially focused on acute hospital episodes, many of the conditions focused upon are indeed chronic. During the latter part of the 1990s, the clinical pathway concept focused on inpatient care was expanded to extended care pathways that included care by an array of long-term care providers.

Professional organizations and consumer groups also have been active in establishing criteria and programs to enhance the quality of long-term care. The Joint Commission on the Accreditation of Hospitals changed its name during the 1980s to the Joint Commission on the Accreditation of Healthcare Organizations. It accredits several major components of the long-term continuum of care: nursing homes, hospital-based step-down units, home health agencies, mental health programs, and hospices. JCAHO continues to refine its evaluation criteria and processes. The PACE program described earlier has created its own organization to develop standards for and to accredit adult day care health programs. During the late 1990s, the HEDIS program, which compares measures of quality for health plans, expanded its initial criteria to include several elements pertaining to chronic care. In all of these public and private endeavors, the emphasis has shifted from measuring process to focusing on patient care and outcomes.

A significant challenge in measuring the quality of long-term care is recognizing that the progression of the condition is likely to be flat or down. Factors such as life satisfaction and functional independence must be considered. Financial limitations must also be acknowledged. In contrast to large acute health care systems, many of the services of the long-term care continuum are relatively small in budget and staff size. With minimum financing, long-term care services simply cannot afford the physical or technological luxuries that acute care services or families can offer. Quality must be balanced with the amount of demand and resource allocation and with realistic expectations about potential outcomes. These become issues for society, as well as individual patients and organizations.

Consumer Rights and Responsibilities

Quality of life becomes closely intertwined with quality of care. Only when individuals have dealt with the first issue can society come to consensus on the second. The nation is becoming increasingly aware of the rights and responsibilities of people with chronic and terminal problems. This is reflected in public policy and, in turn, helps to shape it.

The Patient Self-Determination Act of 1990 was landmark legislation. It requires that health care providers explain to patients their options for treatment and gives patients an opportunity to express their desire for extensive or limited use of high technology to maintain their life. The significance is that it forces individuals—health care providers and patients and families—to confront the quality they desire in their own life and the potentials and limitations of the health care system. Those with multiple, chronic illnesses and severe functional disabilities must decide to what extent they wish to employ available technologies to prolong the normal course of life. It is the health care providers, however, who must assist the consumer in understanding and making these personal choices.

By the late 1990s, living wills and durable powers of attorney for health care are considered essential components of retirement planning. The awareness of the need for such documents preceded the passage of the 1990 Patient Self-Determination Act and helped to promote its passage. As the population ages, the number of people who are functionally disabled and require guardians or conservators increases. Laws have been implemented, primarily at state levels, to regulate the powers one individual can have over another's life and assets. Consumers are increasingly persuaded to consider how they would want their affairs run if they were disabled due to physical or mental health problems, to discuss this with family and physicians, and to articulate their choices prior to the advent of problems. Providers, however, must be educated about how to ask for and respect patients' wishes for end-of-life care.

The Americans with Disabilities Act of 1990 further recognized that institutions must assist those with functional disabilities. While the emphasis of this legislation is nondiscrimination for employment and physical access to facilities, the law also affects access to health care. More recently, the Kennedy-Kasselbaum legislation of 1996 changed the tax law to allow a deduction for long-term care insurance under certain conditions. This law is yet another indication of the increasing awareness of the responsibility of the individual to prepare for their own long-term care needs, and an acknowledgment by the federal government that regulatory measures can encourage consumer choice and responsibility.

Such legislation offers but a few examples of how the nation is becoming aware of the challenges of meeting the needs of the chronically ill and disabled while using scarce resources wisely.

Staffing and Expertise

The majority of staff in formal organizations providing long-term care are low-skilled workers. They receive low pay and have tasks that are physically and emotionally demanding. A high proportion are recent immigrants whose native language and customs differ from those of the majority of frail people for whom they care. Turnover is high, reaching as much as one hundred percent annually in some nursing homes and home health agencies. Aides are particularly difficult to find and keep. OBRA 1987 increased the training required of aides but did not affect the salary levels nor increase payment to providers to meet the expense of implementing the new requirements. Long-term care providers face a major challenge in trying to provide quality care when they do not have the resources to attract and retain quality staff.

A shortage also exists of experts in chronic care, geriatrics, and rehabilitation. Physicians, nurses, social workers, and rehabilitation therapists who specialize in the care of the elderly or chronically ill are in great demand and short supply. For example, in 1996, physicians certified as having a subspecialty in geriatrics numbered fewer than 8,800 (American Geriatrics Society, 1996), and only 3,400 physicians held their primary certification in rehabilitation medicine (American Medical Association, 1997). These numbers are not adequate to meet the needs of the nation's 34 million seniors or 99 million people with chronic conditions.

Payment discourages many health care professionals from going into long-term care. Pay scales are lower than in acute settings. Physicians do not get reimbursed adequately for the time it takes to go to a nursing home or make a home visit, compared to what they get paid for seeing patients in their office. The average pay wage for nurses in nursing homes is lower than the average wage for nurses in a hospital.

Attitudes are also an obstacle to attracting and keeping both skilled and unskilled providers in long-term care. The United States society is one that values youth. Despite attempts to change the image of older adults, many young people still have a negative stereotype of older people. In addition, health professionals, who are trained to "cure," find it difficult to accept chronic illness and an orientation toward maintaining functional independence rather than recovery.

Federal, state, and private organizations have addressed the issues of long-term care manpower shortages. Educators as well as providers have also sought to change attitudes through improved knowledge of the aged and the aging process. Many health care provider organizations now conduct aging sensitivity training as part of their orientation and ongoing inservice education. Nonetheless, developing an adequate pool of health manpower for long-term care remains one of the prerequisite challenges of changing the health care delivery system for the future.

THE LONG-TERM CARE CONTINUUM OF THE FUTURE

Do continuums of long-term care exist? Is it possible to overcome the problems of fragmentation, financing, and access to create an effective, efficient, consumer-oriented, high-quality system of care? Few, if any, complete continuums of long-term care are now in operation. The success of components of a complete continuum of care, however, has been ably demonstrated. Select programs throughout the nation provide encouragement for the future. In contrast to Mrs. Jackson's experience described at the beginning of this chapter, how do extant and future continuums provide long-term care? The following scenario already occurs in exemplary organizations.

Mrs. Smith is an eighty-year-old widow who lives alone. She slips in the bathtub and breaks her hip. She uses her voice-activated emergency response system necklace to call for help. When received, the call automatically asks what the problem is, then calls both a neighbor and emergency assistance. The neighbor comes over to be with Mrs. Smith, having agreed in advance to help in times of emergency.

The paramedics also arrive within minutes, stabilize Mrs. Smith, and take her to the hospital. Mrs. Smith belongs to the hospital-sponsored senior membership program, Silver Services, which was notified automatically via computer when the call came in. A laminated barcoded ID card from Silver Services gives the paramedics and the doctors in the emergency room all the basic administrative and clinical information they need to initiate treatment. The card also contains identification numbers that enable the clinicians to access Mrs. Smith's fully integrated, current medical record through the Internet to obtain more detailed information about her clinical condition and recent treatment history.

While in the hospital, a care coordinator, with whom Mrs. Smith talked when she enrolled in Silver Services, visits her and reassures her that whatever services she needs will be arranged. When Mrs. Smith has recovered enough to be discharged from the acute service, she is transferred to a rehabilitation-oriented skilled nursing facility operated by the hospital. Mrs. Smith never liked the idea of being in a "nursing home," but she does not feel negative about this one because the ambiance is positive, the staff are pleasant and encouraging, and she is confident that her physician and care coordinator will arrange her transfer home.

Indeed, two weeks later Mrs. Smith goes home with home health nursing and rehabilitation. The social worker at the hospital has arranged for Meals on Wheels to bring a hot meal daily, and a homemaker comes in twice a week to help with personal care, shopping, mail, and housekeeping. The emergency response system gives Mrs. Smith the security to remain alone at night, and she knows that she can call the Silver Services number at any time if she has questions or needs non-emergency assistance. Mrs. Smith also knows that her physician is regularly informed of what is happening to her through automated daily updates to her clinical record from all providers. In another couple of weeks, Mrs. Smith is steady enough to leave her second-story apartment and go for additional outpatient therapy. The therapists have automated and immediate access to all of her records through the health system's computerized comprehensive patient record, and thus they know exactly what exercises the home health staff has recommended that she continue.

Mrs. Smith's total spell of illness cost her very little out-of-pocket. The health care providers she used were all participants in the Medicare HMO in which she was enrolled. She made regular monthly payments somewhat above those required for Medicare Part B, and she acknowledged the HMO as her Medicare Part A and B provider. The care coordinator explained to Mrs. Smith that as long as she did not exceed the lifetime allowance and used the providers within the HMO network, she could use whatever levels of institutional or community-based services her physician and care coordinator felt neces-

sary. Mrs. Smith also had the peace of mind of knowing that she had organized her legal and financial affairs well in advance, just in case anything serious happened. A lawyer from Silver Services had helped her prepare a will, designate a sibling to assume durable power of attorney for health care, and express her preferences to her physician about the use of life-sustaining measures.

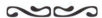

SUMMARY

Long-term care in the United States has undergone major changes in the last thirty years. It has evolved from an insular, isolated potpourri of services bifurcated around nursing homes and social service agencies to a broader, more extensive network of many services available at many locations throughout the community. Its financing sources, coordinating mechanisms, and general outlook have changed greatly as public awareness of its importance has increased.

Long-term care will continue to change as demand grows. The twenty-first century will see the basic structure of the long-term care delivery system shift from one of fragmented services to a comprehensive continuum of care. The future for the continuum of care, while challenged by the forces facing health care in general, is impressive and exciting.

REFERENCES

Adams, P. F., & Marano, M. A. (1995). Current estimates from the National Health Interview Survey, 1994. National Center for Health Statistics. *Vital Health Statistics, 10*(193), 81 (Table 57).

AIDS Hotline, Los Angeles (direct communication, March 1997).

Alzheimer's Association. (n.d.) *Is it Alzheimer's?* (brochure, p. 4). Chicago, IL: Author.

American Association of Retired Persons. (1989). *Veterans and the demand for long-term care* (p. 1). Washington, DC: Author, Public Policy Institute.

American Association of Retired Persons. (1996). *A profile of older Americans* (pp. 1–2). Washington, DC: Author.

American Geriatrics Society. (1996, December 11). *Basic information on the geriatrician workforce.* New York: Author.

American Health Care Association. (1996). *Facts and trends: The nursing facility sourcebook* (p. 57). Washington, DC: Author.

American Hospital Association (1997a). Special data run based on 1995 data.

American Hospital Association (1997b). In 1996–1997 *AHA hospital statistics.* Chicago, IL: Author.

American Medical Association (direct communication, 1997).

Applebaum, R., & Austin, C. (1990). *Long-term case management.* New York: Springer.

Assisted Living Federation of America (1996). *Overview of the assisted living industry.* Fairfax, VA: Author.

Coddington, D., Moore, K., & Fischer, E. (1994). *Integrated health care: Reorganizing the physician, hospital and health plan relationship.* Englewood, CO: Center for Research in Ambulatory Health Care Administration.

Coile, R. (1991). The second "core business" of hospitals in the 1990s. *Health Strategy Report, 3*(5), 1.

Coleman, B. (1991). *The Nursing Home Reform Act of 1987: Provisions, policy, prospects.* Boston: University of Massachuetts.

Cox, N., & Reifler, B. (1994, October). Adult day care: The state of the art. *LTC News & Comment* (p. 5).

The daughter track. (1990, July 16). *Newsweek,* p. 53.

Dey, A. (1997). Characteristics of elderly nursing home residents: Data from the 1995 National Nursing Home Survey. Advance data from *Vital and Health Statistics* (No. 289). Hyattsville, MD: National Center for Health Statistics.

Doty, P., Stone, R., Jackson, M. E., & Adler, M. (1996). Informal caregiving. In C. Evashwick, *The continuum of long-term care* (pp. 129–130). Albany, NY: Delmar.

Evashwick, C. (1987). Definition of the continuum of care. In C. Evashwick & L. Weiss (Eds.), *Managing the continuum of care: A practical guide to organization and operations* (p. 23). Gaithersburg, MD: Aspen.

Evashwick, C. (1997). *Seamless connections.* Chicago: American Hospital Publishing.

Evashwick, C., Rundall, T., & Goldiamond, B. (1985). Hospital services for older adults: Results of a national survey. *The Gerontologist, 25*(6), (631–637).

General Accounting Office. (1987). *VA health care: Assuring quality care for veterans in community and state nursing homes* (Pub. No. GAO/HRD-88-18). Washington, DC: Author.

Gillies, R. R., Shortell, S. M., Anderson D., Mitchell, J. B., & Morgan, K. L. (1993). Conceptualizing and measuring integration: Findings from the health systems integration study. *Hospital and Health Services Administration, 38*(4), 467–490.

Harrington, C., & Newcomer, R. (1990). Social health maintenance organizations as innovative models to control costs. *Generations, 52.*

Health Care Financing Administration. (1991a). *Social health maintenance organization demonstration* (program description). Baltimore: HCFA Office of Demonstrations and Evaluation.

Health Care Financing Administration. (1991b). *Program of all-inclusive care for the elderly (PACE)* (program description). Baltimore: HCFA Office of Demonstrations and Evaluation.

Health Care Financing Administration (1997, March). *Integrated service delivery systems* (fact sheet). Baltimore: HCFA Office of Research and Demonstrations.

Health Care Financing Administration, Health Quality and Standards Bureau. (1980). *Director of adult day care centers.* Washington, DC: U.S. Government Printing Office.

Health data on older Americans: United States, 1992. (1993, January). In *Vital and Health Statistics* (DHHS Pub. No. HS 93-1411, Series 3, No. 27, Table 12).

Health Insurance Association of America. (1995). *Long-term care market survey, 1995.* Washington, DC: Author.

Hoffman, C., & Rice, D. (1996). *Chronic care in America: A 21st century challenge* (pp. 9, 18, 24). Princeton, NJ: The Robert Wood Johnson Foundation.

Hospice Association of America. (1996). *Hospice facts and statistics.* Washington, DC.

Hospital Research and Educational Trust. (1986). *Emerging trends in aging and long-term care services.* Chicago: Author.

Institute of Medicine. (1994). *Training physicians to care for older Americans: Progress, obstacles, and future directions.* Washington, DC: National Academy Press.

Kane, R., & Kane, R. (1982). *Values and long-term care* (p. 2). Lexington, MA: Lexington Books.

Katz, S., Ford, A. B., Moskowitz, R. W., et al. (1985). Studies of illness in the aged. The index of ADL: A standardized measure of biological and psychosocial function. *Journal of the American Medical Association, 94.*

Keenan, M. (1989). *Veterans and the demand for long-term care* (p. 1). Washington, DC: American Association of Retired Persons.

Kemper, P., & Murtaugh, C. (1991). Lifetime use of nursing home care. *New England Journal of Medicine, 324,* 595–600, and Table 2.

Kraus, L., Stoddard, S., & Gilmartin, D. (1996). *Chartbook on disability in the United States, 1996* (pp. 8–9). National Institute on Disability and Rehabilitation Research (No. H133D50017). Washington, DC: U.S. Department of Education.

Lack, S.A. (1978). *The first American hospice—Three years of home care.* New Haven, CT: The Connecticut Hospice.

Lawton, P., & Brody, E. (1969). Assessment of older people, self-maintaining and instrumental activities of daily life. *The Gerontologist, 9,* 179–186.

Levenstein, M. (1995). The Department of Veterans Affairs. In C. Evashwick (Ed.), *The continuum of long-term care.* Albany, NY: Delmar.

Lohr, K. (Ed.). (1986). *Medicare: A strategy for quality assurance* (Vols. I and II). Washington, DC: National Academy Press.

Manton, K. (1989). Epidemiological, demographic and social correlates of disability among the elderly. *The Milbank Quarterly, 67.*

McNeil, J. M. (1992). *Americans with disabilities: 1991–92. Survey of income and program participation* (P 70–33, p. 9). Washington, DC: U.S. Bureau of the Census.

National Adult Day Services Association. (1996). *Adult day services funding fact sheet.* Washington, DC: National Council on Aging.

National Alliance for Caregiving. (1997). *Family caregiving in the U.S.* Bethesda, MD: Author.

National Association for Home Care. (1996). *Basic statistics about home care 1996.* Washington, DC: Author.

National Catholic School of Social Services. (1995). *Hospice care for substance abusing AIDS patients. Final report.* Washington, DC: The Catholic University of America.

National Center for Health Statistics. (1996, June). *Health, United States, 1995* (DHHS Pub. No. PHS 96-1232 6-0250, Table 119, Table 139, Table 140). Hyattsville, MD: Public Health Service.

National Chronic Care Consortium. (1996). *Self-assessment for systems integration tool.* Bloomington, MN: Author.

National Hospice Organization. (1995). *1994–95 hospice statistics.* Arlington, VA: Author.

National Institute on Adult Daycare. (n.d.). *Cost of long-term care.* Washington, DC: National Council on Aging.

National Institute on Adult Daycare. (1994–1995). *Responses from state adult day care association survey.* Washington, DC: National Council on Aging.

Newcomer, R., Harrington, C., & Friedlob, A. (1991). Awareness and enrollment in the social/HMO. *The Gerontologist, 30*(1), 86–93.

Office of Prepaid Health Care Operations and Oversight. (1991). *Monthly report Medicare prepaid health plans* (internal report, Division of Contract Administration). Rockville, MD: Health Care Financing Administration.

Rivlin, A., et al. (1988). *Caring for the disabled elderly: Who will pay?* Washington, DC: The Brookings Institution.

Schroeder, S. (1996). Letter from the Robert Wood Johnson Foundation, Princeton, NJ.

Strahan, G. W. (1996, April 24). An overview of home health and hospice care patients: 1994 national home and hospice care survey (DHHS Pub. No. HS 96-1250 6-0294), *Vital and Health Statistics* Advance Data (No. 274). Washington, DC: National Center for Health Statistics.

Strahan, G. W. (1997, January 23). An overview of nursing homes and their current residents: Data from the 1995 national nursing home survey (DHHS Pub. No. PHS 97-1250 7-0122), *Vital and Health Statistics* Advance Data (No. 280). Hyattsville, MD: National Center for Health Statistics.

U.S. Bipartisan Commission on Comprehensive Health Care (the Pepper Commission). (1991). *A call for action, executive summary.* Washington, DC: U.S. Government Printing Office.

U.S. Department of Health and Human Services. (1991). *Medicare hospice benefits* (Pub. No. HCFA 02154). Washington, DC: U.S. Government Printing Office.

U.S. Department of Veterans Affairs. (1986). *VA in brief* (VA Pamphlet No. 06-83-1). Washington, DC: Author.

U.S. Department of Veterans Affairs. (1989). *Annual Report, 1988.* Washington, DC: Author.

Vladeck, Bruce. (1980). *Unloving care: The nursing home tragedy.* New York: Basic Books.

Von Behren, R. (1986). *Adult day care in America: Summary of a national survey.* Washington, DC: National Institute on Adult Daycare, National Institute on the Aging.

Weissert, W. (1978). *Long-term care: An overview, health, United States, 1978* (DHEW Pub. No. 78-1232). Washington, DC: U.S. Government Printing Office.

White, M., & Gundrum, G. (1996). Case management. In C. Evashwick (Ed.), *The continuum of long-term care.* Albany, NY: Delmar.

Young, A. (1985). *Long-term care: An industry composite* (p. 3). New York: Arthur Young International.

Zawadski, R. (1987). Information systems. In C. Evashwick & L. Weiss (Eds.), *Managing the continuum of care.* Gaithersburg, MD: Aspen.

Zawadski, R., & Von Behren, R. (1990). *The national adult day center census—'89.* San Francisco: University of California Institute for Health and Aging.

Zedlewski, S., et al. (1990). *The needs of the elderly in the 21st century.* Washington, DC: The Urban Institute.

CHAPTER

Mental Health Services

Mary Richardson

Sharyne Shiu-Thornton

CHAPTER TOPICS

Incidence and Prevalence of Mental Disorders
Early Views on Mental Illness
Understanding Mental Illness in the United States
Shaping Mental Health Policy
Delivering Mental Health Services
The Changing Mental Health Service System
Patterns of Mental Health Service Utilization
Mental Health Personnel
Financing Mental Health Care
Managed Mental Health Care
Summary

LEARNING OBJECTIVES

Upon completing this chapter, the reader should be able to:

- Understand the basis for defining mental health services.
- Appreciate the history of mental health.
- Understand the various settings and arrangements for delivering mental health services.
- Appreciate the financing issues in mental health.
- Assess the complex personnel issues in mental health.
- Assess policy alternatives in mental health.

An estimated 30% to 40% of American adults experience one or more psychiatric disorders in their lifetimes (Robins, et al., 1991), while 30% have an active disorder during any given year. Over the last several decades, societal perspectives of mental illness have changed. Mental health research, expanded treatment options, and the civil rights movement have all contributed to a more enlightened social response and greater acceptance of mental health services as a treatment rather than a custodial function.

This chapter describes the development of mental health services in this country, the users and reasons for use, the organization and financing of services, recent trends, and the challenges of providing care. Although related issues of utilization and financing are discussed in other chapters, the unique nature of mental health services is presented in detail in this chapter.

INCIDENCE AND PREVALENCE OF MENTAL DISORDERS

The 1978 President's Commission on Mental Health set the stage for the development and implementation of two epidemiological studies of the prevalence of mental illness: the Epidemiologic Catchment Area (ECA) Program and the National Comorbidity Survey (NCS). The ECA involved interviewing household and institutional residents older than eighteen and was conducted at five sites around the country between 1980 and 1985. More than 20,000 adults were asked about their need for seeking and obtaining mental health services. The NCS, conducted between 1990 and 1992, interviewed a stratified national sample of more than 8,000 adults, using the Composite International Diagnostic Interview. Both studies concluded that approximately 30% of adults will experience a diagnosable mental illness in any given year, but the NCS consistently reports higher rates of mental illness in specific categories, including anxiety disorders (13% versus 17%), alcohol use disorders (7% versus 10%), and major depression (5% versus 10%). The NCS reports a higher lifetime prevalence than the ECA (which reports 30% to 40%), but both confirm a high rate of comorbidity (57% to 60%) (Robins, et al., 1991).

Mental illness affects people differentially, depending on age, sex, and marital status. Ninety percent of all people with psychiatric disorders report onset of first symptoms by the age of thirty-eight while the median age of onset of the first symptom was sixteen. Men experience higher rates of psychiatric disorder over a lifetime than women (36% versus 30%), but they experience about the same rate of active disorder over the course of any single year (30%). The most common disorders, in general, are phobia and alcohol abuse, but their prevalence differs markedly between men and women. The most frequent diagnosis for men aged eighteen to sixty-four is alcohol abuse/dependence followed by antisocial personality, with severe cognitive impairment becoming the most prominent diagnosis for men ages sixty-five and over. Somatization disorders are the most common diagnosis reported for women of all ages, followed by obsessive compulsive disorders. Women between the ages of twenty-five and forty-four often cite major depressive episodes. The rates of mental disorders, except for cognitive impairment, drop after age forty-five for both men and women (Howard, et al., 1996).

Ethnicity and socioeconomic status appear to be correlated to prevalence, but are confounding factors. Persons of color are overrepresented among those in the lowest socioeconomic groups. Blacks generally have a higher lifetime rate of reported psychiatric disorder (38%) than whites or Hispanics. Other differences in lifetime rates, related to socioeconomic status, include people who fail to complete high school (36%), are unemployed (48%), or are working as unskilled laborers (41%). Unemployed individuals report higher rates of mania, schizophrenia, and panic disorder. The lowest rates of psychiatric disorder are among people who are married and never divorced or separated (24% lifetime and 13% active). Unmarried persons report a higher prevalence of drug abuse, mania, and antisocial personality disorders.

Diagnosing Mental Illness

The American Psychiatric Association classifies mental illness within several general categories, including impairment of brain tissue, developmental disorders, and disorders where clinical cause is unknown. A major trend in psychiatric diagnosis is to use more objective, rather than subjective, standards for classification, replicable from one observer to the next. The Diagnostic and Statistical Manual (DSM-IV) published by the American Psychiatric Association contains the classification system used extensively in diagnosing mental illness (Robins, et al., 1991). These classifications are generally used in studies of incidence and prevalence of mental disorder.

In addition, the Epidemiologic Catchment Area (ECA) Program developed a system for assessing mental and addictive disorder prevalence, incidence, and service use rates (Regier, et al., 1984). An interview schedule, the Diagnostic Interview Schedule (DIS), was developed for use by lay interviewers to assess the presence, duration, and severity of symptoms in study participants according to DSM-IV diagnostic criteria. Interviews were subsequently scored by computer according to diagnostic algorithms specified by DSM-IV and other diagnostic systems.

Classification of mental retardation is based on another system, entitled *Mental Retardation: Definition, Classification, and Systems of Support, Special Ninth Edition 1992.* Unique to this classification system is the use of functional rather than clinical definitions and a focus on the interaction between the person, the environment, and the intensities and patterns of needed supports.

Finally, diagnosing mental illness can be further complicated by societal views of mental illness. Defining the overlap between social problems and mental illness is difficult. Are deviations such as delinquency or criminal behavior a mental health problem? What about poverty, discrimination, and unemployment? Mental health caregivers and advocates for persons with mental illness often seek to be inclusive with definitions in order to advocate for societally sanctioned interventions, while others with a more conservative bent are more likely to attribute such social issues to immorality rather than to illness. Under this more conservative approach, individuals are held accountable for the consequences of their illnesses, and society is expected to punish or confine them. Where to draw the line is the fodder for much political debate.

EARLY VIEWS ON MENTAL ILLNESS

Societies have always defined and classified human behavior in ways that differentiated between what was acceptable and what was not. Value systems, which shape social and cultural perspectives, also determine what constitutes deviant behavior. Societal tolerance of deviant behavior partially determines what a particular society believes to be mental illness. Although society now views mental illness in the context of biologic, sociologic, political, and cultural frameworks, there is a history of thought about mental illness and deviant behavior that predates current scientific thought.

During the Middle Ages, aberrant behavior was attributed to demonic influences, evil spirits, and the like. In an agrarian feudal society, people who could not work and sustain themselves were regarded as "mad." Society tolerated such people, who were allowed to wander if they were not too troublesome (Levine, 1981). Communities were able to offer them some basic support; if they became troublesome, they were driven away. With the rise of a mercantile society in Europe and a breakdown of feudal estates, major social and political upheavals occurred, leaving many people homeless, with no means of support. Groups of unemployed, including disbanded soldiers, wandered the countryside joining the ranks of those viewed as mad or insane. Thus a larger social grouping was formed and included people who were considered to be socially destitute. Community resources were quickly overwhelmed.

In England, the Elizabethan Poor Laws of 1601 heralded a recognition of the responsibility of government to society as a whole in addressing the problems of the destitute and the ill. In each community parish, overseers were assigned to provide care for the sick and disaffected members of society.

Later lunatic hospitals were opened throughout England, although their purpose had more to do with protecting society from the misfits than with providing care. Conditions were abominable, and inmates were often chained and provided only the barest essentials of survival.

In 1656, the French Parliament authorized the construction of the Hôpital Générale, where people who were poor, sick, or insane were confined in rather dismal circumstances. The eighteenth century, however, ushered in the Age of Enlightenment. Scientific thought began to replace magic and religion, creating a secular basis for societal debate. In France, Philippe Pinel introduced the idea of mental illness as a medical condition (Weiner, 1979). Pinel, often credited with unchaining the inmates and introducing humanistic treatment, actually worked with Jean Baptiste Pussin, the governor of mental patients who had himself been a patient at the Hospice de Bicetre in Paris. It was Pussin who advocated much of the improved treatment introduced by Pinel. The ideas of both Pinel and Pussin spread throughout Europe and, later, to the United States.

The development of American psychiatry in the nineteenth century was strongly influenced by Dr. Benjamin Rush, long considered the father of American psychiatry. Dr. Rush was also a pioneer in hospital reform. Before the nineteenth century, formal treatment centers in America were nonexistent. Private physician services were available to those with money. The rest faced imprisonment or hospitalization, with one not much different from the other. The hospital reform spearheaded by Pinel in the late 1700s in France was paralleled in this country by Rush's activities. The American Psychiatric Association was started through the efforts of affiliated hospital superintendents who, like Rush, were concerned with hospital conditions. Even into the twentieth century, treatment of mental illness based on medical/clinical approaches occurred in state-supported hospitals which were often located in remote areas and functioned as large human warehouses.

As the scientific revolution gained momentum, Kraepelin, a German physician working in the late 1800s, outlined a concise system of classification establishing mental illness as a separate and distinct disease entity subject to the rules that applied to physical or somatic illness. His work legitimized psychiatry as a branch of medicine. Kraepelin described in detail the symptoms, course of the disease, and prognosis of dementia praecox and manic depressive psychoses. The disease concept, however, implies that the patient can become "well."

Sigmund Freud introduced the psychological view of mental illness, describing the deterministic nature of mental illness, and relating it to disturbances and distortions created by unconscious developmental difficulties, psychic growth and maturation, and conflicts over sexual and self-destructive instincts. His work became the basis for the development of psychoanalysis. The Freudian model leads to long-term and intensive psychotherapy, requiring substantial and expensive therapeutic resources. Thus were born both the biomedical and psychological fields of mental health study and treatment, which continue to exist in a parallel fashion but are not well integrated.

UNDERSTANDING MENTAL ILLNESS IN THE UNITED STATES

Biomedical Advances

The advance of biomedical research in the twentieth century incorporated mental health research, producing substantial evidence for organic causes of mental illness. The discovery of the spirochete that causes syphilis, general paresis, and discoveries of chromosomal aberrations in mental retardation

were cited as evidence. Studies of schizophrenia, defined as a diagnosis by Bleuler in the early 1900s (replacing dementia praecox), and manic depressive syndromes have suggested possible familial tendencies. For example, ten percent of children of schizophrenic patients are also diagnosed as schizophrenic, possibly indicating a genetic basis for this illness.

Transcultural studies of mental illness have demonstrated remarkable uniform prevalence rates for schizophrenia in different countries and cultures. However, techniques for the study of chromosomes that do not isolate genetic differences cause critics to argue that a diagnosis of schizophrenia is highly subjective, and that perception of behavior as being schizophrenic is relative to the environmental context. With the rapid technological sophistication of genetic and other biomedical research, there promises to be substantially more sophisticated mental health research that may assist in determining the relationship between biomedical and social/cultural factors affecting mental illness.

Social Psychiatric and Behavioral Perspectives

During the twentieth century, there has been increasing acceptance of pluralistic determinants of mental illness, including biologic and sociologic factors. Harry Sullivan was the first American psychiatrist to develop a theory stressing the importance of interpersonal relations in disease etiology. Concurrent with the development of social psychiatric definitions were psychological and behavioral concepts of mental illness. Carl Jung broke away from the Freudian approach and formed the field of analytic psychology. Erich Fromme, a psychoanalyst never trained in medicine, and others applied anthropologic and sociologic concepts to Freud's theories. Later, John B. Watson discarded Freudian theory and developed behaviorism, which recognized only observable behavior as critical to diagnosis of mental illness. He believed that all behavior was predictable on the basis of environmental stimuli. Psychologists introduced classic conditioning and learning theory to psychiatrists and other psychopathologists.

Reliance on the disease concept of mental health was reduced. A greater understanding of personality development in the context of social and cultural influences set the stage for the development of a biopsychosocial model. This model recognizes the interaction of biology and psychological development within the context of culture. The development of humanistic psychology had origins in the behavioral movements. The Freudian approach was considered too pessimistic and the behavioral approaches too mechanistic. Carl Rogers developed the technique of client-centered therapy, which recognized the clients' role in affecting their own rehabilitation. According to this approach, client behavior is compared to expected behavior for the culture or environment of the client.

Cultural Concepts of Mental Health

During the 1960s, and continuing throughout the following two decades, a growth in the literature on the significance of culture to the understanding of mental health and illness occurred, reflecting multidisciplinary research contributions from anthropology, psychology, social work, and psychiatry. Various labels have been used to describe these disciplines' focus on the intersection of culture and health/mental health: transpersonal psychology, cross-cultural psychology/psychiatry, and medical and psychological anthropology, to name a few. While the methodological approaches varied, a shared research focus across these disciplines included the description, documentation, and interpretation of mental illness and suffering across cultural groups and languages. Symptom manifestations were described within the larger cultural patterns of kinship, gender roles, health

beliefs and practices, child rearing, and religious/spiritual world views.

Transcultural psychiatry (or cultural psychiatry) incorporates a biopsychosocial approach to understanding the culturally constructed meaning of suffering and illness. The recognition of the complex interplay of biologic, sociologic, and environmental circumstances and the cultural context that shapes and frames meaning stimulated changes in how symptoms need to be interpreted, diagnoses made, and treatment plans developed (Kleinman, 1988; Kleinman & Good, 1985; Sue & Sue, 1990). Juxtaposed with this awareness of the role of culture in symptomatic expressions of illness and suffering was the channeling of funding in the late 1980s to an increased emphasis on the brain and the biological underpinnings of mental illness.

Thus, most of mental health research and practice remains dominated by the mainstream (Eurocentric) perspective of mental illness with the resultant interpretation of what is abnormal or deviant (pathological) behavior a reflection of the values, norms, and belief system of the mainstream. African American patients are more likely to be diagnosed with schizophrenia and substance abuse than similar Caucasian patients (Strakowski, et al., 1995) and receive more psychiatric medication and higher antipsychotic dosages than patients of other races (Bender, 1996). The comorbidity of drinking, depression, and suicide among American Indian populations challenges first assessment, secondly diagnosis, and then meaningful intervention when decontextualized by the diagnostic categories of the DSM-IV (Maser & Dinges, 1992). Mental health services to refugee populations dramatically reflect the challenges of assessment, diagnosis, and treatment and the limitations of mainstream, Western conceptualizations of mental illness as reflected in the DSM-IV when applied with no understanding of the cultural context of the patient. The mainstream provider who is either ignorant or blatantly dismissive of cultural explanations of spirits, ghosts, or ancestors as responsible for one's illness places the provider and the patient at odds at the onset of any encounter. Thus, issues of access and utilization, much less assessment and diagnosis, cannot be fully understood outside the context of a patient's culture (Gong-Guy, et al., 1991; Westermeyer, 1985).

SHAPING MENTAL HEALTH POLICY

Deinstitutionalization

Before World War II, few outpatient mental health facilities existed. Growing federal interest, coupled with advances in psychopharmacology and changing social perspectives of mental illness, began to spur the creation of outpatient facilities. The development of psychopharmacology in the 1950s had a profound impact on the field of mental health. The prognosis for the thousands of patients in mental hospitals—many of whom suffered from schizophrenia, depression, and mania—remained dismal. However, the use of antipsychotic medications for schizophrenia, antidepressants for depression, and lithium in the treatment of mania rapidly improved the prognosis for these patients. Psychotropic drugs led to dramatic breakthroughs in the treatment of mental illness and enabled thousands of patients previously considered incurable to be effectively treated on an outpatient basis.

The use of psychotropic drugs created a climate that encouraged the development of various innovative therapeutic approaches, leading to a radical decline in hospital lengths of stay for patients with psychiatric diagnoses. Patients now could control their behavior through the use of drugs and, it was hoped, with continuing therapeutic support, function within the community. Thus, a mental health system previously based primarily on inpatient facilities had to develop new approaches to serving patients who no longer needed to be hospitalized. The general public, however, remained distrustful of, and misinformed about, the nature of mental illness, and there was little advocacy for improvement except from mental health advocates and professionals. Nevertheless, there was a dramatic increase in outpatient clinics from 400 before World War II to 1,234 by 1954 (Rumer, 1978).

The National Mental Health Act of 1946 (PL 79-487) signified an increased federal interest in the plight of the mentally ill. The law created the National Institute of Mental Health (NIMH) and increased appropriations for therapy and research. In addition, recognition of the psychological problems of soldiers during World War II motivated Veterans Administration (VA) hospitals to provide expanded mental health services.

Civil Rights and Advocacy

Beginning in the late 1950s, mental health services in the United States have been profoundly shaped by a series of important court cases, stimulated by the civil rights movement. Three areas of legal change have had major effects on the chronically mentally ill. They include substantive and procedural alterations in civil commitment laws, the limited implementation of a constitutionally based right to treatment, and the partial recognition of a right to refuse treatment (Lamb & Mills, 1986).

Deinstitutionalization and the way it was implemented were significant factors in the development of civil commitment laws. The influx of previously hospitalized mentally ill people into the community and the lack of consistent residential and treatment services created a large group of people whose lifestyles varied significantly from those of the general population. Philosophical debates raged on the right of an individual to choose this "alternative lifestyle," and the responsibility of society to ensure that individuals who appear unable to care for themselves have protection under the law. Civil commitment laws, initially general in definition, became more definitive and embodied criteria specifying danger to self or others, or the incapacity to care for self, with the presence of mental illness as a requisite for commitment. Laws also became specific regarding the duration of commitment, and the length of time was generally brief. Finally, individuals committed under these laws had rapid access to courts, public defenders, and other elements of the judicial system which ensured due process. Implementation of laws in most states became quite literal, and danger to self or others often became the deciding criterion. Yet, findings suggest that irrespective of commitment criteria, eighty-five percent of those committed are not dangerous. This emphasis may significantly reduce the number of people who could be helped by commitment and, some would argue, contribute to the increase of urban homeless people (Kleinman & Good, 1985).

The right to treatment was first addressed in 1952 in civil commitment cases relating to sexual psychopaths. *Rouse v. Cameron* in 1966, based on arguments of cruel and unusual treatment and the right to due process, found that people judged criminally insane had the right to treatment. Since the early cases did not define criteria for treatment but merely stated that some effort was required, there was little immediate impact. A decision by Judge Frank Johnson of Alabama in 1972, based on a class-action suit (*Wyatt v. Stickney*) related to conditions in state hospitals, required that right to treatment be enforced and implemented. Various courts have subsequently specified minimum standards for treatment. In 1975 the Supreme Court cast significant doubt on a constitutionally derived right to treatment by deciding the case of *Donaldson v. O'Connor* on the narrowest possible grounds. Donaldson, a patient in a Florida hospital for fourteen years, sued for damages and demanded his release. The narrowness of the ruling limited the potential impact of the right-to-treatment litigation on increased support for the chronically mentally ill (Kleinman & Good, 1985).

The right to refuse treatment raises often conflicting interests among society, mental health providers, and patients. The implications of behavior control through the use of behavior therapies, drug therapy, and psychosurgery create problems that have been addressed by the judicial system and by mental health professionals. The first of two right-to-refuse cases considered by the court was *Mills v. Rogers,* a class-action suit brought by patients at Boston State Hospital. In the years since, clinicians have been confronted with a bewildering set of pronouncements from the courts (Applebaum, 1983). Evidence suggests that the right to refuse treatment has significantly increased both use of seclusion and transfers to maximum-security hospitals (Kleinman & Good, 1985) for chronically mentally ill individuals. In *Stensuad v. Reivil* (Reivil, et al., 1985), the court ruled that the purpose of commitment is custody, care, and treatment, and that such treatment reasonably includes psychotropic medication. Confidentiality has long been central to the role of mental health care providers. Over the last decade, exceptions to confidentiality rules have been developed when the life of a third party is endangered by a patient (Eth, 1990). The American Psychiatric Association has proposed a model statute limiting psychiatrists' liability for their patients' violent acts and, at the same time, suggesting that confidentiality may be breached in the context of treating an individual who is infected with the human immunodeficiency virus (HIV) (Westermeyer, 1985). Advocacy for individual rights and the well-being of society is a continuing challenge in the mental health field.

In the late 1980s the federal government passed legislation requiring that states which accept federal funds for mental health services create programs for protecting and advocating the rights of the mentally ill. This legislation is patterned after similar legislation in the field of developmental disabilities. Protection and advocacy agencies for individuals with developmental disabilities are mandated in each state and funded through federal appropriation. Advocates for persons with developmental disabilities have generally been regarded as very successful pioneers in advocacy movements, although their success has met with mixed enthusiasm from professionals and policy makers in the field of developmental disabilities. They remain a significant and powerful force. Legislation establishing similar advocacy systems within mental health built on the developmental disabilities protection and advocacy system by integrating the two.

Impact on Policy

In 1955 the National Mental Health Study Act (PL 84-182) was passed, which authorized $750,000 for a three-year study of the entire mental health system. The result was the Action for Mental Health Report, published in 1961, after President John F. Kennedy had taken office. His continuing interest and support of this new policy direction was responsible for many subsequent changes. Although this report covered many issues in the provision of mental health services, the primary emphasis of the legislation that followed, during the Kennedy administration, was on outpatient services. Concern was increasingly focused on providing comprehensive mental health services to people not requiring hospitalization as well as to those not previously having access to mental health services. The Mental Retardation Facilities and Community Mental Health Centers Construction Act of 1964 (PL 88-164) provided construction

moneys for community mental health centers that were to serve designated catchment areas of 74,000 to 200,000 people. The five basic services that the centers were required to provide included inpatient, outpatient, emergency, day treatment, and consultation and education services. Significantly, the legislation mandated that services be provided regardless of the patient's ability to pay.

Many centers were built with the newly available funding for construction, but money for staffing and operations continued to be scarce. Finally, in 1967, an amendment to the legislation provided the necessary operations money on a matching basis, with funding for each center declining over an eight-year period. This was the "seed money" concept, and it was hoped that the construction and development of a community mental health center would encourage the community to gradually assume financial responsibility for services. Since catchment areas varied in their ability to provide matching funds, the subsidy for services in different areas also varied considerably. And although there was an allowance for poorer communities, the capability to readily obtain local matching funds was a distinct advantage for some centers.

In retrospect, the whole notion of matching local funds ignored the inability of some communities to assume the associated financial burden, especially in areas of greatest need. Since many centers faced closure or significant reduction in services, additional legislation (PL 94-63) was passed in 1975. This law included provision for a one-year distress grant at the end of the eight years of operational support if alternate funding was not obtained. This legislation was designed to overhaul the community mental health center network and also to increase the original five required services to twelve, including care for drug abuse problems, children, and the aged, as well as screening, follow-up, and community living services. Planning and evaluation of local community mental health services were mandated, and two percent of each center's budget was to be used for these purposes. Community mental health centers were also required to operate under the authority of a board of directors structured to represent the local community. These boards, however, were often composed of well-educated, upper-middle-income people who frequently were health care providers, despite the location of many mental health centers in lower-income communities.

Concern for the inadequacies of the mental health system led President Jimmy Carter to establish the President's Commission on Mental Health in 1977. The president's wife, Rosalyn, served as honorary chairperson, continuing an active interest in mental health services that began in Georgia during Carter's tenure as governor. The report produced by this commission influenced policy formation and, in many ways, became the heart of the Carter administration's Mental Health Systems Act, passed by Congress in 1980 (PL 96-398) (Levine, 1981). Although the act authorized continuation of provision to establish additional community mental health centers and authorized spending for many new initiatives, it was never implemented. Under the conservative administrations of Ronald Reagan and George Bush, moneys authorized were never appropriated.

Although the Mental Health Systems Act was never implemented, the national plan, also called for by the President's Commission on Mental Health, was produced and underwent limited distribution (Koyanagi & Goldman, 1991). Titled "Toward a National Plan for the Chronically Mentally Ill," the plan focused on federal mainstream resources, especially those available under the Social Security Act.

Although mental health policy underwent fiscal conservatism during the 1980s, mental health advocates, linked to a doctrine of increased state responsibility, went into action. The National Institute of Mental Health's Community Support Program (CSP), a demonstration program for the care of people with severe mental illness, survived the decade despite repeated attempts by the Reagan administration to eliminate it. In 1986, the State Comprehensive Mental Health Services Plan Act of 1986 (PL 99-660) built on the CSP system by calling on each state to work with the Medicaid agency and prepare a detailed plan for the care of individuals with serious mental illness (Rumer, 1978).

As categorical mental health funds were organized into state block grants, advocates also set about to improve funding in mainstream resources (Rumer, 1978). The four programs upon which these efforts were focused included Supplemental Security Income, Social Security Disability Insurance, Medicaid, and Medicare. The national plan became the blueprint for incremental change. Structural changes were made in each of the four programs that expanded benefits to individuals with mental illness, although full benefit of these changes has yet to be realized.

Mental health policy in the 1990s has been shaped by continuing battles over the role and survival of entitlement programs as well as categorical programs aimed at special populations, such as the mentally ill. In addition, as federal policy makers implement incremental changes in health care financing, mental health services are directly affected as well. Perhaps the two most significant trends of the decade to affect the mental health system are the rapid shift toward managed care, especially market-driven, or for-profit managed care, and the transfer of public funds and accountability by the federal government to the states. National mental health policy has been aimed both at improving access and quality of services and at reducing the variability of services across the country. However, as health care becomes viewed as a marketplace, moves toward greater efficiency through tighter cost controls, and becomes more firmly established in the private sector, Americans who have limited resources, including many who have mental illness, will become dependent upon state-based public services. A move toward state-funded and -managed public services will potentially introduce great variability in public sector mental health services between states. And recent federal legislation to consider mental health benefits to be the same as somatic ones when included in a plan represents the most dramatic effort to date to mainstream these services.

In 1990 the Americans with Disabilities Act (PL 101-336) was passed. This civil rights bill is intended to promote the rights of more vulnerable citizens, including those with mental illness. Primarily it addresses employment and public access, ensuring the rights of individuals to employment without fear of discrimination and access to all public facilities—whether for transportation, recreation, or other similar activities. It generally does not address access to health and mental health care, although it does prohibit employers from providing differential coverage or denying coverage based on disability.

DELIVERING MENTAL HEALTH SERVICES

Prior to 1955, most mental health services were provided in state or county mental hospitals, generally located away from areas of any population density. The policy of deinstitutionalization has created a dramatic reduction in episodes of inpatient treatment since 1955 and a shift away from the use of state and county mental hospitals. Between 1955 and 1980, the resident census of state and county mental hospitals declined from 559,000 to 138,000, or to one-quarter of the previous census (Goldman, et al., 1983). Of the state mental hospitals remaining in operation in the

mid-1980s, thirty were exclusively for children, twelve were security hospitals for the criminally insane, nine were teaching hospitals, and the remaining facilities were not designated for a special program goal or specific clientele.

Despite vigorous efforts at deinstitutionalization, state and county mental hospitals continue to be a locus of care for a wide variety of patient groups, serving as the "floor" of the mental health system, since they are the "source of last resort." They provide acute inpatient treatment to persons who have been unresponsive to treatment in other settings or who have exhausted their financial or other resources. Patient profiles have changed over the years, however. Previously such hospitals were populated by long-stay, predominantly middle-aged and elderly persons with schizophrenia, but now they are serving more young males with schizophrenia, females of all ages with schizophrenia, and elderly females with organic brain syndromes (Holcomb & Ahr, 1987).

Role of the Nursing Home

As long-stay patients were relocated from state and county mental health hospitals, nursing homes became a substitute, providing long-term custodial care functions. Of slightly more than 1.5 million people over the age of eighteen living in nursing homes or personal care homes, approximately 60% have some type of mental disorder (Lair & Lefkowitz, 1990). Approximately 29% have dementia only, including chronic or organic brain syndrome, and 13.7% have dementia in combination with one or more mental disorders. The remainder have a mental disorder but no dementia.

Concern over the numbers of people with mental illness and mental retardation living in nursing homes was the basis for the congressional passage of new laws governing nursing homes as part of the Omnibus Budget Reconciliation Act of 1987 (OBRA 1987). Under these provisions, nursing homes must screen all residents to determine their mental status. If placement in the nursing home is related only to mental status and not justified by the level of nursing care required, the individual is to be moved into a more appropriate treatment setting. In the event an individual is mentally ill with nursing care needs requiring nursing home placement, the nursing home is required to provide treatment appropriate to the mental needs of that patient in addition to the nursing care provided. Great controversy arose with the enactment of the law, and regulatory action has been the subject of considerable lobbying, affecting full implementation of the act.

Deinstitutionalization is undergoing a second-generation effort. During this second phase, court decisions focus on institutions where deinstitutionalization efforts may have already taken place (Geller, et al., 1990). It is likely more difficult to sustain remaining patients in the community, even when adequate services are available. Age, specifically age over sixty, appears significantly related to longer community tenure and a lower likelihood of readmission. The other most consistently significant predictor is prior hospitalization history. Geller and associates found that many people who have displayed a tendency toward frequent hospitalization will persist in that pattern even in the presence of community-based resources.

Questions still remain about whether further reductions in institutional populations are feasible (Gottheil, et al., 1991). Also of interest is the path by which deinstitutionalization is accomplished. If contrasts are drawn between mental health and mental retardation, two areas of service that were initially integrated in federal policy and funding, it is interesting to note their divergence in practice as goals of deinstitutionalization were pursued. Providers of services to individuals with mental retardation and other developmental disabilities argue vehemently that independence, choice, and personal dignity are directly related to living at home in the community. This strongly held belief has been the basis for the development of a network of community-based services over the past three decades, largely financed through state and private sources.

The mental health system, on the other hand, created federally sponsored community mental health centers, intended to form the backbone of community services for persons with severe mental illnesses. As federal funds began to disappear, mental health centers had to seek funding from states and other sources somewhat later in the game. Although financing has become more local in origin, program focus appears to remain heavily oriented toward promoting and preserving federal support. Perhaps coincidentally, the mental health service system continues to place less emphasis on developing natural community supports for integrated living experiences as the disability system is doing. Moreover, mental health services, unlike developmental disabilities services, continue to exist under the influence of medical approaches to treatment, whereas the disability movement has shifted toward education and habilitation models of intervention.

The Homeless Mentally Ill Person

One of the more challenging problems created by deinstitutionalization has been the number of persons released from state and county mental health hospitals who end up on the streets. Critics of the implementation of deinstitutionalization, noting inadequate funding, the failure to develop needed community services, and difficulties in maintaining continuity of care after hospital discharge, cite growing numbers of persons with chronic mental illness among the homeless population. Persons with mental illness make up a substantial percentage of the homeless population of the United States, with estimates ranging from

20% to 40% of the total (Klebe, 1991). Although difficult to quantify, estimates in recent years place the number of homeless people in a range from a quarter million to five million. Consensus has settled on a survey conducted by the Urban Institute in March 1987 over a one-week period, which resulted in an estimate of 496,000 to 600,000 homeless people in the United States. The Urban Institute further estimated that if 600,000 people were homeless during one week, more than one million were homeless at some time during the entire year.

Other studies estimate that 20% to 40% of the homeless population suffer from such serious mental illnesses as schizophrenia, manic-depressive illness, or severe depression. The Urban Institute study indicates that mental illness is most prevalent among single homeless adults, male or female, and is less evident among the typical homeless family of a woman with children, although the prevalence of mental illness among such homeless families is above the average for the general United States adult population. The annual report of the Interagency Council on the Homeless notes that the higher prevalence of mental illness in the homeless population, and, conversely, the rate of homelessness among those who are mentally ill, is not surprising. Noninstitutionalized mentally ill people are less likely to find employment, housing, or other benefits, or assistance to help keep them from becoming homeless than are those who are not mentally ill. Mentally ill people in the community not only are less likely to be able to function or work, but they are also less aware of the services available to them and less willing to seek help. They face frequent discrimination from employers and landlords, and they often face shortages of treatment facilities and housing opportunities in their communities as well. Abuse of alcohol and other drugs has also been a constant problem among the homeless population, often among the same individuals who suffer from mental illness.

The National Institute on Alcohol Abuse and Alcoholism (NIAAA) estimates that 35% to 40% of the homeless population suffers from chronic alcohol problems (Reivil, 1985). The same agency, in conjunction with the National Institute on Drug Abuse (NIDA) and others, estimates that approximately 10% to 20% of the homeless population have chronic problems with drugs other than alcohol. Data from the Urban Institute study indicates that almost half of all severely mentally ill homeless people also have problems with alcohol and other drugs.

There has been quite a bit of talk, but little definitive action, on behalf of homeless persons who are mentally ill (Eth, 1990). In 1984 the American Psychiatric Association (APA) published the results of a Task Force on the Homeless Mentally Ill, and described homelessness as but one symptom of the problems faced by chronically mentally ill people in the United States (Lamb, 1990). The APA Task Force Interagency Council called for a comprehensive and integrated system of care for chronically mentally ill people in order to address the underlying problems that cause homelessness. The task force's recommendations called for an adequate number and range of supervised, supportive housing settings; a well-functioning system of case management; adequate, comprehensive, and accessible crisis intervention in the community and in hospitals; less restrictive laws on involuntary treatment; and ongoing treatment and rehabilitative services, combined with assertive outreach programs when necessary. With few exceptions, these recommendations have not been implemented. In addition to funding problems, a fundamental civil rights issue is being debated. Do the homeless mentally ill have a basic right, irrespective of their mental status and lack of competence, to refuse treatment and appropriate housing and to live on the streets instead? Or does this "right to choice" translate into a life characterized by deprivation, victimization by predators, and the development of life-threatening health care problems or other cruel interpretations of the basic principles of civil rights (Koyanagi & Goldman, 1991)?

THE CHANGING MENTAL HEALTH SERVICE SYSTEM

The total number of mental health organizations in the United States increased steadily from 3,005 in 1970 to 5,284 in 1990. Within that total number, inpatient state and county mental health facilities declined in number, representing only a third of all psychiatric beds in 1990 as compared to four-fifths in 1970. Ironically, despite a major effort to substantially reduce the size and numbers of inpatient state and county mental health facilities, the number of organizations with inpatient settings doubled from 1,734 to 3,430 between 1970 and 1990. Figure 12–1 depicts the increase in organizations with inpatient or residential facilities. This occurred largely as a result of an increase in numbers of private psychiatric hospitals, separate psychiatric services of nonfederal general hospitals, residential treatment centers for emotionally disturbed children (RTCs), and other organizational types with psychiatric beds. Veterans Administration medical centers with psychiatric centers remained relatively unchanged during this same period (Redick, et al., 1994).

The private psychiatric hospital is generally categorized as either nonprofit or for-profit, although few, if any, nonprofit hospitals have been founded in decades. Nonprofit hospital financing comes from a variety of sources, including fees, endowments, grants, government contracts, and private donations. Of the for-profit hospitals, approximately 90% are owned by corporations (Bittker,

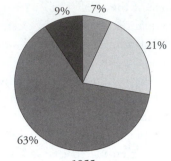

1955
(1.3 million episodes)

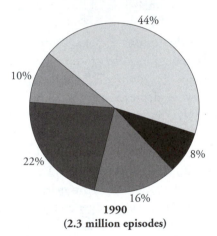

1990
(2.3 million episodes)

Type of Organization

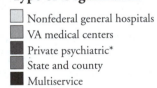

☐ Nonfederal general hospitals
☐ VA medical centers
■ Private psychiatric*
◩ State and county
■ Multiservice

*Includes residential treatment centers for emotionally disturbed children

SOURCE: *Mental Health, United States, 1994* (DHHS Pub. No. SMA 94-3000), edited by R. W. Manderscheid & M. A. Sonnenschein, Washington, DC: U.S. Government Printing Office.

FIGURE 12–1 Inpatient and residential treatment care episodes in mental health organizations, 1955, 1990

1985). The for-profit groups have been characterized by the development of corporate chains. The growth of private psychiatric hospitals and RTCs is believed to be due, in part, to expanded psychiatric hospitalization benefits by a number of insurance carriers. As benefits expanded, the number of inpatient admissions increased between 1970 and 1990 from 1,282,698 to 2,035,245, although the average daily inpatient census in mental health organizations underwent a general decline, dropping from 471,451 in 1969 to 226,953 in 1990 (U.S. Public Health Service, 1980). This is indicative of shorter lengths of stay but higher rates of readmission. These trends have already begun to change, however, with the implementation of managed care. Average length of stay in private psychiatric facilities, for example, is dropping even further as benefit packages become more restrictive and new case management arrangements are being implemented.

Psychiatric outpatient services now constitute a large part of the total mental health services delivery system in the United States, accounting for 74% of the total services provided in 1990 as compared to 1955 when 77% of mental health services were provided in inpatient settings, nearly the reverse (see Figure 12–2). There also has been consistent growth in numbers of organizations providing outpatient services between 1970 and 1990 (1,734 to 3,430), and partial care services (778 programs in 1970 and 2,340 programs in 1990).

PATTERNS OF MENTAL HEALTH SERVICE UTILIZATION

Today, mental health services are organized into separate but overlapping sectors that include both inpatient and ambulatory components. The ECA and NCS data are collected and organized by classifications of service types and include the

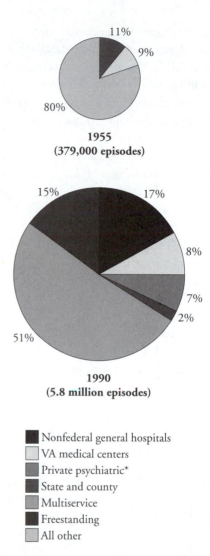

1955
(379,000 episodes)

1990
(5.8 million episodes)

■ Nonfederal general hospitals
▨ VA medical centers
▨ Private psychiatric*
▨ State and county
▨ Multiservice
■ Freestanding
▨ All other

*Includes residential treatment centers for emotionally disturbed children

SOURCE: *Mental Health, United States, 1994* (DHHS Pub. No. SMA 94-3000), edited by R. W. Manderscheid & M. A. Sonnenschein, Washington, DC: U.S. Government Printing Office.

FIGURE 12–2 Outpatient episodes in mental health organizations, 1955, 1990

following sectors: the specialty mental health and addictive disorders (SMA), general medical/nursing home (GM), other human service professionals (HS), and, explicitly recognizing the role of a person's social network, the voluntary support network (VSN) of self-help groups, family, and friends (Regier, et al., 1993).

Information on patterns of use of mental health services is reported from NIMH's ECA and NCS epidemiological studies. Thus data are obtained from two instruments, the ECA's Diagnostic Interview Schedule (DIS), and the NCS's Composite International Diagnostic Interview. The DIS is an instrument for assessing and categorizing mental health problem information for study purposes. The Composite International Diagnostic Interview is based on DSM-III-R diagnoses and includes more categories than the DIS. However, they both provide data unbiased by diagnostic customs of practitioners (Howard, et al., 1996).

Ambulatory Services

Using ECA Program data, Narrow and colleagues (1993) estimated that during a one-year period, 22.8 million persons made 326 million outpatient visits to professional or volunteer sources of care for mental health or substance abuse reasons. Of the 22.8 million persons using services, 12.4 million (54%) met full DIS/DSM-IV criteria for a current mental or addictive disorder during the one-year time frame. An additional 37.4% did not have a one-year diagnosis but met criteria for lifetime psychiatric disorder or a subthreshold condition. Persons with mental health or substance abuse problems using outpatient services averaged 14.3 visits per person per year. The majority (85%) were seen in a professional service, although only 60% of the visits were accounted for in this sector. Nearly 40% of the visits were in the VSN sector, although this sector accounted for only 29% of

persons seeking help. The VSN sector, thus, averaged more visits per person (19.8 versus 10.1) than did the professional sector. SMA sector services accounted for 38.4% of all treated persons, and 37.5% of the visits. The GM sector accounted for 44% of people seeking treatment, but only 11.1% of all mental health/substance abuse visits.

Of the total 22.8 million persons using outpatient services, 3.4 million persons had a substance use disorder and utilized 56.3 million visits during one year. Eighty-three percent of these people were seen in at least one professional setting, while 36% made use of voluntary services. Approximately 1.9 million were persons with a comorbid mental and addictive disorder. More than 62% of the 56.3 million visits made by persons with a substance use disorder (35.1 million visits) were made by persons who also had a comorbid mental disorder. More than 51% of people with comorbid disorders were seen in the specialty mental health sector, and 87% were seen in at least one of the professional settings (Geller, et al., 1990).

There were 6.7 million persons with affective disorder, accounting for 120.2 million visits with an overall annual visit rate of 18 visits per person. Ninety percent were seen in the professional sectors, and more than 28% were seen in the VSN sector. More than 48% were seen in the GM sector, accounting for 12.3% of total mental health and addictions visits to this sector. Bipolar disorders affected 1.1 million persons who utilized 16 million outpatient visits, with more than 80% of these visits made to professional sectors, including 55% to the GM sector.

Persons with anxiety disorders (6.4 million people) utilized 98 million visits, averaging 15.4 visits per person, with 87.3% used in the professional sector and 29% in VSN. Somatization disorders accounted for only 231,000 people utilizing outpatient mental health services during a one-year period, making 5.2 million visits, or 22.3 visits per person. Nearly all visits (96.4%) were in the professional sector. There were 688,000 persons with antisocial disorder who made 18.2 million visits, averaging 26.4 visits per person. Those with antisocial disorders, similar to persons with substance abuse disorders, used the VSN sector more frequently, where 35.9% of treated persons used 54.7% of total visits in this category. Persons with antisocial disorders accounted for only 32% of ambulatory visits in the SMA sector, and 4.1% to the GM sector.

In contrast, persons with severe cognitive impairment, 658,000 persons, were among the highest users of the GM sector where 45% received treatment. A total of 11.2 million visits were made by persons with severe cognitive impairment, with the majority of total visits in a year made to the professional sector (83.6%), and 27.5% to the VSN sector.

More than one million persons with schizophrenia accounted for 16.7 million visits in one year. Approximately 98% of people with schizophrenia received treatment in professional sectors, accounting for 79% of the visits. Persons with schizophrenia were high users of psychiatric outpatient clinics, with 10.6% of all visits made to this setting. Use of services in the GM sector was similar to use by persons with other disorders, but use of the VSN settings was significantly lower.

Inpatient Services

Narrow and colleagues (1993) also report on inpatient service utilization. Approximately 1.4 million people were admitted to an inpatient facility in one year, with 1.1 million having a current DIS/DSM-IV mental disorder at some point in the year. Of the remaining 300,000 persons, nearly all had a lifetime psychiatric disorder or significant psychiatric symptoms. The majority of persons were admitted to general hospitals (43.3%), with an additional 35.2% admitted to state and county

mental hospitals. Private psychiatric hospitals accounted for 10.8% of admissions, VA hospital psychiatric units for 7.1%. The remainder were admitted to community mental health center inpatient services (4.2%) and alcohol/drug treatment units (7.2%).

Persons with substance abuse were particularly high users of general hospital settings, with more than twice as many admitted to general hospitals rather than state and county mental hospitals (50.2% versus 21.4%), as were persons with non-alcoholic drug use disorders (84.7% versus 6.0%). The differences between admissions for persons with substance abuse disorders in general were not reported as statistically significant by the authors, while the differences for persons with nonalcoholic drug use disorders were found to be significant.

Persons with severe cognitive impairment were admitted to state and county mental hospitals more of the time (67.9%) followed by persons with schizophrenia (45.2%), phobia (42.3%), and unipolar major depression (38.7%). Persons with bipolar mental disorder were admitted only 13.4% of the time.

The GM sector in the mental health service system continues to grow in importance. In addition, a large number of people support networks of friends, relatives, and self-help groups which also are of substantial importance. The use of the GM sector underscores the importance of adequate preparation for recognizing, appropriately referring, and treating mental health and addictive disorders within all parts of the health and mental health care systems. Although general hospitals continue to play a major role in providing inpatient mental health services, state and county mental hospitals are still an important sector, serving persons with the most severe mental illness. This is worthy of special concern as the health care system advances toward managed care, leaving state and county mental health hospitals to compete for limited public dollars while serving the most challenging population.

Unmet Needs

In the ECA Program, more than 70% of persons with a recent mental health or addiction disorder received no services, and only 13% reported that they obtained treatment from a mental health professional. The NCS study reported 79% of individuals with a recent disorder who obtained no services, and only about 12% of persons with a recent disorder had obtained some service from a mental health professional during the previous year. Persons with a major depression were the most likely to receive services, and particularly from a mental health professional, while persons with a substance abuse disorder were the least likely to obtain services. Other disorders with wide variation included anxiety disorders for which 33% sought services overall, but considerable variation in source of care was reported within the category. Persons with phobia only reported service utilization approximately one-third of the time while respondents diagnosed with a panic disorder reported use of services almost 60% of the time (Lair & Lefkowitz, 1990).

Other Factors Affecting Use Patterns

People elect to seek mental health services for a variety of reasons including those associated with degree and impact of illness, education, marital status, age, and race (Lair & Lefkowitz, 1990). Other factors contributing to seeking help include consultation with informal help sources, referral by medical providers, supportive family members and friends, and ability to overcome the "stigmatization" society often places on mental illness. Financial and geographic access to services also affects utilization. The concepts of utilization variables and data assessment are relevant to understanding and interpreting mental health data, while specific aspects of use of mental health services are presented in this section.

Figure 12–3 describes the relationship between demographic variables and making a visit to a mental health professional. People with higher education and income are more likely to seek services, although education and income are inversely related to the likelihood of experiencing mental health and addictive disorders. Women are slightly more likely to seek services, although men are more at risk for mental health and addictive disorders over the course of a lifetime. As suggested by utilization patterns, professional intervention for persons with mental health and addiction disorders is substantially influenced by informal help sources and social networks. Medical care providers are another important source of referral to mental health services as well as for the provision of services directly. The degree to which general medical providers are adequately trained to recognize and appropriately intervene in the case of mental illness or substance abuse is still debated. With the growing influence of managed care, help-seeking will be affected by the use of primary care physicians as gate-keepers. It will fall to them to appropriately assess, refer, or intervene. This may prove challenging if they are not trained to conduct and interpret mental health status and psychosocial assessments.

MENTAL HEALTH PERSONNEL

There are many different types of professionals providing mental health services. They involve a number of interesting and complex issues, mostly unique to the mental health field. The number of full-time equivalent (FTE) staff employed in specialty mental health organizations in the United States rose from 375,984 in 1972 to 563,619 in 1990, with the largest increase attributed to professional

Demographic Variable	At Least One Diagnosis in Lifetime	At Least One Visit in Lifetime (Given a Diagnosis)
Gender		
Male	.382	.201
Female	.348	.254
Education		
Grammar school or less	.470	.110
Some high school	.389	.202
High school graduate	.314	.246
Some college	.311	.351
College graduate	.289	.432
Marital status		
Married	.314	.209
Widowed	.362	.101
Separated or divorced	.491	.347
Never married	.375	.273
Race		
White	.329	.274
Nonwhite	.426	.165
Income (in dollars)		
< 10,000	.411	.205
10,000–14,999	.350	.230
15,000–19,999	.331	.250
20,000–24,999	.327	.309
25,000–34,999	.313	.297
> 35,000	.285	.371
Age (in years)		
18–20	.309	.246
21–30	.390	.263
31–40	.398	.367
41–50	.377	.335
51–60	.361	.238
61+	.330	.096

Data from the Epidemiologic Catchment Area survey from 1980 to 1984

SOURCE: *Mental Health, United States, 1994* (DHHS Pub. No. SMA 94-3000), edited by R. W. Manderscheid & M. A. Sonnenschein, Washington, DC: U.S. Government Printing Office.

FIGURE 12–3 Lifetime probability of making a mental health visit given the presence of a diagnosis

patient care staff (from 100,886 to 273,374) (U.S. Public Health Service, 1980). This increase can be attributed in large part to the increase in the number of mental health organizations during this same period. The number of FTE administrative, clerical, and maintenance staff, however, increased by a relatively small amount over the same period, dropping from 36% to 26% of all FTE staff.

Staff patterns varied among the different mental health organizations, due to such factors as differences in types of service programs offered, caseload mix, budgetary factors, and differentials in the supply and accessibility of specific types of staff. For example, in 1986, 35% of the FTE staff in state mental hospitals were classified as "other mental health workers" (holding less than a B.A. degree); by contrast, in other mental health organizations, the proportion of FTE staff in this category ranged downward, from 22% in RTCs to 2% for freestanding psychiatric outpatient clinics. Conversely, state mental hospitals had the smallest percentage of FTE professional patient care staff (30%) (Redick, et al., 1991).

The role and influence of the general medical sector is growing, and approximately 116,642 primary care physicians report that they provide mental health services (Lair & Lefkowitz, 1990). They further report spending 23% of their workweek doing so. Overall, primary care physicians, psychiatrists, social workers, and psychologists provided 53%, 19%, 15%, and 13% of all mental health services, respectively (Knesper & Pagnucco, 1987). This invites further exploration as to the nature and degree of services provided and the preparation for doing so.

The traditional providers of mental health services in the specialty mental health sector, however, continue to be psychiatrists, psychologists, psychiatric nurses, and social workers. The scope of practice amongst the various professionals has changed substantially over the years as social workers and

nurses, in particular, have taken over clinical areas of practice previously claimed by psychiatry. Psychiatry has shifted more toward practice that encompasses the underlying medical issues within mental health practice.

Psychiatrists

Psychiatry is the medical specialty dealing with mental disorders. Traditional psychiatry offers medical/clinical definitions of mental illness. Social psychiatry, in contrast, is concerned with the environmental and societal phenomena involved in mental and emotional disorders and the use of social forces in the treatment of such disorders. Much of the scientific work of social psychiatry has been in the area of epidemiology, particularly estimation of the incidence and prevalence of mental illness in community and hospital settings. Growing concern for the environment in large mental hospitals during and after World War II also added impetus to the social psychiatric movement, and as early as 1946, the American Psychiatric Association adopted a rigid set of standards for mental hospitals and appointed a Central Inspection Board for enforcement of these standards. Social psychiatry, in an effort to transform these large institutions from custodial care to treatment centers, developed the concept of the therapeutic community, the fundamental tenet of which is that patients can assist in their own rehabilitation as well as in the rehabilitation of other patients. Social psychiatry also includes transcultural and community psychiatry. Transcultural psychiatry studies the incidence and prevalence of mental disease across societies and delineates the social forces that affect the manifestations of these illnesses. Community psychiatry has been described as "social psychiatry in action" (Lipton, et al., 1983) and is involved in the development, planning, and organization of community mental health programs and consultation to local agencies.

The number of psychiatrists in the United States increased from approximately 7,000 in 1950 to more than 32,000 by 1985, including those working primarily in administration. By 1994, approximately 44,255 psychiatrists were reported in practice.

Psychologists

Psychology, which struggled to create its own professional identity in the early years of this century, has emphasized scientific research in academic settings. Beginning as a philosophy, psychology has become firmly established as a social science, and psychologists have promoted and conducted research on the functioning of the human mind, especially through development of scientifically validated testing instruments. Beginning in the early twentieth century, psychological testing began to be used in conjunction with psychiatric treatment. Research by psychologists in classic conditioning and behavior theory also aided psychiatrists, who still provided most therapeutic care.

During World War II, psychologists began to be seen in an increased role in clinical practice. With the expansion of mental health services in VA hospitals, the training of clinical psychologists began in earnest. In 1946 the Veterans Administration, in conjunction with the American Psychological Association, began the Veterans Administration Psychology Training Program, which is still a major source of training for clinical and counseling psychologists. The professional application of psychology received further endorsement at the American Psychological Association Vail Conference of 1973, which emphasized the continued training of clinicians and scientists in psychology. Psychologists are licensed or certified in all states and the District of Columbia. In almost all states, the training required for licensure is a doctoral degree, although a few states allow limited licensure for graduates of master's degree programs; however, independent private practice is prohibited. Licensure is not required for practice in some settings, however, and unlicensed psychologists most often practice in school or community mental health facilities.

The American Psychological Association reported a 1986 membership of 63,000. A more recent study reports 56,000 working in the specialty mental health sector specifically (Lair & Lefkowitz, 1990). There are likely more than 70,000 master- and doctorate-level psychologists if nonlicensed psychologists are included (President's Commission, 1978). The pool of clinically trained women psychologists, for the most part, tends to be younger and more diverse in terms of racial and ethnic minority representation. In fact, participation by women in psychology has increased in many ways. Within the practice-oriented subfields, women account for 57% of all new 1989 PhDs, compared to 21% in 1965. By the early 1990s, 62% of all full-time students in doctoral clinical, counseling, and school psychology programs were women.

Psychiatric Nurses

The professional training of nurses in this country began in the 1860s and consisted primarily of apprenticeships. The first training program that prepared nurses to care for the mentally ill was started in 1882 at McLean Hospital, a private psychiatric facility in Waverly, Massachusetts. Although there was a growing appreciation of nurses who received this type of training, poorly funded psychiatric hospitals continued to employ lesser-trained aides at very low pay. Whatever nursing care did exist in these hospitals consisted mainly of custodial care focusing on the physical needs of the patient, and the nurse continued to practice in a dependent relationship with a physician. The development in the 1930s of somatic treatments for mental illness, such as insulin shock therapy, psychosurgery, and electroshock therapy, required the services of highly skilled nurses and established a more significant role for nurses in psychiatric treatment. The advent of the therapeutic community in psychiatric hospitals broadened the role of the nurse even further. As the twenty-four-hour care necessary for developing and maintaining the therapeutic milieu was recognized, the nurse became a valuable member of the therapeutic team. The involvement of nurses in group psychotherapy after World War II resulted in federal appropriations for training nurses. Despite the recognition of psychiatric nursing as a legitimate nursing role, however, the exact function of the nurse in mental health care remained only vaguely delineated.

Nursing education has become much more academically based over the past thirty years as the need for college-level training programs and nursing research was recognized. Graduates of nursing schools obtained an increasingly strong professional and academic education, often training side by side with psychiatrists, psychologists, and social workers. Nurses who earned advanced degrees were often recruited for teaching, however, and the two-year associate degree and diploma nurses were more prevalent in clinical practice. As nurses began to move into the role of psychotherapists, partially in response to the shortage of psychiatrists in most hospitals, interprofessional conflicts developed. But the exploding demand for therapists further legitimated the nurse's role in therapy, and by the late 1960s, the clinical specialty of psychiatric nursing was firmly established. The first organization to certify clinical specialists in psychiatric nursing, in 1972, was the New Jersey State Nurses Association.

Nursing education includes training in psychiatric nursing at all academic levels. The associate degree nurse with two years of training in an academic program and the diploma nurse trained in a hospital program most often provide clinical services. Baccalaureate- and master-level nurses often work in supervisory positions or in teaching, and doctorate-level nurses usually teach rather than provide clinical services. In 1984, approximately 10,034 master's-prepared psychiatric nurses were working in nursing positions (Bittker, 1985), although one study suggests only 3,000 nurses are working in the specialty mental health sector (Knesper & Pagnucco, 1987). A declining number of nurses are entering psychiatric nursing relative to other specialties such as pediatrics and medical surgical nursing. Ninety-six percent of master's-prepared psychiatric nurses are female. As with all mental health professions, psychiatric nursing reflects serious underrepresentation of minorities in its membership. Approximately 96% of all female master's-prepared psychiatric nurses are white; only about 2% each are black and Hispanic, and less than 1% are Asian, Pacific Islander, or Native American.

Social Workers

The history of social work dates back to the late nineteenth century and the volunteer mothers who provided disadvantaged persons with charitable aid through the Charity Organization Societies. Social work began to develop as a profession during the early twentieth century. Reform-minded women struggling for equality became social workers and began working in medical and psychiatric settings, schools, and correctional institutions. The development of social psychiatry also prompted the formation of a professional identity for social workers. Adopting the Freudian psychoanalytic model of many psychiatrists, social workers struggled for increased responsibility in the treatment of mental and emotional disorders.

The practice of psychotherapy expanded the social worker's domain from providing charitable assistance to the poor to providing a therapy that was viewed as legitimate by the middle and upper classes. Since psychoanalysis and psychotherapy remained medical specialties, social workers were less successful in developing a separate professional identity, and their practice continued in the shadow of psychiatry.

Training includes two-year associate degree programs graduating human service workers, baccalaureate programs in social work currently recognized as the beginning professional level, master's-level degrees in social work, and doctoral programs. In addition to the basic training of the discipline, social work education offers specialized training in mental health and in human services administration. The National Association of Social Workers lists about 129,092 members (Bittker, 1985). Of this total, 81,737 are master- or doctoral-level social workers. Eighty-one percent are in full-time practice, and 45,000 are reported to be active within the specialty mental health sector (Lair & Lefkowitz, 1990). Social workers are predominantly female (72%). Social workers are found in the public sector, including health and mental health services, public welfare, and child welfare, and in the private sector, including employee assistance programs and private practice.

Other Mental Health Personnel Concerns

Professionals with expertise in mental health concerns are practicing an increasingly wide range of disciplines. Schools of education are training counseling and guidance personnel as well as special education teachers who work in schools and other settings. The special needs of people recovering from mental and emotional disabilities have been recognized by such professional groups as occupational and recreational therapists and vocational counselors. Practitioners in marriage and family counseling, in art, music, and dance therapy, and in religion provide counseling and therapy in many mental health settings, as do professionals

receiving master of arts (MA) degrees in behavioral sciences with an emphasis on counseling skills.

Training for allied professionals varies tremendously. These personnel serve as mental health workers, alcohol and drug abuse counselors, day care workers, board and home care providers, foster parents, patient advocates, and hospital psychiatric aides. In some mental health centers, half of the positions are filled by these individuals. Community volunteers are another important component of the mental health work force. Thousands of people offer their time and services, performing tasks ranging from assisting with clerical needs to working directly with patients.

Indigenous healers are rarely recognized by traditional mental health service providers. The significance of their role is often poorly understood, underestimated, disparaged, or simply unknown to conventional providers. Depending on the specific culture, healers may be assigned various labels in the literature, for example, indigenous, traditional, or ritual healer; spirit doctor; medicine man/woman; or shaman. These indigenous or traditional healers are distinct from informal caregivers or natural helpers who are found in diverse cultural groups and/or settings. Such individuals may include elders in a community, "natural" leaders, community volunteers, or other individuals who are recognized for particular gifts of helpful caring and compassion.

The extent to which traditional healers and natural helpers may be involved in the care of mentally ill patients varies greatly. Patients and their families may utilize both conventional, mainstream mental health services and traditional healing without the awareness of mainstream providers due to fears that the patients will "offend" their mainstream provider or will lose the services of their mainstream provider. Providers may be completely unaware of the traditional health beliefs and practices of culturally diverse patients or, if they are aware, lack the understanding and skills to integrate the patient's beliefs into their treatment plans. A survey of Canadian family physicians inquiring about the degree to which they supported First Nation patients' utilization of Native healing practices and medicines revealed that while the notion of utilization was broadly accepted, they had limited understanding of how to integrate these practices with their own. Furthermore, the more serious the illness as perceived by the physician, the less likely the physician was to support using other treatment approaches (Zubeck, 1994). There is growing recognition that patients utilize multiple healing approaches along with the conventional, mainstream health system formally available to them. The challenge for integration, much less acceptance, is complex and involves overcoming language barriers, gaining cultural knowledge and information, acquiring skills to broker systems of beliefs between provider and patient, balancing patient safety and well-being, and considering medical, legal, and financial responsibilities.

FINANCING MENTAL HEALTH CARE

Mental health services have historically been financed through the public sector, first by states and their support of state and county mental hospitals and, later, by the federal government with the advent of Medicaid, Medicare, and other federally sponsored mental health programs such as the community mental health centers. Psychiatric insurance under other forms of insurance has traditionally been inconsistent and less comprehensive than coverage for general medical conditions. Coverage for mental illness has been characterized by limitations in the form of caps on total coverage available and higher coinsurance and deductibles. Since the 1970s, however, major United States employers have become increasingly aware of the

need to give greater priority to emotional problems (Goldbeck, 1983). The image of the American worker as being able to cope with any problem drowned in a sea of reports on growing rates of alcoholism, drug abuse, and legal, marital, and financial problems (Howard, et al., 1996). Mental health benefits became more explicitly defined, and benefits were designed and structured in employee assistance programs (EAPs), emphasizing early intervention, particularly when such intervention was viewed as cost-effective. Employee assistance programs, originally focused on alcohol treatment, expanded in scope. Corporate mental health programs began employing staff psychiatrists, psychologists, and social workers. Simultaneously, insurance plans, in general, began to focus more on prevention and early intervention as a means of reducing absenteeism, increasing worker productivity, and managing costs.

Total per capita expenditures for mental health services increased from $3.3 billion in 1969 to $28.4 billion in 1990. If adjustments are made for inflation, however, the total only rose from $3.3 billion to $5.6 billion, an actual increase of $2.3 billion in purchasing power. When measured in constant dollars, state mental hospitals, VA medical centers, and freestanding psychiatric outpatient clinics actually lost purchasing power during this period, although expenditures, measured in current dollars, increased. Private psychiatric hospitals, separate psychiatric services of nonfederal general hospitals, and "all other organizations" showed gains in purchasing power, comprising 22%, 16%, and 20%, respectively, in 1990 compared to 7%, 9%, and 6% in 1969 as depicted in Figure 12–4.

In the 1950s, state psychiatric hospitals accounted for 80% to 90% of expenditures for mental illness care. By the 1970s and 1980s, the introduction of Medicare and Medicaid, coupled with changing federal policy vis-à-vis the community mental health care system, broadened the

Rate per capita civilian population in constant dollars

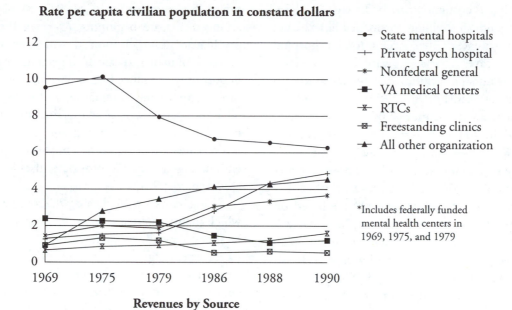

- State mental hospitals
- Private psych hospital
- Nonfederal general
- VA medical centers
- RTCs
- Freestanding clinics
- All other organization

*Includes federally funded mental health centers in 1969, 1975, and 1979

Revenues by Source

SOURCE: *Mental Health, United States, 1994* (DHHS Pub. No. SMA 94-3000), edited by R. W. Manderscheid & M. A. Sonnenschein, Washington, DC: U.S. Government Printing Office.

Figure 12–4 Rate of constant (1969=100) dollar expenditures per capita by type of mental health organization, United States: Selected years, 1969–1990

funding base. Medicare and Medicaid, however, paralleled the principles and coverage typical of health insurance and covered only acute psychiatric inpatient care in general hospitals in the same manner as medical conditions, limiting care in public or private psychiatric hospitals. Outpatient coverage was severely restricted. The greater availability of inpatient coverage skewed the growth of mental health services such that general hospital psychiatric services increased during the period 1960–1980, leaving the financing of state mental hospital systems to state governments. Congress felt that states should continue their responsibility for care of the chronically mentally ill and not shift this cost to the federal government.

In the 1980s, federal dollars accounted for 19% of expenditures for both office-based care and other organized mental health settings as compared to 29% in the general health sector. The reductions in federal support have been absorbed by state and local government, which funded 33% of the total, about three times the corresponding percentage in the health sector. Private insurance and direct patient payments accounted for 52% of mental health expenditures. The federal share of the mental health bill was divided primarily between Medicare and Medicaid. Medicaid payments were more than triple those made through Medicare. In 1986, estimated Medicare mental illness payments were $1.7 billion; about 63% of this total was paid to general hospitals and 19% to psychiatric hospitals, for a total of 82% in hospital inpatient settings. In 1983, Medicaid paid $3.4 billion for mental illness care, with approximately 30% going toward hospital inpatient care, 51% toward intermediate care/skilled nursing facilities, and the remainder to outpatient services (Bittker, 1985).

As America entered the 1990s, health care costs continued to spiral, and the federal government responded by legislating an end to the cost-reimbursement system for Medicare providers predominant in the 1960s and 1970s. Rather, the federal payment for health care became based on payer-determined prices. Psychiatry, however, was excluded from the capitated reimbursement plan under Medicare diagnosis-related groups (DRGs), introduced gradually beginning in 1983. Hospitals defined as rehabilitation, long-term, pediatric, or psychiatric continued to be paid under a cost-based reimbursement system with limits on rate of growth. The exemptions were based on uncertainty about how well a DRG-based payment system would work for specialized facilities and units. Another initiative to contain national health care costs was the resource-based relative value scale (RBRVS) Medicare fee schedule, phased in over a five-year period beginning in 1992, although it had limited impact on psychiatric practice.

As health care costs continued to rise dramatically in the 1990s, outpacing the rate of inflation, employers and insurers found evidence that mental health/substance abuse costs were actually rising faster than were medical surgical costs. Some employers reported 25% or more of their total health care claim dollars were spent toward payment of their mental health/substance abuse claims, which accounted for only 7% of total claims made (Theis, 1994; Winegar & Bistline, 1994). The cost per employee rose from $163 in 1987 to $318 in 1992 (Redick, et al., 1991). By the early 1990s, reports estimated that as much as 40% of all psychiatric hospitalization was inappropriate (Strumwasser, et al., 1991). Managed care arrangements are beginning to bring the rate of psychiatric hospitalization down. One potential outcome of managed care arrangements may be the opportunity to reduce overall medical care costs by more appropriately integrating and utilizing mental health services. A growing literature is beginning to report that appropriate use of mental health care can reduce other medical expenses by eliminating some inappropriate use of services (Mechanic, 1995).

Rising costs of Medicaid, the program upon which many Americans with the most severe mental illness depend, coupled with increases in private sector spending under a typical fee-for-service structured mental health benefit package led to a concerted effort to seek more effective means for managing mental health care. This set the stage for integrating mental health benefits into the growing managed care movement.

MANAGED MENTAL HEALTH CARE

Prepaid health plans such as health maintenance organizations (HMOs), utilization review organizations (UROs), and comprehensive case management all began to emerge as organizational types in response to reducing costs and improving the integration of the differing parts of the health care system. Insurers and employers have also collaborated with fee-for-service practitioners and hospitals to create preferred provider organizations (PPOs) and exclusive provider organizations (EPOs) intended to offer care at a discounted rate. These types of comprehensive prospective payment systems have begun to play an important role in the delivery of psychiatric services, often termed behavioral health care within these new arrangements.

By 1994, half of the membership of the National Association of Psychiatric Health Systems (representing private sector psychiatric systems) utilized some form of capitated payment, and 20% reported risk-sharing arrangements (Covall, 1995). Within the public sector, at least thirty-five states have implemented some form of capitated payment system for Medicaid clients with severe mental illness, and the Health Care Financing Administration (HCFA), which oversees the Medicaid program, has awarded more than seventeen waivers allowing states to change the types of services provided, the method of delivery, and the population to be served (Shera, 1996).

Implemented on a state-by-state basis, Medicaid managed care strategies vary. For example, some states have integrated people with severe mental health problems into the total population under management while others have elected to use a managed care carve-out, a special financing arrangement where persons needing mental health services are targeted separately from those in the general health service system. Others have devised their own systems or utilized reinsurance mechanisms to minimize the financial risk of provider organizations (Durham, 1994).

Psychiatric practice in HMOs, concurrently the most common model of prospective payment, has been shown to be cost-effective, and differing models of mental health service delivery have emerged. Psychiatric services, or behavioral health care services, are often included in other alternative provider organizations, although often with modest coinsurance payments and strict limits on the duration of services.

Improved integration between medical care and psychiatric services or behavioral health care is growing in importance for several reasons. Possibilities for costs offsets, created by new models incorporating medical and psychiatric care, provide an impetus, as does the growing role of medical providers and the general health sector in mental health service utilization. Mental health problems may present initially as somatic complaints. Reasons for somatization may include: (1) culturally held perceptions that less stigma is attached to a medical encounter as compared to a mental health encounter, (2) culturally shaped expressions of emotional or psychological distress that are reflected in body/physical sensations, and (3) the legitimization of the medical visit over the mental health visit where the medical encounter is financially covered.

Improved integration also increases the likelihood of identifying and effectively treating comorbidities between physical and mental disorders. Effective integration, however, requires a broad spectrum of service choice and flexible financing mechanisms in order to meet the needs of people with both mild and severe mental illness. HMOs have shown the ability to manage mental health care with significant cost savings, but enrolled populations traditionally have not included those with the most severe mental illness (Mechanic, 1994). It remains to be seen how effectively and efficiently people with severe mental illness will fare under such arrangements.

Integrating persons with severe mental illness into managed financing and care schemes is a daunting task. The chronicity of the condition and the likelihood that its severity will affect individual ability to seek and appropriately utilize care are significant challenges within a system that emphasizes outpatient treatment and aims for short-term recovery. These conditions are exacerbated by high rates of poverty and dependence among this population. Durham (1994) cautions that within managed care systems that view capitation financing mechanisms as a "quick fix" for out-of-control budgets, persons with severe mental illness are at risk for inappropriate, perhaps naive, approaches to care. The emphasis, rather than financing, should be on informed and well-supported clinical providers, flexible service networks, clinical guidelines and outcome measurements specifically addressing the care needs of persons with severe mental illness, and financial incentives that do not put physicians at odds with pursuing care that is in the best interest of the patient (Durham, 1994).

As the management of care more closely links mental health and the larger health services system, concerns for patient care and treatment are raised. Confidentiality, considered an essential component of the therapeutic process, may be compromised as computer-based patient record systems become more widespread and access to records becomes expanded (Parsi, et al., 1995). The contractual relationship between managed care organizations and their enrollees has been called into question. Psychiatrists and other providers express concern that clinical goals and concern for the patient will become subsumed by organizational concerns and cost-reduction goals, promoting reduced utilization of care in situations where such reductions are not warranted, and may produce ill-intended consequences. These concerns have become heightened with the rapid expansion of for-profit managed care systems and the emphasis on shareholder return.

Courts have ruled, however, that cost-containment methods that adversely impact a physician's medical judgment and result in injury to a patient may result in liability (*Wickline v. State*, 1986). Breach of contract (*Williams v. HealthAmerica*, 1987), breach of warranty (*Boyd v. Albert Einstein Medical Center*, 1988), and fraud have all been successfully litigated (Chittenden, 1991; Hall, 1994; Manderscheid & Sonnenschein, 1990).

Recent research has shown that outcomes of care can be improved through effective system and service integration, however. Von Korff and Simon (1996), reporting on a study of 25,916 enrolled members of a large, nonprofit HMO, found significant improvement in patients with major and minor depression when provided a redesigned,

more structured intervention and follow-up program, although initial costs of care were reported to be higher (Theis, 1994). They hypothesize that nonprofit HMOs are particularly suited for improving the management and outcome of patients with mental illness because of their public domain research capabilities, in addition to their experience in organizing and managing integrated care. Wagner and colleagues (Wagner, et al., 1996) suggest the following guidelines, based on experiences in developing and implementing clinical guidelines for common psychological disorders: a need for structured treatment programs; provider training programs; automated case registries; restructured primary-specialty care relationships; new assessment and care technologies; and care incentives that reward optimal long-term outcomes and proactive follow-up (Goldbeck, 1983).

SUMMARY

The mental health system is working vigorously to catch up with current knowledge and philosophy, but its efforts are warped by a confusing mixture of economic and political constraints. Previous philosophy that heralded the ability of all people to live in the community has not been realized. Many people who need mental health services and have no financial or social resources find only limited, or possibly no, services. Mental health services for those who do have resources have expanded and changed considerably, leaving even greater evidence of a two-tiered system of care. Despite the many problems that remain in the system, mental health professionals, citizen advocates, and consumers continue to labor toward greater access to financial resources, more and improved services, and less stigma for mental illness. Custodial treatment still exists, but we are learning how to use all of our treatment resources better. Many people do go unserved or inappropriately treated, but the problems of the mentally ill continue to receive attention and concern. In short, the mental health system continues to gain credence and legitimacy as a significant and important part of health care.

REFERENCES

American Association on Mental Retardation. (1992). *Mental retardation: Definition, classifications, and systems of support* (special 9th ed.).

Applebaum, P. (1983). Refusing treatment—The uncertainty continues. *Hospital and Community Psychiatry, 34,* 11–12.

Bender, K. J. (1996, September). Study finds higher antipsychotic dosages given to Blacks. *Psychiatric Times,* 3–4.

Bittker, T. (1985). The industrialization of American psychiatry. *American Journal of Psychiatry, 142,* 149–154.

Chittenden, W. A. (1991). Malpractice liability and managed health care: History and prognosis. *Tort and Insurance Law Journal, 26,* 451–496.

Covall, M. (1995). Fine-tuning psychiatric health care. *Health Systems Review, 29*(4), 30–34.

Durham, M. (1994). Healthcare's greatest challenge: Providing services for people with severe mental illness in managed care. *Behavioral Sciences and the Law, 12,* 331–349.

Eth, S. (1990, April). Psychiatric ethics: Entering the 1990s. *Hospital and Community Psychiatry, 41*(4), 384–386.

Geller, J. L., Fisher, W. H., Wirth-Cauchon, J. L., & Simon, L. J. (1990, August). Second-generation deinstitutionalization, 1: The impact of Brewster vs. Dukakis on state hospital casemix. *American Journal of Psychiatry, 147*(8), 982–987.

Goldbeck, W. (1983). Psychiatry and industry: A business view. *Psychiatry Hospital, 13,* 11–14.

Goldman, H., Adams, N., & Taube, C. (1983). Deinstitutionalization: The data demythologized. *Hospital and Community Psychiatry, 34,* 129–134.

Gong-Guy, E., Cravens, R. B., & Patterson, T. E. (1991, June). Clinical issues in mental health service delivery to refugees. *American Psychologist,* 642–648.

Gottheil, D., Winkelmayer, R., Smoyer, P., & Exine, R. (1991, July). Characteristics of patients who are resistant to deinstitutionalization. *Hospital and Community Psychiatry, 42*(7), 745–748.

Hall, R. C. W. (1994). Legal precedents affecting managed care: The physician's responsibilities to patients. *Psychosomatics, 35,* 105–117.

Holcomb, W. R., & Ahr, P. R. (1987). Who really treats the severely impaired young adult patient? A comparison of treatment settings. *Hospital and Community Psychiatry, 38,* 625–631.

Howard, K. I., Cornille, T. A., Lyons, J. S., Vessey, J. T., Lueger, R. J., & Saunders, S. M. (1996, August). Patterns of mental health service utilization. *Archives of General Psychiatry, 53*(8), 696–703.

Interagency Council on the Homeless. (1991). *The 1990 annual report of the Interagency Council on the Homeless.* Washington, DC: Author.

Klebe, E. R. (1991, April 12). *Homeless mentally ill persons: Problems and programs.* CRS Report for Congress (Pub. No. 91-344). Washington, DC: Library of Congress.

Kleinman, A. (1988). *Rethinking psychiatry: From cultural category to personal experience.* New York: Free Press.

Kleinman, A., & Good, B. (1985). *Culture and depression.* Berkeley, CA: University of California Press.

Knesper, D. J., & Pagnucco, D. J. (1987). Estimated distribution of effort by providers of mental health services to U.S. adults in 1982 and 1983. *American Journal of Psychiatry, 144,* 883–888.

Koyanagi, C., & Goldman, H. H. (1991). The quiet success of the national plan for the chronically mentally ill. *Hospital and Community Psychiatry, 42*(9), 899–905.

Lair, T., & Lefkowitz, D. (1990, September). Mental health and functional states of residents of nursing and personal care homes. In *Agency for health care policy and research. National Medical Expenditure Survey research findings 7* (DHHS Pub. No. 1990-3470). Washington, DC: U.S. Government Printing Office.

Lamb, H. R. (1990, May). Will we save the homeless mentally ill? *American Journal of Psychiatry, 147*(5), 649–651.

Lamb, H., & Mills, M. (1986). Needed changes in law and procedure for the chronically mentally ill. *Hospital and Community Psychiatry, 37,* 475–480.

Levine, M. (1981). *The history and politics of community mental health.* Oxford: Oxford University Press.

Lipton, F., Sabatini, A., & Katz, S. (1983). Down and out in the city—The homeless mentally ill. *Hospital and Community Psychiatry, 43,* 817–821.

Manderscheid, R. W., & Sonnenschein, M. A. (Eds.). (1990). *Mental health, United States, 1990* (DHHS Pub. No. ADMI 90-1708). Washington, DC: U.S. Government Printing Office.

Maser, J. D., & Dinges, N. (1992). Comorbidity: Meaning and uses in cross-cultural clinical research. *Culture, Medicine, and Psychiatry, 16,* 409–425.

Mechanic, D. (1994). Integrating mental health into a general health care system. *Hospital and Community Psychiatry, 45*(9), 893–897.

Mechanic, D. (1995). Management of mental health and substance abuse services: State of the art and early results. *The Milbank Quarterly, 73*(1), 19–55.

Narrow, W. E., Regier, D. A., Rae, D. S., Mandersheid, R. W., & Locke, B. Z. (1993, February). Use of services by persons with mental and addictive disorders. *Archives of General Psychiatry, 50*(2), 95–107.

Parsi, K. P., Wislade, J. D., & Corcoran, J. D. (1995). Does confidentiality have a future? The computer based patient record and managed mental health care. *Trends in Health Care Law, 10*(½), 78–82.

President's Commission on Mental Health. (1978). *Final report Vol. II, Task panel reports.* Washington, DC: U.S. Government Printing Office.

Redick, R. W., Witkin, M. J., Atay, J. E., & Manderscheid, R. W. (1991, April). *Staffing of mental health organizations, United States, 1986 (Mental Health Statistical Note No. 196).* Washington, DC: U.S. Department of Health and Human Services, U.S. NIM.

Redick, R. W., Witkin, M. J., Atay, J. E., & Manderscheid, R. W. (1994). Highlights of organized mental health services in 1990 and major national and state trends. *Mental Health* (U.S. NIM Rep. No. 77-99).

Regier, D., Myers, J., Kramer, M., et al. (1984). The NIMH epidemiological catchment area (ECA) program: Historical context, major objectives and study population characteristics. *Archives of General Psychiatry, 41,* 934–941.

Regier, D. A., Narrow, W. E., Rae, D. S. Manderscheid, R. W., Locke, B. Z., & Goodwin, F. K. (1993,

February). The de facto US mental and addictive disorders service system. *Archives of General Psychiatry, 40*(2), 85–94.

Reivil, S.R., et al., No. 84-C-383-S (W.D. Wis., Jan. 10, 1985).

Robins, L. N., Locke, B. Z., & Regier, D. A. (1991). An overview of psychiatric disorders in America. *Psychiatric Disorders in America.* New York: Free Press.

Rumer, R. (1978). Community mental health centers: Politics and therapy. *Journal of Health Politics, Policy and Law, 3,* 531–558.

Shera, W. (1996). Managed care and people with severe mental illness: Challenges and opportunities for social work. *Health and Social Work, 21*(3), 196–201.

Strakowski, S. M., & Lonczak, H. S., et al. (1995, March). The effects of race on diagnosis and disposition from a psychiatric emergency service. *Journal of Clinical Psychiatry, 56*(3), 101–107.

Strumwasser, I., Paranjpe, N. V., Udow, et al. (1991). Appropriateness of psychiatric and substance abuse hospitalization. *Medical Care, 29*(Suppl.), AS77–AS90.

Sue, D. W., & Sue, D. (1990). *Counseling the culturally different* (2nd ed.). New York: Wiley.

Theis, G. A. (1994). Considerations under capitated behavioral health care services. *Medical Interface, 7*(10), 123–129.

U.S. Public Health Service, U.S. Department of Health and Human Services Steering Committee on the Chronically Mentally Ill. (1980). *Toward a national plan for the chronically mentally ill.* Washington, DC: Author.

Von Korff, M., & Simon, G. (1996). *Mental illness in the general medical sector: Prevalence, burden, utilization, management and outcomes.*

Wagner, E. H., Austin, B. T., & Von Korff, M. (1996). Improving outcomes in chronic illness. *Managed Care Quarterly, 4,* 12–25.

Weiner, D. B. (1979). The apprenticeship of Philippe Pinel: A new document, "Observations of Citizen Pussin on the Insane." *Psychiatry, 736,* 1128–1134.

Westermeyer, J. (1985, July). Psychiatric diagnosis across cultural boundaries. *American Journal of Psychiatry, 142*(7), 790–805.

Winegar, N., & Bistline, J. L. (1994). *Marketing mental health services to managed care* (pp. 14–15). New York: Haworth.

Zubeck, M. (1994, November). Traditional native healing. *Canadian Family Physician, 40.*

PART V

NONFINANCIAL RESOURCES FOR HEALTH CARE

CHAPTER

The Role of Pharmaceuticals in the Health Care System*

Stuart O. Schweitzer

William S. Comanor

CHAPTER TOPICS

The Structure of the Pharmaceutical Industry
Market Conduct
Government Regulation
Industry Performance
Public Policy Questions

* The contents of this chapter are based on two previous publications by the authors: (1) "Pharmaceuticals," by W. S. Comanor & S. O. Schweitzer, in *The Structure of American Industry* (9th ed.), edited by W. Adams & J. Brock, 1995, Englewood Cliffs, NJ: Prentice Hall; and (2) *Pharmaceutical Economics and Policy,* by S. O. Schweitzer, 1997, New York: Oxford University Press.

LEARNING OBJECTIVES

Upon completing this chapter, the reader should be able to:

- Understand the structure and operation of the pharmaceutical industry.
- Appreciate the scope and importance of pharmaceuticals in health care.
- Understand many economic issues of this industry.
- Comprehend the complex public policy issues and concerns involving this industry.

The American pharmaceutical industry is the envy of the world. It leads in the development of new technology and for decades has achieved a rapid pace of innovation. It pays high wages to its employees and offers advanced products to its customers, not only in the United States but throughout the world.

Nevertheless, the industry has been subject to continual criticism from American political leaders. For decades politicians from both parties have asserted that its products are overpriced and its profits are excessive. The arguments reached a high point forty years ago in lengthy hearings before the Senate Subcommittee on Antitrust and Monopoly during the 1950s and early 1960s. And in 1993, Senators David Pryor (Arkansas) and William Cohen (Maine), Democratic chair and ranking Republican member of the Senate Committee on Aging, respectively, wrote: "This pattern of excessive inflation by drug manufacturers has made it extremely difficult for millions of Americans to afford life-saving medications. . . . [And it is time therefore] for pharmaceutical cost containment" (U.S. Senate, 1993).

Why should such a successful industry be subject to such attack? Are these senators merely responding to political pressures and failing to acknowledge other industry dimensions in which its performance is exemplary? Are pharmaceutical prices truly high and increasing, and if they are, is this the expected cost of a rapid pace of pharmaceutical innovation? Or does this industry function as a traditional monopolist with its performance claims merely overstated? Should we perhaps view the pharmaceutical industry's performance in a more negative light?

Although the debate has become better informed and more knowledgeable over the years, it still centers on how to characterize the performance of the industry and on what policy actions should be taken, if any, to improve its performance.

Though new laws were enacted in 1962 and again in 1984 to reform the regulatory process, controversy surrounding the pharmaceutical industry has not diminished. Evidently whatever problems existed have not been solved by past legislative efforts.

This chapter explores the economic and policy issues raised in the continuing debate. To do so, the structure of the pharmaceutical industry is studied. We consider how firms are organized, what functions are carried out by them, and how the various firms interact to comprise the larger industry. We note especially how multinational the industry is, with world-leading firms representing many countries. Next, typical patterns of firm conduct among both leading firms and smaller rivals are addressed. In particular, we explore how pharmaceutical prices are set and research priorities determined. Next we consider the ways that government regulates the industry, especially as it affects the introduction of new products. Lastly, we turn to the major policy issues that receive both government and public attention.

THE STRUCTURE OF THE PHARMACEUTICAL INDUSTRY

All firms in the United States economy are vertically integrated to some extent, meaning that they combine functions at various stages of the production or service process. Specific input that could be purchased is sometimes produced by the firms. Thus the firm's output could be limited to a single product but, in fact, is a series of intermediate products. The extent of integration within firms is a distinguishing characteristic of firms and industries.

In the pharmaceutical industry, the leading companies are engaged in three distinct activities that characterize this industry: manufacturing and production, research and development, and selling and promotion. In principle these could be carried out separately. Together they determine the products that are sold, the prices that are set, and the levels of output. They also determine the total costs of member firms.

Although production costs comprise a substantial proportion of total costs, they still account for less than half. As indicated in Table 13–1, they represent less than 30% of sales revenues for a sample of large, United States–based companies and less than 40% of total costs. The next largest category is advertising and promotion, although the actual amounts are not reported by most companies. The third is research and development outlays, which in the early 1990s were approximately 12% of revenues. This percentage allocation is nearly double that reported for earlier years.

The Manufacturing Function

In their manufacturing function, pharmaceutical firms engage in two fairly distinct activities. The first is similar to that carried out in other segments

TABLE 13–1 Revenue allocation (%) for leading pharmaceutical companies

	1958	*1966*	*1991*
Production costs	32.1	35.0	27.7
Research and development	6.3	6.5	12.1
General and administrative	10.9	35.0[a]	35.0[a]
Advertising and promotion	24.8	—	—
Income taxes	12.8	10.0	7.1
Net profits	13.0	13.5	16.0
Number of companies sampled	22	17	10

a   These figures include advertising and promotion as well as general administrative expense.

SOURCE: "Pharmaceuticals," by W. S. Comanor & S. O. Schweitzer, in *The Structure of American Industry* (9th ed.), edited by W. Adams & J. W. Brock, 1995, Englewood Cliffs, NJ: Prentice Hall.

of the broader chemical industry: the generation and production of basic chemicals that serve as the active and inert ingredients in their final products. In most cases, these substances are generated from basic materials by means of chemical reactions, although some products, such as antibiotics, are produced through biological processes.

In the second stage of the manufacturing process, the resulting chemicals are combined with other chemicals and with inert materials to make the final product. For the most part, this involves purifying and mixing the materials and then encapsulating the resulting substance. In many instances, the basic materials are purchased from others so that manufacturing activities are limited to the second-stage processes.

Research and Development

In sharp contrast with its manufacturing function, the research and development function of the pharmaceutical industry provides its special characteristic. Before World War II, this function was almost entirely absent. The leading firms of that time produced a limited number of well-known products that did not change much from year to year. These firms typically sold active drug ingredients through wholesalers to retail pharmacies. In many cases, pharmacists made their own pills, filled capsules, and prepared liquid suspensions and tinctures. Because the pharmacist's skill was critical to making the products, the brand name of the manufacturer of the ingredients was less important.

Then, at the end of the war, when industry leaders realized that their future depended on research and development, the pharmaceutical industry underwent a veritable revolution. Indeed, the introduction of the first antibiotics demonstrated that more effective drugs could be discovered that would generate high consumer demand. The pharmaceutical companies saw that new and improved products could be highly profitable, and so they began to invest large and increasing sums into creating them.

What occurred in these years was a major technological breakthrough that had important ramifications for the future of the industry. The advance was not in the development of a single product or in the manner by which pharmaceuticals are produced. Rather, it was an advance in the process by which new pharmaceuticals were discovered. As Peter Temin (1980) noted, the technological revolution that created the modern pharmaceutical industry "was a method of research rather than a method of production." The firms that grew and prospered were those that rapidly adopted the new technology.

In the years that followed, expenditures on research and development continued to increase. By the early 1990s, the member firms of the Pharmaceutical Manufacturers Association (PMA) spent $8.9 billion for research on and development of drugs designed for humans, of which 18% was

spent abroad and the rest in the United States (Pharmaceutical Manufacturers Association, 1991).

This research effort led to a vast array of new pharmaceuticals. Between 1946 and 1991, as reported in Table 13–2, the industry introduced

TABLE 13–2 New single-entity drug introductions to U.S. markets, 1946–1991

Year	Number of Entities	Year	Number of Entities
1946	19	1970	16
1947	26	1971	14
1948	29	1972	10
1949	38	1973	17
1950	32	1974	18
1951	38	1975	15
1952	40	1976	14
1953	53	1977	16
1954	42	1978	23
1955	36	1979	15
1956	48	1980	13
1957	52	1981	19
1958	47	1982	26
1959	65	1983	22
1960	50	1984	15
1961	45	1985	20
1962	24	1986	24
1963	16	1987	20
1964	17	1988	19
1965	25	1989	24
1966	13	1990	24
1967	25	1991	30[a]
1968	12		
1969	9	Total	1,215

a   This figure is the number of new entities approved by the FDA in 1991 rather than the number of actual introductions.

SOURCE: "Pharmaceuticals," by W. S. Comanor & S. O. Schweitzer, in *The Structure of American Industry* (9th ed.), edited by W. Adams & J. W. Brock, 1995, Englewood Cliffs, NJ: Prentice Hall.

over 1,200 new entities, or 27 per year on average. This figure, however, disguises some important differences. In the seventeen years between 1946 and 1962, before new regulatory requirements were imposed, 684 entities were introduced, which is more than half the total number introduced during the entire forty-five-year period. In the seventeen years after 1962, however, only 275 entities were introduced, which represents a decline of about 60%. A new regulatory regime, described later, had changed the ease with which new drugs could be developed and introduced. Still, the introduction of new products has remained a major feature of this industry, and the rate of drug development has even accelerated in more recent years.

Although research spending rose throughout the postwar era, the number of new products dropped from its early heights as the research costs per new product exploded. In the years before 1962, these costs are estimated to have been $6.5 million per product (Hutt, 1982), but they then jumped to between $65 million and $75 million per successful new product by the end of the decade. When capitalized to the date of the Food and Drug Administration's (FDA) approval, these costs ranged from $108 million to $124 million per new chemical entity (U.S. Congress, Office of Technology Assessment, 1993). And they have continued to rise. For new drugs first entering human testing in the 1970s, capitalized after-tax research and development costs were reported at between $140 million and $194 million per product. The development and introduction of new pharmaceuticals had become a very costly enterprise.

The industry's response, however, was not to withdraw from the research enterprise but to expand its efforts. The rapid pace of new product introduction has continued. New drugs are introduced to replace older ones, a process that has given the pharmaceutical industry very different characteristics than it would have had if products had changed very slowly or even remained the same from year to year. This pattern has determined the structure, behavior, and performance of the industry.

Advertising and Promotion

The marketing function is the third essential task performed by leading firms in the pharmaceutical industry. Since new products are introduced at a rapid pace and older ones are quickly discarded, physicians need information about them. Indeed, for physicians even a few years beyond training, many, if not most, of the leading products were introduced after they started to practice, so the pharmaceutical companies must have some means of telling them about the new drugs.

The leading pharmaceutical companies have long accepted this role and accordingly have spent large sums on it. In 1958, the principal companies spent approximately one-quarter of their total revenues on advertising and promotion, and they most likely spend similar proportions today. Of the 185,900 people employed by PMA-member firms in 1989, fully 55,500, or nearly 30%, were in marketing (Pharmaceutical Manufacturers Association, 1991).

Since pharmaceuticals are prescribed only by health professionals, the industry's products do not have a broad distribution but, rather, are directed specifically at medical personnel. These efforts traditionally have taken two forms: first, the companies recruit a class of specialized sales personnel, called detailmen and -women, who call on physicians individually to present the products offered by their firms; and second, the companies spend substantial sums on advertising in professional journals and through presentations at medical conferences.

To a large extent, these advertising and promotional efforts are directed toward new products. These expenditures, for both firms and therapeutic categories, typically are greatest in a product's early years but fall steadily after that (Comanor, 1986). Since physicians and other health professionals decide whether to use a new product in their practice soon after it has been introduced, the pharmaceutical companies have a strong incentive to promote their products heavily at that time. Subsequently, when physicians' prescribing patterns have become established, their marketing expenses often decline.

Although sales personnel usually emphasize new products, some older products also carry large detailing expenditures. For example, in 1971, Abbott Laboratories spent over $2 million detailing Erythromycin, which had been introduced in 1952 (Leffler, 1981). Such efforts suggest that pharmaceutical advertising and promotion are designed to gain physicians' loyalty as well as to provide information.

Most firms continue to push products still protected by patent, then their efforts fall sharply when that protection is removed. Branded advertising and promotion decrease by roughly 10% per year for the two years before the patent expires and then drop even more when the patent actually does expire: 20% with the entry of the first generic rival and another 40% when the number of generic rivals reaches five. Apparently these efforts are designed to expand the market for the product, and the original supplier no longer finds it profitable to do so when it must share the product with others (Caves, et al., 1991).

Whatever the impact of these expenditures, the accuracy of the information provided along with the advertising and promotion remains in dispute. Critics argue that a substantial share of the industry's advertising and promotion is misleading. One study found that most of the pharmaceutical advertising in medical journals did not meet the FDA's criteria for scientific quality and, moreover, did not have much educational value (Wilkes, et al., 1992).

In effect, the authors found that journal advertising did not give physicians full information about the characteristics and uses of new drugs.

Leffler (1992), however, disagreed with this view, arguing that the study overstated the purpose and function of advertising. He has "serious doubts whether the purpose of medical journal advertisements is to inform the reader about the details of the product rather than simply to announce the availability and/or remind the physician of the product's name." Also, he argued, "one would certainly hope that physicians are reasonably knowledgeable about pharmaceuticals, that they are reasonably skeptical about the self-serving claims of advertisers and that journal ads are not the main source of their information about the specific details of the drugs."

Organizational Characteristics

Just as the pharmaceutical industry has a variety of functions, it also consists of a variety of firms that together make up the industry. Although before World War II, there were several traditional drug manufacturers, the revolutionary changes that took place after the war changed this structure. It still includes many of these old-line firms, but a steady process of consolidation has joined many of them together. In addition, many of the major European companies have entered the United States market and established subsidiaries that have become important parts of the American industry. The latter include the American subsidiaries of Ciba-Geigy and Hoffman-LaRoche, which are major Swiss companies; Glaxo-Wellcome, a British company; and Beecham Laboratories, also British, which entered the United States market through a merger with SmithKline to form SmithKline Beecham.

One important factor leading to the consolidation process was the greatly increased cost of introducing a new product. A firm had to be big to support an extensive research establishment that could undertake many projects at the same time, so that the research successes and failures could balance out to reduce the firm's overall risk. For small firms and small laboratories, therefore, research can be exceedingly risky, but that risk is diminished substantially through diversification across a number of projects. A second factor was the desire to reduce the costs of marketing, leading firms to seek partners in order to "fill in" gaps in a firm's portfolio of products.

Not only have new pharmaceutical firms from abroad entered the industry, but an entirely new technology has given birth to still more new firms. During the latter part of the 1980s and into the 1990s, the number of biotechnology firms has increased rapidly. This new technology applies genetic engineering to pharmaceuticals, in which a gene from one organism is inserted into another and the result is made into a usable product. But the new technology refers not only to the production of individual products but substantially to the process by which new products are discovered. In effect, this type of technological change is analogous to what occurred in the 1950s, in that it deals with the research rather than only manufacturing.

Regardless of their novel means of discovery and manufacturing, the pharmaceuticals discovered and produced in this manner still must compete with those developed and produced using more conventional methods; the products are sold in the same markets.

During the latter part of the 1980s and early 1990s, an area of pharmaceutical growth occurred. Many small generic pharmaceutical manufacturers entered the industry. Regulatory barriers to approval of generic drugs were greatly removed in 1984, and generic producers have poured into the industry. Unlike the leading manufacturers, these firms do little or no research and have only minimal marketing expenditures. Rather, they rely on

the research and marketing efforts of others, with their own activities generally limited to manufacturing. But for many of these firms, even this is abbreviated. Instead, their activities are limited to the second stage, encapsulating the basic chemicals or otherwise producing the final products. Such firms often buy the basic chemicals from large pharmaceutical companies or other fine-chemical manufacturers. Usually, however, they produce products that meet the standards set by the FDA and do so at a cost that is not much higher than that of the major companies.

The presence of generic drugs in the marketplace has expanded quickly in recent years. In 1980, before the new legislation, they accounted for only a small share of pharmaceutical sales in the United States, but by 1992, that share had risen to approximately 37%, based on industry data. It includes generic prescriptions for single-source drugs and is not limited to those sold by generic manufacturers.

Throughout the 1980s, this process of consolidation continued, as did the entry of foreign and United States firms. For the most part, these trends have offset each other, but at the same time, the share of generics has grown. The market concentration of prescription drug sales is shown in Table 13–3. Although the aggregate share of the largest companies has fallen somewhat, the share of the fifty largest companies, including many generic manufacturers, has not. To be sure, these aggregate concentration ratios are not conclusive evidence of changes in competitive conditions in this industry.

The Global Industry

Although the United States has the largest national market for pharmaceuticals and accounts for 27% of the total sales in the developed world (current share of United States sales in the twenty-four-nation Organization for Economic Cooperation and Development), it is nonetheless an

TABLE 13–3 Aggregate share of U.S. prescriptions, 1982–1990 (%)

Company Group	1982	1986	1990
Leading company	8.4	6.7	7.6
Four largest companies	29.5	25.0	24.5
Eight largest companies	48.9	43.4	41.6
Twenty largest companies	79.4	74.9	74.7
Fifty largest companies	96.7	97.5	95.1

Note: These data report new and refilled prescription dollars as dispensed at the pharmacy-cost level.

SOURCE: "Pharmaceuticals," by W. S. Comanor & S. O. Schweitzer, in *The Structure of American Industry* (9th ed.), edited by W. Adams & J. W. Brock, 1995, Englewood Cliffs, NJ: Prentice Hall.

international industry. Precisely because research has become so expensive, it is essential for firms to recoup their investments over as large a territory as possible. Because most countries have their own drug regulations, the largest companies have formed subsidiaries throughout the world, and those without such subsidiaries often sign cross-licensing agreements with those that have them. Indeed, the major companies have become so visible in each important market that it is often difficult to identify a company's "home."

Because the marginal production costs of most drugs are fairly low, it is profitable for a firm to sell its products even where national regulations, incomes, or practices force relatively low prices. As long as prices exceed marginal costs, some contribution is made to the research and development overhead, and as a result, there can be large differences among the prices charged for the same drugs in different countries.

Not only do prices differ among countries, but there also are substantial differences in the availability of products. Because the government agencies responsible for approving pharmaceuticals function differently in different countries, not all drugs are approved at the same time. Although some countries are more likely to approve drugs developed at home, this is not true for the United States, which instead is more likely to approve drugs after they have been introduced elsewhere.

Another question first raised by Wardell (1973) is whether the United States lags behind other countries in approving new drugs. It is slow in approving some new drugs, but recent evidence has shown that all countries are slow in approving some new products (Schweitzer, 1993) and that no country is consistently ahead in approving all new drugs (Schweitzer, et al., 1996).

MARKET CONDUCT

After examining the structure of the pharmaceutical industry, we look at the actions of pharmaceutical firms in regard to both their price-setting behavior and their research and development investment decisions. The activity of these firms in the national economy and in health care is exceedingly important.

Price Behavior

Pricing of pharmaceuticals is perhaps the most controversial aspect of the industry. Consumers, and their elected legislative representatives, are highly attuned to drug prices. It appears that consumers are more sensitive to the prices of pharmaceuticals than they are to the cost of other health services that are far more expensive. With the relatively low level of insurance coverage for pharmaceuticals, and their appearance as a "product" rather than a sophisticated "service," it is not surprising that consumers are more likely to complain about a $50 bottle of tablets than a $500 radiology procedure or a $5,000 hospital stay.

How Are Pharmaceutical Prices Determined?

Although the research costs required to introduce a new drug are substantial, they are usually incurred before the product is sold to even one single consumer. As a result, research costs are fixed costs in that they are required to sell the product but do not vary with the amount sold. Similarly, most marketing costs are incurred in the early years of a product's life cycle and are designed to introduce it to the medical community. Like research costs, they do not vary with output and also are fixed costs. For the most part, therefore, the only variable costs in this industry are at the manufacturing stage. For large research-intensive companies, variable costs represent only about 30% of the product's value. The marginal costs for these products are quite low and reveal little about the prices charged for pharmaceuticals.

Research, marketing, and manufacturing costs all reflect conditions on the supply side of the market. None of them has a major impact on pharmaceutical pricing behavior. In contrast, prices depend on demand-side considerations. That is, the prices charged for pharmaceuticals are determined largely by how valuable or therapeutically useful they are and what consumers are willing to pay for them. Also important are the prices charged for rival products. The seller of a new or old pharmaceutical cannot sell its product for more than the price charged by its rivals unless it is therapeutically superior. If it is not, the seller usually prices its product no higher than those of its rivals and, indeed, sometimes must offer a discount.

When a new product is introduced, whether it offers a small or great therapeutic advance, usually there are existing products that are used for the same or similar indications. These alternative products are what physicians would prescribe in the absence of the new product and thus are the rivals with which the new one must compete. Note that this concept of relevant market, resting on specific therapeutic indications, is far narrower than the conventional standard of a therapeutic category. On the other hand, it is narrower than classifications such as antibiotics or hypertensives, which are so broad that they include pharmaceuticals with very different indications.

Why should the prices charged for rival products be relevant, since physicians only prescribe the pharmaceuticals, whereas their patients must actually pay for them? The answer is that many physicians do pay attention to the prices charged for the drugs they prescribe, particularly physicians in rapidly growing managed care settings. Especially when insurance companies or health maintenance organizations (HMOs) pay for pharmaceuticals, the relative prices of rival products influence prescribing decisions. Price behavior in this industry cannot be explained, therefore, by assuming that prescribing physicians pay little attention to actual prices. Demand factors, and especially relative prices, do matter.

The demand-side factor most important in determining the price charged for a new pharmaceutical is its therapeutic advance compared with older products already on the market. To explore the importance of this factor, one study examined the amount by which new products are priced above their existing substitutes (Lu & Comanor, 1996). The results are given in Table 13–4 for new products, divided between those used for acute and for chronic ailments. As indicated, the average price premiums for more therapeutically advanced products are substantially greater than those offering only modest gains, and largely imitative products are generally priced at or below the levels set for existing products. A second factor is the number of existing substitutes. The more substitutes that are available, the lower the introductory price will be.

TABLE 13–4 Relative prices at time of introduction

Primary Use	Important Therapeutic Gain[a]	Modest Therapeutic Gain[a]	Little or No Therapeutic Gain[a]
Acute	2.97/3.22	1.72/3.09	1.22/1.37
Chronic	2.29/3.12	1.19/1.58	0.94/1.07

a These categories are determined by the Food and Drug Administration at the time of introduction. These price relatives report both median and mean values in each class of products from a sample of 135 new products introduced between 1978 and 1987.

SOURCE: "Pharmaceuticals," by W. S. Comanor & S. O. Schweitzer, in *The Structure of American Industry* (9th ed.), edited by W. Adams & J. W. Brock, 1995, Englewood Cliffs, NJ: Prentice Hall.

Another dimension of pharmaceutical price behavior is the rate of price advance following a product's introduction. For the most part, largely imitative products follow a penetration strategy, in which the introductory price is fairly low but then increases steadily over time. On the other hand, more innovative products are introduced at a higher price but then have few price increases and sometimes even small price declines over time. Moderately innovative products follow an intermediate path. The price levels for highly innovative products are fairly stable after they have been introduced, although this is not true for more imitative products.

A third milestone in the picture of pharmaceutical prices occurs when patents expire, enabling generic producers to enter the market, generally offering the products at much lower prices. Even if their manufacturing costs are higher than those of the original producers, they still set their prices much lower than those of the original seller.

The prices set by generic producers are greatly affected by the number of entrants that sell the product. As that number increases, the price competition becomes more vigorous, and prices fall below the level found when there is only a single entrant.

Average prices fall even though the prices charged for the original branded products are *increased* and not *reduced* when another firm enters. The original manufacturers do not usually compete with the new generic entrants on the basis of price but, rather, find it more profitable to concentrate on the segment of the market that includes brand-loyal customers. Such buyers are physicians and patients who prefer a particular brand and so continue to use it despite the presence of a lower-priced substitute. When generic manufacturers enter production, the price differential widens as the prices charged for the original branded products increase.

Price variation is extremely high in the pharmaceutical industry, with some buyers paying much more for the same drug than other buyers. The buyers who are best able to negotiate substantial discounts from list prices are health maintenance organizations (HMOs) and other managed care plans because they are able to control prescribing decisions by their participating physicians. Retail pharmacies, which are passive in the product selection decision, are unable to obtain the same discounts. Economic theory describes this phenomenon as "price discrimination," and today it is described as "tiered pricing."

Since demand conditions can vary greatly among different sets of buyers, with each having its own price elasticity, one would expect firms to charge different prices to different buyers. Although pharmaceutical companies establish a list price for each drug, many sales are made by discounting that price, and these discounts can be substantial. These discounts may differ between individual and chain-store pharmacies and between hospitals and HMOs. A critical fact about this market is that there is no single price for an individual product even at a specific time; instead, prices depend on the demand conditions presented by particular buyers. Such price differences are not unusual in American industry. For example, airline prices differ greatly between trips that do and do not extend over a Saturday night. The airlines apparently believe that this is the principal factor distinguishing business from vacation travel, and they set their prices accordingly. It should be noted that the National Association of Retail Druggists has sued major drug manufacturers in order to obtain the same discounts (or rebates) that they give to chain pharmacies and managed care providers (Genuardi, et al., 1996). The decision in this case will have important implications for managed care.

Pharmaceutical prices are not determined by costs but by demand and competitive factors. Since marginal costs are only a small share of total costs, it is not surprising that prices exceed marginal costs and also that the extent of these differences varies greatly among buyers. The most important demand-side factor affecting price is the therapeutic advance embodied in the product, which is precisely what competitive processes should enforce. In addition, the number of substitute products leads to lower prices at the time of introduction and afterward. Both results indicate that competitive forces play important roles in determining pharmaceutical prices.

Another difficulty in interpreting price trends for drugs is that our way of measuring price change is better suited to tracking price changes of products than it is to measuring the price effect of new products that enter a market and replace older products. When these new products are better than the old ones, as is often the case for pharmaceuticals, we need price measures that account for quality change. This technique is hardly ever used now.

Are United States Drug Prices Too High Compared to Those in Other Countries?

The issue of drug pricing in an international context has recently been raised in the United States, since drugs appear to be more expensive in the United States than in other countries. For example, a General Accounting Office (GAO) study compared the prices of the two hundred top-selling drugs in the United States with the prices of those drugs in the United Kingdom and Canada. The finding was that Americans pay substantially more for drugs than patients pay in the other two countries (United States General Accounting Office, 1992, 1994).

But price comparisons are more complex than they would appear to be on the surface. Should one merely compare prices of identical products, as the GAO did, or should one take into account differences in consumption patterns in different countries? If one country's price for a product is much higher than another's, but that product is only rarely used in the first country, the price comparison has little meaning. Consumption patterns also become important when one considers the role of generic drugs. Countries differ in their reliance on generics. The market share for generics in the United States is relatively large. To compare the prices of a branded product in the United States and Canada, for example, is less meaningful if that product is subject to more generic substitution in the United States than in Canada because of American reliance on cheaper generic versions. Another question, more technical, is whether international comparisons should be based upon official exchange rates or upon an adjusted rate of exchange that more accurately reflects the value of a nation's currency in purchasing similar products.

Research Behavior

As noted earlier, the leading pharmaceutical companies are continuing to increase their investment in research and development. Like other investments, these expenditures are made because the net present value of future returns is positive, even with the enormous costs associated with bringing a new product to market. Unlike other investments, however, competitive factors can be important.

Some economists have suggested that pharmaceutical companies use research as a competitive weapon to capture markets ahead of their rivals and, in effect, "race" to develop new products. The research programs of major companies, however, are determined mainly by three criteria: unmet medical need, scientific potential, and the capabilities of their researchers. Research efforts are not so easily shifted among therapeutic areas that research directors can readily redirect their programs to compete with others.

The leading pharmaceutical companies are not mirror images of one another but have developed special expertise in certain research areas. Despite the role of existing medical needs in determining research directions, such capabilities are very important. The leading pharmaceutical companies are heterogeneous organizations with their own strengths and capacities, thereby making competitive research and development difficult.

GOVERNMENT REGULATION

The technological revolution that created the modern pharmaceutical industry also led to a new regulatory structure, which eventually became full government supervision of the research process. In 1938, Congress established the Food and Drug Administration (FDA), whose mission was to ensure the safety of drugs sold in the United States. Before a new drug could be marketed, its seller was required to submit both animal and clinical studies that demonstrated its safety for human consumption. The FDA was given the power to reject this application, but had to do so within six months.

The FDA's mission was broadened in 1962 to include assurance of effectiveness as well. The FDA now was required to rule on therapeutic efficacy as well as safety before permitting a new product to be marketed, and the time constraint previously imposed was removed.

Although the new requirement to demonstrate efficacy seemed at first like a harmless and sensible regulatory provision, its consequences were enormous. The FDA now specified what tests were required and what data records must be collected and kept. To rule on the effectiveness of a new product, the regulators required a considerable amount of new information from both animal and clinical trials. Furthermore, these trials had to meet rigorous scientific standards, for otherwise how could it be shown that a new product was truly efficacious? Demonstrating efficacy is far more complex than demonstrating safety.

The review process starts when a manufacturer files an Investigational New Drug (IND) application that is based on preclinical studies. The FDA's approval of these preclinical studies is signaled when it grants an IND, allowing human testing. Clinical trials are then conducted in a series of phases. Phase I trials assess the drug's safety among a relatively small number of normal, healthy subjects. Phase II trials are the first opportunity to test the new drug on patients having the medical condition that the product is designed to treat. Because safety has not been firmly established, Phase II trials are limited in size. Phase III trials build on past experience and are larger and of longer duration, often lasting several years. Phase IV and V trials follow and are used to determine the drug's long-term effects and to compare the new drug with alternatives already available.

The approval process concludes when the firm is granted a New Drug Approval (NDA) and can begin marketing the drug. The time from IND to NDA typically takes five to seven years. Compared with the 1970s, there has recently been a drop in approval rates, but also in the average time required by the FDA to approve new drugs (U.S. Congress, 1993).

A direct result of this regulatory delay has been a substantial decline in effective life of a patent. The great majority of new pharmaceuticals are patented, which gives their developers a form of protection from competition. To ensure their position as inventor, companies apply for a patent early in the development process, even though the introduction of the product must await the FDA's approval. As a result, effective patent lives are much shorter than the statutory period, now twenty years. In part to correct for the regulatory delay, the Drug Price Competition and Patent Term Restoration Act of 1984 was enacted, which extended the term for up to five years but no more than fourteen years. It also granted three-year periods of exclusivity, regardless of patent status, for new or supplementary NDAs on which new clinical trials were required. In recent years, therefore, these periods of exclusive marketing have recovered somewhat.

The regulatory delays have attracted considerable attention and many complaints. In response, in 1987, the FDA established the Treatment Investigational New Drug program to deal with life-threatening diseases for which no alternative therapy exists. In such circumstances, the FDA permits physicians to use, on a case-by-case basis, drugs still being tested. Although manufacturers are permitted to charge for these drugs, they rarely have done so.

The 1984 law extended the period of patent protection for all new products whose market introduction was impeded by regulation delay, but it also facilitated generic competition when that period ended. Although previously the FDA had required that generic producers duplicate the studies and tests carried out by the original developer, the 1984 act permitted these firms to file an Abbreviated New Drug Application (ANDA), which requires them only to demonstrate bioequivalency between their product and the original drug. On average, an ANDA requires only eighteen months for approval. As a direct result of this law, there has been a major expansion in the number and sales of generic producers.

In 1983, Congress passed the Orphan Drug Act, the purpose of which was to stimulate the development of drugs with limited market potential, because either the condition was so uncommon or the drug's development and manufacturing costs were too high. It authorized the FDA to assist manufacturers in designing research protocols, to subsidize clinical and preclinical drug studies, and, finally, to grant seven years of marketing exclusivity to the first firm to receive NDA approval for a drug for a particular medical condition.

INDUSTRY PERFORMANCE

An industry's market power is conventionally measured by differences between prices and marginal costs. Drug prices typically exceed marginal costs, but the pharmaceutical industry does not function as a standard competitive industry. Its leading firms enjoy substantial degrees of market power; at the same time, however, industry performance is not adequately measured by the conventional criteria of a competitive industry. If the pharmaceutical industry were highly priced/competitive, there would be little investment in research and development; few if any new products would be introduced; and the companies would have little need to spend large sums on marketing their products. That was the status of the industry before World War II. In the modern pharmaceutical industry, however, the appropriate criteria for industry performance are more broadly stated, since few industry watchers believe that returning the industry to its prewar status would improve its performance.

The dominant characteristic of the modern industry is the substantial allocation of resources to research and development and the extensive array of new therapeutic agents that have resulted. To be sure, not every research project is successful; there are more "wrong turns" than "right ones." Many research dollars are spent on projects for which no new products result, and the average research costs of new products include this work as well. Consequently, as noted earlier, millions of dollars are spent on each new product introduced. In addition, all new products are not equally successful or innovative; instead, the revenues received are highly skewed.

The critical dilemma for evaluating the performance of the pharmaceutical industry has long been the conflict between static and dynamic efficiency. Low prices are desired not only because they benefit consumers but also because higher prices limit patients' ability to buy and use essential drugs. Although the theoretical standard for the maximum economic welfare of marginal cost pricing is too stringent for this industry, society still prefers the lowest possible prices that are consistent with intensive research and the rapid introduction of beneficial new drugs. Unfortunately, this criterion is not precise because high prices and profits stimulate research spending and because therapeutically better products are priced above their current substitutes. In effect, there is a trade-off between static and dynamic efficiency.

If public policy actions are taken that reduce prices too severely, the prospective returns from investing in research and development will decline; there will be less investment in product introduc-

tion; and fewer new products will be developed. On the other hand, if the rewards from pharmaceutical innovation expand too much, then consumers will suffer, and important new products will not be as accessible as they might be. The main issue is balancing these competing objectives.

Ideally, society would gain most from a mechanism that permitted it to achieve both objectives at the same time, through an institutional change that permitted intensive research along with low prices for the fruits of that research. But that would require an industry substantially different from the one that now exists, and such a change would raise many new issues.

With the existing industrial structure, there is a conflict between society's two objectives. At the same time, it is apparent that we have decided that relatively high prices are worth the benefits that flow from major new investments in pharmaceutical research and development. We have made our choice, but through our political representatives, we nonetheless complain about it.

PUBLIC POLICY QUESTIONS

Pharmaceuticals constitute only a small share of health expenditures in the United States, under 9% of national health expenditures (U.S. Department of Health and Human Services, 1995). But they are a much larger share in other countries, and the proportion is especially large in the developing world. In addition, pharmaceuticals raise the productivity of other health care inputs, such as physician visits and hospitals, so this sector is vitally important in every country. Although topics in pharmaceutical economics and policy are frequently discussed in policy circles, comprehensive examinations of the entire sector are surprisingly rare. This is an especially serious problem because the health care system is complex and its components interact with one another. Policies affecting one segment will have an impact on the others. Therefore, health reforms designed with the best of intentions have frequently had serious unintended consequences.

The pharmaceutical sector is, of course, a component of any health care *system;* drugs are but one of many inputs, which include physician services and hospital and ambulatory based capital equipment. In many instances, pharmaceuticals complement these other inputs, as in the case of antibiotics. And there are other examples of a *substitution effect,* in which one input, in this case drugs, replaces other inputs. For instance, in the 1970s, psychoactive drugs permitted ambulatory care of patients with mental illness who had previously required hospitalization. But Martin and McMillan (1996) have observed that reduced insurance coverage for drugs leads to increased use of hospital care.

This *system* view of the health sector is necessary to understand many policy issues concerning pharmaceuticals. In this section we discuss five of these: the adequacy of pharmaceutical research and development, financial access to new drugs, pharmaceutical prices, international drug price comparison, and government intervention in the pharmaceutical market.

Is Pharmaceutical Research and Development Adequate?

The foundation of the pharmaceutical industry is its research and development (R&D). The Office of Technology Assessment of the United States Congress reported that research and development spending by United States pharmaceutical companies was between $5.7 billion and $6.6 billion in 1990, having grown at an annual rate of between 7.6% and 9.4% per year since 1976 (U.S. Congress, 1993). Ninety percent of pharmaceutical R&D is done by the private sector. Although the direct government share of R&D expenditures is small, it is

targeted to specific needs. For example, where commercial rewards of research are too small to elicit private sector investment, two federal programs attempt to stimulate private sector activity. In 1983 Congress passed the Orphan Drug Act to create incentives for private pharmaceutical companies to engage in research and development into drugs without a large commercial market. And in 1986 Congress enacted the Federal Technology Transfer Act, which established Cooperative Research and Development Agreements (CRADAs) (U.S. Congress, 1993). Through CRADAs, a federal laboratory directly transfers research resources to a private developer to facilitate cooperative research. These programs subsidizing noncommercially viable research also suggest a model whereby R&D could be directed to problems of developing countries, where incidence and prevalence of diseases infrequently seen in industrialized countries, such as malaria, may be enormous, but incomes of those afflicted are so low that the commercial market is small.

Can Consumers Afford New Pharmaceuticals?

The demand for pharmaceuticals, of course, derives from the demand for health. While most markets have two participants, the producer and the consumer, demand for health care is also determined by so-called "third-party intermediaries," the insurers or other payers who stand behind the patient ready to pay for whatever he or she decides to purchase. But the picture for health care is even more involved because the physician frequently has two roles as decision maker: as a provider of care and as the consumer's agent. This "agency relationship," in which the professional acts in the consumer's best interest, has been the subject of intense debate for decades, primarily because of the incentives built into fee-for-service medical care. Fee-for-service payment rewards the practitioner for performing additional services. A disquieting, inherent conflict of interest faces the physician who is paid according to the quantity of services performed.

Health insurance creates an odd division between professional advice, service delivery, consumption, and payment. Health services are traditionally selected by the physician, who neither consumes the service nor pays for it. The patient receives the service but, for approximately 80% of expenditures, does not pay for it directly (U.S. Department of Health and Human Services, 1995). Payment is left to government or private insurers—third-party payers. Of course, patients ultimately pay, but only indirectly, and as part of a greater pool of insurance beneficiaries and taxpayers. In the pharmaceutical market, another professional also participates—the pharmacist. The role of pharmacists is changing rapidly, and we will look particularly at some of the forces shaping the future of this profession.

But the diffusion of managed care is making the picture even more complicated because treatment decisions, formerly arrived at jointly between the physician and the patient, are increasingly being made by third-party payers. Both the privately insured and those insured by public programs such as Medicare and Medicaid are joining managed care plans, which combine the insurance function with medical-care decision making. Treatment plans are frequently established by the managed care plan as a way of improving quality of care while reducing the use of unnecessary care and lowering the cost of necessary care. In the case of pharmaceuticals, these treatment protocols, or guidelines, frequently specify which drugs are to be used or denote when generic versions of a drug are to be prescribed.

But third-party insurance coverage is far less comprehensive for pharmaceuticals than it is for many other health services. While insurance (both government and private) covered 96% of hospital services in 1992 and 82% of physician services, it covered only 72% of the cost of pharmaceuticals (Health Insurance Association of America, 1994). As a result, pharmaceuticals comprise over 30% of all out-of-pocket expenditures for health services (Health Insurance Association of America, 1994). For the elderly, this situation is even more pronounced, for they consume some 35% of all drugs, a disproportionately large share. The situation is exacerbated by the greater health care needs of the elderly and the lack of insurance coverage for ambulatory drugs by their major source of health insurance, Medicare. Long (1994) estimates that 45% of the elderly have no insurance coverage for pharmaceuticals. Thus, patients are more sensitive to prices charged for pharmaceuticals than for other services. They "demand" pharmaceuticals in the true economic sense, both consuming the product and paying for it out of pocket, to a greater extent than they do for most other health services.

Pharmaceutical demand is influenced by the fact that drugs are both a traditional product, in the sense of other manufactured goods, and also a service, because of the professional component in selection and dispensing. Another important consideration is the degree of market concentration or competition in the industry, and how consumers—and their physician agents—receive information about therapeutic alternatives.

How Does the Government Intervene in the Pharmaceutical Market?

Few industries in industrialized countries are subject to as much direct regulatory control as the pharmaceutical industry. Every product produced for the prescription market is subject to intense scrutiny and government-mandated testing. The direct cost of these clinical trials is high, but more expensive is the indirect cost—time. Premarketing approval in the United States often takes as long as five to seven years, delaying the future revenue stream even for those drugs that successfully pass the trials and prove to be safe and effective. The United States' national drug approval agency is the Food and Drug Administration (FDA), part of the Department of Health and Human Services. Once a drug is approved by the FDA for a specific indication, the introducing firm is free to distribute and market the product for that use. But the FDA continues to closely regulate marketing activities, and firms are prohibited from marketing a drug for indications for which FDA approval has not been granted, even if scientific literature and customs use validate these other uses.

Increasingly, drugs must also be approved for use by a multitude of third-party payers who agree to cover the cost of pharmaceuticals for their subscribers or beneficiaries. Most states have used formularies in their Medicaid programs as the basis for authorizing reimbursement to pharmacies for drugs dispensed to indigent patients in the respective states. Congress attempted to deal with the problems produced by restrictive formularies in passing the Omnibus Budget Reconciliation Act (OBRA), which guaranteed a state's Medicaid recipients access to all drugs manufactured by any company that agreed to grant to that state's Medicaid program the greatest price discount it offered to any other purchaser.

Today managed care is growing rapidly, and most of these health plans cover drugs as part of their benefit package. The influence of managed care coverage decisions on the pharmaceutical industry has grown to become a critical factor determining industry strategy and marketing tactics. Formularies are frequently used by managed care plans to reduce pharmaceuticals cost by restricting drug utilization to those products that are viewed as cost-effective.

Another important government intervention in the pharmaceutical sector is the granting of patent protection. Both the approval process and patent protection are barriers to entry purposely established to protect the innovative process. But both are intensely debated because their effects on patients are frequently unfavorable as well as favorable. While many argue, for example, that patent protection is essential if the pharmaceutical industry is to recoup its enormous investment in R&D, others note that this protection comes at a price. It restricts access to markets by less expensive generic products, often depriving patients of cheaper, essentially identical products. Generic drugs are typically manufactured by firms that have not engaged in any of the original R&D work and therefore have only modest fixed costs.

While patents limit competition from generic products, competition also comes from similar (but not identical) products produced by other R&D firms, so it is easy to overstate the benefit that patent protection creates for drug companies. The pharmaceutical industry is highly competitive in many markets so that being first in a market has distinct advantages; success tends to attract competition from other firms.

This brief overview of pharmaceutical economics and policy highlights a number of health policy choices that face both the public and private sectors in the United States and other countries. In fact, these choices must be faced by countries with widely differing health systems, whether they are socialized, based on social insurance, or largely market-oriented. The following questions are illustrative of the issues that must be discussed by health care policy makers everywhere.

- Can the rapid growth in technological development of drugs be maintained while assuring that the benefits are widely accessible to the population?
- Are physicians provided sufficient information at reasonable cost regarding drug therapy

alternatives to enable them to make informed, cost-effective treatment decisions?

- Can a financing program for pharmaceuticals be developed that will provide access to new drugs, encourage drug compliance by patients, and lead to efficient allocation of resources among drug alternatives?
- Are United States drug prices close enough to those in other countries to assure American patients that they do not bear a disproportionate burden of the worldwide costs of R&D for each product?
- Can the drug approval process be streamlined so that the burden it imposes on both pharmaceutical firms and potential patients is held to the minimum level necessary to assure both safety and access?
- Is market exclusivity protection sufficient to provide for an acceptable rate of return to R&D investment, while offering the consuming public the lowest possible price for their medication?
- Can wealthy countries, perhaps through multilateral arrangements, encourage the diffusion of pharmaceutical technology to developing countries, where the burden of disease is enormous but the commercial market for drugs is small?

Each of these policy issues is best framed in terms of choices, which are made all the more difficult because society frequently makes inconsistent demands: consumer safety *and* access, or low prices *and* corporate incentives to invest. Regardless of the difficulty, the choices must be carefully explored.

REFERENCES

Bezold, C. (1981). *The future of pharmaceuticals.* New York: Wiley.

Bowman, M. A. (1994). Pharmaceutical company-physician interaction. *Archives of Family Medicine, 152*(4), 317–318.

Caves, R. E., Whinston, M. D., & Hurwitz, M. A. (1991). Patent expiration, entry and competition in the U.S. pharmaceutical industry. *Brookings paper on economic activity: Microeconomics* (pp. 39–40). Washington DC: Brookings Institution.

Comanor, W. S. (1986, September). The political economy of the pharmaceutical industry. *Journal of Economic Literature, 24,* 1178–1217.

DiMasi, J. A., Hansen, R. W., Grabowski, H. G., & Lasagna, L. (1991). The cost of innovation in the pharmaceutical industry. *Journal of Health Economics, 10,* 107–142.

Genuardi, J. S., Stiller, J. M., & Trapnell, G. R. (1996). Changing prescription drug sector: New expenditure methodologie. *Health Care Financing Review, 17*(3), 191–204.

Health Insurance Association of America. (1994). *Source book of health insurance data.* Washington, DC: Author.

Hutt, P. B. (1982, Spring). The importance of patent term restoration to pharmaceutical innovation. *Health Affairs,* 9.

Kessler, D. A., Rose, J. L., Temple, R. J., Shapiro, R., & Griffin, J. P. (1995). Therapeutic class wars—Drug promotion in a competitive marketplace. *New England Journal of Medicine, 331,* 1350–1353.

Leffler, K. B. (1981, April). Persuasion or information? The economics of prescription drug advertising. *Journal of Law and Economics,* 62.

Leffler, K. B. (1992, December 10). Assessing prescription drug advertising: Is information the proper criterion? UCLA Seminar on Pharmaceutical Economics and Policy (pp. 4–5), Los Angeles, CA.

Long, S. (1994, Spring). Prescription drugs and the elderly: Issues and options. *Health Affairs, (II),* 157–174.

Lu, J. Z., & Comanor, W. S. (1996). Strategic pricing of new pharmaceuticals. *UCLA research program in pharmaceutical economics and policy* (Working Paper 95-1).

Martin, B. C., & McMillan, J. A. (1996). The impact of implementing a more restrictive prescription limit on Medicaid recipients: Effects on cost, therapy, and out of pocket expenditures. *Medical Care, 34*(7), 686–701.

Pharmaceutical Manufacturers Association. (1991, September). *Statistical fact book* (Fig. 2–1). Washington, DC: Author.

Schweitzer, S. O. (1993). Comparison France-Etats Unis de l'autorisat on de mise sur le marche do nouveaux produits pharmaceutiques. *Journal d'economic medicale, 11,* 33–34.

Schweitzer, S. O., Schweitzer, M. E., & Sourty-LeGuellec, M.-J. (1996). Is there a United States drug lag? The timing of new pharmaceutical approvals in the G-7 countries and Switzerland. *Medical Care Research and Review, 53*(2), 162–178.

Silverman, M., & Lee, P. R. (1974). *Pills, profits and politics.* Berkeley, CA: University of California Press.

Temin, P. (1980). *Taking your medicine: Drug regulation in the United States* (p. 87). Cambridge, MA: Harvard University Press.

U.S. Congress, Office of Technology Assessment. (1993, February). *Pharmaceutical R&D: Costs, risks and rewards* (OTA-H-522). Washington, DC: U.S. Government Printing Office.

U.S. Department of Health and Human Services. (1995). *Health United States.* Washington, DC: Author.

U.S. General Accounting Office. (1992, September). *Prescription drugs: Companies typically charge more in the United States than in Canada* (CAO/HRD-92-110).

U.S. General Accounting Office. (1994, January). *Prescription drugs: Companies typically charge more in the United States than in the United Kingdom* (GAO/HEHS-94-29).

U.S. Senate. (1993, February). *Staff report to the special committee on aging.* Washington, DC: U.S. Government Printing Office.

Wardell, W. M. (1973). Introduction of new therapeutic drugs in the United States and Great Britain: An international comparison. *Clinical Pharmacology Therapeutics, 14,* 773–790.

Weekend Edition/Saturday. (1995, September 30). *Thalidomide use by AIDS, cancer patients a controversy.* Washington, DC: National Public Radio.

Wilkes, M. S., Doblin, B., & Shapiro, M. (1992). Assessing prescription drug advertising. *Annals of Internal Medicine, 116*(11), 912–919.

CHAPTER

Health Care Professionals

Stephen S. Mick

CHAPTER TOPICS

LEARNING OBJECTIVES

Upon completing this chapter, the reader should be able to:

- Appreciate the growth in and changes in the composition of the health profession workforce during the twentieth century.
- Understand the key role of physicians and osteopaths in the workforce, and account for the growth in physician supply.
- Account for the various trends and changes in dentistry, public health, nursing, and pharmacy, and the forces affecting these health professionals.
- Comprehend the importance and potential of physician assistants and nurse practitioners in the health care system.
- Understand the various major transitions occurring in the health care workforce, particularly the impact of managed care.

Health care professionals play a key role in the provision of health services to meet the needs and demands of the population. This chapter highlights health care professional trends and discusses issues of provider supply, education and training, distribution, specialization, and the impact of managed care on the health professions workforce.

EMPLOYMENT TRENDS IN THE HEALTH CARE SECTOR

As the twenty-first century approaches, observers will look back at the twentieth century and be struck by the dramatic growth in the number and types of personnel employed in the health care sector. Table 14–1 shows the large gains in health sector employment in the United States, starting with a pool of about 624,000 employed persons in 1920 and growing to more than 8 million by 1994. These figures include primarily those people with training and skills unique to the health care sector and exclude clerical staff, artisans, laborers, and others who have supporting roles in the delivery of health services. Almost one-third of all those employed in the health sector probably fall into this supporting category. Although these approximately 1.5 million nonclinical workers are not discussed in this chapter, they are important because they evidence the role the health care sector has played for new employment opportunities in the service-oriented economy that now characterizes the United States.

The health care sector has maintained a steadily increasing proportion of all persons employed, and it currently includes about 6.5% of the United States labor force. Thus, growth in employment in the health care sector (1,182% increase between 1920 and 1994) has outpaced growth in overall employment in the economy (196% increase) as well as total population growth (145% increase). This growth is underscored by the 424% increase in the rate of health care personnel per 100,000 population, from a low of 586 in 1920 to a high of 3,069 in 1994 (Table 14–1).

At least as extraordinary as the increased supply of health care personnel has been the emergence of a wide variety of new categories of personnel, including physicians' assistants (PAs), nurse practitioners (NPs), dental hygienists, laboratory technicians, nursing aids, orderlies, attendants, home health aids, occupational and physical therapists, medical records technicians, X-ray technicians, dietitians and nutritionists, social workers, and the like. The Department of Labor recognizes about four hundred different job titles in the health sector. Some of the most rapid growth in the supply of health care personnel has occurred in these recently developed categories.

The traditional health care occupations of physician, dentist, and pharmacist have generally experienced declines, some dramatic, in their relative

TABLE 14–1   The health sector as a proportion of all employed persons, by decade: 1920–1994

	1920	*1930*	*1940*	*1950*	*1960*	*1970*	*1980*	*1991*	*1994*
Employment in health sector (thousands)[a]	624	859	972	1,394	1,966	3,130	5,030	6,981	8,001
Total number of persons employed (thousands)[b]	41,614	48,829	44,888	56,225	64,639	78,627	97,270	116,877	123,060
Health sector as a proportion of all occupations	1.5%	1.8%	2.2%	2.5%	3.0%	4.0%	5.2%	6.0%	6.5%
Total U.S. population (millions)	106.5	123.1	132.6	152.3	180.7	205.1	227.7	252.7	260.7
Number of health personnel per 100,000 population	586	698	733	915	1,088	1,428	2,209	2,763	3,069

a   These figures do not include secretarial and office workers, craftsmen, laborers, and other personnel such as cooks, janitors, and so on who work in supporting roles in the health care sector.

b   Figures for 1980 and 1990 include employed persons 16 years of age and over; figures from 1940 to 1970 include employed persons 14 years of age and over; earlier data are based on persons 10 years of age and over.

SOURCES: Adapted from "Understanding the Persistence of Human Resources Problems in Health," by S. Mick, 1978, *The Milbank Quarterly, 56,* pp. 463–499, Table 3; *Statistical Abstract of the United States: 1992* (112th ed.), U.S. Bureau of the Census, 1992, Washington DC: U.S. Government Printing Office; *Statistical Abstract of the United States: 1995* (115th ed.), U.S. Bureau of the Census, 1995, Washington, DC: U.S. Government Printing Office.

proportion of all health care personnel. For example, physicians (including osteopaths) constituted 30% of all persons in health occupations as the decade of the 1920s began, but had declined to about 9% by 1990. Over the same period, dentists declined from 8% to about 2%, and pharmacists from 11% to about 3%. Registered nurses have fluctuated up, then down during this seventy-year period: about 20% in 1920 to a high of 36% in 1940, then a steady decline to about 25% in 1990. The group of health care workers that has gained the largest share of the overall number includes allied health technicians, technologists, aides, and assistants: they composed a mere 1–2% in 1920, but in 1990, they made up over 50%. These figures should not mask the fact that *all* groups of health care personnel have increased in absolute number from year to year, as inspection of any of the tables in this chapter will show. What the data emphasize is the higher rate of growth of nontraditional allied health and support personnel, who now constitute more than two-thirds of all personnel employed in the health care sector.

The primary reasons for the increased supply and wide variety of health care personnel in the twentieth century are the interrelated forces of technological growth, specialization, health insurance coverage, the aging of the population, and the emergence of the hospital as the central institution of the health care system. The hospital became the setting where new technology could be used and where medical, nursing, and other health professional students could be educated. The technological revolution has led to diagnostic and treatment procedures that, in turn, have led to an increased use of hospitals, with a corresponding concentration of health personnel. The rise of private health insurance in the 1940s, plus enactment of the publicly funded insurance systems in the mid-1960s (Medicare and Medicaid), fueled hospital growth because reliable payment mechanisms provided hospitals with assured revenues.

Current concerns with escalating health care costs, however, have led to a substantial increase in the use of health care facilities outside the hospital. These facilities include urgent care centers, ambulatory surgery centers, hospices, freestanding diagnostic centers, and others. Furthermore, the number of people cared for in their own homes has increased, leading to a demand for such personnel as home health aides and inhalation or respiratory therapists as well as nursing personnel. Whereas all this has been a pressure for new employment opportunities, a general emphasis on efficiency—often associated with managed care systems—has created a counterpressure in favor of a more limited use of health professionals. What the net effect of these pressures will be is one of the unanswered questions of the mid-1990s. Thus, the hospital sector, although critical to the growth in health care personnel throughout most of this century, is giving way to these systems, and they will probably do much to shape the size and structure of employment in health care well into the twenty-first century, a topic addressed throughout this chapter.

Technological innovation has also led to increased specialization of health care personnel, primarily during the last thirty-five years. This specialization has resulted in new categories of health care providers within the traditional professions (for example, pediatric nephrologists and gastroenterologists in medicine, periodontists in dentistry, and intensive care unit [ICU] specialists in nursing). There has also been the advent of new types of allied health professions (for example, occupational and radiological technicians and speech pathologists).

Health care personnel will be discussed in greater detail by focusing on five of the more traditional groups of professions—physicians and osteopaths, dentists, public health professionals, nurses, and pharmacists—and two of the more recently developed categories of personnel—PAs and NPs.

THE EXPANDING SUPPLY OF PHYSICIANS

The Continuing Fear of a Surplus

The number of physicians in the United States has increased rapidly in the last twenty-five years, with an estimated 665,250 active physicians, including osteopaths (described more fully in a later section) practicing in 1995 (Table 14–2). Between 1970 and 1995, there was a 104% increase in the supply of active physicians, resulting in an average of approximately 252 physicians per 100,000 population. In 1980, the Graduate Medical Education National Advisory Committee (GMENAC) reported to the Secretary of the United States Department of Health and Human Services that there would be a surplus of physicians of 70,000 in 1990, and roughly 140,000 in 2000, underscoring the belief that the nation could substantially reduce its subsidization of medical education (Graduate Medical Education National Advisory Committee, 1980). In 1994, the Council on Graduate Medical Education (COGME), an advisory group to the federal government, noted that despite the warning of a surplus made more than fifteen years ago, United States physician supply was still growing one and a half times faster than the general population (Council on Graduate Medical Education, 1994).

Why has physician supply grown so much? To answer this question, one must understand that the United States physician workforce consists of two different groups: first, persons who are United States citizens and who are trained in United States

TABLE 14–2 Number of active physicians: 1970, 1980, 1990, 1995

Health Occupation	1970		1980		1990		1995[a]	
	Number	Personnel per 100,000 Population	Number	Personnel per 100,000 Population	Number	Personnel per 100,000 Population	Number	Personnel per 100,000 Population
Physicians	326,200	156.0	457,500	197.0	601,060	240.0	665,250	252.5
MDs	314,200	150.0	440,000	189.5	543,310	228.9	630,770	239.4
DOs	12,000	6.0	17,100	7.5	27,750	11.1	34,480	13.1

a   Projected figures

SOURCES: *Fourth Report to the President and Congress on the Status of Health Personnel in the United States* (DHHS Pub. No. HRS-P-0084.4), May 1984, Washington, DC: U.S. Government Printing Office; *Seventh Report to the President and Congress on the Status of Health Personnel in the United States* (DHHS Pub. No. HRS-P-OD-90-1), March 1990, Washington, DC: U.S. Government Printing Office; *Health Personnel in the United States: Eighth Report to Congress* (DHHS Pub. No. HRS-P-OD-92-1), 1992, Washington, DC: U.S. Government Printing Office.

medical schools; second, persons who are foreign-trained physicians (known as International Medical Graduates, or IMGs).

As for United States medical graduates (USMGs), Table 14–3 shows the substantial increase in both the number of medical schools and the number of medical students (first-year and total enrolled) over the last thirty years. By 1995–1996, the yearly number of graduates had more than doubled the 1965–1966 number. This increase can be directly attributed to massive federal outlays for training, research, and construction in the 1960s and 1970s. By the early 1970s, 40–50% of medical school support came from federal sources. However, the retreat of the federal government from an active role in the financial support of medical education was initiated in the early 1980s as a result of pressures to reduce federal spending, of the perception that there was an adequate supply of physicians in the United States, and of a conservative administrative ideology regarding federal intervention in medical education. By the early 1990s, the federal government provided about 20–25% of medical school finan-

cial support through direct subsidies and research, down from about 44% in 1970. In short, dramatic growth in the domestically educated supply of physicians occurred between the mid-1960s and 1980s. Thereafter, the domestic supply of newly graduated physicians has been relatively constant, hovering around 17,000 new MDs annually.

The second important factor in the increased supply of physicians has been the influx of IMGs into the United States. In 1992, 139,086, or 23%, of the total active physician population of 605,685 physicians were IMGs. The inflow of IMGs began after World War II when the United States Congress passed legislation that made it relatively easy for professionals from foreign countries to come to this country to obtain advanced graduate training. This effort was in response to the need for skilled personnel in many developing countries and to other countries' rebuilding after the war's destruction to educate a new cadre of professional personnel. It was also an attempt to inculcate the values of democracy into a new generation of young professionals who were offered advanced

TABLE 14–3 Number of allopathic medical schools, applicants, students, graduates, and ratio of first-year students to applicants: Selected academic years 1965–1966 through 1995–1996

Academic Year	Number of Schools	Number of Applicants	Number of Students		Number of Graduates	Ratio of First-Year Students to Applicants
			Total	First Year		
1965–1966	88	18,703	32,835	8,759	7,574	1:2.4
1970–1971	103	24,987	40,487	11,348	8,974	1:2.2
1975–1976	114	42,303	56,244	15,351	13,561	1:2.8
1980–1981	126	36,100	65,497	17,204	15,667	1:2.0
1985–1986	127	32,893	66,604	16,929	16,125	1:1.9
1990–1991	126	29,243	64,986	16,803	15,481	1:1.7
1995–1996	125	46,591	66,906	17,024	16,029	1:2.7

SOURCES: Adapted from the following: "Undergraduate Medical Education, 1980," *Journal of the American Medical Association, 243,* pp. 849–866; "Educational Programs in U.S. Medical Schools," by H. Jonas, S. Etzel, & B. Barzansky, 1991, *Journal of the American Medical Association, 226,* pp. 913–923; "Educational Programs in U.S. Medical Schools, 1995–1996," by B. Barzansky, H. Jonas, & S. Etzel, 1996, *Journal of the American Medical Association, 276,* pp. 714–719.

education in Communist Bloc countries and exposed to Communist ideological positions.

By the mid-1960s, favorable immigration policies for physicians had encouraged this movement; there was, in addition, an unceasing demand for interns and residents in United States hospitals as measured by the existence each year of unfilled house officer positions. By the early 1970s, IMGs accounted for more than 40% of new physician licentiates, 30% of filled residency positions, and 20% of the active physicians in the United States. One-third of the growth in physician supply in the 1970s was due to increases in the number of physicians trained outside the United States.

As the 1980s began, the number of IMGs filling residency positions was in decline, having decreased from 18,395 in 1972–1973 to 12,259 in 1980–1981. Throughout the decade of the 1980s, the number of IMGs stabilized between 12,000 and 13,000 (Table 14–4). Then, most unexpectedly, the number of IMGs begin to increase: in 1990, there were 14,914 IMGs undertaking residency

training, a jump from 12,259 in the preceding year, or a growth of 22%. This compared to 73,071 and 67,988 USMGs in residency training in 1989 and 1990, respectively, an actual drop of nearly 1%. By 1995, the trend had continued: 24,982 IMGs in residency training, a number greater than in any preceding year in history and a 67.5% increase over the 1990 figure.

The question is, how can it be that so many IMGs are entering United States medicine when there is a supposed "surplus" of physicians as announced by the GMENAC in 1980 and reaffirmed by the important federal advisory group, the Council on Graduate Medical Education (COGME) in its various reports from the late 1980s to the present day (Council on Graduate Medical Education, 1994)? Although there is no clear and proven answer to this question, there are a number of probable reasons. First, although the United States may have a surplus of physicians, that is, more physicians than there are requirements for their services, these physicians have

TABLE 14–4 International medical graduates (IMGs) in residency positions: Selected years 1980 through 1995

	1980	*1982*	*1984*	*1986*	*1988*	*1990*	*1992*	*1995*
Total IMG residents	12,259	13,123	13,525	12,207	12,433	14,914	19,264	24,982
Percentage of total residents	19.9%	18.6%	18.0%	15.7%	15.3%	17.9%	20.0%	25.5%
U.S. citizen IMG residents	4,814	6,388	7,386	5,845	5,131	5,026	5,015	4,030
U.S. citizen IMGs as a percentage of all IMGs	39.3%	48.7%	54.6%	47.9%	41.3%	33.7%	26.0%	16.1%

SOURCES: Adapted from the following: "Graduate Medical Education in the United States, 1984–1985," by A. Crowley, 1985, *Journal of the American Medical Association, 254,* pp. 1585–1593; "Graduate Medical Education in the United States," by S. Etzel, R. Egan, M. Shevrin, & B. Rowley, 1989, *Journal of the American Medical Association, 262,* pp. 1029–1037; "Graduate Medical Education in the United States," by B. Rowley, D. Baldwin, M. McGuire, S. Etzel, & C. O'Leary, 1990, *Journal of the American Medical Association, 264,* pp. 822–832; "Selected Characteristics of Graduate Medical Education in the United States," by B. Rowley, D. Baldwin, & M. McGuire, 1991, *Journal of the American Medical Association, 266,* pp. 933–943; "Graduate Medical Education, 1993," *Journal of the American Medical Association, 270,* pp. 1116–1122; "Graduate Medical Education, 1996," *Journal of the American Medical Association, 276,* pp. 739–748.

continued to be distributed too often in non–primary care specialties; in urban and suburban locations, and not in rural and inner-city locations; and in practice settings that are desirable, for example, group practices, well-established HMOs, and the like, and not in less desirable settings, for example, public hospitals, state mental hospitals, and prison health services. Thus, IMGs who have entered the United States health care system "fill gaps" to some extent, frequently practicing in specialties, geographic locations, and employment settings avoided by USMGs.

Table 14–5 shows the magnitude of this problem regarding federally designated physician shortage areas in the United States in 1994. The bars in Table 14–5, representing the states, show the difference in proportions between active USMGs and IMGs in shortage and partial shortage counties within each state. That is, the number of IMGs in shortage counties is divided by the total number of IMGs in the entire state, and the same operation is done for USMGs. By subtracting the resulting proportion of IMGs from the resulting proportion of USMGs, one can compare the relative propensity

of IMGs (or USMGs) to be found in shortage counties. Thus, for any state beneath the 0.0% line, relatively more IMGs than USMGs were located in shortage counties, whereas for any state above this line, relatively more USMGs were so located. States with an extreme overrepresentation of IMGs (5–15%) in shortage counties included Mississippi, South Dakota, North Dakota, Michigan, Wisconsin, Texas, Vermont, and Arkansas. Nineteen other states had a less extreme overrepresentation of IMGs (between 0% and 5%). These data are just one way to measure the "gap filling" roles in which many IMGs have been engaged.

A second reason for the large IMG presence in the United States has been that teaching hospitals, that is, those in which physicians, nurses, and most other health professionals are trained, continue to enjoy relatively generous funding via the Medicare program to underwrite the costs of graduate medical education (Council on Graduate Medical Education, 1995a). The result has been that many more residency positions exist than there are USMGs to fill them. This acts as a sort of "suction"

TABLE 14–5 Percent difference between proportion of active USMGs and IMGs in shortage and partly shortage counties, U.S. states, 1994*

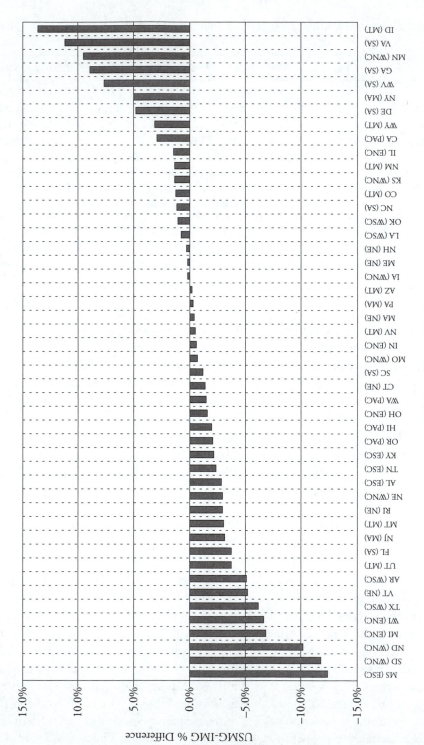

U.S. State (Census Division)

USMG-IMG % Difference

* Omits AK, DC, and MD either for lack of data or no shortage or partly shortage counties

SOURCE: Unpublished data from the Area Resource File, Bureau of Health Professions, DHHS.

or "pull" factor to bring IMGs to the United States. Often, these hospitals serve large numbers of persons who are poor or without health insurance, or both, as well as those on Medicaid. Estimates of the number of hospitals that are "dependent" on IMG residents *and* that serve the poor vary between 77 and 276, many concentrated in New York, Texas, New Jersey, Michigan, and Illinois (Whitcomb & Miller, 1995). However, the number of hospitals falling into this category is probably greater than these figures indicate because the authors used conservative criteria to determine "IMG dependence."

A third reason for the IMG presence has been brought on by the increased market penetration of managed care plans in urban areas. These plans generally are not linked to teaching hospitals and therefore do not train residents or any other health professionals. Nor do they incur the costs of research, as do the teaching hospitals. The managed care plans can therefore charge lower premiums and offer lower cost services to employers and other groups anxious to cut their rising health care costs. Teaching hospitals, in order to compete, have searched for lower-cost substitutes, and residents (often IMGs) actually may provide a lower-cost substitute than skilled nurse, NP, or PA services because the latter work fixed hours per week and generally are paid higher overtime rates. A resident works longer hours, is paid a fixed salary, and is a physician. Thus, as managed care has spread in urban markets where IMG residents are traditionally located, there has been more pressure on teaching hospitals to increase the residency complement.

Other factors undoubtedly have played a role in the recent increase of IMGs. Whatever the case, the medical community and groups such as the Institute of Medicine have evinced concern about the IMG situation. The Institute of Medicine (1996) and others such as the Pew Health Professionals Commission have called for limits on the number of residency slots available each year.

Such limits on residency positions, if somehow implemented, would make it exceedingly difficult for most new IMGs to compete for training opportunities in the United States, such that the international component of physician supply would be severely curtailed.

In summary, there was a marked increase in the supply of United States physicians in the 1970s and 1980s due to an increased number of United States medical schools and the number of United States medical graduates. The immigration of IMGs supplemented this increase during the 1970s but contributed to an increasingly smaller proportion of this increase during the 1980s. In the 1990s, a new cycle of IMG growth is now the major factor contributing to the increase in physician supply. The obvious question related to the dramatic increase in supply over the last twenty-five years is why it was necessary to use a dual—domestic and foreign—strategy to achieve this. The answer is twofold: first, before the 1970s, policy makers and medical experts strongly believed that there was a serious shortage of physicians in the United States, with several studies estimating the shortage in 1975 to be in the range of 10,000 to 50,000. This set in motion unprecedented public and private spending to increase the capacity of the nation's medical education establishment.

Second, our nation has never had a coordinated physician personnel policy as has, for example, France or Canada; in particular, undergraduate and graduate medical education systems have operated largely independently of each other. Thus, the policy of increasing the number of United States medical schools and United States medical graduates has not been closely connected to the graduate medical training system. The result has been that students graduating from United States medical schools have filled a smaller proportion of available residencies positions, often leaving, as noted earlier, the less desirable positions (both for residencies and permanent employment) for IMGs (Mick, 1992; Mick & Worobey, 1984).

As the physician shortage was perceived to turn into a surplus, the number and proportion of IMGs fell to lower levels. Specialties once heavily populated by IMGs gained appreciable numbers of USMGs, and the number of unfilled residency positions almost disappeared. Most observers believed that IMGs were less able to compete against USMGs for scarcer residency slots. However, the nation has witnessed a reversal of all these trends. As noted, although the number of IMGs has soared, these foreign-trained physicians continue to serve in areas that USMGs continue to avoid; furthermore, in 1993, for example, the proportion of IMGs undertaking primary care residencies was about 54%, whereas the proportion of USMGs undertaking this kind of residency was about 32%. The argument that IMGs have used primary care as a base from which to subspecialize is not evident: in each of the residency training years between 1991 and 1994, the proportion of IMGs in internal medicine subspecialties was consistently less than the comparable proportion of USMGs. For instance, in the training year 1994–1995, 25% of IMGs were in the various subspecialties of internal medicine whereas 30% of USMGs were in these subspecialties. Still, an overall primary care specialty shortage appears to exist, and we now turn to this topic.

Trends in Specialty Distribution

Simply increasing physician supply has not guaranteed that necessary medical services would be readily available to the general population. Of particular interest is the availability of primary care—the entry level into the health care system where basic medical services are provided. Primary care includes the diagnosis and treatment of common illness and disease, preventive services, home care services, and uncomplicated minor surgery and emergency care.

The increased supply of physicians has not resulted in major changes in the proportion of physicians in primary care specialties—general practice, family practice, general internal medicine, and general pediatrics (Table 14–6). There has been substantial growth in primary care specialties both in absolute numbers and in percent: from 1980 to 1995, the number of primary care physicians has grown to over 45,000, an increase of 28%. But, the growth in *other* specialty groupings has been greater: over the period of 1986 to the year 2000, estimates are that, whereas primary care will increase by about 22%, other specialties will enjoy greater growth—the specialties of internal medicine, 50%; general surgery and surgical subspecialties, 27%; and all other specialties, 39%. Efforts in the 1970s to increase support for primary care residencies appear to have helped increase the proportion of all active primary care physicians only slightly to a little more than 38% in 1980. Since then, however, the proportion in primary care fell to 34% in 1986, and to 32.5% in 1995; it is estimated to drop to 32% by 2000. This decline is a major concern in view of the amount of public and private funding that has occurred during the last twenty-five years to increase the number and proportion of primary care physicians.

Despite these trends, there are those who argue that the nation is not in any urgent need for more primary care physicians or for any radical public policy effort to educate more (Whitcomb, 1995). Challenged is the proposition that the United States should have 50% of all physicians in primary care specialties (Council on Graduate Medical Education, 1994), and the rationale for the challenge is that in the early 1990s, the United States already had a physician to population ratio of about 69 per 100,000 population, which compared favorably with ratios in Canada, England,

TABLE 14–6 Number of active physicians (MDs) and percentage distribution by specialty groups: Selected years, 1980, 1986, 1995, 2000

Specialty	1980		1986		1995[b]		2000[b]		Percent Change 1986–2000
	Number	*Percent*	*Number*	*Percent*	*Number*	*Percent*	*Number*	*Percent*	
All specialties	414,916	100.0%	521,010	100.0%	630,670	100.0%	684,850	100.0%	31.4%
Primary care specialties[a]	159,922	38.5%	179,410	34.4%	205,200	32.5%	219,190	32.0%	22.2%
Other medical specialties	25,882	6.2%	62,530	12.0%	83,170	13.2%	93,940	13.7%	50.2%
Surgical specialties	110,778	26.7%	134,140	25.7%	158,970	25.2%	170,340	24.9%	27.0%
All other specialties	118,334	28.5%	144,930	27.8%	183,330	29.1%	201,380	29.4%	38.9%

a   Includes general practice, family practice, general internal medicine, and general pediatrics
b   Estimated

SOURCES: *Fifth Report to the President and Congress on the Status of Health Personnel in the United States* (DHHS Pub. No. HRS-P-OD-86-1), March 1986, Washington, DC: U.S. Government Printing Office; *Seventh Report to the President and Congress on the Status of Health Personnel in the United States* (DHHS Pub. No. HRS-P-OD-90-1) March 1990, Washington, DC: U.S. Government Printing Office; *Health Personnel in the United States: Eighth Report to Congress* (DHHS Pub. No. HRS-P-OD-92-1), 1992, Washington, DC: U.S. Government Printing Office.

and Germany, countries in which experts believed that an adequate number of primary care physicians existed. One conclusion is that it is not so much the number of primary care physicians that is the problem but rather the number of specialist physicians. The latter group should be reduced in number while the former group should be left alone.

Observers of the managed care phenomenon note that high market penetration of such plans is already producing change in the specialty composition of physicians in these markets. As managed care plans use more primary care "gate-keeper" physicians to care for patients and to make referrals to specialists, the demand for the former grows and for the latter decreases. Evidence of this is found in recruitment advertising for physicians: a study of seven medical journals from 1984 through 1995 showed a doubling of advertised positions for family medicine physicians and declines in positions for internal medicine specialists, pediatric specialists, anesthesiologists, pulmonologists, and ortho-

pedic surgeons, among others (Seifer, et al., 1996). Furthermore, many specialists find it to their advantage to redefine themselves as primary care providers, abandoning their specialty practices, and even going so far as to take "refresher" courses in basic patient care medicine. These market experiences have already sent signals to medical schools and residency training programs that a shift in training emphasis toward primary care is a major element in the ability of medical graduates to find employment opportunities.

Geographic Distribution of Physicians

One of the assumptions underlying federal health personnel policy in the 1960s and early 1970s was that a significant increase in the overall supply of physicians would both resolve the problem of a serious shortage and improve the geographic distribution of physicians. But although there is now debate between adherents of the surplus and shortage hypotheses, there is less debate about the persistent chronic shortages in rural and inner-city areas.

With the output of physicians from medical schools outpacing the growth of the United States population, the population/physician ratio declined from one physician per 840 people in 1960 to one per 513 people in 1980 and to one per 415 people in 1990. From 1960 to 1970, the vast majority of these physicians located in urban and suburban areas. However, the supply of physicians increased in both metropolitan statistical areas (MSAs) and non-MSAs after 1970 to the present day. Among the total population living in both MSAs and non-MSAs, there was a 28% decrease in the population/physician ratio during the period 1970–1983. Thus, there was some evidence in favor of the market "diffusion" theory that argued that an abundance of physicians in urban areas would cause movement of physicians in these crowded areas to less densely populated rural areas, provided that demand for medical services was present.

Policy makers have traditionally assumed that physicians, particularly specialists, would not locate in rural areas. Market forces have caused some change in the distribution of those specialists who were certified by one of twenty-three specialty boards, that is, medical societies that confirm via a number of procedures whether a physician is especially qualified to engage in his or her specialty. By the late 1970s, locales with populations of more than 20,000 had at least one board-certified physician in each of a variety of specialties, but communities with populations of fewer than 20,000 were not as likely to have physicians such as these, and counties with smaller populations still had difficulties in attracting physicians of any kind, be they board-certified or not. Rural counties with the smallest populations have gained a few new physicians, but today, in some states, counties without a primary care physician continue to exist.

The impact of specialization on the geographic distribution is not surprising. Until recently, general practitioners were the majority of physicians in rural areas. The supply of general practitioners has since almost disappeared, to be replaced in the late 1970s and 1980s by recently trained family medicine practitioners. Graduates of family medicine residency programs have located in non-MSA areas more frequently than other specialists, with, for example, 27% of family medicine residents who graduated in 1991 locating in towns of 25,000 people or fewer that were not within twenty-five miles of a large city. When one adds those graduate family medicine residents in the same size towns but within twenty-five miles of a large city, the proportion jumps to 42% (American Academy of Family Physicians, 1991). Family medicine practitioners appear to have become the new core of rural physician supply, particularly in smaller towns.

Physicians have been reluctant to locate in rural areas for reasons like lack of adequate medical facilities; professional isolation; limited support services; inadequate organizational settings including lack of group practices; excessive workloads and time demands; limits on earnings; lack of social, cultural, and educational opportunities; and spouse's influence (Gordon, et al., 1992). Efforts to improve the distribution of physicians have tried to address some of these factors.

Federal efforts to improve the distribution of physicians have included loan forgiveness, the National Health Service Corps, Area Health Education Centers (AHECs), and extensive support for the development of family practice training programs, among others (Ricketts, 1994). These programs have experienced a number of difficulties over the last fifteen years; many were severely cut back during the Reagan era and were only partially refunded during the Clinton administration. The Republican-dominated United States Congress has called for the dismantlement of most of these programs, including the successful AHECs. What the future holds for federal policy to improve physician distribution remains to be seen.

At the state level, there have been efforts to improve physician distribution through the authority of Offices of Rural Health in states like North Carolina, North Dakota, and Nevada. State-level policy has been aimed at increasing the recruitment and retention of health care providers in rural areas as well as cooperative ventures of consortia of states to decentralize medical education programs and coordinate placement of graduates.

Despite the variety of approaches to alter the urban/rural location of physicians, unequal distribution persists. Market forces have altered distribution to some degree, but many rural communities still find it difficult to recruit and retain physicians. The same is true for inner-city locations. Often those locales with the greatest need continue to have the biggest problems attracting physicians. As mentioned earlier, national bodies like the Institute of Medicine (1996) have called for a cutback in IMGs, and the Pew Health Professions Commission (1995) has even proposed a reduction in the number of United States medical schools. However, without specific programs aimed at increasing the number of physicians in underserved areas, it is difficult to see how a reduction in the overall number of physicians can do anything but worsen the historic problem of physician maldistribution.

Developing policies to alter physician distribution, therefore, has turned out to be a difficult undertaking. The limited impact of previous attempts suggests that broader policy options should be considered. The possibilities include changing reimbursement systems to provide a financial reward for physicians practicing in underserved areas. Another remedy might be to modify even more than has been done the admissions policies of medical schools in order to place more emphasis on applicants interested in primary care practice. Or undergraduate and graduate medical education systems could be changed to ensure that the curriculum, counseling, clinical setting, and role models presented are better related to health needs of the underserved. A revitalized and expanded National Health Service Corps might be one of the best short-term solutions to the distribution problem. Whatever steps are taken, a balance must be found between changing the size and composition of the physician workforce so that goals of improving physician distribution are not forgotten.

Changes in Medical Education

The past twenty-five-year period has been one of change for both undergraduate and graduate medical education. Change has occurred and is occurring in two general realms: the size and composition of students and the organization of medical education itself. In the first case, the stereotype of the typical medical student—a white urban male who will eventually practice a medical or surgical specialty in a large urban setting—has changed. In the second case, the relationship of medical schools to the rest of the health care sector has changed.

On the undergraduate level, from 1970–1971 to the current time, the first-year medical school class size increased by over 50%, with the 1994–1995 entering class totaling 17,048. First-year enrollments hovered in the 17,000 range throughout the 1980s and into the 1990s. Compared to the early 1970s, there is no question that United States medical schools responded to the call to increase the supply of physicians.

The undergraduate medical curriculum remains broad-based, with the first two years consisting of lectures and laboratory work in the basic sciences, followed by two years of work in the clinical sciences through seminars and work in hospital wards and clinics. The role models and values in most medical schools continue to emphasize acute care for hospitalized patients. This is changing, however, with the increase in ambulatory and noninstitutional services: more and more medical students are experiencing out-of-hospital training experiences. The professional socialization of medical students shows signs of changing, with more emphasis on preceptorships in primary care settings and shifts in the focus of a growing number of medical school faculty from research to the provision of patient care. The latter has occurred due to changes in the distribution of medical school funding resulting from a deemphasis on federal funding and greater reliance on state and local support as well as revenues from faculty practice plans.

Another important issue in the system of medical education concerns women and minority students. Concerted efforts to increase their enrollment have borne fruit: over the past twenty-five-year period, the first-year enrollment of female medical students has increased from 11.1% to 43.2%; total female enrollment increased from 9.6% to 41.8% (Table 14–7). A more modest, but significant, increase in minority students has been registered: from 1970–1971 to 1995–1996, the percentage of minority students in allopathic medical schools increased from about 9% to over 34% of all first-year students (Table 14–8). The greatest increase in minority students has been among Asian Americans, Native Americans, Hispanic Americans, and African Americans, in that order. For example, although African Americans increased their number by 119% over the twenty-five-year period just noted, Asian Americans increased over fourteen-fold. The presence of minority physicians is extremely important because it has been shown that minority patients are four times more likely to receive care from minority physicians than nonminority ones. Low-income, Medicaid recipients, and uninsured patients are also more likely to receive care from minority physicians (Moy & Bartman, 1995).

The graduate medical education "pipeline" has also undergone major changes in the last twenty-five years. The total number of residency positions increased significantly, from 65,615 in 1971 to 102,615 in 1995. The percentage of positions filled had increased until 1985 when only 1,696 posts, or 2% of the total, remained vacant. Since 1986, however, there has been an increasing percentage of unfilled posts to 5% in 1989 where it has stabilized

TABLE 14–7 Students in allopathic medical schools, by gender: Selected academic years, 1970–1971, 1980–1981, 1990–1991, 1995–1996

Academic Year	All First-Year Students	First-Year Female Students	Percent Female of First-Year Students	Total Students Enrolled	Total Female Students	Percent Female of Total Students
1970–1971	11,348	1,256	11.1%	40,487	3,894	9.6%
1980–1981	17,204	4,970	28.9%	65,497	17,373	26.5%
1990–1991	16,803	6,499	38.7%	64,986	24,164	37.2%
1995–1996	17,024	7,351	43.2%	66,906	27,976	41.8%

SOURCES: Adapted from the following: "Undergraduate Medical Education," by A. Crowley, S. Etzel, E. Petersen, et al., 1985, *Journal of the American Medical Association, 254,* pp. 1565–1572; "Educational Programs in U.S. Medical Schools," by H. Jonas, S. Etzel, & B. Barzansky, 1991, *Journal of the American Medical Association, 226,* pp. 913–923; "Programs in U.S. Medical Schools," by B. Barzansky, H. Jonas, & S. Etzel, 1996, *Journal of the American Medical Association, 276,* pp. 714–719.

through 1994 (5,408 unfilled positions, or 5%). As noted earlier, the declining proportion of IMGs in residency slots reversed itself about the same time as unfilled slots began to rise: the percent of IMGs in United States residency positions increased from 16% to 24%.

As for the organization of medical schools and their relationship to the rest of the health care sector, notable shifts have occurred. First and foremost, medical schools and their affiliated hospitals have been forced to compete for patients—both ambulatory and inpatient—by managed care plans. These plans, as noted earlier, do not bear the costs of medical education, nor do they sponsor basic clinical research; hence, they are able to underbid the prices that medical school–affiliated hospitals and health systems must charge to recover their costs. This phenomenon has produced both the downsizing of many medical schools and their affiliated hospitals as well as the merger of some others. For example, a number of medical school mergers have taken place in New York City and Philadelphia. Certain medical schools in California have considered mergers.

Another result of the increased competition felt by university medical centers is the willingness of some to affiliate with national for-profit hospital systems. For instance, in a number of states, the medical schools have developed leasing arrangements with for-profit systems to run teaching hospitals, to refurbish outdated facilities, to institute efficient management techniques, and generally to bring a new infusion of capital to hard-pressed teaching institutions. In return, the for-profit systems gain a foothold into the very heart of the United States medical education establishment. Observers view medical school and for-profit hospital system affiliations with mixed feelings. On the one hand, the for-profit systems bring a wealth of management expertise to often antiquated organizational arrangements and procedures; they also provide a means of allowing the medical centers to compete more effectively with the growing number of managed care plans. In fact, the teaching

TABLE 14–8 Minority students in the first year of allopathic medical school: Selected academic years, 1970–1971 through 1995–1996

Academic Year	All First-Year Students	Racial/Ethnic Category					Total Minority	Percent Minority of First-Year Students
		African American	Native American	Hispanic American	Asian American	Other Minority[a]		
1970–1971	11,348	697	11	100	190	—	998	8.8%
1975–1976	15,295	1,036	60	461	282	73	1,912	12.5%
1980–1981	17,186	1,128	67	818	572	—	2,585	15.0%
1985–1986	16,929	1,030	61	953	1,164	—	3,208	18.9%
1988–1989	16,868	1,210	76	949	2,100	—	4,335	25.7%
1995–1996	17,024	1,527	153	1,192	2,925	—	5,797	34.1%

a Data were not provided for the category "Other Minority" for certain years. Where data were provided, they include some persons counted under "Hispanic American."

SOURCES: *Minorities and Women in the Health Fields, 1990 Edition* (DHHS Pub. No. HRSA-P-DV-90-3), 1990, Washington, DC: U.S. Government Printing Office; Adapted from: "Educational Programs in U.S. Medical Schools, 1995–1996," by B. Barzansky, H. Jonas, & S. Etzel, 1996, *Journal of the American Medical Association, 276,* pp. 714–719.

hospitals often become part of a preexisting managed care plan that has already proven itself effective in the market. On the other hand, it was over eighty-five years ago that the famous Flexner Report urged the medical education community to rid itself of institutions that were run on a for-profit basis, arguing that the for-profit motive was inconsistent with the thorough and scientific training of physicians (Flexner, 1910). The mid-1990s is not the early part of the twentieth century, and conditions have changed such that the worry of the Flexner Report may be inappropriate today. However, there will probably be increasing discussion and debate about the propriety of for-profit organizations' involvement in medical education and to what degree the profit motive is compatible with the social welfare function of health care delivery.

In summary, undergraduate and graduate medical education has changed in the last twenty-five years. Even with a warning of a surplus of physicians, some of the recommendations of the final report of the GMENAC, such as a decrease in the size of medical school classes by 10% by 1984, were largely ignored. It is therefore not surprising that in the latter part of the 1990s, there should once again be renewed calls for reductions in the number of physicians in training and a greater emphasis on primary care specialization. Managed care competition may end up producing the reduction in medical education capacity at both the undergraduate and graduate levels that numerous blue-ribbon committees with their downsizing recommendations have been unable to achieve. These issues, joined to the debate engendered by the presence of IMGs in United States residencies, promise to keep the fundamental problems of the training and deployment of the physician workforce a number one policy issue as the country moves toward the twenty-first century.

OSTEOPATHY

Often neglected in discussions of medical personnel is the small but significant number of osteopaths in the United States. Osteopathy differs from allopathic medicine in that osteopaths traditionally emphasize treatments that involve corrections of the position of joints or tissues, and they stress diet or environment as factors that might destroy natural resistance. Allopathic medicine views the physician as an active interventionist attempting to neutralize effects of disease by using treatments that produce a counteracting effect. Despite these differences, osteopaths are licensed to practice medicine and perform surgery in all states, are eligible for graduate medical education in either osteopathic or allopathic residencies, and are reimbursed by both Medicare and Medicaid, the two major federal financing programs.

The growth in osteopaths has been great, but this is partially due to the small base number to begin with: in 1970, there were 12,700 osteopaths; in 1991, there were about 29,200, an increase of about 130%. The ratio of osteopaths to population was 11.6 to 100,000 (refer to Table 14–2). This figure is deceptive, however, because osteopaths are unevenly distributed around the country. Four of five osteopaths were located in just sixteen states, led by Michigan, Pennsylvania, Ohio, Florida, Texas, and New Jersey, in descending order. Hence, in states like these, osteopaths make a contribution to health care disproportionate to their overall number. Finally, although there were only 5 doctors of osteopathy per 100,000 in metropolitan areas in 1986, the rate in rural areas was six times as great, or 30 per 100,000 in nonmetropolitan areas. This is, of course, the opposite of allopathic physicians, whose ratio is larger in metropolitan than nonmetropolitan areas.

There are fifteen schools of osteopathy, and they are located, not surprisingly, in the states with the largest number of osteopaths. From 1975–1976 to

1992–1993, there was an increase in first-year class size of 96% (Table 14–9). There has been an increasing proportion of first-year female students over the same period (14% to 35%) as well as an increase in minority first-year students (5% to 20%). Since 1987, there have been more osteopaths in allopathic residency programs than in osteopathic programs, underlining the narrow difference between the two groups. Nearly 40% of osteopaths train in the primary care specialties of general internal medicine and general practice, although in 1990, of those osteopaths in actual practice, about 55% were in primary care. Combining these facts with osteopaths' location in specific states underscores their importance to health care delivery of primary care medicine.

In short, osteopathic medicine is a small but important form of medical practice that shares the burden of care with allopathic physicians. It has experienced the same changes, for example, increasing proportions of women and minorities and increasing numbers of applicants, as its larger cousin has undergone.

DENTISTRY: A PROFESSION IN TRANSITION

In 1991, there were approximately 155,000 active dentists practicing in the United States. The supply of dentists has been increasing during the past decade, and so has the ratio of active dentists to population: in 1960, the ratio was 49.4 per 100,000 population, and in 1991, 61.3 per 100,000 (Table 14–10). As in medicine, the increases that occurred can be attributed to federal legislation passed in the 1960s and early 1970s that directly attempted to remedy the perceived shortage. This legislation resulted in increases in the number of dental schools from 47 to 60 in the period 1960 to 1980 and an increase in the number of first-year dental students from 3,600 to more than 6,000 in the same period (Table 14–11). However, since 1980, the total number of dental schools and the first-year class dropped to 55 and 4,001, respectively, by 1990. In the 1992–1993 academic year, these numbers were virtually the same.

TABLE 14–9 First-year students by gender and minority status, graduates of osteopathic medical schools: Selected academic years, 1975–1976, 1980–1981, 1985–1986, 1987–1988, 1989–1990

Academic Year	First-Year Students Enrolled	First-Year Female Students	Percent Female of First-Year Students	First-Year Minority Students[a]	Percent Minority of First-Year Students	Total Number of Graduates
1975–1976	1,038	140	13.5%	55	5.3%	809
1980–1981	1,496	329	22.0%	99	6.6%	1,151
1985–1986	1,737	489	28.2%	185	10.7%	1,560
1990–1991	1,950	667	34.2%	385	19.7%	1,534
1992–1993	2,035	715	35.1%	398	19.6%	1,609

a   Includes African, Hispanic, Native, and Asian Americans

SOURCES: *Minorities and Women in the Health Fields, 1990 Edition* (DHHS Pub. No. HRSA-P-DV-90-3), 1990, Washington, DC: U.S. Government Printing Office; *Minorities and Women in the Health Fields, 1994 Edition* (HRSA-P-DV-94-2), 1994, Washington, DC: U.S. Government Printing Office.

TABLE 14–10 Total and active dentists and dentist/population ratios: Selected years, 1960 through 1991

Year	Number of Dentists[a]		Total Population (Thousands)	Active Dentists per 100,000 Population
	Total	Active		
1960	105,200	90,120	182,287	49.4
1970	116,250	102,220	206,466	49.5
1975	126,590	112,020	217,095	51.6
1980	147,280	126,240	228,831	55.2
1991	—	155,000	252,700	61.3

a   Includes dentists in federal service

SOURCES: *Fourth Report to the President and Congress on the Status of Health Personnel in the United States* (DHHS Pub. No. HRS-P-0084.4), May 1984, Washington, DC: U.S. Government Printing Office; *Seventh Report to the President and Congress on the Status of Health Personnel in the United States* (DHHS Pub. No. HRS-P-OD-90-1), March 1990, Washington, DC: U.S. Government Printing Office; *Health Personnel in the United States: Ninth Report to Congress,* 1993, Washington, DC: U.S. Government Printing Office.

Some of the recent trends that are descriptive of medical schools are also descriptive of dental schools. The percentage of female first-year students has soared from a mere 2% in 1970 to 35% in 1992 (Table 14–11). The proportion of minority students has also increased dramatically—from 3% in 1970 to 30% in 1992. Dental schools have started to deemphasize their support from federal sources and have increased their state support, dental clinic revenues, and fees from tuition. Also, as with medicine, there was a sizable decrease in the number of applicants to dental school in the 1980s, although the decline started earlier and was steeper for dentistry. Since 1975, when dental school applications peaked at 15,734, there was a steady decline until 1989 when 4,996 persons applied, yielding an applicant-admission ratio of only 1:3. Since then applications have increased so that for the 1991–1992 academic year, 5,632 persons applied for dental school. The decline, smaller class sizes, reductions in federal support, and increased costs have reduced the number of dental schools from 60 to 54.

Unlike their physician counterparts, dentists typically work in solo or small group private practices. Current economic pressures on the dental profession, however, have initiated changes in the delivery of dental services. During the 1980s, a variety of nontraditional practice settings emerged for dentists, including HMOs and retail locations in malls, stores, and plazas. Although only a small proportion of dental services is provided in these settings, this organizational innovation is an indication of the more competitive environment dentistry is facing in the mid-1990s.

The vast majority of dentists are in general practice. Only about one-seventh of all dentists are specialists, and the proportion of specialists has remained stable in recent years. Orthodontists comprise roughly one-third of all dental specialists, with oral surgeons totaling almost another one-fourth of the specialist population.

There is significant variation in the distribution of dentists across the regions of the United States and metropolitan versus nonmetropolitan areas. This variation is caused by the same factors that have led to physician maldistribution, as well as by

TABLE 14–11   Number of dental schools, students, including female and minority students, and graduates: Selected academic years, 1960–1961 through 1989–1990

Academic Year	Number of Schools	Number of Students[a] Total	First-Year	First-Year Female Students	Percent Female of First-Year Students	Total Minority Students	Percent Minority of Total Students	Total Number of Graduates[b]
1960–1961	47	13,580	3,616	—	—	—	—	3,290
1970–1971	53	16,553	4,565	94	2.1%	552[c]	3.3%	3,775
1980–1981	60	22,842	6,030	1,194	19.8%	2,453	10.7%	5,550
1990–1991	55	15,951	4,001	1,522	38.0%	4,766	29.9%	3,995
1992–1993	54	15,980	4,072	1,413	34.7%	4,794	30.0%	3,918[d]

a   Includes African, Hispanic, Native, Asian American, and, for 1970, "Other Minorities"
b   Excludes graduates of the University of Puerto Rico for 1960–1961 and 1970–1971
c   Estimated minority enrollment
d   Data for 1991–1992

SOURCES: *Minorities and Women in the Health Fields, 1990 Edition* (DHHS Pub. No. HRSA-P-DV-90-3), 1990, Washington, DC: U.S. Government Printing Office; *Health Personnel in the United States: Eighth Report to Congress, 1991* (DHHS Pub. No. HRS-P-OD-92.1), 1992, Washington, DC: U.S. Government Printing Office; *Health Personnel in the United States: Ninth Report to Congress, 1993*, Washington, DC: U.S. Government Printing Office; *Minorities and Women in the Health Fields, 1994 Edition* (DHHS Pub. No. HRSA-P-DV-94-2), 1994, Washington, DC: U.S. Government Printing Office.

the lack of reciprocity in the licensing of dentists across states. More than one-half of all dentists practice in the state in which they were trained, yet at least eighteen states have no school of dentistry. Those portions of the country that are most rural have the lowest dentist/population ratios: for example, in 1992, an urban state like Massachusetts had 79.9 dentists per 100,000 population whereas a rural state like Alabama had 44.2 per 100,000. In the late 1980s, there were over 700 federally designated dental shortage areas, approximately three-quarters of which were in nonmetropolitan areas.

In addition to the traditional maldistribution of dentists, there is concern that there may be a growing gap between the availability of dentists and the need for their services, especially since the financing of dental services is on a much smaller scale than that for physician services. Currently, less than

one-half of the United States population has dental insurance, and federal funds pay for less than two percent of all dental care (*Health Personnel in the United States: Ninth Report to Congress*, 1993). For example, Medicare pays for no dental services whatsoever. Other factors contributing to the gap include the following: (1) whereas fluoridation of water has reduced the number of dental caries and fillings needing replacement, about 75% of dental caries in children are concentrated in about 25% of the population, with disease levels higher among minority populations; (2) minority populations where dental problems appear to be concentrated and which have little, if any, dental insurance are expected to grow between the mid-1990s and 2020, thus potentially widening the gap between ability to pay and receipt of services; and (3) the ever-growing adult population, at greater risk for gingivitis and adult-onset periodontis (a major contributor to tooth loss), will need more dental services.

Auxiliary Personnel

The practice of dentistry has undergone major technological and organizational changes in the past several decades. Of particular importance has been the increased use of dental auxiliary personnel. The three major types of dental auxiliaries are dental hygienists, dental assistants, and dental laboratory technicians. Dental hygienists provide oral prophylaxis services and dental health education and comprise the only group of auxiliaries that is licensed. Dental assistants have generally supported the dentist at chairside and have had the opportunity in some states to perform expanded functions under the dentist's supervision. Dental laboratory technicians make oral appliances following the written prescriptions of dentists. In 1992, there were about 74,000 full- and part-time active dental hygienists, and roughly 200,000 dental assistants and 70,000 dental laboratory technicians.

Most dentists employ some dental auxiliary on a full- or part-time basis. The government has supported the training of expanded-function dental auxiliaries (dental hygienists or dental assistants who receive additional education and training that enable them to perform a broader array of clinical functions), as well as the training of dental students to help improve their administrative and organizational skills in managing multiple auxiliary team practices. Support for the auxiliary concept has been largely due to an increase in the productivity of dental practices that employ such persons.

Increasing educational and professional requirements for dental hygienists (they must carry their own malpractice insurance) have made them able to practice without the physical presence of a dentist, something allowed in forty states. There is evidence that these hygienists can provide greater access to dental services in underserved areas, at lower cost and without overall reduction in the quality of care. However, state regulations and the opposition of professional dentists' organizations do not favor the use of dental hygienists, and there is currently a struggle between dentists and dental hygienists over self-regulation and autonomy. This controversy will continue as long as the maldistribution of dentists persists and evidence continues to appear that dental hygienists can perform a variety of functions independently and inexpensively with no loss of quality.

Thus, the dental professions are in transition. The growth of dentists will continue but probably at a lower rate than other health professions. The financial condition of a number of the remaining fifty-four dental schools, especially private ones, is poor, and there may be more closures in the next several years, further reducing the growth of dentistry. The role of the expanded function dental auxiliary is still unclear. The demand for dental care is very sensitive to economic conditions (because dental insurance covers only two-fifths of the population and one-third of dental expenditures) and can decrease during recessionary periods. Hence, a shortage one year can quickly turn to a surplus the next. Yet, these economic conditions mask the epidemiological and demographic changes that are slowly altering the need for services. How these many factors combine to affect the future of dentistry should be watched closely.

PUBLIC HEALTH: NEW ROLES, NEW POSSIBILITIES

Traditionally, health professionals trained in public health have been sharply demarcated from those involved in the direct delivery of personal health services. Even so, the Institute of Medicine, in its landmark publication, *The Future of Public Health,* stated that the goal of public health activities was nothing less than assuring the conditions for people to be healthy (Institute of Medicine, 1988). In theory, then, there is a natural affinity between health professionals in public health and those in direct health care delivery.

In practice, public health roles have been centered on, among others, administration of local, state, and national public health agencies; planning, implementing, and evaluating prevention, screening, and health education programs; surveillance and control of environmental hazards and pollutants; and the epidemiological description and explanation for the incidence and prevalence of disease and trauma in populations. In certain settings, for example, municipal or county health departments, public health professionals have worked closely with other health professionals such as public health nurses in the delivery of primary care services to special populations such as indigent families, migrant workers, and groups of uninsured persons. In general, however, public health professionals have been a relatively "unseen" group of persons working to maintain a fundamental infrastructure allowing an understanding of and an implementation of health-promoting activities at the population level: safe drinking water, adequate sanitary systems, control of infectious diseases, and prevention of disease and injury-producing behavior such as smoking, high speed driving, and the like.

The principal training programs for careers in public health are located in the twenty-six accredited schools of public health, seven accredited health education programs, and eleven community medicine programs. Nearly four hundred other nonaccredited programs exist that offer training in the various subfields of public health such as health administration and environmental health. The primary academic degree is either the Master of Public Health (MPH) or the Master of Science in Public Health (MSPH). Other common avenues for careers in public health include the study of medi-

cine, with emphasis on and board certification in preventive medicine, and the study of public health nursing, dentistry, nutrition, industrial hygiene, or social work, among others. Advanced graduate training in some of the fields of public health, for example, epidemiology, environmental health sciences, health services research, health behavior and health education, and biostatistics, is normally obtained through the accredited schools of public health leading to the Doctor of Philosophy (Ph.D.), the Doctor of Public Health (Dr.P.H.), or the Doctor of Science (Sc.D.).

Total enrollment in schools of public health has nearly doubled over the period 1975–1976 to 1991–1992, growing from 6,461 to 12,032, respectively, an 86.2% increase. In 1990–1991, there were 3,903 graduates from these schools. Of the total of the students enrolled during the 1981–1982 academic year, 9.9% were members of underrepresented minority groups (African, Hispanic, and Native Americans); by the 1991–1992 academic year, this proportion had grown to 15.7%. The percent of women in the 1981–1982 total enrollment was 55.4%, whereas this percent was 65.9% by 1991–1992 (Bureau of Health Professions, 1993). Thus, during a period of major expansion in the number of students studying public health (public health ranked fourth in total enrollment after allopathic medicine, pharmacy, and dentistry), there was significant growth of opportunity for historically underrepresented minorities (116% increase) and women (63%) during the decade of the 1980s.

New Roles for Public Health Professionals

The melding of public health functions with those of professionals in the direct delivery of personal health services is now underway with the expansion of managed care plans. As explained in other chapters in this text, managed care plans assume the responsibility for the health care of defined populations of enrollees within a budgetary system constrained by capitation arrangements, that is, a prospectively fixed payment for each enrollee for a defined period of time, usually one year. Because the financing system no longer permits an open-ended cost-based billing for services to insurers, the managed care plan has clear incentives to find ways to deliver health care services efficiently and, more to the point here, to find ways to keep the covered population healthier in the first place.

This function is part of the fundamental mission of public health: collect information on and monitor disease incidence and prevalence of the plan's enrollees; monitor the outcome of the health care delivery process; and develop, implement, and monitor programs of prevention and other forms of positive intervention into the health habits and behavior of the plan's enrollees, for example, smoking and diet, receipt of prenatal care, immunization against infectious diseases, and the like. To the extent that managed care plans emphasize these traditional public health roles, the plans may well be the catalysts for the integration of public health and personal health services that has long been called for in the United States. But because of traditional insurance schemes based on retrospective cost-based reimbursement and because of deep professional fissures between some health professionals and public health professionals, among other reasons, this integration has proceeded very slowly.

In short, more than ever, future careers in public health promise to join community-based practice—the historical purview of public health—and the institutional practice of the healing arts. The task of disease prevention and health maintenance promises to force integration of these two domains. However, if universal entitlement to health care via a comprehensive health insurance program fails to

materialize, there will continue to be a need for traditional community-based public health specialists involved in meeting needs of disadvantaged groups.

NURSING

Registered nurses are the largest group of licensed health care professionals in the United States. The supply of registered nurses (RNs) grew from 1,662,382 in 1980 to over 2,033,032 in 1988, an increase of 22%. By 1992, the *active,* that is, employed, supply of RNs was 1,853,042, a number considerably less than the overall figure four years earlier. This reflects a major feature of the nursing workforce: a substantial number of nurses not working in nursing or inactive in the economic workforce.

Profiles show that most nurses are women, with less than 5% of the RN workforce being male. About seven of ten nurses are married, and less than 10% are from minority groups. Over 40% of RNs are diploma school graduates, usually from hospital-based programs. The shifting education pattern of RNs, with increasing emphasis on a four-year baccalaureate degree, is discussed in greater detail below.

Despite the overall absolute increase in the number of nurses employed in nursing, there has been until recently a consensus that a shortage of nurses existed relative to demand. Data from the early 1990s indicated that the shortage may have been easing: in 1991, for example, the national average RN vacancy rate in hospitals was 8.7%; the previous year it had been 11% (*Health Personnel in the United States: Ninth Report to Congress,* 1993). And, as will be discussed, with the increased employment of RNs in nursing homes and in home health agencies, the general picture shows improvement compared with what it was in the late 1980s. Understanding the causes of the apparently cyclical nature of the imbalance between supply and demand for nurses is not easy. Some have pointed to the large number of inactive nurses as the main reason for the fluctuation: economic forces cause nurses to enter and leave the workforce when required. The labor force participation of nurses, however, is similar to that of women in comparable professions, and so the existence of a pool of inactive nurses may not in itself be the key reason. What may be more fundamental are the personal characteristics and the persistent position of women in society as influences on nurses' ability and desire to work. Only about 8% of unemployed nurses actively seek nursing employment; the vast majority of unemployed nurses are over fifty years of age or are married with children at home (Levine & Moses, 1982). One job characteristic that does appear to influence nurse employment is salary (Aiken, 1982). Nurses are not paid well relative to their training and responsibilities, and thus when there has been a shortage, it has been termed a shortage due to lagging salaries.

Approximately one-third of employed nurses work part-time, and the majority of these are married with children at home. Although concern has also been focused on nursing attrition due to "burn-out" or poor working conditions, or both, surveys indicate that only a small number of nurses work in other professions. Thus, the shortages of nurses cannot simply be attributed to increases in the number of part-time workers or attrition from the profession.

In any event, there has been an easing of the nursing shortage. For example, nearly 83% of RNs were employed in nursing in 1992, up from 77% in 1980, 79% in 1984, and 80% in 1988. The total number of nursing graduates, while having fallen throughout the 1980s, has registered increases in the 1990s. Unpublished data for 1991–1992 show about 82,000 graduates, a 13% increase from the 1990–1991 figure. The annual number of nursing graduates was much lower in the late

1980s, reaching a low of 61,660 in 1988–1989. The demand for nursing services from the non–acute care sector, for example, long-term care for the growing number of chronically ill persons, home health care services, and preventive care, seems to have abated somewhat. Coupled with the downsizing and merging activities of many acute care facilities which often entail cutbacks in nursing personnel, the supply of nurses may, for the moment at least, have moved toward an equilibrium with demand.

Like most health care professionals, nurses are not distributed evenly throughout the United States. For example, in 1991, the RN/population ratio in the United States was 697/100,000 population. New York state's ratio was 823/100,000, whereas Arkansas's ratio was 506/100,000. The maldistribution appears to be due to the geographic immobility of women who are married and second wage earners in a family, as well as the inability of rural and inner-city hospitals and other facilities to offer an adequate range of incentives (for example, flexible working hours, increased salaries, fringe benefits, and safe working conditions) to attract nurses.

Rural institutions have found that urban-based education and training programs often have not been relevant to rural needs. Rural hospitals must frequently hire recent nursing graduates with limited skills and often resort to dependence on pool nurses from temporary employment agencies. This problem is of particular concern because of the increased responsibilities and range of skills needed by rural nurses. In the near future, rural providers are not likely to improve their chances of attracting well-trained nurses with a broad range of skills. Still, cooperative efforts by state government and local providers can often make a difference in the presence of RNs. South and North Dakota, rural states with traditional shortages of physicians, have managed to achieve nurse/population ratios well above the national average: 910 and 976 per 100,000, respectively.

Nursing Education and Role Changes

The federal government was largely responsible for the increases in nursing school class size over the period 1960–1980, having spent about $2.0 billion for nursing education. The more than doubling of the admissions to nursing schools over this period is eloquent testimony to this (Table 14–12). The growth in admissions slowed considerably between

TABLE 14–12 Admissions to schools offering initial programs in registered nursing by type of program, 1960–1961, 1970–1971, 1980–1981, 1984–1985, 1989–1990, 1990–1991

Academic Year	Baccalaureate[a]	Diploma	Associate Degree	Total
1960–1961	8,674	38,460	2,085	49,219
1970–1971	20,299	28,792	29,433	78,524
1980–1981	35,808	17,494	56,899	110,201
1984–1985	39,573	14,875	63,776	118,224
1990–1991	33,437	10,220	69,869	113,526
1991–1992	37,886	10,691	74,079	122,656

a Includes students in a few generic programs leading to a masters' or doctoral degree

SOURCES: *Fourth Report to the President and Congress on the Status of Health Personnel in the United States* (DHHS Pub. No. HRS-P-0084.4), May 1984, Washington, DC: U.S. Government Printing Office; *Seventh Report to the President and Congress on the Status of Health Personnel in the United States* (DHHS Pub. No. HRS-P-OD-90-1), March 1990, Washington, DC: U.S. Government Printing Office; *Health Personnel in the United States: Eighth Report to Congress, 1991* (DHHS Pub. No. HRS-P-OD-92-1), 1992, Washington, DC: U.S. Government Printing Office; *Factbook Health Personnel United States* (DHHS Pub. No. HRSA-P-AM-93-1), 1993, Washington, DC: U.S. Government Printing Office; *Minorities and Women in the Health Fields, 1994 Edition* (DHHS Pub. No. HRSA-P-DV-94-2), 1994, Washington, DC: U.S. Government Printing Office.

1980 and the early 1990s, but there continues to be growth nonetheless. Of particular interest, however, is the switch that has occurred in the control of nursing education from the hospital to nursing educators in colleges and universities.

Three forms of training lead to licensure as an RN: three-year diploma programs that are hospital-based, two-year associate degree programs that are generally in community colleges, and four-year baccalaureate nursing programs in universities or four-year colleges. As Table 14–12 indicates, in 1991–1992, only 10,691 (9%) of new nursing students were enrolled in diploma programs; in 1960–1961, the percentage had been 78.

In contrast to the other health professions discussed in this chapter, for reasons that are not clear, the supply of RNs has not included as great a proportion of minority group members. Table 14–13 shows that in recent years, from 15–16% of RN students were members of minority groups. From 1989 through 1991, the percentage has actually declined slightly, despite the dramatic increase in students from 201,458 to 257,983 persons. The largest minority group—African Americans—grew from about 7% in 1980 to a peak of over 10% in 1989; however, this percentage has declined ever since. Why the field of nursing should lack the appeal to minorities that other health professions appear to have remains an unanswered question, deserving inquiry and remedy.

The major employment patterns now and in the future are shown in Table 14–14. The hospital is and will remain the major locus of employment for RNs, sectioning off about two-thirds of the nursing workforce. Nursing home employment is expected to increase in importance, whereas other areas of employment will show stability over the period 1995–2005. These figures may appear to contradict the notion that non–hospital-based employment is gaining in popularity; however, since many hospitals are themselves involved in owning and

TABLE 14–13   Students in nursing schools (RN only), by minority status, 1980–1981 and 1989–1990

Academic Year	All Students	African American	Percent African American of Total	Hispanic American	Percent Hispanic American of Total	Asian American	Percent Asian American of Total	Native American	Percent Native American of Total	Percent Minority of Total
1980–1981	219,188	14,365	6.6%	5,785	2.6%	—	—	—	—	—
1989–1990	201,458	20,789	10.3%	6,046	3.0%	5,201	2.6%	1,064	0.5%	16.4%
1990–1991	237,598	21,529	9.1%	7,349	3.1%	6,947	2.9%	1,700	0.7%	15.8%
1991–1992	257,983	22,147	8.6%	7,667	3.0%	8,306	3.2%	1,685	0.7%	15.4%

SOURCES: *Health Personnel in the United States: Eighth Report to Congress* (DHHS Pub. No. HRS-P-OD-92-1), 1992, Washington, DC: U.S. Government Printing Office; *Minorities and Women in the Health Fields, 1994 Edition* (DHHS Pub. No. HRSA-P-DV-94-2), 1994, Washington, DC: U.S. Government Printing Office.

TABLE 14–14   Estimated and projected requirements for full-time equivalent registered nurses by employment setting, 1990, 1995, 2000, 2005

Field of Employment	Estimated 1990	Percent	Estimated 1995	Percent	Projected 2000	Percent	Projected 2005	Percent
Registered nurse total	1,466,000	100.0%	1,610,200	100.0%	1,735,400	100.0%	1,854,300	100.0%
Hospital	1,009,700	68.9%	1,086,600	67.5%	1,155,700	66.6%	1,224,700	66.0%
Nursing home	105,300	7.2%	130,300	8.1%	157,300	9.1%	183,100	9.9%
Home health	53,000	3.6%	57,000	3.5%	60,900	3.5%	64,400	3.5%
Other community/ public health	111,900	7.6%	136,700	8.5%	149,000	8.6%	157,600	8.5%
Ambulatory care	101,200	6.9%	107,200	6.7%	111,500	6.4%	115,600	6.2%
Other	84,900	5.8%	92,400	5.7%	101,000	5.8%	108,900	5.9%

SOURCE: *Health Personnel in the United States: Eighth Report to Congress* (DHHS Pub. No. HRS-P-OD-92-1), 1992, Washington, DC: U.S. Government Printing Office.

operating non–hospital-based services (such as home health services and ambulatory care sites), these figures may not reveal the true picture. Within these settings, new roles have emerged for the RN. These include clinical nurse specialist, nurse practitioner, nurse anesthetists, and nurse clinician. These positions involve employment in new ambulatory cares settings (for example, managed care plans, ambulatory surgery centers, freestanding urgent care centers, and the like), nursing homes, and home care programs providing care for the elderly and others with chronic illness. Nurses are also finding opportunities in statewide, regional, and hospital-level utilization and quality review roles in which they participate in inspection of clinical records describing patient care.

The nursing profession is attempting to change its broader role in the health care system, calling for an expansion of the *independent* role of the nurse within institutional settings and the creation of new professional roles outside them. Nurses are seeking to clarify their relationship to physicians, particularly within the context of clinical decision making in the hospital. They have developed new delivery modes, such a primary nursing, in which the nurse assumes direct responsibility for comprehensive care for a group of patients over a given period of time.

Nursing professionals want to control their future. They are trying to shed the traditional stereotype of the nurse as underpaid female hospital laborer. In the process, considerable controversy has been created both inside and outside the profession. This is often most visible when labor collective bargaining groups attempt to unionize nurses, forcing to the surface the ambivalence many nurses feel between being a highly skilled professional delivering personalized services versus an underpaid employee in a bureaucratic health care organization. Associate degree and diploma graduates want to continue to function in viable roles within the nursing profession. Institutions want to employ combinations of nursing personnel suitable to their particular environments. These forces, as well as the current restrictive interpretation of state nurse practice acts, suggest that there will be no easy solutions to changing and, one hopes, strengthening the future relationships among nurses, physicians, and health care organizations.

PHARMACISTS

As is the case for all of the health professional groups discussed so far, pharmacists are also undergoing extensive change. Until recently, pharmacists performed the traditional role of preparing drug products and filling prescriptions. In the 1980s and 1990s, pharmacists expanded that role to include acting as an expert for clients and patients about the effects of specific drugs, drug interaction, and generic drug substitutions for brand-name drugs.

This role has even expanded to include selecting, monitoring, and evaluating appropriate drug regimens and providing information not only to patients but also to other health care professionals. Finally, in their role as businessmen and women, pharmacists have had to learn more about the managerial and financial aspects of working in a retail trade.

There has been steady growth in the number of pharmacists during the last quarter-century, although the percentage growth has not been as great as in other health care professions (Table 14–15). From 1973–1974 to 1991–1992, there was a 45% increase in the overall number. First-year enrollment in pharmacy schools leveled off during the 1980s, although there was a major increase in the proportion of female first-year students, from about 30% in 1973–1974 to about 63% in 1991–1992. The growth of minorities in pharmacy, although not as great, has been steady, increasing from about 12% in 1980–1981 to 21% in 1991–1992. Another phenomenon of note is the popularity of Doctorate in Pharmacy programs, which lead not only to research and teaching positions but also to levels of higher administrative responsibility, often in health care organizations and managed care plans.

Pharmacists are employed in a number of settings, but the growth of chain drugstores has had a notable impact. As the 1990s began, about 40% of all pharmacists were employed in chains. Over the decade of the 1980s, the proportion of new pharmacy graduates hired by chains increased from about 27% to 42%. About 40% of the remainder of graduates worked in hospitals and independent pharmacies.

Forces that may contribute to an increase in the need for pharmacists include the increased use of drugs, especially among the growing aged population, and pharmacy's expanded role under changes in the Medicaid program that require review of

TABLE 14–15   Number of active pharmacists and number of pharmacy students, by gender and minority status: Selected academic years, 1973–1974, 1980–1981, 1990–1991, 1991–1992

Academic Year	Total Active Pharmacists	First-Year Students[a]	First-Year Female Students[a]	Percent Female of First-Year Students[a]	Total Graduates	Total Minority Graduates	Percent Minority of Total Graduates
1973–1974	112,600	8,342	2,508	30.1%	5,957	—	—
1980–1981	142,400	7,551	3,655	48.4%	7,323	891	12.2%
1990–1991	161,900	8,356	4,926	59.0%	7,122	1,461	20.5%
1991–1992	163,600	8,664	5,470	63.1%	7,113	1,501	21.1%

a   Includes students in the first year of the three years of pharmacy education, excluding any students in prepharmacy years

SOURCES: *Minorities and Women in the Health Fields, 1990 Edition* (DHHS Pub. No. HRSA-P-DV-90-3), 1990, Washington, DC: U.S. Government Printing Office; *Health Personnel in the United States: Eighth Report to Congress* (DHHS Pub. No. HRS-P-OD-92-1), 1992, Washington, DC: U.S. Government Printing Office; *Minorities and Women in the Health Fields, 1994 Edition* (DHHS Pub. No. HRSA-P-DV-94-2), 1994, Washington, DC: U.S. Government Printing Office; *Factbook: Health Personnel in the United States* (DHHS Pub. No. HRSA-P-AM-93-1), 1993, Washington, DC: U.S. Government Printing Office.

patient drug use and patient counseling. Nevertheless, making projections about the future supply of pharmacists in relation to future need or demand is difficult because of the rapidly changing employment circumstances in the field. Further, the aging of the American population would suggest that more medication prescriptions will be written and more work for pharmacists will result. At the same time, because pharmacists are expanding their role to include nontraditional activities, as mentioned, the amount of time an individual pharmacist might spend in traditional "druggist" activities will probably decline. With computerized information processing systems, assistance from pharmacy technicians, and mail order approaches that pharmacists will be using in increasing numbers, one would expect a positive gain in productivity, and perhaps a diminished need for an increased supply. In short, a number of factors make predicting the future balance of supply and demand difficult, and given the importance of drug therapies for modern medical care, policy makers should watch this important health profession closely.

PHYSICIAN ASSISTANTS (PAs) AND NURSE PRACTITIONERS (NPs)

The perceived shortage of physicians in the mid-1960s led to the development of two types of health care providers: physicians assistants (PAs) and nurse practitioners (NPs). PAs are qualified by academic and practical training to provide patient services under the direction and supervision of a licensed physician who is responsible for the performance of the PA. PAs are able to diagnose, manage, and treat common illnesses; provide preventive services; and respond appropriately to common emergency situations. Laws and regulations in all states (except Mississippi) and the District of Columbia now authorize the use of PAs under a physician's supervision. Thirty-four states, as well as the District of Columbia, allow delegation by a physician to the PA the authority to prescribe certain medications. The typical PA training program consists of two years of didactic study followed by clinical training. Programs vary widely, however, in terms of admission requirements, curriculum, and site of educational training. There were fifty-nine accredited PA programs in the early 1990s, and of the 27,000 persons having received PA training, 23,300 were in practice as of mid-1993.

After declining slightly from 2,600 to 2,400 students enrolled in PA training programs during most of the 1980s, the number of students has surged dramatically to over 3,800 during the academic year 1992–1993. There is a tendency for PAs more often than physicians to serve in rural and medically underserved areas, with about 34% of PAs working in communities of less than 50,000. Although men represent more than one-half (58%) of practicing PAs, women now make up more than one-half of all newly graduating PAs. Most PAs are white, non-Hispanic (91%) with the remainder consisting mostly of underrepresented minorities.

In 1983, there were 3,807 PAs employed in United States hospitals, and by 1990, there were 5,315, a 40% increase. Still, only one-third of PAs work in hospitals, with the majority located in ambulatory care settings; however, the percentage of PAs in hospital settings varies widely by state, with, for example, Connecticut having over 50% of PAs versus California, with 9%, in hospitals. Most PAs work in the private sector (81%), and about 12% work for the federal government including the Veterans Administration, the armed forces, and the United States Public Health Service. Finally, the proportion of PAs working in primary care settings has declined over the period 1978 to 1991, from 67% to 43%. General surgery, surgical subspecialties, orthopedics, and emergency medicine all registered increases. There appears to be a correlation between specialization of this sort and states that do not allow physician delegation of prescription writing to PAs.

NPs are registered nurses who have completed formal programs of study preparing them for expanded roles and responsibilities. These roles include obtaining comprehensive health histories, assessing health status, performing physician examinations, formulating and managing a care regimen for acute and chronically ill patients, teaching, and counseling (Abdellah, 1982). As of 1992, there were some 48,200 NPs in the United States.

There are a range of training programs for NPs, including pediatric, nurse-midwife, family, adult, psychiatric, and geriatric programs. At the beginning of the 1990s, there were 212 NP training programs with enrollments approaching 23,000 persons, nearly three-fourths of whom were part-time students. The focus of training for about 63% of students has been advanced clinical practice, with nearly one-fourth in medical-surgical specialties, 15% in maternal and child specialties, and the remainder in psychiatric–mental health, community health, and gerontological specialties. Of the 37% not in advanced clinical practice, 13% focused on teaching and nearly one-fourth on administration and management (*Health Personnel in the United States: Ninth Report to Congress*, 1993).

There are important differences in the perceptions of the roles of PAs and NPs. PAs are viewed by the medical profession as physician "extenders" who can perform many of the usual functions completed by physicians. Nurses view NPs as registered nurses in an expanded role. This includes greater supervision of and responsibility for primary patient care, with extra emphasis on the traditional nursing values of prevention and counseling. Despite these perceptual differences, as well as differences in education, training, and outlook, many of the performance characteristics of PAs and NPs appear to be similar.

Issues in PA and NP Use

Among the issues that need to be resolved before PAs and NPs can be used to their full capacity and original promise are legal restrictions concerning practice, reimbursement policies, and relationships with physicians. The legal status of PAs and NPs varies considerably across states. As noted in the case of PAs, many states permit considerable delegation of tasks and responsibilities, including prescribing certain drugs. State legislation expanding medical delegation has been unduly restrictive with regard to the scope of practice of qualified nonphysicians, although progress is being made.

Laws and regulations governing the expanded role of the nurse practitioner are also changing rapidly but inconsistently. Although the majority of states have altered their nurse practice acts to facilitate expanded roles, the constraints on the scope of NP practice continue to vary from state to state. A particular barrier is whether an individual state will authorize prescription practices of NPs. Although more than forty states have explicit regulatory provision for limited prescriptive authority, these authorizations vary in the degree of independence and in the types of drugs and devices that may be prescribed. There may also be geographic limitations, for example, more NP discretion in rural than urban settings.

Third-party reimbursement imposes another constraint on the use of PAs and NPs. Current policies generally link their reimbursement directly to the employing physician or institution. Since 1989, federal law requires direct Medicaid reimbursement for pediatric NPs and family NPs whether or not the NP is directly supervised by a physician. Many states, however, are not yet in compliance with federal legislation. As for the private health insurance sector, some states have laws allowing reimbursement to NPs, but this coverage is usually optional and is not widespread. Some progress has been made in reimbursement of NPs

and PAs through the Medicare program. For example, in 1989, the United States Congress, in its mandate that a Resource-Based Relative Value Scale (RBRVS) fee schedule supplant the usual and customary schedule for physician payment under Medicare Part B, called for study of including "nonphysician providers" in the fee schedule. Experimental programs are under review and may lead to a special reimbursement schedule.

A final area of concern is current and future relations with physicians. In the past, physicians were reasonably accepting of these personnel. Yet, about the time that these mid-level practitioners were becoming popular among those seeking a lower-cost substitute for physician services, the physician surplus was discovered, and physicians were wary of employing personnel who might take away their work. Further, there was, as noted earlier in this chapter, a tendency for some physicians to move into previously medically underserved areas.

Yet, slowly, there has been an increase in NPs and PAs, and much of the current demand has been generated by managed care plans whose efforts to cut costs, find flexibility in deployment of caregivers, and emphasize primary care and prevention coincide with the lower salaries, the broad skill set, and the training that are typical of NPs and PAs. Further, there are many roles that these mid-level professionals have been filling and continue to fill: providing primary care to underserved populations often in underserved areas as well as care to the elderly and the mentally ill, providing preventive care and health education, and delivering specialty services in hospitals in lieu of house staff. New practice settings for NPs and PAs include schools, industrial settings, prisons, and nursing homes.

The outcome of the current debate about the physician surplus and the role of IMGs in the physician workforce will be consequential for PAs and NPs. If efforts are successful in reducing the growth of physician supply, the employment of these mid-level health professionals will be enhanced throughout the health care system. If the physician workforce is not reduced in number, the historic barriers to PAs and NPs will continue to provide difficulty for attainment of the full promise of PA and NP service delivery.

THE CHANGING NATURE OF HEALTH PROFESSIONALS

This chapter has summarized trends in the supply of health professionals. From the 1960s into the early 1980s, federal and state support resulted in large increases in the number of graduates of most health professional occupations. From the mid-1980s to the present time, the growth of some occupational groups, for example, PAs and NPs, has probably been affected as much by the workforce requirements of managed care plans as by any public policy effort. Simultaneously, women and minorities have greatly benefited from this overall growth. During much or part of the 1980s, there was stability and even decline in the number of applicants to various health professional training programs (for example, medicine, nursing, and dentistry), but these trends have been reversed in many instances, with a new phase of growth in a number of fields.

The federal and state investment in health care personnel improved access to health care and helped schools training health professionals to remain financially viable. The reduction of government spending for the health professions has been caused by the reallocation of these funds to other portions of federal and state budgets and by the belief that a surplus of many types of health professionals existed. Many of the major trends affecting the United States health care system, such as restrictive public and private sector reimbursement and the growth of alternative delivery systems and managed care plans, portend continuing pressures against health professions growth. Still, as noted, the demand for training in almost all the health professions has increased dramatically from the downturn of the mid- to late-1980s, all of which suggests a restrictive labor market with employment opportunities less abundant than in the past decade.

The increasing number of women in all of the health professions also suggests that, on balance, with the rise of single-parent households and the continued disproportionate household and child-rearing responsibilities that married or single working mothers bear, female health professionals, particularly physicians, will probably work fewer hours per week and fewer weeks per year than men. This could add up to a need for more personnel to make up desirable levels of full-time equivalent labor. For example, if the proportion of women entering medicine continues at the current pace, the effective full-time equivalent supply of physician services will decline by about 4% between 1986 and 2010, other things being equal (Kletke, et al., 1990). On the other hand, the increase in managed care plans with their efficient use of health care personnel will produce a countervailing force in relation to overall numbers of health care professionals. Such conflicting forces make predicting the balance between need and demand versus supply of health professionals a very difficult enterprise.

THE IMPACT OF MANAGED CARE

Managed care deserves the final comment in this chapter's conclusion. More than perhaps would have been predicted even four or five years ago, the rapid growth of managed care plans and in the number of Americans enrolled in these plans has become a major force reshaping the size and composition of the health care professions work-force. In the immediate future, there are at least four important consequences of managed care on the workforce (Council on Graduate Medical Education, 1995b). First, more and more health professionals will have some sort of relationship with managed care. For example, most physicians are now involved in managed care either as full-time employees or as contractors with one or more plans. Over three-fourths of all physicians are esti-mated to have at least one managed care contract. This trend appears irreversible.

Second, many observers feel that continued managed care growth will only magnify and exac-erbate the problem of a provider surplus, particu-larly among physicians. Furthermore, there is worry that the historical imbalance between prima-ry care and specialization will be worsened. However, market pressures from the plans are already having an impact in favor of medical stu-dent and resident choice of primary care medicine and away from other specialties.

Third, many educational institutions will expe-rience severe financial difficulty as managed care plans erode their patient bases. That is, managed care plans that historically have had little if any involvement with education and training are underbidding educational institutions such as uni-versity medical schools which have had higher per patient expenses because of the costs of training. What the impact of this pressure will be is hard to predict. Some likely results include lower clinical income for teaching organizations, and, hence, lower health professional income. There may be a reduction in the number of training sites for health professional students. Educational institutions will move to employ the lowest-paid health profession-als who can practice within a given level of patient care. The open-ended growth of clinical diagnostic and treatment capacity will surely be dampened.

Fourth, the education that health professionals receive will probably witness a shift to the kind of clinical practice that health plans require. Those educational institutions that have not already adapted to these new demands are showing them-selves to be obsolete and are placing themselves at risk for organizational failure. This emphasis will consist of prevention, treatment of the whole per-son and not simply one or the other organ systems, prudent exercise of diagnostic and treatment approaches in which efficiency and cost-effective-ness are key, emphasis on "evidence-based" care in which preferred treatment approaches will have predictably positive and clear-cut outcomes, reliance on provider teams with more integration of different skill sets, and the like.

Until the time that such education becomes the norm, some health professionals will be ill-equipped to provide services in managed care plans. Further, the cost-savings pressures on man-aged care plans may lead some to overload primary caregivers with more work than they can handle and to pressure primary caregivers to accept clinical responsibilities that are beyond their purview and training. Taken together, the educational content and work requirements that managed care plans demand will place a heavy challenge on health pro-fessional training programs of all types.

In the longer run, these problems will probably be addressed by all the health professions because the market pressure that managed care plans exert is perhaps stronger than even the combined lobby-ing ability of organized medicine, medical schools, nursing, and the like. Adaptation will occur, but its shape is hard to anticipate. One intriguing hypoth-esis that must be entertained is whether attempts already underway in the medical profession to limit growth in physician supply will eventually work against managed care plans as they are currently controlled. Steady growth in physician supply did not begin until the early 1970s, about the same time that steady growth in managed care began. Although certainly not the only factor that has spurred managed care growth, an increase in the supply of physicians has been a key component of managed care success: more physicians finding it difficult to start private practices and, once started, to attract sufficient patient bases have turned to managed care employment. If medicine reduces its growth and thus moves toward relative scarcity, it may well be able to exert its control over its employers. Although this particular scenario is speculative, what is not speculative is the interactive nature of all the health professions and delivery organizations and the often surprising outcomes of that interaction. The future presents a vastly different possibility than that predicted when the 1990s began, and the trends that emerge will be of the greatest interest.

REFERENCES

Abdellah, F. (1982). The nurse practitioner 17 years later: Present and emerging issues. *Inquiry, 5,* 470–497.

Aiken, L. (1982). The impact of federal health policy on nurses. In L. Aiken (Ed.), *Nursing in the 1980s: Crises, opportunities, challenges.* Philadelphia: Lippincott.

American Academy of Family Physicians. (1991). *Report on survey of 1991 graduating family practice residents.* Washington, DC: Author.

Bureau of Health Professions, Health Resources and Services Administration. (1993). *Factbook: Health personnel in the United States* (DHHS Pub. No. HRSA-P-AM-93-1). Washington, DC: U.S. Government Printing Office.

Council on Graduate Medical Education. (1994). *Fourth report to Congress and the Department of Health and Human Services secretary: Recommendations to improve access to health care through physician workforce reform.* Washington, DC: U.S. Government Printing Office.

Council on Graduate Medical Education. (1995a). *Seventh report to Congress and the Department of Health and Human Services secretary: Recommendations for Department of Health and Human Services' programs.* Washington, DC: U.S. Government Printing Office.

Council on Graduate Medical Education. (1995b). *Sixth report to Congress and the Department of Health and Human Services secretary: Managed health care: Implications for the physician workforce and medical education.* Washington, DC: U.S. Government Printing Office.

Flexner, A. (1910). *Medical education in the United States and Canada: A report to the Carnegie Foundation for the Advancement of Teaching* (Bull. No. 4). New York: The Carnegie Foundation.

Gordon, R. J., Meister, J. S., & Hughes, R. G. (1992). Accounting for shortages of rural physicians: Push and pull factors. In W. M. Gesler & T. C. Ricketts (Eds.), *Health in rural North America: The geography of health care services and delivery* (pp. 153–178). New Brunswick, NJ: Rutgers University Press.

Graduate Medical Education National Advisory Committee. (1980). *Report to the Secretary, DHHS, Vol. I; GMENAC summary report* (DHHS Pub. No. HRA 81-653). Washington, DC: U.S. Government Printing Office.

Health personnel in the United States: Ninth report to Congress, 1993 edition (DHHS Pub. No. P-OD-94-1). (1993). Washington, DC: U.S. Government Printing Office.

Institute of Medicine. (1988). *The future of public health*. Washington, DC: National Academy Press.

Institute of Medicine. (1996). *The nation's physician workforce: Options for balancing supply and requirements*. Washington, DC: National Academy Press.

Kletke, P. R., Marder, W. D., & Silberger, A. B. (1990). The growing proportion of female physicians: Implications for U.S. physician supply. *American Journal of Public Health, 80,* 300–304.

Levine, E., & Moses, E. (1982). Registered nurses today: A statistical profile. In L. Aiken (Ed.), *Nursing in the 1980s: Crises, opportunities, challenges*. Philadelphia: Lippincott.

Mick, S. S. (1992). *The 1987 career characteristics of foreign and U.S. medical graduates who entered the U.S. medical system between 1969 and 1982.* Report to the Educational Commission for Foreign Medical Graduates, Philadelphia, PA.

Mick, S. S., & Worobey, J. L. (1984). Foreign and United States medical graduates in practice: A follow-up. *Medical Care, 22,* 1014–1025.

Moy, E., & Bartman, B. A. (1995). Physician race and care of minority and medically indigent patients. *Journal of the American Medical Association, 273,* 1515–1520.

Ricketts, T. C. (1994). Health care professionals in rural America. In J. E. Beaulieu & D. E. Berry (Eds.), *Rural health services: A management perspective.* Ann Arbor, MI: AUPHA Press/Health Administration Press.

Seifer, S. D., Troupin, B., Rubenfeld, G. D. (1996). Changes in marketplace demand for physicians: A study of medical journal recruitment advertisements. *Journal of the American Medical Association, 276,* 695–699.

Whitcomb, M. E. (1995). A cross-national comparison of generalist physician workforce data. *Journal of the American Medical Association, 274,* 692–695.

Whitcomb, M. E., & Miller, R. S. (1995). Participation of International Medical Graduates in graduate medical education and hospital care for the poor. *Journal of the American Medical Association, 274,* 696–699.

PART VI

ASSESSING AND REGULATING HEALTH SERVICES

CHAPTER

Health Policy and the Politics of Health Care

Philip Lee

A. E. Benjamin

CHAPTER TOPICS

LEARNING OBJECTIVES

Upon completing this chapter, the reader should be able to:

- Understand the impact of health policies on health care.
- Understand the political system in the United States as it pertains to the development of health policy.
- Gain knowledge of the development of health policy in the United States.
- Appreciate the actual and potential roles of government in health care.
- Appreciate the competing political, economic, and social goals of health policy objectives.
- Understand political pressures between public and private forces in health care.

Political considerations have significantly affected nearly all of the developments discussed in this book. However, the importance and central role of health care policy analysis and politics can best be highlighted by directly discussing these issues. That is the purpose of this chapter. While many of the topics mentioned here have been discussed from a variety of perspectives in other chapters, the policy and politics of changes in health care in the nation are the focus here, and examples of developments in health care serve as illustrations of the central role of political forces in shaping our health care system. The philosophies and processes discussed in other chapters are further analyzed here.

Government plays a major role in planning, directing, and financing health services in the United States. The significance of the public sector is apparent as one considers the following: public programs account for approximately 40% of the nation's personal health care expenditures; most physicians and other health care personnel are trained at public expense; over 50% of all health research and development funds are provided by the government; and most nonprofit community and university hospitals have been built or modernized with government subsidies. The bulk of government expenditures are federal, with state and local governments contributing significant, but much smaller, amounts.

Health policies and programs of the United States government have evolved piecemeal, usually in response to needs that were not being met by the private sector or by states and local governments. The result has been a proliferation of federal categorical programs administered by more than a dozen government departments. Over the years, new programs have been added, old ones redirected, and numerous efforts made to integrate and coordinate services. In the 1980s a major effort was made by the Reagan administration to significantly diminish the federal role in domestic social policy through the transfer of some programs to the states, reduced federal funding, or elimination of federal support entirely. The effort has been only partially successful and has not changed the basic configuration of publicly supported health programs, although the burden of financing now falls more heavily on state and local governments. Functions of the public and private sectors have become increasingly interrelated, and roles are often poorly delineated. There can be little argument that the primary function of most government programs in health has been to support or strengthen the private sector (for example, hospital construction, subsidy of medical student training, Medicare) rather than to develop a strong system of publicly provided health care.

Although United States government policies have evolved over a two-hundred-year period, most of those affecting health services have developed since the enactment of the Social Security Act of 1935. Many federal health programs evolved because of failures in the private sector to provide necessary support—for example, biomedical research; others arose because results of the free market were grossly inequitable—for example, hospital construction; and some programs, such as Medicare and Medicaid, developed because health care was so costly that many could not afford to pay for necessary health services. Some federal health programs, such as biomedical research, potentially benefit everyone, while others, such as the Indian Health Service, reach only a small but needy segment of the population. Some programs, such as poliomyelitis immunization and health personnel development, have been effective in achieving their goals; others, such as health planning, have probably not realized even limited objectives; still others, such as Medicare, have reached some goals, although at a much higher cost than originally anticipated.

The process by which health policy is made in this country can be best understood by considering a fundamental paradox in American health care: government spends more and more money to support a wide range of health programs, services, and agencies, yet the role of government in the reform of our health care system remains limited and halting. Government is faced with a crisis in health care, defined primarily in terms of rising costs to public treasuries, while proposed solutions are framed in terms that do not address in a comprehensive fashion the sources of demand on the public purse. Indeed, solutions to the cost crisis have combined withdrawing benefits from those very recipient populations whose health care needs justify government intervention with attempts to reduce costs by either stimulating competition or regulating (reducing) payment to hospitals, nursing homes, and physicians. While federal policies may move in one direction, state policies may move in another. To understand this paradox, it is necessary to consider several characteristics of public policy making and thus to explore the sources of

the paradox and the nature of policy processes in health.

DIMENSIONS OF POLICY MAKING IN HEALTH

Policy making in health care crosses several levels of government and hundreds of programs and is complex; no single analytical scheme can do it sufficient justice. Still, public policy students have identified five dimensions of the policy process: (1) the relationship of government to the private sector, (2) the distribution of authority within a federal system of government, (3) pluralistic ideology as the basis of politics, (4) the relationship between policy formulation and administrative implementation, and (5) incrementalism as a strategy of reform. Each will be considered in detail.

Public and Private Sector Politics

Although the role of government in health care has grown considerably in recent years, that role remains relatively limited. The United States government is less involved in health care than are the governments of many other industrialized countries (Jonas & Banta, 1981). This circumstance derives primarily from a persistent ideology that identifies the market system as the most appropriate setting for the exchange of health services and from a related belief that private sector support for public sector initiatives can be acquired only through accommodation to the interests of health care providers. The significance of the market ideology has been elaborated in analyses of the passage of Medicare and Medicaid in 1965 (Marmor, 1973; Vladeck, 1980). The persistence of doubts about the appropriate role of government is certainly apparent in the renewed vitality of neoconservatism, in which it is argued that the market can better respond to the economic and social problems of our time if it is unfettered by government intervention (Wade, 1982).

Uncertainty about the role of government in health care has numerous consequences. The primary concern is the absence of any design or blueprint for governmental reform (Ginzberg, 1978). Instead, the public sector (with its relatively immense capacity to raise revenues) is called on periodically to open and close its funding spigots to stimulate the health care market. Hospital construction and physician education are prominent examples of public activity. Not only is there no blueprint for public sector action, but governments in America harbor grave doubts about the appropriateness of regulation as a public sector activity. Dependence at the federal level on "voluntary approaches," such as the reduction of hospital costs in the late 1970s, delayed serious consideration of more stringent measures even as the costs to government of hospital care continued to rise dramatically (Pechman, 1979).

A Federal System

The concept of federalism has evolved dramatically in meaning and practice since the founding of the republic more than two hundred years ago. Originally, federalism was a legal concept that defined the constitutional division of authority between the federal government and the states. Federalism initially stressed the independence of each level of government from the other, while incorporating the idea that some functions, such as foreign policy, were the exclusive province of the central government, while other functions, such as education, police protection, and health care, were the responsibility of regional units—state and local government. Federalism represented a form of governance that differs both from a unitary state, where regional and local authority derive legally from the central government, and from a confederation, in which the national government has limit-

ed authority and does not reach individual citizens directly (Hale & Palley, 1981; Reagan & Sanzone, 1981).

Shifts in responsibilities assigned to various levels of government do not pose a serious problem for health policy if at least two conditions are met: (1) administrative or regulatory responsibilities and financial accountability are consonant, and (2) the various levels of government possess the appropriate capacities to assume those responsibilities assigned to them. Important questions can be raised regarding whether either of these conditions has been met in the development of health policy during the last two decades.

Analysis of federal-state relationships in programs as divergent as Medicaid, provider licensure, and family planning under Title X of the Public Health Service Act have suggested that the structure of these relationships produces outcomes widely held to be dysfunctional (for example, Medicaid cutbacks) because one level of government (for example, the states) can do nothing else under the conditions established by another (for example, the federal government). The disjunction between administrative responsibilities and financial accountability (that is, the term of federalistic arrangements) in these cases has yielded results for which governments and the recipients of health care ultimately have paid a price. What seems to matter most in the structure of relationships within federalism is not so much the distribution of activities but the relationships among levels of government (Vladeck, 1979).

For allocations of authority among levels of government to work, it is important that governments possess those capacities appropriate to the responsibilities they confront. Governments must possess the capacity to generate revenue, the capability to plan and manage policies and programs, and the political will to plan and implement needed reform. State and local governments have been found wanting in each of these respects. Because state governments do not tax as heavily as the federal government (Reagan, 1972), their capacity for generating new revenues is limited. Many states, moreover, are viewed as having inadequate administrative infrastructures, lacking sufficient sophisticated management techniques, and having limited capabilities in the conduct of policy analysis and planning.

Finally, there is evidence that state and local governments may have less political will to make decisions in the public interest than the federal government. Wide variations among states in program outputs (for example, Medicaid) suggest significant inequities. The argument is not that every state, if freed from federal constraints, would establish standards for health programs that are certain to fall below former federal standards. Rather, it is that some states will surely exceed some federal standards and others will fall far below what is generally considered adequate. At the heart of this problem, many argue, is the reputedly greater susceptibility of state governments to interest group pressures and narrow conceptions of the public good.

Perhaps the most significant instance of the failure of the states to provide their citizens equal rights and equal protection has been in the area of civil rights. In education, housing, health care, and virtually every area of domestic social policy, it has been necessary for the federal government, particularly the federal courts, to require compliance with federal laws and regulations.

There is some countervailing evidence that the capacity and will to govern is becoming more widely diffused within the federal system. States (taken as a group) have spent a higher percentage of their budgets on health care than the federal government has, even though absolute federal expenditures for health have grown to more than double state and local health expenditures combined (Clarke,

1981). A considerable increase at the state level in the conduct of policy analysis and its use in policy deliberations is one indication that state capacity to plan and manage is improving (Lee & Staffeldt, 1977). Regarding inequities and political will, on the other hand, little counterevidence has emerged to challenge the argument that the states are more vulnerable to interest groups (for example, provider groups in health) and that the result is a wide program variation among states in response to provider, not consumer, interests. The structure of federalism enables provider groups to maximize their power at the expense of consumer interests (Estes, 1980; Vladeck, 1979).

In a recent monograph on federalism and the national purpose, Brizius (n.d.) groups the arguments favoring centralization into eight clusters of related principles: (1) national purpose, (2) national security, (3) equity, (4) guaranteeing rights, (5) efficiency, (6) competence, (7) uniformity, and (8) unity. In contrast to the principles tending toward centralization are those that support greater decentralization and the maintenance of a truly federal system. Brizius groups twelve arguments for decentralization into seven principles: (1) diversity, (2) political sovereignty, (3) guaranteeing rights, (4) limits on power, (5) accountability, (6) efficiency and competence, and (7) competition.

The argument regarding centralization and decentralization has not been settled, despite a vigorous debate in the past decade. No agreement has been reached on the vital question of the distribution of authority and responsibility among various levels of government. The federal government finances hospital and medical services for the elderly through Medicare; it contributes at least 50% of health care costs for Medicaid beneficiaries, is the major supporter of biomedical research, provides a limited amount of support for a variety of health services (for example, mental health, family planning, crippled children's services, AIDS, substance abuse), is the sole regulator of the entry of new drugs into the market, and plays a critical role in the regulation of environment and occupational health.

States spend a large portion of their general fund budgets on health care for the poor (Medicaid), on mental health services, on the support of a range of public health programs, and on the education and training of health professionals.

Local governments remain an important provider of health care, particularly hospital, outpatient, and emergency care for the poor, mental health and substance abuse services, and a variety of public health services. Both state and local governments are mandated by higher levels of government (by either regulation or court order) to provide services or implement various environmental health or occupational health and safety regulations.

Pluralistic Politics

Pluralism is a term used by political theorists to describe a set of values about the effective functioning of democratic governments. Pluralists argue that democratic societies are organized into many diverse interest groups, which pervade all socioeconomic strata, and that this network of pressure groups prevents any one elite group from overreaching its legitimate bounds. As a theoretical framework for explaining the political context of policy making, this perspective has been criticized relentlessly and appropriately (Bachrach, 1967; Schattschneider, 1960). As an ideology that continues to influence the way elites and masses view government, pluralism becomes a basis for considering some essential elements of the process of public decision making in this country.

Interest groups play a powerful role in the health policy process. Most federal and state laws designed to address the health care needs of the population are shaped by the interaction among interest groups, key legislators, and agency representatives.

Ginzberg (1977) has identified four power centers in the health care industry that influence the nature of health care and the role of government: (1) physicians, (2) large insurance organizations, (3) hospitals, and (4) a highly diversified group of participants in profit-making activities within the health care arena.

The influence of these power centers is evident in policies at all levels of government. The development of Medicare and Medicaid policies reflects the powerful influence of physicians, hospitals, and nursing homes as well as their allies in the health insurance industry. For example, in enacting Medicare, Congress ensured that the law did not affect the physician-patient relationship, including the physician's method of billing the patient. The system of physician reimbursement adopted by Medicare was highly inflationary because it provided incentives to physicians to raise prices and to provide ancillary services, such as laboratory tests, electrocardiograms, and X-ray films. Hospital reimbursement historically has been based on costs incurred in providing care, creating strong incentives to provide more and more services. Despite the impact of steadily rising Medicare costs on the Social Security trust fund, on Social Security taxes (paid by employers and employees), and on the elderly, until recently, Congress has steadfastly refused to alter Medicare's methods of payments to physicians and hospitals. It was not until 1989 that the United States Congress adopted a set of policies to reform payments for physicians' services in the Medicare program. Also, many features of the program, patterned on principles developed by the medical industry, have had remarkable staying power.

The passage of a hospital prospective payment system (PPS) for Medicare by Congress in 1983 signaled a potential shift in the power of key interest groups in health. Recent history has made it clear that an apparent legislative defeat (for example, the passage of Medicare) can subsequently become an important source of benefits and power for ostensibly losing interests (for example, the medical lobby). The implementation of PPS has not been a fiscal disaster for hospitals, as some predicted, and it remains to be seen whether federal payment reforms will effect any fundamental alteration in the role of major power centers in health care.

As the case of Medicare suggests, health policy in the United States has been a product largely of medical politics (Silver, 1976a). Marmor et al. (1976) describe the political "market" in health (that is, institutional arrangements among actors in the political system) as imbalanced. In an imbalanced market, participants have unequal power, and those with concentrated rather than diffuse interests have the greater stake in the effects of policy. At least until recently, provider interest groups have had a far greater stake in shaping health policy than have consumer interests. Recently, large employers have become increasingly important in the health policy debates at the federal and state levels, particularly on issues related to health care cost containment.

Some observers argue that the rising costs of health care may be changing the configuration of interest groups seeking to influence health policy. In recent years, steadily escalating costs have stimulated other interests, especially labor, business, and governments themselves into giving greater attention to health policy and its implications. Polls of public attitudes show a growing dissatisfaction with health care financing in the United States and a strong desire for major reforms (Blendon, et al., 1990; Blendon & Taylor, 1989). In other words, the public's interests may be shifting from diffuse to concentrated. The result may be that increased competition in the political marketplace from a more diverse set of participants will lessen the dominance of medical provider groups (Feldstein, 1981). The pluralist dream of effective interest groups that prevent any one group from overreaching its legitimate bounds continues to influence our thinking about health care.

Policy Implementation

The nature of the health process is determined not only by the balance between provider and consumer interests but also by the relationships of these interests to government actors. Public policy students have observed that policy making moves through at least three stages: (1) agenda setting, the continuous process by which issues come to public attention and are placed on the agenda for government action; (2) policy adoption, the legislative process through which elected officials decide the broad outlines of policy; and (3) policy implementation, the process by which administrators develop policy by addressing the numerous issues unaddressed by legislation (Estes, 1980; Sabatier & Mazamania, 1979). An important element of the health policy process involves the relative roles of elected officials and professional administrators. As one moves from agenda setting to policy adoption and implementation, it can be argued that the role of elected officials becomes more remote and that of administrators more crucial.

No policy theorist has pressed this argument with more conviction than Lowi (1979). A central theme in what he calls interest-group liberalism is the growing role of administrators in politics. According to Lowi, in a period of resource richness and government expansion, such as the 1960s, government responded to a range of major organized interests, underwrote programs sought by those interests, and assigned program responsibility to administrative agencies. Through this process, the programs became captives of the interest groups because the administrative agencies themselves were captured. Interest groups dominate the policy process, he argues, not only through their influence on the legislative process (policy adoption) but also through control of administration (policy implementation). In effect, governments in the United States make policies without laws, and they leave the law making to administrators.

The study of policy implementation in health has received increased attention in recent years (Kingdon, 1984; Oliver, 1991; Sabatier, 1988; Silver, 1978). Not surprisingly, the landmark legislation creating Medicare and Medicaid in 1965 has been the subject of much of this analysis. A study of Medicare by Feder (1977) is especially enlightening. She describes a number of crucial decisions related to the nature of the federal role that were not addressed by the legislation and discusses the process by which the Social Security Administration subsequently addressed these decisions. Feder argues that the agency could have pursued two fundamentally different strategies. Using a cost-effectiveness strategy, the agency could have assessed the impact of alternative approaches to a problem (for example, hospital payment) on cost and quality and selected a course that would achieve maximum health care value per dollar spent. As an alternative, with a balancing strategy, the agency could have sought to identify relevant political actors (for example, the American Hospital Association), weighed their capacity to aid or threaten program survival, and selected those policies that would minimize political conflict (Feder, 1977).

Feder makes a persuasive argument that the Social Security Administration selected a balancing strategy. She traces the various consequences for the public interest of an approach that administratively transfers policy discretion to those provider groups with the greatest stake in the contents of that policy. For those directly involved in the implementation of the Medicare program, the primary motivation was not only to minimize political conflict but also to ensure access for elderly Social Security beneficiaries to hospital and physician services. At one point, access was jeopardized because of the vigorous enforcement of the Civil Rights Act by the United States Public Health Service and the Social Security Administration on instructions of the Secretary of Health, Education, and Welfare. When compliance with the Civil Rights Act was assured in hospitals, particularly in the South and Southwest, access barriers disappeared. Reimbursement policies followed the intentions of Congress and achieved the initial objective of ensuring high levels of hospital and physician participation in Medicare.

Incremental Reform

The powerful role of administrators in the implementation of policy is derived in part from the broad and ambiguous nature of much federal and state health legislation. Despite dramatic improvements in the capacity of congressional staff to conduct policy analysis, the constraints of politics are such that ambiguity frequently is employed to ensure the passage of legislation.

The public policy process in American government can best be described in terms of an incremental model of decision making (Lindblom, 1959; Wildavsky, 1964). Simply stated, this model posits that policy is made in small steps (increments) and that policy is rarely modified in dramatic ways. Major actors in the political bargaining process, whether legislators, interest groups, or administrators, operate on the basis of certain rules, and these rules are founded in adherence to prior policy patterns. Because the consequences of policy change are difficult to predict and because unpredictability is risky in the political market, policy makers prefer reform in small steps to more radical change.

An example of incremental change was the gradual evolution of the National Institutes of Health from a small federal laboratory conducting biomedical research in the 1930s to a multibillion-dollar research enterprise. The addition of new institutes took place over a fifty-year period. Budgets also grew gradually, beginning after World War II. Even when major health policy initiatives were adopted, such as Medicare and Medicaid, the change was in the source of funds to pay for medical care for the elderly and the poor, not in the organization or provision of medical care.

The incremental model was elaborated by decision theorists concerned with ways that policy makers manage a large information load and the uncertainty of their political environment. Quite a different view, but one that is compatible with this perspective, has been developed by Alford (1975). Alford addresses the nature of reform in health care and its ideological basis. He identifies three approaches to reform, including market reformers, who call for an end to government interference in health care delivery and the restoration of market competition in health care institutions, and bureaucratic reformers, who blame market competition for defects in the system and call for increased administrative regulation of health care. What these perspectives share, notes Alford, is that each leads to incremental reform and the extent to which they challenge fundamental patterns of policy is limited. A third approach, the structural interest perspective, begins with an analysis of the ways in which the other two accept and benefit from current arrangements in health care. This perspective is formulated to challenge the effective, institutional control exercised by dominant structural interests that benefit from continuance of the system in its present form. As Alford makes clear, the market and bureaucratic approaches are descriptive of the limits of health care reform, and they underlie resistance to change in the health system.

Relatively little research in the United States has examined the institutional and class basis of public policy, including health policy (Estes, 1982). Those who hold that defects in health care are rooted deeply in the structure of a class society would radically alter the present health care system, creating a national health service, with decentralization of administration and community control over health care institutions and health professionals. Those who view defects in health care as having a class basis believe that tinkering with the health care system itself cannot achieve the desired outcomes but that these will follow major structural changes in society.

European countries that practice a parliamentary rather than representative democracy can effect larger changes more swiftly. In the parliamentary form of government, party policies are implemented speedily because the winning party practices bloc voting. Delay is caused only by the inability to achieve power. In representative governments, the parties cannot manage the discipline necessary to enforce party loyalty to programs or policies because elected representatives owe more, or at least as much, to their personal appeal as to party designation. The party discipline of parliamentary government is replaced by the quest for consensus in representative government, and consensus is most readily achieved when proposed reforms involve only modest changes.

A HISTORICAL FRAMEWORK: THE DEVELOPMENT OF HEALTH POLICY FROM 1798 TO 1988

Although the federal system in the United States has evolved continuously, at certain periods in our history, the relationship among the federal, state, and local governments has undergone dramatic change. The major shifts in intergovernment relations were often the result of a crisis (the Civil War, the Great Depression, civil rights issues) rather than the result of a critical examination of the issues.

Public health and health care did not loom large in the policy debate about federalism until the late 1940s, when President Truman advocated a program of national health insurance, and again in the 1960s, when implementation of Medicare transformed the role of the federal government in health care. Over the years, however, health policy issues (for example, federal regulation of food and drugs, federal support for biomedical research, hospital construction, and health professions education) have raised critical issues about the role of government in health care, intergovernmental relations, and the role of the private sector.

The private sector in the United States has always maintained a larger role in health care than it has in most other industrial nations. This has been true in both the financing and delivery of services. While it is not possible to do full justice to the rich history of health care policy here, an effort is made to present highlights in the development of health policy that reflect the manner in which much has changed and much has stayed the same.

The slow emergence of public policies and programs related to health and health care in the United States has generally followed the pattern of other industrial countries, particularly those in western Europe (Lee & Silver, 1972). At least three stages in the process have been identified:

1. Private charity, including contracts between users and providers, and public apathy or indifference.
2. Public provision of necessary health services that are not provided by voluntary effort and private contract.
3. Substitution of public services and financing for private, voluntary, and charitable efforts.

Although these three stages have been identified within many nations, different patterns have been observed among industrial countries. Political parties in the United States have been more reluctant than those in European countries or Canada to challenge the medical profession, hospitals, and the health insurance industry to promote health care reform.

The role of government at the federal, state, and local levels in public health and health care evolved partly in response to changes occurring in the health care system (Torrens, 1988). With the major changes in health care that have occurred over the past two hundred years, particularly those in the past fifty years, has come a transformation in the role of government.

THE EARLY YEARS OF THE REPUBLIC: A LIMITED ROLE FOR THE FEDERAL GOVERNMENT (1798–1862)

During the early years of the republic, the federal government played a limited role in both public health and health care, which were largely within the jurisdiction of the states and the private sector. Private charity shouldered the responsibility of care for the poor. The federal role in providing health care began in 1798, when Congress passed the Act for the Relief of Sick and Disabled Seamen, which imposed a twenty-cent-per-month tax on seamen's wages for their medical care. The federal government later provided direct medical care for merchant seamen through clinics and hospitals in port cities, a policy that continues to this day. The federal government also played a limited role in imposing quarantines on ships entering United States ports in order to prevent epidemics (Lee & Silver, 1972). It did little or nothing, however, about the spread of communicable diseases within the nation, a problem that was thought to lie within the jurisdiction of the individual states.

Through the eighteenth, nineteenth, and early twentieth centuries, the major diseases in the United States, as in Europe, were infectious diseases, as discussed in Chapter 1. Tuberculosis, pneumonia, bronchitis, and gastrointestinal infections were the major killers. As the sanitary revolution progressed in the nineteenth century, social and economic conditions advanced, nutrition improved, reproductive behavior was modified, the burden of acute infection declined, and the burden of chronic illness began to rise. National health policies during the eighteenth and nineteenth centuries were limited to the imposition of quarantines to prevent epidemics and the provision of medical care to merchant seamen and members of the armed forces. In laws beginning with the Act Relative to Quarantine of 1796, Congress preempted state and local authority and put an end to long-standing federal-state disagreements regarding the authority to prevent and control epidemics of yellow fever and cholera, as well as recurring outbreaks of plague and smallpox (Lewis & Sheps, 1983).

States first exercised their public health authority through special committees or commissions. Most active concern with health matters was at the local level. Local boards of health or health departments were organized to tackle problems of sanitation, poor housing, and quarantine. Later, local health departments were set up in rural areas, particularly in the South, to counteract hookworm, malaria, and other infectious diseases that were widespread in the nineteenth and early twentieth centuries.

THE EVOLUTION OF HEALTH POLICY: THE EMERGENCE OF DUAL FEDERALISM AND THE TRANSFORMATION OF AMERICAN MEDICINE (1862–1935)

The Civil War brought about a dramatic change in the role of the federal government. Not only did the federal government engage in a war to preserve the union but it also began to expand its role in other ways that significantly altered the nature of federalism in the United States. This changing federal role was reflected in congressional passage of the first program of federal aid to the states, the Morrill Act of 1862, which granted federal lands to each state. Profits from the sale of these lands supported public institutions of higher education, known as "land-grant colleges" (Hale & Palley, 1981). Toward the end of the nineteenth century, the federal government began to provide cash grants to states for the establishment of agricultural experiment stations. While the federal role generally was expanding, the change had little impact on health care. An important exception occurred in the late 1870s when the Surgeon General of the Marine Hospital Service was given congressional authorization to impose quarantines within the United States.

While the first state health department was established in Louisiana in 1855, it was not until after the Civil War that the states began to assume a more significant role in public health. Massachusetts established the first permanent board of health in 1869. By 1909, public health agencies were established in all the states. During this period, there also was rapid development of local health departments; state and local governments based their policy changes and management practices on the rapid advances in the biological sciences. Drawing on these advances, state and local health departments moved beyond sanitation and quarantine to the scientific control of communicable diseases (Miller, et al., 1981).

The basic policies that created both state and local health departments derived from the police power of state governments (Miller, et al., 1977). Thus, the states, and not the federal government, were the key to translating the scientific advances of the late nineteenth century into public health policy and the dramatic improvements in public health that followed.

The most significant role played by state governments in personal health care during this period was in the establishment of state mental hospitals. These first developed as a result of a reform movement in the mid-nineteenth century led by Dorothea Dix. Over the next century, state mental institutions evolved into isolated facilities for custodial care of the chronically mentally ill. The development of these asylums reinforced the stigma attached to mental illness and placed the care of the severely mentally ill outside the mainstream of medicine for more than a century (Foley, 1975).

Hospitals began to evolve in the nineteenth century from almshouses that provided shelter for the poor. Hospital sponsorship at the local level was either public (local government) or through a variety of religious, fraternal, or other community groups. Thus, the nonprofit community hospital was born; this institution, rather than the local public hospital, gradually became the primary locus of medical care. Physicians provided voluntary services to the sick poor in order to earn the privilege of caring for their paying patients in the hospital (Silver, 1976b). Hospital appointments became important for physicians in order to conduct their practices. Hospitals increased in number in the late-nineteenth century and began to incorporate new medical technologies, such as anesthe-

sia, aseptic surgery, and later, radiology. Although charity was the major source of care for the poor, public services also began to grow in the nineteenth century. Gradually, local government assumed responsibility for indigent care. The development of the hospital is discussed further in Chapter 10.

After the Morrill Act, the next major change in the role of the federal government came more than forty years later in the regulation of food and drugs. After twenty years of debate and much public pressure, Congress enacted the Federal Food and Drug Act in 1906 to regulate the adulteration and misbranding of food and drugs, a responsibility previously exercised exclusively by the states. The law was designed primarily to protect the pocketbook of the consumer, not the consumer's health. While it provided some measure of control over impure foods, it had little impact on impure or unsafe drugs (Silverman & Lee, 1974). The legislation not only represented a major change in the role of the federal government but also provided the constitutional basis for present-day regulation of testing, marketing, and promotion of prescription and over-the-counter drugs.

A number of other important developments in the early decades of the twentieth century had a strong impact on health care and health policy. Among the most significant were reforms in medical education that transformed not only education but also professional licensing and, eventually, health care itself. The American Medical Association and the large private foundations (for example, Carnegie and Rockefeller) played a major role in this process. Voluntary hospitals also grew in number, size, and importance. Medical research produced new treatments. Infant mortality declined as nutrition, sanitation, living conditions, and maternal and infant care improved. Health care changed in significant ways, but it was little affected by public policy.

THE EVOLUTION OF HEALTH POLICY: FROM DUAL FEDERALISM TO COOPERATIVE FEDERALISM (1935–1961)

The Great Depression brought action by the federal government to save banks, support small businesses, provide direct public employment, stimulate public works, regulate financial institutions and business, restore consumer confidence, and provide Social Security in old age. The role of the federal government was transformed in the span of a few years. Federalism evolved from a dual pattern, with a limited role in domestic affairs for the federal government, to a cooperative one, with a strong federal role.

The Social Security Act of 1935 was certainly the most significant domestic social legislation ever enacted by Congress. This marked the real beginning of what has been termed "cooperative federalism." The act established the principle of federal aid to the states for public health and welfare assistance. It provided federal grants to states for maternal and child health and crippled children's services (Title V) and for public health (Title VI). It also provided for cash assistance grants to the aged, the blind, and destitute families with dependent children. This cash assistance program provided the basis for the current federal-state program of medical care for the poor, initially as Medical Assistance for the Aged in 1960 and then as Medicaid (Title XIX of the Social Security Act) in 1965. Both later programs linked eligibility for medical care to eligibility for cash assistance. More important, however, the Social Security Act of 1935 established the Old Age, Survivors' and Disability Insurance (OASDI) programs that were to provide the philosophical and fiscal basis for Medicare, a program of federal health insurance for the aged, also enacted

in 1965 (Title XVIII of the Social Security Act). Passage of the Social Security Act of 1935 was significant, for it provided the basis for direct federal income assistance to retired persons and established the basis for federal aid to the states in health and welfare; however, this legislation did not include a program of national health insurance. This was due principally to the opposition of the medical profession to any form of health insurance, particularly publicly funded insurance.

In 1938, after the death of a number of children due to the use of Elixir of Sulfonamide, consumer protection became an important issue for policy makers. This disaster resulted in the enactment of the Food, Drug and Cosmetic Act of 1938, which required manufacturers to demonstrate the safety of drugs before marketing. This law was a further extension of the federal role and was consistent with other major changes in that role that occurred during the 1930s. After the passage of this act, little change was made in drug regulation law until the thalidomide disaster in the early 1960s.

Growing attention to maternal and child health, particularly for the poor, was reflected in grants to the states and in a temporary program instituted during World War II to pay for maternity care of wives of Army and Navy enlisted men. This means-tested program successfully demonstrated the capacity of the federal government to administer a national health insurance program. With rapid demobilization after the war and opposition by organized medicine, the program was terminated, but it was often cited by advocates of national health insurance, particularly those who accorded first priority to mothers and infants.

Introduction of the scientific method into medical research at the turn of the century and its gradual acceptance had a profound effect on national health policy and health care. The first clear organizational impact of the growing importance of research was the transformation of the United

States Public Health Service Hygienic Laboratory, established in 1901 to conduct bacteriologic research and public health studies, into the National Institutes of Health (NIH) in 1930, with broad authority to conduct basic research. This was followed by enactment of the National Cancer Act of 1937 and the establishment of the National Cancer Institute within the framework of NIH. There followed multiple legislative enactments during and after World War II that created the present institutes, focused primarily on broad classes of disease, such as heart disease, cancer, arthritis, neurologic diseases, and blindness. In the fifteen years immediately after World War II, NIH grew from a small government laboratory to the most significant biomedical research institute in the world. NIH became the principal supporter of biomedical research, quickly surpassing industry and private foundations. Indeed, in the period after World War II until the 1960s, federal support for biomedical research represented one of the few areas of health policy in which the federal government was active. The influence of organized medicine was a critical factor in limiting the federal role in other areas during this period.

In addition to federal support for biomedical research, largely through medical schools and universities, and a limited program of grants to states for public health and maternal and child health programs, federal policy related to hospital planning and construction became of primary importance. After World War II, it was evident that many of America's hospitals were woefully inadequate, and the Hill-Burton federal-state program of hospital planning and construction was launched in response in 1942. Its initial purpose was to provide funds to states to survey hospital bed supply and develop plans to overcome the hospital shortage, particularly in rural areas. The Hill-Burton Act was amended numerous times as its initial goals were met. This legislation provided the stimulus for a massive hospital construction program, with federal and state subsidies primarily for community, nonprofit, and voluntary hospitals. Public hospitals, supported largely by local tax funds to provide care for the poor, received little or no federal support until the needs of private institutions were met. The program became a model of federal-state-private sector cooperation in the distribution of substantial federal resources. It was a prime example of cooperative federalism and the major force—until enactment of Medicare and Medicaid—behind modernization of the voluntary community hospital system.

After World War II, President Truman urged Congress to enact a program of national health insurance, funded through federal taxes. President Truman's efforts and those of his supporters in Congress and organized labor were thwarted, again largely as a result of opposition by the American Medical Association. No progress was made in extending the federal role in financing of medical care because the medical profession argued that voluntary health insurance, such as Blue Cross, and commercial insurance could do the job.

By 1953, when the Department of Health, Education, and Welfare (DHEW), now the Department of Health and Human Services, was created, the federal government's role in the nation's health care system, although limited, was firmly established. This role was designed primarily to support programs and services in the private sector. Biomedical research, research training, and hospital construction were the major pathways for federal support. The Food and Drug Administration also became part of DHEW and was its primary regulatory agency. Traditional public health programs, such as those for venereal disease control, tuberculosis control, and maternal and child health, were supported at minimal levels through categorical grants to the states. Federal support for medical care was restricted to military personnel, veterans, merchant seamen, and Native Americans until 1960, when enactment of the Kerr-Mills law authorized limited federal grants to states for medical assistance for the aged. This program proved short-lived, but it highlighted the need for a far broader federal effort in medical care for the poor and the aged.

THE TRANSFORMATION OF HEALTH POLICIES: THE NEW FRONTIER, THE GREAT SOCIETY, AND CREATIVE FEDERALISM (1961–1969)

A number of major federal health policy developments took place between 1961 and 1969, during the presidencies of John F. Kennedy and Lyndon B. Johnson. Although federal support was extended directly to universities, hospitals, and nonprofit institutes conducting research, most federal aid in health was channeled through the states. The term *creative federalism* was applied to policies developed during the Johnson administration that extended the traditional federal-state relationship to include direct federal support for local governments (cities and counties), nonprofit organizations, and private businesses and corporations to carry out health, education, training, social services, and community development programs (Reagan & Sanzone, 1981). The primary means used to forward the goals of creative federalism were grants-in-aid. More than two hundred grant programs were enacted during the five years of the Johnson administration.

The first major health policy changes after the election of President Kennedy again were the result of a crisis. The thalidomide disaster in Europe had little direct impact in the United States because the Food and Drug Administration had not approved the drug for marketing here. The disaster nonetheless focused renewed attention on the problems of drug safety, efficacy, and promotion and led to the most sweeping reforms of federal drug laws in twenty-four years. The 1962 amendments to the Food, Drug and Cosmetic Act specified that a drug must be demonstrated to be effective, as well as safe, before it could be marketed. Advertising also was strictly regulated, and more effective provisions for removal of unsafe drugs from the market were included (Silverman & Lee, 1974).

The categorical programs that developed during the period of creative federalism were numerous and varied. Some programs were based on disease (heart disease, cancer, stroke, and mental illness), some on public assistance eligibility (Medicaid), some on age (Medicare, crippled children), some on institutions (hospitals, nursing homes, neighborhood health centers), some on political jurisdiction (state or local departments of public health), some on geographic areas that did not follow traditional political boundaries (community mental health centers, catchment areas, the Appalachian Regional Commission), and some on activity (research, facility construction, health professionals training, and health care financing) (Lewis & Sheps, 1983).

Among the more important new laws enacted during the Johnson administration were the Health Professions Educational Assistance Act of 1963, which authorized direct federal aid to medical, dental, pharmacy, and other professional schools, as well as to students in these schools; the Maternal and Child Health and Mental Retardation Planning Amendments of 1963, which initiated comprehensive maternal and infant care projects and centers serving the mentally retarded; the Civil Rights Act of 1964, which prohibited racial discrimination, including segregated schools and hospitals; the

Economic Opportunity Act of 1964, which provided authority and funds to establish neighborhood health centers serving low-income populations; the Social Security Amendments of 1965, particularly Medicare and Medicaid, which financed medical care for the aged and the poor receiving cash assistance; the Heart Disease, Cancer and Stroke Act of 1965, which launched a national attack on these major killers through regional medical programs; and the Comprehensive Health Planning and Public Health Service Amendments of 1966 and the Partnership for Health Act of 1967, which reestablished the principle of block grants for state public health services (reversing a thirty-year trend of categorical federal grants in health). This legislation also created the first nationwide health planning system, which was dramatically changed in the 1970s to focus on regulation of health care as well as health planning (U.S. Department of Health, Education, and Welfare, 1976). It should be noted that not until the Nixon and Reagan administrations was the block grant concept widely applied to federal grants-in-aid to the states. Of the many new health programs initiated during the Johnson presidency, only Medicare was administered directly by the federal government.

The programs of the Johnson presidency had a profound effect on intergovernmental relationships, the concept of federalism, and federal expenditures for domestic social programs. Grant-in-aid programs alone (excluding Social Security and Medicare) grew from $7 billion at the beginning of the Kennedy and Johnson administration in 1961 to $24 billion in 1970, at the end of that era. In the next decade, the impact was to be even more dramatic as federal grant-in-aid expenditures for these programs grew to $82.9 billion in 1980. "Grants-in-aid,"

note Reagan and Sanzone (1981), "constitute a major social invention of our time and are the prototypical, although not statistically dominant [they now constitute over 20% of domestic federal outlays], form of federal domestic involvement."

The programs of the Johnson administration not only had a significant effect on the nature and scope of the federal role in domestic social programs but also had important consequences for health care. Federal funds for biomedical research and training, health personnel development, hospital construction, health care financing, and a variety of categorical programs were designed primarily to improve access to health care and secondarily to improve its quality. Increased attention during this period was given to the notion of health care as a right, a concept similar to the principle of the "earned right" that underlies the Social Security System (Callahan, 1977; Lee & Jonsen, 1974).

Although there was a profound change in the role of the federal government, many policies adopted during this time reflected the interests of the medical profession, the hospitals, and the health insurance industry. Medicare and Medicaid hospital reimbursement policies were designed to ensure hospital participation. Adoption of the cost-based method of reimbursement proved a boon for hospitals but was very costly for the taxpayer. Policies designed to meet the physician shortage of the 1960s eventually developed full support from organized medicine. Designed to strengthen the capacity of the nation's medical schools to respond to a nationally perceived need, these policies also provided direct benefit to an interest group of growing power—medical schools.

HEALTH POLICY IN AN ERA OF LIMITED RESOURCES: FROM CREATIVE FEDERALISM TO NEW FEDERALISM AND A RETURN TO DEPENDENCE ON COMPETITION AND THE PRIVATE SECTOR (1969–1992)

During the 1970s, President Nixon coined the term *new federalism* to describe his efforts to move away from the categorical programs of the Johnson years toward general revenue sharing, through which federal revenues were transferred to state and local governments with as few federal strings as possible, and toward block grants, through which grants were allocated to state and local governments for broad general purposes. During the Nixon and Ford administrations (1969–1977), considerable conflict developed between the Republican-controlled executive branch and the Democrat-controlled Congress with respect to domestic social policy, including the new federalism strategy originally advocated by President Nixon. Congress strongly favored categorical grants, with their detailed provisions, and was opposed to both revenue sharing and block grants. This period also witnessed an erosion of trust between federal middle management and congressional committees and subcommittees (Walker, 1981).

President Nixon also differed sharply from President Johnson in his explicit support for private rather than public efforts to solve the nation's health problems. On this fundamental issue, the Nixon administration made its position clear:

Preference for action in the private sector is based on the fundamentals of our political economy—capitalistic, pluralistic and competitive—as well as upon the desire to strengthen the capability of our private institutions in their effort to provide health services, to finance such services, and to produce the resources that will be needed in the years ahead (Richardson, 1971).

Although Nixon was a strong advocate for private sector leadership, he did propose a national health insurance plan based on an employer mandate. The proposal lost in Congress because the liberals felt that they would soon be able to enact a single-payer program, based on the Medicare model.

Although the Nixon administration attempted to implement its new federalism across a broad front, progress was made primarily in the fields of community development, personnel training, and social services. Categorical grant programs in health continued to expand despite attempts by both the Nixon and Ford administrations to transfer program authority and responsibility to the states and to reduce the federal role in domestic social programs. During the period 1965–1975, more than seventy-five major pieces of health legislation were enacted by Congress, indicating continued support for the categorical approach by the legislative branch of the federal government (U.S. Department of Health, Education, and Welfare, 1976).

Although categorical health programs proliferated in the 1960s and 1970s, the expansion of two programs—Medicare and Medicaid—dwarfed the others. While those programs contributed to medical inflation, their growth was due largely to the rising costs of medical care. Federal and state governments became third parties that underwrote the costs of a system that had few cost-constraining elements, and the staggering expenditures had profound effects on health policy.

The federal government's response to skyrocketing health care costs (and thus government expenditures) assumed a variety of forms. Federal subsidies of hospitals and other health facility construction were ended and replaced by planning and regulatory mechanisms designed to limit their growth. In most cases, these proved to be short-lived and ineffective because they were not directly linked to Medicare or Medicaid. In the mid-1970s, health personnel policies focused on specialty and geographic maldistribution of physicians rather than physician shortage, and by the late 1970s, concern was expressed about an over-supply of physicians and other health professionals (Lee, et al., 1976). Direct subsidies to expand enrollment in health professions schools were cut back and then eliminated. Funding for biomedical research began to decline in real dollar terms when an abortive "war on cancer" launched by President Nixon appeared to produce few concrete results and when Medicare and Medicaid preempted most federal health dollars.

An additional regulatory initiative enacted during President Nixon's second term was the National Health Planning and Resource Development Act of 1974 (PL 93-641). This law incorporated some of the planning principles from the Partnership for Health Act of 1967 and the Heart Disease, Cancer and Stroke Act of 1965, both of which were terminated with the enactment of PL 93-641. In addition to the health planning responsibility assigned to state health planning and development agencies (SHPDAs) and to local health systems agencies (HSAs), the law required that health care facilities obtain prior approval from the state for any expansion, in the form of a "certificate of need" (CON). The impact of this new approach to health planning and regulation was limited (Salkever & Bice, 1976), and the program was eliminated early in the Reagan administration.

More important than the constraints placed on resources allocated for health care were regulations instituted to slow the growth of health care costs in the Medicare and Medicaid programs. Two direct actions were taken by the federal government: (1) a limit on federal and state payments to hospitals and physicians under Medicare and Medicaid (included in the 1972 Social Security amendments), and (2) a period of wage and price control applied to the general economy when the Economic Stabilization Program was introduced to dampen increasing inflation. Wage and price controls on hospitals and physicians were continued after the general restrictions were removed. When controls were lifted in 1974, health care costs again began to climb.

Another regulatory initiative was designed to control costs through limiting the use of hospital care by Medicare and Medicaid beneficiaries. Although the original Medicare and Medicaid legislation required hospital utilization review committees, these appeared to have little effect on hospital use or costs. In 1972, amendments to the Social Security Act (PL 92-103) required the establishment of professional standards review organizations (PSROs) to review the quality and appropriateness of hospital services provided to beneficiaries of Medicare, Medicaid, maternal and child health, and crippled children programs (paid for under authority of Title V of the Social Security Act). PSROs were composed of physicians who reviewed hospital records in order to determine whether length of stay and services provided were appropriate. Results of these efforts have been mixed. In only a few areas where PSROs have been in operation is there evidence that cost increases have been restrained, and in these areas, it is not clear that the PSRO has been a critical factor.

An attempt was also made to control costs through major changes in the organization of medical care, as discussed throughout this book. Efforts were made to stimulate the growth of group practice repayment plans, which provide comprehensive services for a fixed annual fee. These capitation-based prepayment organizations were defined in federal legislation enacted in 1973 as health maintenance organizations (HMOs). Studies had demonstrated that HMOs could provide comprehensive care at significantly less cost than fee-for-service providers, primarily because of lower rates of hospitalization (Luft, 1980). Predictably, the federal stimulus for development of HMOs encountered strong resistance from organized medicine. Nevertheless, the program successfully enhanced professional and public awareness of HMOs and assisted in the development of a number of small prepaid group practices. The impact on costs at the national level, however, remained minimal until the 1990s.

Although the new federalism advocated by President Reagan was a dramatic departure from previous policies and trends because of the scope of his proposals, the roots of these policies were first evident in the comprehensive Health Planning and Public Health Service amendments enacted in 1966 during the presidency of Lyndon Johnson. They were increasingly evident in both the policy initiatives and the budgetary decisions of Presidents Nixon and Ford. Not only were Nixon and Ford's new federalism policies similar to those later advocated by President Reagan, but their fiscal and monetary policies also were designed to reduce the growth of federal spending and program responsibility.

During the presidency of Jimmy Carter (1977–1981), there were few health policy initiatives that were successful. The Carter administration tried without success to get Congress to enact hospital cost-containment legislation. Special interests, particularly hospitals and physicians, again prevailed. They were able to convince Congress that a voluntary effort would be more effective. Escalating health care costs did moderate during the debate in Congress, but when the threat of mandatory controls was no longer present, costs rose at a record rate. The picture in the late 1970s was one of frustration with efforts to control health care costs. Concern about access to care became a secondary consideration.

Following the Clinton effort at health care reform in 1993–1994, the most significant development of the 1990s has been the rapid growth of managed care. Managed care has cast a wide net and means different things to different observers. Included under this umbrella is the integration of health insurance and the delivery of care. Health services can be provided either directly or through another entity, possibly including the management of that practice.

While growth in both public sector and private sector supporting HMOs was slow during the 1970s and 1980s, it was building the base for explosive growth in the 1990s. Medicare has been the slowest to take advantage of the potential savings in shifting from a payer to a purchaser. Beginning in 1972 (the year before the HMO Act passed), Medicare initiated a risk-sharing contract option for HMOs. The program did not begin, however, until 1978 with a five-site demonstration program. Because of the slow growth in the original risk-sharing demonstration, Congress authorized a managed care capitated-payment option based on prospective payment methodologies. This option was implemented in 1985. Medicare HMO enrollment has increased steadily since risk contracting began in 1985. Growth in the private sector, however, far outpaced the Medicare growth of managed care in the late 1980s and in the 1990s. The congressionally mandated Physician Payment Review Commission (PPRC), in its 1996 report to Congress, noted:

The changes in managed care during the past three years have been extraordinary. What were once considered "alternative delivery systems" have emerged as mainstream methods of financing and delivering medical care in the U.S. (Physician Payment Review Commission, 1996).

The PPRC survey found three major types of managed care plans: (1) staff/group model HMOs; (2) network/independent practice associations (IPAs); and (3) preferred provider organizations (PPOs). The plans are also offering a point of service (POS) option that permits an enrollee to seek care outside the plan network for an added charge.

The number of Medicare beneficiaries enrolled in risk-contracting HMOs reached almost 9% in 1996, with an additional 2% in cost-reimbursed HMOs. In recent years, the growth has been accelerated, particularly in a few states. Enrollment in risk-contracting HMOs is particularly significant in California (36%), Oregon (34%), Arizona (31%), and Hawaii (31%) (Health Care Financing Administration, 1996).

Medicaid growth in managed care, driven largely by the states' desire to control rapidly rising costs, has been far more rapid than has Medicare's growth. The two mechanisms used by the states have been section 1915(b) and section 1115 waiver authority. In recent years, states have turned increasingly to the section 1115 waivers. The section 1115 waiver authority was enacted in 1962 to authorize research and demonstration projects that are "likely to assist promoting the objectives" of the Social Security program (including Medicaid since 1965). By mid-1997, a total of thirty-three states were either developing, operating, or had applied for approval of statewide Medicaid waivers under section 1115 authority (Kaiser Commission on the Future of Medicaid, 1995). The waivers have included expansion of eligibility, limited cost-sharing mandatory enrollment in managed care systems, eliminating provider reimbursement protections, program monitoring, and delivery systems innovations (Kaiser Commission on the Future of Medicaid, 1995). Currently over a quarter of Medicaid beneficiaries are enrolled in managed care, and the number is likely to continue to grow well into the twenty-first century.

In the private sector, growth in the numbers enrolled in managed care has been rapid in the past decade. Currently, about 90 million people are enrolled is managed care plans. Often employers choose a single managed care plan and give their employees no choice of plan. By contrast, federal employees who are privately insured (for example, federal employees health benefits) may choose among a number of managed care plans, as well as indemnity fee-for-service plans.

While there has been a sharp drop in the rate of increase in medical care costs since the rapid growth of managed care, in some states (for example, California) premiums have actually declined. Many questions remain, however, whether the initial savings can be sustained. The savings have derived largely from dramatic reductions in hospital admissions, with a consequent reduction in hospital occupancy and hospital costs. The next step is to reduce the number of hospital beds available. As hospital length-of-stay beds are reduced in number, less and less can gained in this area. At the same time, technology continues to advance and to be one of the primary drivers of lost increases.

The failure to pass national health care reform in 1993–1994, as well as the political trauma of the adoption and repeal of Medicare catastrophic coverage in 1988–1989, has produced much reflection about the political forces that doomed these efforts and about the prospects for substantial reform in the foreseeable future (Blendon, et al., 1995; Heclo, 1995; Skocpol, 1995). Informed observers provide us with little ground for optimism. A host of reasons are cited, among them a governmental system of separated institutions that routinely frustrates major policy change and the growing power of politics and ideology over health services research and policy analysis (Mann & Ornstein, 1995). Most daunting, perhaps, is the fact that policy making at the federal level has become budget-driven to a degree that opportunities for legislating new programs have all but vanished (Mann & Ornstein, 1995). Deficit pressures and the imperatives of the budget process have effectively driven out serious attention to substantive policy issues and focused policy making on cost-cutting revisions of existing programs (Mann & Ornstein, 1995). If 1993–1994 represented a rare window of opportunity for reform (and some argue that the window was barely ajar), then that opportunity has clearly passed, and the prospects for any major reform in the near future are few.

As bleak as that scenario may seem, there is also reason to believe that government will remain deeply involved in the business of health care policy for the foreseeable future and that occasions for policy change will continue to emerge as the latest incremental policy solutions fall short of the mark and themselves generate new policy problems. The politics of health care reform and the continuing debate about managed care have significantly raised the awareness of the American public about issues in the organization and financing of health care. This new salience combined with a stronger economy and some possible tempering of antigovernment sentiment suggest that efforts at modest policy reform will continue and that universal coverage, while still a dream, has not disappeared from the American policy agenda.

The Reagan administration accelerated the degree of pace of change in policy that had been developing since the early Nixon years. The most prominent shifts in federal policy advanced by the Reagan administration that directly affected health care were (1) a significant reduction in federal expenditures for domestic social programs, including the elimination of the revenue-sharing program initiated by President Nixon; (2) decentralization of program authority and responsibility to the states, particularly through block grants; (3) deregulation and greater emphasis on market forces and competition to stimulate health care reform and

more effective control of health care costs; (4) tax reductions, despite significant increases in the national debt, with a resulting decline in the fiscal capacity of the federal government to fund domestic social programs; and (5) Medicare cost containment through the implementation of a prospective payment system for hospitals based on costs per case, using diagnosis-related groups (DRGs) as the basis for payment.

An important consequence of the block grants enacted by Congress at the urging of the Reagan administration is that the wide discretion that these grants provide to the individual states fosters inequities in programs among the states. This, in turn, makes it impossible to ensure uniform benefits for target populations, such as the poor and the aged, across jurisdictions or to maintain accountability with so many varying state approaches (Estes, 1980). Because the most disadvantaged individuals are heavily dependent on state-determined benefits, they are especially vulnerable in periods of economic flux. These policies also have increased pressure on state and local governments to underwrite program costs at the same time that many states, cities, and counties are under mounting pressure to curb expenditures.

Although the Reagan administration strongly favored deregulation and stimulation of competitive market forces, this had little impact on federal health care policies except in the health planning area. The federal health planning legislation was not renewed in the 1980s, but a number of states continue to operate certificate of need programs in an attempt to control the proliferation of expensive technologies.

In contrast to eliminating health planning as a means of regulation, the Reagan and Bush administrations used regulations to limit hospital reimbursement and physician fees in the Medicare program.

At the state level, however, major changes were underway in the 1980s that responded to the growing influence of the free-market ideology. In California, major reforms were enacted in 1982 in an attempt to increase competition among hospitals and reduce the costs of Medicaid in that state. Private insurance companies were authorized to contract directly with hospitals through preferred provider contracts in an attempt to stimulate price competition among hospitals.

Congress has considered a number of procompetitive proposals related to Medicare, Medicaid, and private health insurance. Although the proposals differ in detail, several elements characterize the procompetitive approach: (1) changes in tax treatment for employers, employees, or both, regarding employer contributions to health insurance plans (not supported by Congress) in the 1980s or the 1990s even though costs continued to escalate; (2) establishment of incentives or requirements for employers to offer employees multiple choices of health insurance plans, subject to certain limitations with respect to coverage of services and cost sharing, including catastrophic illness benefits and preventive care (in many states, employers have provided employees with fewer choices of managed care plans in the 1990s); and (3) establishment of Medicare voucher systems under which elderly and disabled individuals would receive a fixed payment instead of a defined benefit.

Although recent federal procompetition-deregulation policies have attracted the greatest attention, it was the dramatic reduction in federal fiscal capacity due to tax cuts and the growing federal deficit that had the most immediate effect on health services. While the federal government was limiting Medicare payments to hospitals and physicians and giving modest encouragement to HMOs, a number of states moved to restrict expenditures for Medicaid beneficiaries because of the continued impact of high costs on Medicaid expenditures at the state and federal levels. Several states, including California, have enacted dramatic policy changes,

restricting patients' freedom to choose providers, reducing levels of hospital and physician reimbursement, and shifting the burden of large numbers of poor patients back to local government.

The politics of limited resources in the 1970s continued into the 1980s and 1990s. The prolonged period of postwar economic growth, based on productivity gains, came to a halt in the early 1970s and was not reviewed until the mid-1990s. The additional resources needed in domestic social programs and defense were more and more constrained as a result. Controlling the costs of health care became a critical need at the federal and state levels. In the 1970s, policy efforts focused more on limiting federal and state expenditures in Medicare and Medicaid than they did on dealing with the root causes of the problem—the growing supply of physicians, the rapid growth in biomedical technologies in health care, and reimbursement incentives in Medicare, Medicaid, and private insurance mediated through the fee-for-service health system that have led to enormous inflation in health care costs.

Whether these approaches to restraining hospital and physician expenditures are effective remains to be seem. To date, the Medicare cost-containment strategies based on regulating hospital and physician payments have not been applied broadly to the private sector. It is likely that they will restrain the rate of increase in Medicare expenditures but increase those in the private sector due to cost shifting, unless the managed care strategies prove effective. Given a policy process characterized by limited government roles, federalism, pluralism, administrative bargaining, and incrementalism, prospects remain relatively dim for controlling expenditures in ways that protect vulnerable groups such as the poor and the elderly. It is increasingly evident that those groups whose needs originally inspired special programs are relinquishing the gains achieved in access to care.

The cost-containment strategies of the past decade, particularly those since 1981, combined with the effects of the recessions of 1981–1982 and 1990–1992 on unemployment and access to private health insurance, contributed to lower priority accorded access to care for the poor, as did the growth of the undocumented alien, immigrant, and refugee populations and the diminishing commitment to provide for the near poor and the working poor with private health insurance through employment. This has led to a significant increase in the number of uninsured and underinsured. Census Bureau data for 1994 revealed that 17% of the population under age sixty-five (over 40 million people) lacked any health insurance, an increase of more than 20% since 1979 (Blendon, et al., 1986). Despite the improved economy and low levels of unemployment, the number of uninsured, particularly among low-wage workers and their dependents, continues to grow.

Federal policies related Medicare and Medicaid, taxes, and refugees and undocumented aliens; state policies related to health care cost containment and Medicaid; and the policies of private insurance companies and employers related to private health insurance, competition, and cost containment have all contributed to the rising number of uninsured and underinsured. Because the working poor, the disabled, refugees, new immigrants, undocumented aliens, and workers in small businesses do not have the influence of the large employers, the insurance industry, physicians, hospitals, and other influential participants in health policy, it is unlikely that their voices will be heard unless the costs of their care impose such a burden on state and local governments and community hospitals (that is, bad debt and charity care) that these groups will gain allies willing to advocate on their behalf. Because the interests of these groups remain diffuse in terms

of potential for political action, it is unlikely that they can compete effectively in the policy process with the interest groups that have long influenced the shape of public policy in health.

The rise in health care costs continued as the dominant health policy issue of the 1990s. Between 1970 and 1990, the share of gross national product (GNP) spent on health care rose from 7.3% to 12.3%. National health spending in 1991 rose 11% over 1990, to $738 billion. This was the fifth consecutive year of double-digit annual increases (U.S. General Accounting Office, 1991). The United States Department of Commerce projected increases in 1992 to $817 billion, a record 14% of GNP. While the rate of health cost increases has slowed dramatically in recent years, there is evidence in late 1997 that health insurance premiums will again begin to rise. Estimates for the year 2000 imply that the percentage of GNP devoted to health care will likely reach 16%.

Families and businesses pay for health care directly through health insurance premiums and out of pocket (for example, deductibles, copayments) and indirectly through payroll, income, and other taxes that pay for public programs. According to a 1991 report by Families USA Foundation, the United States spent $5,535 per family for health care in 1991; approximately two-thirds of health care costs are paid by families and one-third is paid by businesses (Families USA Foundation, 1991).

For two decades health care spending in the United States outpaced the growth of the rest of the economy, with consequences for workers (depressed wages), business (a growing share of profits to health care), families (rising out-of-pocket costs and rising taxes to pay for public programs), and government (increasing share of government expenditures for health care). This began to change in the 1990s.

HEALTH POLICY: NEW SOLUTIONS, OLD PROBLEMS (1993–2002)

As the Clinton administration took office in 1993, there was talk in health care circles of federally driven reform on the scale of that produced by the Social Security Act legislation of 1935 and 1965. To the surprise of most, the election campaign of candidate Bill Clinton in 1992 not only raised health care as a salient national issue but also set the stage for a major health care reform process in 1993–1994. President Clinton and his team proposed comprehensive financing reform based on a strategy he called "managed competition," orchestrated by government and designed to stimulate private sector decisions that would expand coverage and control costs. The president initiated an elaborate process that developed a plan that he presented to Congress and the American people in September 1993. The thirteen hundred pages that translated this plan into legislative specifics were introduced in Congress in early 1994. The essential elements included universal coverage, purchasing cooperatives, budget caps, employer-mandated coverage, and no tax increase to expand coverage. The proposal was translated by its opponents into limited choice for consumers, loss of benefits and increased costs for many of the insured, government interference with the market and consumer choice, the addition of new government bureaucracies, and limits on professional autonomy. The public was confused. Congress could not reach agreement on any reform, and the proposal died in the spring of 1994. The failure of health care reform was yet another example of "American exceptionalism" when compared to other industrialized democracies. Indeed, even Taiwan and Korea had enacted programs of universal health insurance while the United States failed again. It also illustrated the difficulty of enacting comprehensive, as opposed to incremental, reforms in the United States.

If this period began with the promise of comprehensive reform at the federal level, by late 1994, the tables were turned once again as policy attention shifted back to reliance on competitive forces and the market with selective interference from government. In the Fall 1994 election, the Republicans gained control of both the United States House of Representatives and the United States Senate. The result was prolonged stalemate, with little accomplished in any area of health policy, except for the enactment of the Kennedy-Kassenbaum bill which extended health insurance protection for individuals who were changing jobs or were temporarily unemployed. In addition, the Ryan White Care Act (AIDS services) was extended, but no other significant health legislation was even reauthorized. After the 1996 presidential and congressional elections, President Clinton was returned to office, but the Republicans strengthened their control in the Senate and maintained their majority, somewhat diminished, in the House. The result was to be a dramatic shift from the confrontation and deadlock of 1995–1996 to a consensus on a play to balance the federal budget by 2002, including the most significant reforms in the Medicare program since 1965. The Balanced Budget Act of 1997 calls for a reduction in Medicare spending increases of $115 billion by 2002 and a dramatic increase in the choice of managed care plans, including HMOs, independent practice associations (IPAs), preferred provider organizations (PPOs), provider service organizations (PSOs), and even medical savings accounts. Medicare's basic fee-for-service option would continue.

Various forces will affect future policies: some, such as the aging of the population, are beyond the control of policy makers; others, such as the rapid increase in physician supply and the use of an increasing number of new technologies in health care, are amenable to more direct policy interventions. One of the keys will be to reach agreement on the nature and scope of cost containment. The Balanced Budget Act of 1997 was a major step forward in reaching consensus on health care cost containment in the future—it combines both managed care strategies and regulatory policies that focus on limiting provider payments rather than restricting consumer choice.

While two fundamentally different approaches to cost containment have been advocated and applied in the past fifteen years—regulation and competition—it appears that a mixed system will continue in the United States because of the strong role of the private sector, a federalist system of government, the dominance of pluralistic politics, and a penchant for incremental reform.

In the excellent review of health care reform, *Intensive Care,* edited by Mann and Ornstein (1995), the three key factors affecting health policy at the federal level were discussed in detail: (1) the budget, (2) information, and (3) oversight.

The budget has become the prime driver of policy, for both entitlement programs (for example, Medicare) and discretionary programs (for example, all the programs of the United States Public Health Service). Mann and Ornstein noted:

In an era of large deficits and the fiscalization of policy debate, the institutions within Congress for exercising its power of the purse affect the way health care policy is made. Largely in response to pressure to do something about the deficit, these institutions have been expanded in recent years to include budget resolutions, reconciliations, scorekeeping, discretionary spending caps, and "paygo" roles in addition to normal authorizing and appropriations process (p. 4).

They also observed:

In an era of large budget deficits and continuous fiscal constraints, opportunities for legislating new programs have all but vanished . . . policy making increasingly consists of shaping the administration and revision of existing programs, which heightens the importance of oversight to members of Congress (p. 5).

During the past decade, two new support agencies created by Congress to advise of hospital payment in the Medicare program have played very important advisory roles. In 1997, Congress merged the two commissions in order to link the analysis of Part A (hospital) and Part B (physician and related services) in Medicare.

Incrementalism appeared to be returning to the issue of extending coverage to the uninsured. In spite of the difficulties and complexities, Congress provided limited additional resources to states to expand health insurance coverage to children either through Medicaid or the private sector (Thorpe, 1997).

While health care financing and cost containment are not the dominant domestic social policy issues that they were in the early 1990s, they are likely to remain on the national policy agenda until the process of incremental reform really deals with the twin problems of rising health care costs and access to health insurance. The next chapters in health care reform will reflect the same factors that have affected health policy during the past sixty years.

REFERENCES

Alford, R. R. (1975). *Health care politics: Ideological and interest group barriers to reform.* Chicago: University of Chicago Press.

Bachrach, P. (1967). *The theory of democratic elitism: A critique.* Boston: Little, Brown.

Blendon, R. J., et al. (1990). Satisfaction with health systems in ten nations. *Health Affairs, 9,* 185–192.

Blendon, R. J., Aiken, L. H., Freeman, H. E., et al. (1986). Uncompensated care by hospitals or public insurance for the poor. *New England Journal of Medicine, 314,* 1160–1163.

Blendon, R. J., Brodie, M., & Benson, J. (1995, Summer). What happened to support for the Clinton plan? *Health Affairs, 14,* 7–23.

Blendon, R. J. & Taylor, H. (1989). Views on health care: Public opinion in three nations. *Health Affairs, 8,* 149–157.

Brizius, J. A. *Federalism and national purpose* (pp. 72–98). (n.d.). Working paper 2, Project on the Federal Social Role, National Conference on Social Welfare, Washington, DC.

Callahan, D. (1977). Health and society: Some ethical imperatives. *Daedalus, 106,* 1.

Clarke, G. J. (1981). The role of the states in the delivery of health services. In S. C. Jain (Ed.), *Role of state and local governments in relation to personal health services.* (Reprinted from *American Journal of Public Health, 71,* 59–69, 1981).

Estes, C. L. (1980). *The aging enterprise.* San Francisco: Jossey-Bass.

Estes, C. L. (1982). Austerity and aging in the United States: 1980 and beyond. *International Journal of Health Services, 12,* 573.

Families USA Foundation. (1991, December). *Health spending: The growing threat to the family budget.* Washington, DC: Author.

Feder, J. M. (1977). *The politics of federal hospital insurance.* Lexington, MA: Lexington Books.

Feldstein, P. J. (1981). The poltics of health. In P. R. Lee, N. Brown, & I.V.S.W. Red (Eds.), *The nation's health: Article booklet* (pp. 40–42). San Francisco: Boyd & Fraser.

Foley, H. A. (1975). *Community mental health legislation.* Lexington, MA: Lexington Books.

Ginzberg, D. (1978). Health reform: The outlook for the 1980s. *Inquiry, 15,* 311–326.

Ginzberg, E. (Ed.). (1977). *Regionalization and health policy.* Washington, DC: U.S. Government Printing Office.

Hale, G. E., & Palley, M. L. (1981). *The politics of federal grants.* Washington, DC: Congressional Quarterly Press.

Health Care Financing Administration. (1996). *1996 profiles of Medicare, 30th Anniversary, Health Care Financing Administration fiscal report for 1996.* Washington, DC: Author.

Heclo, H. (1995, Spring). The Clinton health plan: Historical perspective. *Health Affairs, 14,* 86–98.

Jonas, S., & Banta, D. (1981). Government in the health care delivery system. In S. Jonas (Ed.), *Health care delivery in the United States.* New York: Springer.

Kaiser Commission on the Future of Medicaid. (1995, September). *Medicaid and the elderly, policy brief.* Washington, DC: Author.

Kingdon, J. W. (1984). *Agendas, alternatives, and public policies.* Boston: Little, Brown.

Lee, P. R. & Jonsen, A. R. (1974). The right to health care. *American Review of Respiratory Diseases, 109,* 591–593.

Lee, P. R., LeRoy, L., & Stalcup, J. (1976). *Primary care in a specialized world.* Cambridge, MA: Ballinger.

Lee, P. R., & Silver, G.A. (1972). Health planning—A view from the top with specific reference to the USA. In J. Fry & W. A. J. Farndale (Eds.), *International medical care.* Oxford, UK: Medical and Technical Publishing.

Lee, R. D., & Staffeldt, R. J. (1977). Executive and legislative use of policy analysis in the state budgetary process. *Policy Analysis, 3,* 395–405.

Lewis, I., & Sheps, C. (1983). *The sick citadel: The American academic medical center and the public interest.* Cambridge, UK: Oelgeschlager, Gunn & Hain.

Lindblom, C. E. (1959). The science of "muddling through." *Public Administration Review, 10,* 79–88.

Lowi, T. J. (1979). *The end of liberalism: The second republic of the United States.* New York: Norton.

Luft, H. S. (1980). *Health maintenance organizations: Dimensions of performance.* New York: Wiley-Interscience.

Mann, T. E., & Ornstein, N. J. (Eds.). (1995). *Intensive care: How Congress shapes health policy.* Brookings Institute.

Marmor, T. R. (1973). *The politics of Medicare.* Chicago: Aldine.

Marmor, T. R., Wittman, D. A., & Heagy, T. C. (1976). The politics of medical inflation. *Journal of Health Politics, Policy and Law, 1,* 69–84.

Miller, C. A., Gilbert, B., & Warren, D. G. (1977). Statutory authorizations for the work of local health departments. *American Journal of Public Health, 67,* 940–946.

Miller, C. A., Moos, M. K., & Kotch, J. B., et al. (1981). Role of local health departments in the delivery of ambulatory care. In S. C. Jain (Ed.), *Role of state and local governments in relation to personal health services.* Chapel Hill: University of North Carolina Press.

Oliver, T. R. (1991, July). *A conceptual guide to policy implementation.* Unpublished manuscript. University of California, Institute for Health Policy Studies, San Francisco, CA.

Pechman, J. A. (Ed). (1979). *Setting national priorities: The 1980 budget.* Washington, DC: The Brookings Institution.

Physician Payment Review Commission. (1996). *Annual report to Congress, 1996.* Washington, DC: Author.

Reagan, M. D. (1972). *The new federalism.* New York: Oxford University Press.

Reagan, M. D., & Sanzone, J. G. (1981). *The new federalism* (2nd ed.). New York: Oxford University Press.

Richardson, E. L. (1971). *Towards a comprehensive health policy in the 1970s.* Washington, DC: U.S. Department of Health, Education and Welfare.

Sabatier, B., & Mazamania, D. (1979). Conditions of effective implantation. *Policy Analysis, 5,* 481–504.

Sabatier, P. A. (1988). An advocacy coalition framework of policy change and the role of policy-oriented learning therein. *Policy Sciences, 21,* 129–168.

Salkever, D. S., & Bice, T. W. (1976). The impact of certificate-of-need controls on hospital investment. *Milbank Memorial Fund Quarterly, 54,* 185–214.

Schattschneider, E. E. (1960). *The semisovereign people.* New York: Holt, Rinehart & Winston.

Silver, G. A. (1976a). Medical politics, health policy, party health platforms, promise and performance. *International Journal of Health Services, 6,* 331–343.

Silver, G. A. (1976b). *A spy in the house of medicine.* Germantown, MD: Aspen.

Silver, G. A. (1978). *Preface: The uncertainties of federal child health policies.* Hyattsville, JD: National Center for Health Services Research.

Silverman, M., & Lee, P. (1974). *Pills, profits, and politics.* Berkeley, CA: University of California Press.

Skocpol, T. (1995, Spring). The rise and resounding demise of the Clinton plan. *Health Affairs, 14,* 66–85.

Thorpe, K. E. (1997, July–August). Incremental approaches to covering uninsured children: Design and policy issues. *Health Affairs, 16*(4), 64–78.

Torrens, P. R. (1988). Overview of the health services system. In S. J. Williams & P. R. Torrens (Eds.), *Introduction to health services* (3rd ed.). New York: Wiley.

U.S. Department of Health, Education, and Welfare. (1976). *Health in America 1776–1976.* (DHEW Pub. No. HRA 76-616). Washington, DC: U.S. Government Printing Office.

U.S. General Accounting Office. (1991, November). *Health care spending control: The experience of France, Germany, and Japan* (GAO Pub. No. HRD-92-9). Washington, DC: U.S. Government Printing Office.

Vladeck, B. C. (1979). The design of failure: Health policy and the structure of federalism. *Journal of Health Politics, Policy and Law, 4,* 522–535.

Vladeck, B. C. (1980). *Unloving care: The nursing home tragedy.* New York: Basic Books.

Wade, R. C. (1982, August 1). The suburban roots of new federalism. *The New York Times Magazine,* pp. 20, 21, 39, 46.

Walker, D. (1981). *Toward a functioning federalism.* Cambridge, MA: Winthrop.

Wildavsky, A. (1964). *The politics of the budgetary process.* Boston: Little, Brown.

CHAPTER

16

Assessing and Improving Quality of Care*

Scott Weingarten

CHAPTER TOPICS

* This chapter is adapted from "Implementing Clinical Practice Guidelines," by S. Weingarten & S. Deutsch, Chapter 6 in *Internal Medicine* (5th ed.), Stein, 1997, St. Louis, MO: Mosby.

LEARNING OBJECTIVES

Upon completing this chapter, the reader should be able to:

- Appreciate the complexity of defining and measuring the quality of care.
- Understand how measuring and monitoring quality can result in improved outcomes.
- Define how quality is assessed and assured.
- Appreciate strategies that now exist for influencing physician behavior.
- Review illustrative scenarios of quality improvement programs.

The debate on quality of health care has taken center stage. On one hand, advances in medical care proceed at an astronomical pace. The populations' life span has been steadily increasing. New medical technologies and procedures abound. American medical care has produced some of the most sophisticated technologies in the world.

The paradox of health care, however, is that while there have been unprecedented advances in medical technology, concerns about quality of care not only continue but intensify. For example, recent studies have documented compromised outcomes for patients who have reduced access to medical care. Furthermore, there are concerns that the proliferation of managed care will promote the underutilization of necessary medical resources and compromise quality of patient care.

WHAT IS QUALITY?

This debate on quality has forced us to ask some very basic questions. What is quality of patient care? Can quality of care be measured? Purchasers of health care are asking these questions about the quality of care provided by health plans, hospitals, and health care providers. As they spend an increasing amount of money on health care and public concern about health care quality receives greater attention, they are searching for objective information on the quality of care that patients are receiving.

An Illustration of Quality

An example of the difficulty of making judgments about quality of care could be illustrated through the experience of a patient undergoing coronary artery bypass surgery. A patient with significant coronary artery disease consults with a cardiac surgeon prior to surgery. The cardiac surgeon spends little time with the patient during the preoperative visit. She makes little effort to educate the patient about what will happen before, during, and after surgery. One week later, the surgery is performed without complications. The length of stay for the patient in the acute care hospital is eleven days, which is five days longer than the average length of stay for patients undergoing coronary artery bypass surgery in that particular hospital. The total hospital costs for that patient are $10,000 more than for an average patient in that particular hospital. After adjusting the length of stay and cost for case complexity, the cost and length of stay is still much greater than for comparable cases in that hospital and region. The patient, however, survived the operation and had an uncomplicated hospital course and was free from postoperative complications. Three months later, the patient's health is excellent, and he is able to enjoy tennis free from symptoms.

From a technical standpoint, the operation went flawlessly and the clinical outcome was excellent. The "art" of caring for the patient, however, was questionable, as the patient received little information about the care that he was going to receive before, during, and after surgery. The physician exhibited poor communication skills. And if utilization were considered a measure of quality, the prolonged length of stay and increased costs associated with the operation might be considered indicative of suboptimal quality of care.

Did this patient receive excellent or poor quality medical care? Judgments of this type depend on many different factors, and the importance attached to each of those factors. Some patients might believe that the quality of care was excellent as evidenced by the clinical outcome (the patient had an uncomplicated hospital course and was able to resume an active lifestyle). Some patients, however, especially those who place a higher value on the "art of care" and desire a more personalized approach, might have a more negative opinion about the quality of care that they received. Finally, if one examines the "economic outcome," the care would not have compared favorably to the care provided to other patients. To a certain extent, quality is in "the eyes of the beholder," and it may not always be perfectly clear whether an individual patient received good or poor quality medical care. This principle can also apply to evaluating the care provided to populations of patients.

Measurement Issues

Competition and market forces have taken hold of health care delivery. In the past, competition in health care was largely based on cost. As in many other sectors of the economy, there is a strong desire to base competition on both quality and cost, or the value of care. To achieve this goal, it is necessary to have valid and reliable measures of quality of care that can be measured relatively cost-effectively.

In the past, physicians have often felt comfortable ordering tests, prescribing treatments, and advising patients relatively free from scrutiny regarding the care that they provided. The focus of providing care was on individual patients rather than populations of patients. Assessments of quality of care were usually made only the most egregious of cases, such as by peer review committees and through medical malpractice litigation. Furthermore, research investigations question the ability of peer review committees to accurately assess quality of care; the validity of this method for assessing quality has been shown to be poor. Review of medical malpractice cases is also considered to be an insensitive and nonspecific measure of quality of care, since poor quality of care may not be associated with litigation and not all medical malpractice cases are caused by poor quality of care.

As a result of quality measurement, "report cards" and other expressions of quality of care information have become commonplace. Physicians often are concerned that accountability and "report cards" intrude into the care that they provide to patients. However, physicians' and other health care providers' concern about this intrusion seems to be outweighed by the sentiments of the purchasers who are demanding to understand the care provided to their employees or beneficiaries through the inspection of objective data.

In many industries, purchasing decisions are made based on cost and quality. In health care, however, this has not been the case. Purchasing decisions have been largely based on the cost of care. Cost has been the predominant factor driving health care purchasing, in part because cost has been easier to measure than quality of care. Information on quality, if available, could be used to direct value-based purchasing decisions. The alternative is that competition in health care would be based entirely on the cost of care; this could lead to a downward price spiral where care is provided by those who offer medical care at the lowest cost. In the most extreme case, this could mean that clinicians and health care organizations providing the least care to patients would have the opportunity to care for the most patients.

One of the most notable attempts to measure quality of care provided at different hospitals is published annually by *U.S. News and World Report.* These reports, which have been published since 1990, are based on the opinion of physicians who have been identified as leaders in the field of medicine. The ratings are based on "clinical expertise," technology, teaching status, experience, and outcome (mortality rates). Recent critiques of this effort, however, suggest that the data included in this analysis preclude valid and meaningful comparisons of quality. Furthermore, an analysis of the information suggests that the ratings reflect hospital reputation rather than objectively measured information about quality of patient care.

Assuming that quality rankings are based on reputation rather than objective measures of quality, a hospital providing excellent quality of care, without a matching reputation, might not be publicly acknowledged as a high-quality institution. Furthermore, a hospital with an excellent reputation might continue to be regarded as high quality regardless of whether there are data that support or refute that finding.

VARIATIONS IN CARE

Variations in care have been demonstrated in different regions throughout the country, in different hospitals in the same region, and even among different physicians practicing at the same hospital. Increasingly, questions are being asked regarding the cause of these variations (Wennberg & Gittelsohn, 1973). One possible explanation is that many clinical decisions cannot be supported by scientific evidence and, instead, are determined by an individual physician's experience and training, along with the "art of medicine." Of those clinical decisions that are based on scientific evidence, the scientific knowledge is at times inconsistent and difficult for physicians and other health care providers to access in real time while they are caring for patients. Variations in care may be further

accentuated by differences in patient preferences, since patients may choose different options when informed about alternative treatments.

Another factor affecting variations in patient care is the explosion of available medical information. It has been said that there are more than 20,000 biomedical journals and more than 2,000,000 medically related articles published each year. An individual physician could be expected to read and retain a relatively small fraction of the published medical literature. The proliferation of medical information has led to the concern that physicians will not be able to keep current with the latest medical literature. Without a method of organizing and summarizing available, current, and relevant clinical information, it may be impossible for an individual clinician to remain current and to apply available clinical information to each patient's care. Failure to remain current with the literature may lead to delays in translating important new medical advances into widespread clinical practice.

OPPORTUNITIES TO IMPROVE CARE

There are many reasons to measure quality of care. Perhaps the most compelling reason is to attempt to improve quality of care. It has been said, "if you cannot measure it, you cannot manage it." Measurement of quality can illuminate opportunities to improve quality of care. For example, one might discover missed opportunities to immunize children against infectious diseases and to offer mammograms to women. Measurement of quality is also important to determine whether there are gaps between actual medical practice and optimal medical practice as defined by review of the scientific literature. The measurement of quality may be particularly important when the scientific evidence demonstrates that there is a "best practice" or an optimal method of caring for patients. In this case, one could compare the actual provision of therapy with best practice. For example, beta-blockers have been shown to improve the outcomes of patients with an acute myocardial infarction. Therefore, because there is a process (provision of beta-blockers) and outcome (survival) link, the discovery of underutilization of this treatment could be associated with compromises in patient care.

Additional research has disclosed a significant gap between optimal medical care (care that would lead to the best patient outcomes) and care that is being provided on a widespread basis (Ellerbeck, et al., 1995; Krumholtz, et al., 1995; Weiner, et al., 1995). Whether examining influenza immunization of elderly patients, the performance of mammograms, or childhood immunizations, studies consistently have demonstrated opportunities to improve the quality of patient care. For example, the published literature demonstrated that thrombolytic therapy was associated with a reduction in mortality long before it was widely recommended for clinical practice for patients suffering with acute myocardial infarction. In addition, aspirin is an inexpensive, safe, and effective medication for treating patients with acute myocardial infarction. To determine the use of aspirin in patients with acute myocardial infarction, a retrospective study was performed on hospitalized patients sixty-five years of age and older (Krumholtz, et al., 1995). Among those patients without contraindications to aspirin, more than one-third did not receive aspirin during the first two days of hospitalization. Those patients who received aspirin had a lower mortality rate than those who did not. Increasing the use of aspirin for elderly patients after acute myocardial infarction may be a cost-effective and simple strategy to improve quality of care and to reduce the mortality rates for elderly patients suffering from acute myocardial infarction (Krumholtz, et al., 1995).

Research has also demonstrated a significant opportunity to improve the quality of care provided to elderly diabetic patients (Weiner, et al., 1995). A majority of patients did not receive regular glycosylated hemoglobin levels (which is important for monitoring the control of blood sugar in diabetic patients). Furthermore, many patients did not receive cholesterol screening. These findings demonstrated a significant opportunity to improve quality of care provided to diabetic patients.

Health services researchers have discovered a significant rate of inappropriate care, including the use and application of invasive procedures (Brook, 1989). Inappropriate care can be determined using many different definitions, including the provision of care when risks are greater than the potential benefits. Furthermore, it is believed that the provision of inappropriate care may contribute to rising health care costs, and curbing this care may be an excellent method of reducing costs without sacrificing, and with possibly improving, quality of patient care.

Benchmarking

Many of the early efforts to measure quality were primitive and not felt to be reflective of quality of care by many clinicians. Some of these efforts included the measurement of hospital admission rates and hospital lengths of stay. "Benchmarking" was performed to compare a hospital's admission rate with admission rates at "best performing" hospitals. The problem with these analyses is the difficulty in achieving consensus around what constitutes an appropriate hospital admission rate. For example, a hospital with a higher admission rate may have a lower rate of discharging patients from the emergency department to their home inappropriately. "Benchmarking" has traditionally been based on utilization, rather than on quality of care or patient outcome. Furthermore, utilization data that cannot be linked to patient outcomes is of limited value. Utilization data have often come from administrative data systems that were not designed to collect information to evaluate the quality of care.

FRAMEWORK FOR MEASURING QUALITY

Donabedian was an early pioneer in developing a framework for evaluating the quality of care. He defined quality as having at least three dimensions, including structure, process, and outcome of care. He said that "it is possible to divide this management into two domains: technology of medicine, and of the other health sciences, to the management of a personal health problem. Its accompaniment is the management of the social and psychological interaction between client and practitioner. The first of these has been called the science of medicine and the second its art." He also defined "a third element in care which could be called its 'amenities.'" The Institute of Medicine later defined quality as the "degree to which health services for individuals and populations increase the likelihood of desired health outcomes and are consistent with current professional knowledge." Quality of care can be measured in patients who are ill and also in patients who are well.

The locus of quality measurement can vary. Quality of health care can be measured in a community, health plan, physician organization (such as a medical group or independent practice association), hospital, or even care provided by an individual physician. Another key issue affecting outcome measurement has to do with the timing of measurement. For example, for patients discharged following hospitalization for community-acquired pneumonia, one month after discharge may be an adequate amount of time to assess patient outcome. However, for patients recovering after total hip replacement surgery, it may be necessary to wait one to two years after surgery to fully understand a patient's recovery (reduction in pain and improvement in physical functioning), and possibly five to ten years or longer to determine whether a repeat operation was required.

Assessment of quality can also be performed through implicit and explicit measurement. Explicit measurement entails comparing the quality of care against some predetermined standard, for example, the number of patients who sustained a myocardial infarction and who were treated with a beta-blocker. Implicit measurement is usually subjective, without a comparison with a predetermined performance criteria.

Quality of care studies have also been influenced by recent attempts to better understand the impact of patient preferences on clinical decision making and the role of shared medical decision making. Patient involvement in the care process has assumed greater importance in recent years.

Structure of Care

The dimensions of quality of care include structure, process, and outcome. The structure of care includes information on the facilities and people caring for patients. Information on the facilities may include hospital bed size or the procedures performed in a hospital. Information on the caregivers might include the percentage of doctors who are board-certified. Studies on the structure of care often show a weak correlation between these characteristics and the quality of care provided to patients and patient outcomes. Therefore, the evaluation of structure as a measure of quality is often not regarded as clinically meaningful.

Process of Care

In contrast, process of care relates to what is done to particular patients (such as diagnostic tests or procedures). Measuring the process of care is clinically credible when there is a proven link between process (performing that test or procedure) and a clinically important outcome measure (mortality, quality of life, patient satisfaction). If there is not a link between the process of care and outcome, process measurement may not yield meaningful results.

Attempts have been made to detect underutilization of medical care by measuring the processes of care (for example, an individual patient either did or did not have a mammogram). Process of care measurement may also be applied to a population of patients. For example, the annual mammography rate for women fifty years of age and older is 75%. This is clinically meaningful, since there are randomized controlled clinical trials that have shown that mammography can reduce long-term mortality from breast cancer in women of an appropriate age range. Other process measures might include PAP smear rates and childhood immunization rates.

There is some concern about attempting to utilize process measures to evaluate quality of care. For example, results of such analyses have shown that a health plan may score very well in one area while scoring poorly in another area, making overall judgments about quality of care difficult. If a health plan had a high mammography rate and a low PAP smear rate, would this health plan be considered a good or poor quality health plan? If a consumer considering the selection of a health plan had access to these data, how would these rates, if at all, influence his or her decision? Finally, since health plans are not directly responsible for the performance of mammograms or PAP smears, would this information be considered a valid measure of the health plans' performance?

Outcome of Care

Patient outcome can be measured to evaluate quality of patient care. An outcome is the result of the care provided to patients. Inadequate process of care, however, may not always result in poor patient outcome. For example, many children who are not immunized will not die from communicable diseases. In this case, the outcome is favorable even though most clinicians would regard the care as being of poor quality.

In the past, quality of care has been largely measured through the examination of clinical and physiologic variables. Such measures might include whether a patient recovering after total hip replacement develops a postoperative infection. For a patient recovering from a total hip replacement, the patient's severity of pain and ability to physically function might also be considered very important measures of quality. And the rapidity with which a patient is able to return to work can potentially relate to the quality of care.

The following are examples of patient outcome measures. These measures include clinical (survival), patient-centered (quality of life), and satisfaction measures:

- The five-year mortality rate from breast cancer
- The mean quality-of-life score for patients with stage II breast cancer
- The percentage of patients receiving a mammogram who were very satisfied with the care that they received in the radiology suite

Mortality Rates

There is controversy regarding whether hospital mortality rates are a valid measure of quality of care. Validity is enhanced when the rates are adjusted for severity of illness and the volume and severity of comorbid conditions. There are some studies that indicate that hospitals with higher severity-adjusted mortality rates have more preventable deaths, which could infer that quality of care relates to mortality rates. Issues about the validity of this information, however, led to concerns about publishing hospital mortality rates as a measure of quality.

One of the most visible efforts to measure the quality of care provided by physicians has been measuring severity-adjusted mortality rates for physicians who perform coronary artery bypass surgery. Since mortality is an important outcome measure for patients, mortality rates, assuming that there has been adequate adjustment for case severity, may relate to quality of care. Mortality rates, however, would be an insensitive measure of the quality of care provided to patients undergoing cataracts surgery or to patients in the outpatient setting.

The most significant concern about attempting to infer information about quality of care from mortality rates is that there must be adequate adjustment for severity of patient illness. For example, if one hospital treats patients who are more severely ill than another hospital, a higher mortality rate may not reflect worse quality of care, but rather that patients in that hospital are more severely ill and therefore have a higher probability of dying. In order to use outcome information to judge quality of care, adjustment must be made for patient severity of illness. Severity-of-illness measures have been used to predict probability of death, morbidity, or a prolonged length of hospital stay. Severity measures can incorporate variables related to diagnosis, physiological variables, and laboratory variables.

Comorbidity

Comorbidity relates to the volume and severity of existing illnesses. Comorbidity may also be predictive of adverse outcomes. For example, a patient suffering an acute myocardial infarction with severe diabetes mellitus and chronic obstructive pulmonary disease may have a higher probability of an adverse outcome than patients with acute myocar-

dial infarction without any comorbid illnesses. Therefore, understanding the volume and severity of comorbid illnesses may be essential for relating the results of outcome measurement studies to the evaluation of the quality of care rendered to individual patients.

Health Status

Recently, there has been increasing interest in measuring patient-centered outcomes such as health status (and health-related quality of life). Recent studies have shown that there are valid, reliable, and responsive instruments to measure outcomes from the patient's perspective. The acceptance of these measures has increased as they have been shown to correlate with physiological measures (for example, a patient's physical functioning score correlates with their ability to perform on a treadmill). Since many procedures are performed to reduce pain and improve functioning, such as total hip replacement and cataracts surgery, measurement of health-related quality of life and health status may better reflect quality of care than many clinical measures. Research efforts in measuring patient-based outcomes has led to improvements in these measures, including instrument reliability (in test and retest studies), validity (the results correlate with physiological measures of health), and responsiveness (the measures change over time in a manner consistent with changes in physiological health).

Patient Satisfaction

Along with other measures of quality, significant attention has been devoted toward the measurement of patient satisfaction. Satisfaction relates to the quality of service provided to patients. The validity of patient satisfaction as a measure of technical quality of care (technical aspects of medical care) is uncertain. Employer groups, however, view patient (employee) satisfaction as an important indicator for assessing the performance of health plans, hospitals, and physician organizations. Furthermore, certain organizations have attempted to understand patient ratings of individual physicians. Physician reimbursement and other incentives have been linked to patient satisfaction ratings.

Access to Care

Another important measure of quality of care is access to necessary health care services. Access may relate to care provided by physicians and/or subspecialists or the availability of tests and procedures. The recent interest in measuring access to care reflects the public's concern that necessary and appropriate health care services may be underutilized in a capitated environment (an environment that provides a financial incentive to provide less medical care).

ATTEMPTS TO STANDARDIZE QUALITY MEASURES

One of the most significant challenges in the field of quality improvement is the need to standardize performance measures. If physician organizations must respond frequently to multiple queries about quality of care, the financial burden of measurement may exceed the benefits. This could occur if the resource requirements necessary for reporting quality diverted significant resources away from caring for patients and negatively impacted quality of patient care. This would be especially true if efforts to measure quality do not result in documented benefits in patient care.

The National Committee for Quality Assurance (NCQA) is responsible for coordinating the development of HEDIS (Health Plan Employer and Data Information Set) as a measure of the quality of care provided by health plans. Employer groups helped sponsor the development of these measures

to monitor the care provided to their employees. The measures, largely developed by clinical and methodological experts, initially emphasized outpatient process of care measures (such as childhood immunization rates, mammography rates, and PAP smear rates). HEDIS has been expanded to include the measurement of patient outcomes. The outcome measures in HEDIS 3.0 include patient satisfaction and health status.

COST CONTAINMENT AND QUALITY

Health care costs have been rising at an unsustainable pace. As concerns about rising health care costs escalate, numerous efforts have been initiated to curb costs. These efforts include shortening hospital lengths of stay, decreasing hospital admission rates, reducing the use of expensive tests and procedures, and decreasing referrals to specialists. Some cost-containment strategies probably maintain and possibly enhance quality of care. Some efforts, however, may compromise quality of care, especially when necessary and appropriate care is eliminated.

A number of studies have demonstrated that when access to medical care is reduced for poor patients, quality of care is compromised and patient outcomes may worsen. Furthermore, some efforts to control costs for specific aspects of care may lead to an increase in costs in other sectors. For example, an effort to limit the number of drugs made available to mentally ill patients was found to increase the number of emergency department visits and partial hospitalizations for psychiatrically related conditions. This effort to reduce costs was associated with an increase in overall health care costs (the reduction in drug costs was offset by an increase in costs associated with patient care visits).

MANAGED CARE AND QUALITY

Outcome studies have been conducted to compare quality of care in managed care and fee-for-service health systems. In the aggregate, no system consistently demonstrated better quality of care, although differences in care have been reported in some studies. No clear differences are seen when comparing most quality of care and outcome measures.

Quality of preventive care has been shown in some studies to be better in managed care organizations than in fee-for-service medicine. Other studies have shown better patient satisfaction among patients cared for in a fee-for-service setting when compared with a managed care organization. A recent study, which received considerable attention, showed a greater decline in physical functioning among elderly patients enrolled in managed care organizations when compared to fee-for-service medicine (Ware, et al., 1996). However, studies have not consistently documented this finding. Additional research will be required before it can be determined whether quality of care is better or worse in managed care organizations.

Furthermore, not all managed care organizations are equal, and it is possible that quality of care may vary with the organization. Many of the previous studies have examined care provided in mature managed care organizations, and the results may not be generalizable to managed care organizations with less experience.

PRACTICE GUIDELINES

Health services research studies left a trail of observations regarding the delivery of medical care services, including unexplainable variations in medical care, the provision of inappropriate medical care, and gaps between optimal medical practice and widespread clinical practice (Wennberg & Gittelsohn, 1973). Some have promoted the idea that practice guidelines may remedy this situation (Woolf, 1993). Medical practice guidelines, otherwise known as practice parameters or protocols, are a means of providing organized medical knowledge to clinicians that could potentially influence the care delivered to individuals and populations of patients. Practice guidelines have been defined as "systematically developed statements to assist practitioner decisions about appropriate health care for specific clinical circumstances." The guidelines are often derived from systematic reviews of the scientific evidence, and the information is condensed into documents to assist clinicians and patients. The guidelines consolidate available scientific knowledge about the best and most appropriate treatments for patients with common diseases and conditions (Brook, 1989). The expression of guidelines may vary from relatively simple statements, such as mammography should be offered to all women over a certain age, to more comprehensive and complicated patient care management strategies.

Proponents of clinical guidelines believe that they have the potential to improve clinical decision making, decrease undesirable variations in medical care, improve quality of care, and decrease health care costs (Woolf, 1993). Enthusiasm for guidelines, however, is tempered by concerns that guidelines oversimplify the practice of medicine, devalue the "art of medicine," and infringe upon physician autonomy and clinical freedom. There is also a concern that they may be used in a punitive manner or by plaintiffs' attorneys against health care providers in medical malpractice cases. In addition, some clinicians believe that the primary motivation behind the development of practice guidelines is to contain costs rather than to improve quality of care (Tunis, et al., 1994).

There are a number of organizations either producing or sponsoring the development of practice guidelines. Those organizations include the United States federal government (United States Preventive Services Task Force, the Agency for Health Care Policy and Research), specialty societies (American College of Cardiology, American College of Physicians), academic medical centers, health plans, and commercial organizations. As a testimonial to the number of organizations producing practice guidelines, the American Medical Association's Directory of Practice Parameters lists and catalogues more than two thousand different guidelines. These guidelines, however, are of variable quality, ranging from scholarly syntheses of the available scientific evidence (for example, American College of Physicians, Agency for Health Care Policy and Research) to guidelines that are less rigorous and comprehensive.

Although many different guidelines are in circulation, the impact of many of these guidelines on patient care is unknown. Furthermore, the acceptability, credibility, and quality of guidelines vary. Recent studies have demonstrated that professional society guidelines receive a higher level of confidence from some physicians than guidelines produced by other sources (Tunis, et al., 1994). One study showed that practice guidelines developed by health plans are often viewed as less credible than guidelines developed by other organizations.

With the large number of guidelines in existence, it may be a daunting task for clinicians to decide which guidelines are most appropriate for their patients, and which guidelines offer the greatest opportunity to improve medical care. Guidelines vary widely in the method used to create them, the rigor with which the scientific evidence is reviewed and organized, the background of the individuals creating the practice guidelines, and the resources devoted toward their development.

For many conditions, there are multiple guidelines available on the same topic. Given the variability in the process used to create guidelines, it is not surprising that conflicts have been identified between different guidelines on the same topic. These conflicts can create confusion among clinicians contemplating using them to assist in the care of their patients. Furthermore, it may be perceived that some developers of guidelines have conflicts of interest that may influence guideline recommendations. An example of this concern is the development of guidelines with the perceived goal of promoting subspecialty consultation.

There are different methods of developing practice guidelines. A preferred method includes the rigorous integration of all available and relevant scientific evidence (for example, randomized controlled clinical trials and meta-analyses) (Cook, et al., 1992). Guidelines developed in this manner are often called "evidence-based" guidelines. Many guidelines, however, are based on expert opinion alone, unsubstantiated by higher levels of scientific evidence. Some people believe that evidence-based guidelines may be more acceptable to clinicians, most of whom were trained in the application of the scientific method. (The scientific method is a basic foundation for medical, nursing, and pharmacy training.)

Some desirable attributes of practice guidelines include the following.

1. The purpose of the guideline should be clearly expressed. For example, the guideline was developed to improve the appropriateness of providing mammography to women.
2. The content of guidelines must be frequently reviewed and updated regularly. For example, a two year-old guideline to assist clinicians who are caring for patients with AIDS that does not incorporate the latest scientific evidence could

lead to suboptimal medical care. Ideally, guidelines should have an expiration date.

3. The guidelines must be flexible enough to account for the nuances of clinical medicine. The clinical nuances of medicine are often subtle; therefore, it is unrealistic to expect to apply a guideline to every conceivable patient.

4. Guidelines should be easy to follow. Complicated guidelines with multiple branch points are often difficult to remember. These guidelines may not be adopted into practice in the absence of sophisticated information technology.

5. The guidelines should be applicable in a variety of geographic and health care settings.

6. Guidelines should be linked to demonstrable improvements in patient outcomes, which may include morbidity, mortality, health status, quality of life, satisfaction, and cost of care. Outcome validation is especially important when scientific support for the recommendations is uncertain. It is often easier to achieve clinician support for guidelines that have been shown to improve patient outcomes.

Although an evidence-based approach to guideline development is appealing for eventual physician acceptance of the guidelines, there are limitations of this approach. One of the most notable limitations is a paucity of scientific evidence to support many common clinical practices. In other cases, the available evidence may be incomplete, contradictory, or of insufficient quality or credibility to be used to develop a guideline.

Despite the explosive growth in the number of medical practice guidelines, until recently, there has been relatively limited evidence that they have had an impact on medical care. There has been a disproportionate amount of time spent on their development as compared with time spent on their implementation and evaluation. A systematic review of the published literature on practice guidelines, however, demonstrated that guidelines have significant potential to improve patient care (Grimshaw & Russell, 1993). Of fifty-nine published studies on practice guidelines, fifty-five demonstrated at least one significant change in care associated with the introduction of a guideline. The magnitude of the effects was variable. Moreover, of the eleven studies that examined patient outcomes, nine demonstrated beneficial changes in patient care. A more recent update of this work continues to demonstrate that the majority of guideline studies demonstrate at least one improvement in care. Although the clinical significance is not always large, overall available research would suggest that there is continued reason to pursue practice guideline development, implementation, and evaluation.

If a guideline is not adopted into practice, it will have relatively little impact on patient care. Many studies have demonstrated that dissemination of guidelines alone fails to produce widespread adoption, including guidelines published by prestigious scientific organizations such as the National Institutes of Health (Kosecoff, et al., 1987). Many barriers to physician adoption of guidelines must be overcome for guidelines to have the opportunity to improve patient care (Goldman, 1990; Greco & Eisenberg, 1993). The literature has convincingly demonstrated that a carefully crafted implementation plan is requisite for the adoption of guidelines; otherwise, there may be no sustained change in clinical practice (Corey & Merenstein, 1987; Eisenberg, 1986; Goldman, 1990).

Physician attitudes and beliefs about practice guidelines may influence their adoption (Tunis, et al., 1994). A recent survey of physician attitudes showed that a majority of physicians believed that guidelines would be used for disciplinary actions. This same survey showed that a significant number of physicians believed that guidelines will increase health care costs even although their development is motivated by a desire to reduce costs.

Many different implementation strategies have been employed to encourage clinician adoption of guidelines (Figure 16–1). For example, any one of these strategies, or several of them, could be employed to implement the United States Preventive Services Task Force (USPSTF) guidelines regarding mammography. The USPSTF guidelines state that "routine screening for breast cancer every 1–2 years, with mammography alone or mammography and annual clinical breast examination (CBE), is recommended for women aged 50–69."

A systematic overview was performed to determine the relative effectiveness of different strategies to modify physician behavior (Davis, et al., 1995). The results showed that information dissemination and education alone usually fail to change physician practice or patient outcomes. However, more comprehensive and multifaceted implementation strategies (for example, use of physician opinion leaders, "academic detailing") were effective in producing change in physician practice. These strategies were accompanied by up to 20–50% reduction in the provision of inappropriate care. This information should cause a loss of confidence in dissemination strategies that depend on education alone and call for renewed enthusiasm for strategies that include multiple simultaneous approaches toward implementing guidelines.

Implementation Strategies

Some of the implementation strategies used with practice guidelines include the following.

Traditional Education. Published studies have demonstrated that traditional continuing medical education programs fail to produce sustained changes in clinical practice (Davis, et al., 1995; Oxman, et al., 1995). Although educational programs may appear to be a cost-effective method of

I. Traditional education
II. Retrospective feedback
III. Concurrent feedback (reminders)
IV. Incentives
V. Administrative solutions
VI. "Academic detailing"
VII. Opinion leaders
VIII. Patient education
IX. Application of information technology
X. Physician (clinician) involvement in the development and implementation process

FIGURE 16–1 Implementation strategies to encourage adoption of practice guidelines

gaining widespread acceptance of guidelines, available information on the effectiveness of education as a dissemination strategy suggests that expectations should be low, except when education is used in conjunction with other implementation strategies. A Grand Rounds or continuing medical education program could be used to inform clinicians about the USPSTF guidelines on mammography; however, little sustained change should be anticipated.

Retrospective Feedback. Results are mixed regarding the effects of retrospective feedback and physician profiling on physician practice (Balas, et al., 1996). Although changes in patient care have been demonstrated in studies employing retrospective feedback and profiling, the magnitude of the effect is often small. Therefore, enthusiasm for physician profiling and retrospective feedback may not always be supported by proven changes in patient care.

Retrospective feedback could be used to provide clinicians with feedback about their mammography rates (for example, 75% compliance with USPSTF mammography guidelines). Also, each clinician's mammography rates could be compared with those of his or her peers.

Concurrent Feedback (Reminders). Studies have demonstrated that real-time feedback of guideline information to physicians, while they are caring for patients, can be associated with a significant increase in their adoption of the guidelines (Mugford, et al., 1991). Reminders enable physicians to decide whether a particular guideline is appropriate for their individual patient at the time they are providing care. However, some studies have shown that the effects of guidelines on clinical practice diminish when reminders are discontinued.

To encourage adherence to USPSTF mammography guidelines, checklists, written reminders, or cues could be used to prompt physicians to perform mammograms in appropriate patients at the time of the visit (also see information technology).

Incentives. Many studies have shown that incentives, monetary and otherwise, may significantly influence clinical decision making (Eisenberg, 1986). It stands to reason that incentives, or removal of disincentives, may promote adoption of practice guidelines. Linking physician reimbursement to adoption of USPSTF mammography guidelines would be considered a method of incentives for physicians to follow the guidelines.

Administrative Solutions. In general, administrative rules have been shown to produce changes in physician practice (Eisenberg, 1986). Therefore, administrative mandates may be used to enforce adoption of guidelines, although the safety of this approach is largely unproved. An administrative solution to promote the adoption of guidelines could best be illustrated by the exclusion of a particular drug from a formulary. An administrative fiat might be less appropriate for increasing adoption of USPSTF mammography guidelines.

"Academic Detailing." "Academic detailing," a method involving one-on-one educational interactions, has been shown to change physician behavior (Soumerai & Avorn, 1990). Face-to-face sessions may prove to be successful when the message is brief and repetitive. During these encounters, the educator attempts to understand each clinician's approach to a particular clinical situation. The "detailer" explains the guideline to the physician who then has the opportunity to raise questions and concerns about the application of the guideline to patient care. Although this approach has proven effective, it can be costly and labor-intensive.

Using the "academic detailing" model, the educator might schedule a meeting or series of meetings with each clinician to better understand their beliefs and attitudes about the USPSTF mammography guidelines. Using that information as background, the "detailer" could explain the potential benefits of following USPSTF mammography guidelines.

Opinion Leaders. Studies have shown that the visible support of practice guidelines by "opinion leaders" may promote adoption of the guidelines (Eisenberg, 1986). Using a "social influence" model of changing clinician behavior, local peer pressure and influence may affect practice patterns. Therefore, recruiting local and influential "physician champions" to promote guidelines may prove to be effective. Respected opinion leaders could be used to promote the USPSTF mammography guidelines.

Patient Education. Patient education and outreach programs can be used to promote patient understanding of the rationale behind guidelines. Patients may initiate questions with their physician that lead to adoption of the guideline. Patient education could be used to directly inform women about the potential benefits of mammography with the hope that women who are overdue would contact their physician and request a mammogram.

Application of Information Technology. Recent technological advances in clinical information systems have been accompanied by studies examining the use of computerized reminders to implement practice guidelines (Pestotnik, et al., 1996; Rind, et al., 1994). Several of these studies have shown that real-time computer reminders can lead to increased adoption of guidelines. The desire to implement multiple practice guidelines, and the application of guidelines to patients with multiple conditions and comorbid illnesses, will also increase the potential benefits of using computerized reminders as an implementation strategy. Furthermore, when physicians interact with practice guidelines on a dynamic basis (such as with computerized order entry systems), computer technology may prove to be a cost-effective method of implementing several guidelines at the same time. Finally, information technology may enable the performance of cost-effective outcome studies. Intranet-based strategies to disseminate guidelines will undoubtedly receive significant attention as integrated delivery networks refine their attempts to disseminate and implement guidelines.

Busy physicians and clinicians may be less likely to seek out guidelines if they either detract from the patient encounter or reduce time with patients. Time constraints may limit the adoption of paper-based guidelines, especially if they require a physician to search out guidelines while the patient waits in the office or in the examining room. In the future, practice guidelines and other clinical decision support tools may be embedded in clinical decision support software housed in an electronic medical record. The key decision points, and the guidelines to support the most appropriate clinical decisions, may be linked to diagnoses, diagnostic tests, treatments, symptoms, or signs. The widespread deployment of this type of system may significantly advance attempts to implement complicated guidelines and allow for the capture of patient outcome data and the use of this information to improve medical care. With each patient encounter, a clinical information system could be used to process the age, gender, date of last mammogram (if appropriate), breast cancer risk factors (if appropriate and available), and the date of the visit to determine if the patient is overdue for a mammogram. If the patient is overdue, the physician would be prompted to speak to the patient about the potential benefits of mammography.

Physician (Clinician) Participation in the Development and Implementation Process. Social influence models suggest that the involvement of key individuals in the development of guidelines, especially those individuals involved with patient care, may encourage the eventual adoption of guidelines (Eisenberg, 1986). Therefore, many health care organizations encourage the involvement of a diverse group of health care practitioners to develop, adapt, and update guidelines. A multidisciplinary team might be assembled to review and adopt the USPSTF mammography guideline and to discuss possible strategies for effectively implementing the guideline.

The most effective guideline implementation efforts often involve several different approaches to implementation; the use of a single strategy may prove to be less effective (Eisenberg, 1986; Goldman, 1990; Greco & Eisenberg, 1993). However, studies have shown that guidelines are imperfect and may not be relevant to many patients. In fact, a recent study demonstrated that preserving each physician's ability to override guidelines is important for maintaining the quality of patient care. Therefore, with very few exceptions, guidelines should be used to complement rather than substitute for clinical decision making. Coercive implementation strategies, such as tying compliance with guidelines to physician incentives, may become problematic when the scientific evidence supporting a guideline is uncertain.

After a guideline has been implemented, especially guidelines based on uncertain scientific evidence, the effects on patient care should be evaluated (Weingarten, et al., 1994). Although there have been many different evaluations of guidelines, unfortunately, there have been relatively few considering the large number of guidelines that have been disseminated as part of a comprehensive effort to evaluate guidelines. Measured effects could include the acceptance of the guidelines by physicians, the impact on clinical outcomes (for example, mortality, morbidity), the effect on patient-centered outcomes (for example, patient health status, patient satisfaction, return to work), and economic outcomes (for example, cost of outpatient care and inpatient care). Finally, there is a definable cost associated with developing, updating, implementing, and evaluating guidelines. The true economic impact of any guideline should account for the cost of the guideline program. The cost savings attributed to the guideline, if any, should be offset by the program costs.

The importance of evaluating certain practice guidelines in clinical practice cannot be overestimated. In a study of patients with congestive heart failure, it was hypothesized that providing physicians with information on the timing of transfer of patients with congestive heart failure and pulmonary edema out of the coronary care unit or intermediate care unit would lead to better quality and less costly medical care (Weingarten, et al., 1994). This hypothesis was then tested in a controlled study. That study showed that although lengths of stay in intermediate care units for patients with congestive heart failure were reduced, total length of stay actually increased. Therefore, the failure to address the continuum of medical care resulted in a probable increase in total health care costs following implementation of a strategy designed to reduce health care costs.

The Importance of Practice Guidelines

In conclusion, practice guidelines, and other systematic approaches to clinical decision making, are being promoted to reduce undesirable variations in care, reduce health care costs, and improve the quality of medical care. There is early evidence to suggest that guidelines based on available scientific evidence, and implemented in an effective manner, may improve patient care. Some dissemination and implementation strategies, however, may prove to be effective while others may incur cost without benefit. Given the current enthusiasm for guidelines and the resources devoted to their development, the promise of guidelines may best be realized through careful attention to their implementation and evaluation in clinical practice. In this new era of physician accountability for clinical decisions and greater attention to improving the health of populations of patients, systematic approaches to clinical decision making, including the use of practice guidelines, are likely to continue to play an important role in the practice of medicine.

DISEASE MANAGEMENT

"Disease management," also known as "health care management," is a concept that has been promoted to address the comprehensive management of patients across the continuum of care. Disease management programs reduce the emphasis on treating acute episodes of care while seeking a more comprehensive approach to the total care of a patient. The approach emphasizes preventive care and care that prevents or delays complications from a disease. Practice guidelines and clinical decision support tools are often developed to identify the primary determinants of both the quality and cost of care for patients enrolled in a disease management program.

CLINICAL PATHWAYS

Clinical pathways have emerged as recent strategies for improving the quality and cost-effectiveness of medical care. Clinical pathways have been used in industry for decades, and their purpose is to sequence work to maximize efficiency of the work flow. Unfortunately, there are very few available data examining the effect of clinical pathways on patient care; most of the literature on this topic comes from outside of the health care field.

Clinical pathways have been developed and implemented at many hospitals across the United States in an effort to improve the quality of care and to reduce health care costs safely. Clinical pathways often include information about the most appropriate treatment and timing of treatment (as well as sequencing different forms of therapy). There are recent examples of using clinical pathways to improve patient care.

INFORMATION TECHNOLOGY AND QUALITY

Many processes of care measures, such as mammography rates, PAP smear rates, and childhood immunization rates, are easier to measure in a managed care population with sophisticated information systems. Organizations with less sophisticated information systems may struggle to cost-effectively determine process measures.

Information technology is critical for measuring and improving the quality of patient care. First, in order to cost-effectively measure quality of patient care, patients must be identified accurately and efficiently. For example, to measure the quality of care provided to patients with diabetes (for example, the level of blood sugar control), one must be able to rapidly identify all patients with diabetes.

Second, the data must be gathered efficiently and cost-effectively. In order to monitor quality of care, data needs to be ascertained quickly and with little labor and cost involved. The use of information systems allows the rapid determination of the numerator and denominator for many different variables. This could be most efficiently performed by employing information technology. For example, glycosylated hemoglobin levels reflect the control of blood sugar in patients with diabetes. If glycosylated hemoglobin levels could be determined cost-effectively from clinical information systems, then cost-effective monitoring could occur.

Finally, patients who receive the greatest benefit from quality improvement projects, such as those with the highest probability of developing complications, could be rapidly identified. For example, patients with the poorest blood sugar control might derive the greatest benefit from being enrolled in a structured program for diabetic patients (the opportunity for improvement is greatest).

The Internet will be used for a variety of medical applications. First, it will be used by patients to gather medical information. Second, intranet technologies will be used to disseminate practice guidelines and protocols by provider organizations and to cost-effectively disseminate clinical strategies to improve the quality of patient care. Information on quality of care will be disseminated over the Internet to consumers and providers. A business coalition has already experimented with using a Web site as a vehicle for disseminating information about quality of care provided by different health plans. Finally, Internet technology may be used to gather patient outcome data. For example, information on patient outcomes (health status, satisfaction, and return to work) presumably could be obtained by querying patients via the Internet.

HAZARDS OF QUALITY MEASUREMENT

A hazard of measuring quality of care is that the data could be misused and adversely affect health care providers. If a measure is purported to reflect quality, yet truly reflects factors unrelated to quality, the information could be potentially misleading. The Health Care Financing Administration (HCFA) previously disseminated information on hospital mortality rates publicly. Although detailed efforts were made to adjust mortality rates for case complexity (severity of patient illness), there was sufficient concern about the validity of the data to cause concern that the rates provided little insight about the quality of care provided at hospitals.

EXAMPLES OF SUCCESSFUL QUALITY IMPROVEMENT PROGRAMS

Hypertension

Studies have examined whether the use of practice guidelines can improve the care provided to patients in the outpatient setting and to patients with chronic diseases such as hypertension (Aucott, et al., 1996). The guidelines were implemented using a strategy that included education, a "clinical champion," a pharmacist intervention, and physician feedback. The use of guideline medications was greater in the intervention (guideline) group than in the control group. Moreover, blood pressure control was better in the intervention group. In conclusion, intensive implementation of hypertension guidelines probably reduced costs and improved quality of patient care.

Depression

Disease management has been promoted as a strategy to improve the care of patients with depres-sion. In a disease management study, patients with major or minor depression, treated by primary care physicians, were randomized to receive intensive treatment based on guidelines and patient education or usual care (Katon, et al., 1995). Patients with major depression in the disease management group were more adherent to medication, more likely to believe that their medications were beneficial, and more likely to be satisfied with their medical care. Moreover, for patients with major depression, the intervention improved their symptoms. Patients with minor depression also were more adherent to medications and more likely to believe that their medications were helpful. A "disease management" approach to the care of patients with depression (with education, attention to patient adherence, and guidelines) can improve the care of patients with depression.

Diabetes Mellitus

A study was performed to determine the effectiveness of a disease management approach to the care of patients with diabetes mellitus (Peters, et al., 1995). Care was provided by physician-supervised nurse specialists who followed computer-assisted protocols. Dietary counseling and patient education was also provided. After implementation of this program, there was a significant reduction in the glycosylated hemoglobin levels (studies have demonstrated that lower glycosylated hemoglobin levels are associated with improved patient outcomes). Moreover, the hospitalization rate for acute complications from diabetes mellitus was much lower than the national average. This study demonstrated that a systematic approach to the provision of preventive care for diabetic patients can improve patient care.

Congestive Heart Failure

Disease management is a comprehensive approach to patient care that addresses care for patients across the continuum (including the hospital, subacute, and outpatient settings). A study examined whether this approach could improve the quality of care for patients with congestive heart failure (Rich, et al., 1995). A multidisciplinary approach (an approach involving physicians, nurses, pharmacists, and other health care providers) of providing health care was studied in patients hospitalized for congestive heart failure. The care included an educational intervention by a nurse, instruction by a dietitian, review of medications, social service, and home visits. The intervention was associated with a statistically significant reduction in the hospital readmission rate. The cost of health care also was reduced by $460 per patient, and there was a greater improvement in quality of life in patients in the intervention group. The multidisciplinary approach to the care of patients with congestive heart failure improved quality of care and patient outcome, and reduced health care costs. Therefore, a disease management approach appears to have improved quality of care and outcome for patients with congestive heart failure.

Coronary Artery Bypass Surgery

There are a limited number of scientifically rigorous studies that have demonstrated objectives and improvements in patient outcome from quality improvement projects. In one report, cardiac surgeons performing coronary artery bypass surgery in New England proposed an intervention that included physician training in continuous quality improvement, site visits to "benchmark" hospitals, feedback of data, protocols, clinical pathways, and many other techniques (O'Connor, et al., 1996). Following this intervention, there was a 24% reduction in hospital mortality rate. This study shows an association between a well-organized quality improvement program and a reduction in hospital mortality. A more recent study, however, demonstrated reductions in mortality rates from coronary artery bypass surgery in a state without a planned quality improvement program. Future investigation should examine whether the reduction in mortality rates is related to the quality improvement program.

SUMMARY: THE FUTURE ROLE OF QUALITY MEASUREMENT

Efforts to measure quality of care have accelerated during the past decade. The race to measure quality is fueled by the belief that valid and reliable measures of quality could be used to base health care competition on value (quality and cost) rather than just cost. This would allow patients and purchasers to select health care providers, physician organizations, hospitals, and health plans by reviewing information including objective measures of quality of care.

Most important, there have been some very exciting efforts involving the use of quality measures to identify areas for improvement of patient care. These opportunities have been identified in almost every aspect of health care. Moreover, through the use of quality improvement tools and techniques such as practice guidelines, clinical pathways, disease management programs, and information technology, significant strides have been made that have resulted in demonstrable improvements in patient care. As the field of quality measurement and improvement matures, the opportunities to improve the health of individuals and populations may prove to be boundless and should result in significant improvements in the quality of care and outcomes for patients around the world.

REFERENCES

Aucott, J. N., Pelecanos, E., Dombrowski, R., et al. (1996). Implementation of local guidelines for cost-effective management of hypertension. A trial of the firm system. *Journal of General Internal Medicine, 11,* 139–146.

Balas, E. A., Austin Boren, S., Brown, G. D., Ewigman, B. G., Mitchell, J. A., & Perkoff, G. T. (1996). Effect of physician profiling on utilization. Meta-analysis of randomized clinical trials. *Journal of General Internal Medicine, 11,* 584–590.

Brook, R. H. (1989). Practice guidelines and practicing medicine. Are they compatible? *Journal of the American Medical Association, 262,* 3027–3030.

Cook, D. J., Guatt, G. H., Laupacis, A., & Sackett, D. L. (1992). Rules of evidence and clinical recommendations on the use of antithrombotic agents. *Chest, 102*(Suppl.), 305S–311S.

Corey, G. A., & Merenstein, J. H. (1987). Applying the acute ischemic heart disease predictive instrument. *Journal of Family Practice, 25,* 127–133.

Davis, D. A., Thomson, M. A., Oxman, A. D., et al. (1995). Changing physician performance: A systematic review of the effect of continuing medical education strategies. *Journal of the American Medical Association, 274,* 700–705.

Eisenberg, J. M. (1986). *Doctors' decisions and the cost of medical care.* Ann Arbor, MI: Health Administration Press.

Ellerbeck E. F., Jencks S. F., Radford M.J., et al. (1995). Quality of care for Medicare patients with acute myocardial infarction. A four-state pilot study from the Cooperative Cardiovascular Project. *Journal of the American Medical Association, 273,* 1509–1514.

Goldman, L. (1990). Changing physicians' behavior: The pot and the kettle. *New England Journal of Medicine, 322,* 1524–1525.

Greco, P. J., & Eisenberg, J. M. (1993). Changing physicians' practices. *New England Journal of Medicine, 329,* 1271–1273.

Grimshaw, J. M., & Russell, I. T. (1993). Effect of clinical guidelines in medical practice: A systematic review of rigorous evaluations. *Lancet, 342,* 1317–1322.

Katon, W., Von Korff, M., Lin, E., et al. (1995). Collaborative management to achieve treatment guidelines: Impact on depression in primary care. *Journal of the American Medical Association, 273,* 1026–1031.

Kosecoff, J., Kanouse, D. E., Rogers, W. H., et al. (1987). Effects of the National Institutes of Health Consensus Development Program on physician practice. *Journal of the American Medical Association, 258,* 2708–2713.

Krumholtz, H. M., Radford, M. J., Ellerbeck, E. F., et al. (1995). Aspirin in the treatment of acute myocardial infarction in elderly Medicare beneficiaries. Patterns of use and outcomes. *Circulation, 92,* 2841–2847.

Mugford, M., Banfield, P., & O'Hanlon, M. (1991). Effects of feedback of information on clinical practice: A review. *BMJ, 303,* 398–402.

O'Connor, G. T., Plume, S. K., Olmstead, E. M., et al. (1996). A regional intervention to improve the hospital mortality associated with coronary artery bypass graft surgery. The Northern New England Cardiovascular Disease Study Group. *Journal of the American Medical Association, 275,* 841–846.

Oxman, A. D., Thomson, M. A., Davis, D. A., & Haynes, R. B. (1995). No magic bullets: A systematic review of 102 trials of interventions to improve professional practice. *Canadian Medical Association Journal, 153,* 1423–1431.

Pestotnik, S. L., Classen, D. C., Evans, R. S., et al. (1996). Implementing antibiotic practice guidelines through computer-assisted decision support: Clinical and financial outcomes. *Annals of Internal Medicine, 124,* 884–890.

Peters, A. L., Davidson, M. B., & Ossorio, R. C. (1995). Management of patients with diabetes by nurses with support of subspecialists. *HMO Practice, 9,* 8–13.

Rich, M. W., Beckham, V., Wittenberg, C., et al. (1995). A multidisciplinary intervention to prevent the readmission of elderly patients with congestive heart failure. *New England Journal of Medicine, 333,* 1190–1195.

Rind, D. M., Safran, C., Phillips, R. S., et al. (1994). Effect of computer-based alerts on the treatment and outcomes of hospitalized patients. *Archives of Internal Medicine, 154,* 1511–1517.

Soumerai, S. B., & Avorn, J. (1990). Principles of educational outreach ("academic detailing") to improve clinical decision making. *Journal of the American Medical Association, 263,* 549–556.

Tunis, S. R., Hayward, R. S. A., Wilson, M. C., et al. (1994). Internists' attitudes about clinical practice guidelines. *Annals of Internal Medicine, 120,* 956–963.

Ware, J. E., Jr., Bayliss, M. S., Rogers, W. H., Konsinski, M., & Tarlov, A. R. (1996). Differences in 4-year health outcomes for elderly and poor, chronically ill patients treated in HMO and fee-for-service systems. Results from the Medical Outcomes Study. *Journal of the American Medical Association, 276*(13), 1039–1047.

Weiner, J. P., Parente, S. T., Garnick, D. W., et al. (1995). Variation in office-based quality. A claims-based profile of care provided to Medicare patients with diabetes. *Journal of the American Medical Association, 273,* 1503–1508.

Weingarten, S., Riedinger, M., Conner, L., Johnson, B., & Ellrodt, A. G. (1994). Reducing lengths of stay in the coronary care unit with a practice guideline for patients with congestive heart failure. Insights from a controlled clinical trial. *Medical Care, 32,* 1232–1243.

Wennberg, J., & Gittelsohn, A. (1973). Small area variations in health care delivery. *Science, 182,* 1102–1108.

Woolf, S. H. (1993). Practice guidelines: A new reality in medicine. III. Impact on patient care. *Archives of Internal Medicine, 153,* 2646–2655.

CHAPTER

Ethical Issues in Public Health and Health Services

Pauline Vaillancourt Rosenau

Ruth Roemer

CHAPTER TOPICS

LEARNING OBJECTIVES

Upon completing this chapter, the reader should be able to:

- Appreciate the central role of public health ethical concerns in health policy and management.
- Understand ethics issues with regard to the development and distribution of, and payment for, services, and with regard to the organization, management, assessment, and delivery of services.
- Acquire a framework for ethical analysis of issues within health services systems.
- Be a humanistic as well as technically adept participant in the health services field.

The cardinal principles of medical ethics (Beauchamp & Childress, 1989; Beauchamp & Walters, 1994)—autonomy, beneficence, and justice—apply in public health ethics but in somewhat altered form. Personal autonomy and respect for autonomy are guiding principles of public health practice as well as of medical practice. In medical ethics, the concern is with the privacy, individual liberty, freedom of choice, and self-control of the individual. From this principle flows the doctrine of informed consent. In public health ethics, autonomy, the right of privacy, and freedom of action are recognized insofar as they do not result in harm to others. Thus, from a public health perspective, autonomy may be subordinated to the welfare of others or of society as a whole.

Beneficence, which includes doing no harm, promoting the welfare of others, and doing good, is a principle of medical ethics. In the public health context, beneficence is the overall goal of public health policy and practice. It must be interpreted broadly, in light of societal needs, rather than narrowly, in terms of individual rights.

Justice—whether defined as equality of opportunity, equity of access, or equity in benefits—is

the core of public health. Serving the total population, public health is concerned with equity among various social groups, with protecting vulnerable populations, with compensating persons for suffering disadvantages in health and health care, and with surveillance of the total health care system. As expressed in the now classic phrase of Dr. William H. Foege, "Public health is social justice" (Foege, 1987).

THE CONCERN OF PUBLIC HEALTH ETHICS

This chapter is concerned with public health ethics as distinguished from medical ethics. Of course, some overlap exists between public health ethics and medical ethics, but public health ethics, like public health itself, applies generally to issues affecting populations, whereas medical ethics, like medicine itself, applies to individuals. Public health involves a perspective that is population-based, a view of conditions and problems that gives preeminence to the needs of the whole society rather than exclusively to the interests of single individuals.

Public health ethics evokes a number of dilemmas, many of which may be resolved in several ways depending on one's standards and values, that is, one's normative choices (ours are indicated). Data and evidence are relevant to the normative choices involved in public health ethics. The reader is referred to the health services research wherever appropriate.

In order to illustrate the concept of public health ethics, several general questions to be considered in different contexts are raised. It should also be noted that another public health question is how threats to the environment are reconciled with the need for employment. Issues in environmental control have an enormous impact on public health. Here, however, the focus is on the ethical issues in policy and management of personal health services.

Equity and environmental matters are discussed in Paehlke and Vaillancourt Rosenau (1993).

- What tensions exist between protection of the public health and protection of individual rights?
- How should scarce resources be allocated and used?
- What should be the balance between expenditures and quality of life in cases of chronic and terminal illness?
- What are appropriate limits on the use of expensive medical technology?
- What obligations do health care insurers and health care providers have to meet the "right to know" of patients as consumers?
- What responsibility exists for the young to finance health care for older persons?
- What obligation exists for government to protect the most vulnerable sectors of society?

There is no clear, definitive answer that is universally applicable to any of these questions. Context and circumstances sometimes require qualifying even the most straightforward response. In some cases, differences among groups and individuals may be so great and conditions in society may be so diverse and complex that no single answer to a question is possible. In other instances, a balance grounded in a public health point of view is viable. Sometimes there is no ethical conflict at all because one solution is optimal for all concerned: for the individual, the practitioner, the payer, and society. For example, few practitioners would want to perform an expensive, painful, medical act that was without benefit and might do damage. Few patients would demand it, and even fewer payers would reimburse for it. A likely societal consensus would suggest that public health would be better served if scarce health resources were used for better purposes (Eddy, 1994). But in

other circumstances, competition for resources would pose a dilemma as between providing a new, effective, but expensive drug of help to only a few, on one hand, and use of a less expensive but less effective drug for a larger number of persons, on the other. Such a dilemma was posed for the Medicaid program in 1988 when an expensive heart medicine became available that was only slightly more effective than a much less expensive product. In fact, drug formularies are based on the resolution of such problems.

Even in the absence of agreement on ethical assumptions and facing diversity and complexity that prohibit easy compromises, mechanisms are suggested for resolving the ethical dilemmas in health care that do exist. These are explored in the conclusion.

A word of caution: space is short and our topic complex. Every dimension of every relevant topic cannot be explored to the satisfaction of all readers. What is offered here, instead, is an introduction with a goal to awaken readers, be they practitioners, researchers, students, patients, or consumers, to the ethical dimension of public health. The reader is reminded of the ethical assumptions that underlie their own public health care choices. This chapter, then, is limited to considering selected ethical issues in public health and the provision of personal health services. The topic is examined by components of the health system: (1) development of health resources, (2) economic support, (3) organization of services, (4) management of services, (5) delivery of care, and (6) assurance of the quality of care (Roemer, 1991).

Overarching Public Health Principles: Our Assumptions

It is argued that the following are the general assumptions of a public health ethic.

1. Provision of care on the basis of health need without regard to race, religion, gender, sexual orientation, or ability to pay
2. Equity in distribution of resources, giving due regard to vulnerable groups in the population, for example, ethnic minorities, migrants, children, pregnant women, the poor, the handicapped, and others
3. Respect for human rights, including the right to autonomy, privacy, liberty, and health and well-being, keeping in mind social justice considerations

ETHICAL ISSUES IN THE DEVELOPMENT OF RESOURCES

Discussion of the development of resources refers to health *personnel, facilities, drugs, equipment, and knowledge.* The choices among the kinds of personnel that are trained, the facilities that are made available, and the commodities that are produced are not neutral. The production and acquisition of each of these involve ethical assumptions, and they in turn have public health consequences.

The number and types of personnel required and their distribution are critical to public health. The nation needs to have an adequate supply of personnel and facilities for a given population in order to meet the ethical requirements of providing health care without discrimination or bias. The proper balance of primary care physicians and specialists is essential to the ethical value of beneficence so as to maximize health status (Cooper, 1994). Also, quality of care declines where specialists are not available (Ayanian, et al., 1994).

The ethical imperative of justice requires special measures to protect the economically disadvantaged, such as primary care physicians working in health centers. The imperfect free market mechanisms employed in the United States to date have resulted in far too many specialists relative to generalists. Canada has achieved some balance, but this has involved closely controlling medical school enrollments and residency programs.

At the same time, the ethical principle of autonomy urges that resource development also be diverse enough to permit consumers some choice of providers and facilities. Absence of choice is a form of coercion. It also reflects an inadequate supply. But it results, as well, from the absence of a range of personnel. Patients should have some, though not unlimited, freedom to choose the type of care they prefer. Midwives, chiropractors, and other effective and proven practitioners should be available if health resources permit it without sacrificing other ethical considerations. The ethical principle of autonomy here might conflict with that of equity, which would limit general access to specialists in the interest of a better distribution of health care access to the whole population. The need for ample public health personnel is another ethical priority, necessary for the freedom of all individuals to a healthful, disease-free environment.

Physician assistants and nurses are needed, and they may serve an expanded role, substituting for primary care providers in some instances to alleviate the shortage of primary care physicians, especially in underserved areas. State regulation impacts significantly on the success of such programs (Sekscenski, et al., 1994). But too great a reliance on these providers might diminish quality of care when they are required to substitute entirely for physicians, particularly with respect to differential diagnosis (Roemer, 1977). The point of service is also a significant consideration. For example, more effective and expanded health care and dental care for children could be achieved by employing the school as a geographic point for monitoring and providing selected services (U.S. General Accounting Office, 1994).

Health personnel are not passive commodities, and freedom of individual career choices may conflict with public health needs. Here autonomy of the individual must be balanced with social justice and beneficence. In the past, the individual's decision to become a medical specialist took precedence over society's need for more generalists. A public health ethic appeals to the social justice involved and considers the impact on the population. A balance between individual choice and society's needs is being achieved today by restructuring financial compensation for primary care providers.

Similarly, in the United States, an individual medical provider's free choice regarding where to practice medicine has resulted in underserved areas, and ways to develop and train health personnel for rural and central-city areas are a public health priority (Braden, 1994; Helms, 1991). Progress has been made in the complex problem of providing rural health clinics, but more needs to be done (Fogel & MacQuarrie, 1994). For example, one option is to increase funds for the National Health Service Corps (NHSC) (Wolfe, 1991). When needs and preferences of the NHSC doctors and their families are taken into consideration, these doctors remain at their posts longer and have higher morale (Pathman, et al., 1994).

Similar ethical public health dilemmas are confronted with respect to health facilities. From a public health point of view, the need for equitable access to quality institutions and for fair distribution of health care facilities takes priority over an individual real estate developer's ends or the preferences of for-profit hospital owners. Providing a range of facilities to maximize choice would suggest the need for both public and private hospitals, community clinics and health centers, inpatient and outpatient mental health facilities, as well as long-term care facilities and hospices. The financial crisis facing public hospitals throughout the nation poses an ethical problem of major proportions

(Sack, 1995). At stake is the survival of facilities that provide an enormous volume of care for the poor, that train large numbers of physicians and other health personnel, and that provide specialized services—trauma care, burn units, and so on—for the total urban and rural populations they serve.

Research serves a public health purpose too. For example, research has advanced medical technology, and its benefits in new and improved products should be accessible to all members of society. Public health ethics also focuses on the importance of research in assessing health system performance including equity of access and medical outcomes.

The Joint Commission on Accreditation of Healthcare Organizations is going to provide consumers with information about provider performance or outcomes. The National Committee on Quality Assurance, a national agency located in Washington, D.C., will undertake similar activities (Winslow, 1994). Only if what works and is medically effective can be distinguished from what does not work and is medically ineffective will public health interests be best served. Health care resources need to be used wisely and not wasted. Health services research can help assure this goal.

Research is central to the development of public health resources. Equity mandates a fair distribution of research resources among the various diseases that affect the public's health because research is costly, resources are limited, and choices have to be made. Research needs both basic and applied orientation to assure quality (Comroe & Dripps, 1976). There is a need for research on matters that have been neglected in the past, as has been recognized in the field of women's health (Council on Ethical and Judicial Affairs, 1991; Hafner-Eaton, 1994; U.S. Public Health Service, 1985). Correction of other gross inequities in the allocation of research funds is urgent. Recent reports indicate that younger scientists are not sufficiently consulted in the peer review process, and they do not receive their share of research funds. Ethical implications involving privacy, informed consent, and equity affect targeted research grants for AIDS, breast cancer, and other special diseases. The legal and ethical issues in the human genome project involve matters of such broad scope—wide use of genetic screening, information control, privacy, and possible manipulation of human characteristics—that Annas has called for "taking ethics seriously" (Annas, 1989).

The orphan drug law, through tax exemption, focuses enormous resources on diseases that affect a very few individuals (Wagner, 1992). This law may be an instance where society assumes that beneficence takes precedence over equity and social justice. The apparent exaggerations in pricing and profitability have led to regulatory efforts to limit abuse (Coster, 1992). By contrast, in some instances, discoveries made while researching diseases that impact on only a few individuals, as with basic research, can lead to findings that benefit broader populations.

Conduct of biomedical research involving human subjects is governed by federal law in the United States. Ethical issues are handled by ethics advisory boards convened to advise the Department of Health and Human Services on the ethics of biomedical or behavioral research projects and by institutional review boards of research institutions seeking funding of research proposals. Both kinds of board are charged with the responsibility of reviewing clinical research proposals and assuring that the legal and ethical rights of human subjects are protected. A new section, Protection of Human Subjects of Biomedical and Behavioral Research, was added to the Public Service Act, Title IV, Part 1 (Ladimer & Newman, 1963; U.S.C.A., 1995). Among the principal concerns of these boards is assurance of fully informed and unencumbered consent by patients competent to give consent in order to assure the autonomy of subjects. They are also concerned with protection of the privacy of human subjects and the confidentiality of their relation to the project. An important legal and ethical duty of researchers, in the event that a randomized clinical trial proves beneficial to health, is to terminate the trial immediately and make the benefits available to the control group and to the treated group alike.

While the ethical principles that should govern biomedical research involving human subjects are a high priority, criticism has been leveled at the operation of some institutional review boards as lacking objectivity and as being overly identified with the interests of the researcher and the institution (Annas, 1991). At the same time, United States institutional review boards would object to studies carried out in Europe on the ground that they are not adequately protective of subjects (Patriarca, 1994).

Recommendations to correct these defects include: appointing patient and consumer advocates to review boards in addition to physicians and others affiliated with the institution and in addition to the sole lawyer who is generally a member of the review board; having advocates involved early in the drawing up of protocols for the research; having third parties interview patients after they have given their consent to make sure that they understood the research and their choices; requiring the institution to include research in its quality assurance monitoring; and establishing a national human experimentation board to oversee the four thousand institutional review boards in the country (Hilts, 1995).

Correction of fraud in science and the rights of subjects are important ethical considerations in developing knowledge. Ethical conflict between the role of the physician as caregiver and as researcher is not uncommon inasmuch as what is good for the patient is not always what is good for the research project. Certainly, in some instances, society stands to benefit at the expense of the research subject, but respect for the basic worth of the individual means that an individual has a right to be informed before agreeing to participate in an experiment. Only when consent is informed, clear, and freely given can altruism for the sake of advancing science and humanity be authentic. Still, exceptions to informed consent are sometimes justified. For example, because of the need for medically trained emergency personnel, a convincing case can be made for using deceased patients to teach resuscitation procedures. There is "no risk to the dead person, and families could not realistically be expected to discuss consent at such a difficult time" (Burns, et al., 1994; Orlowski, et al., 1988).

Policy makers concerned with the development of resources for health care thus confront tensions between protection of public health and protection of the rights of individual patients and providers. They face issues concerning the allocation of scarce resources and the use of expensive medical technology. In resolving these issues, their decisions need to be guided by the principles of autonomy, beneficence, and justice as applied to the health of populations.

ETHICAL ISSUES IN ECONOMIC SUPPORT

Nowhere is the public health ethical perspective clearer than on issues of economic support. Personal autonomy and respect for privacy remain essential, as does beneficence. But a public health orientation suggests that the welfare of society merits a close regard for justice. It is imperative that everyone in the population have equitable access to health care services with dignity, so as not to discourage necessary utilization, and in most cases this means universal health insurance coverage. Lack of insurance makes for poorer medical outcomes even

though individuals without health insurance do receive care in hospital emergency rooms (Braveman, et al., 1994; Haas, et al., 1993; Weissman & Epstein, 1994).

From a public health perspective, financial barriers to essential health care are inappropriate. If each and every human being is to develop to his or her full potential, to participate fully as productive citizens in our democratic society, then preventive health services and the alleviation of pain and suffering due to health conditions that can be effectively treated must be provided without financial barriers. Removing economic barriers to health services will not mean that the difference in health status between rich and poor will disappear. But the removal of economic barriers is a necessary, if not a sufficient, condition for this goal.

From a public health point of view, the economic resources to support health services should be fair and equitable. Any individual's contribution should be progressive, based on his or her ability to pay. While some individual contribution is appropriate, no matter how small, as a gesture of commitment to the larger community, it is also ethically fitting for the nation to take responsibility for a portion of the cost. The exact proportion may vary across nation and time, depending on the country's wealth and the public priority attributed to health services (Roemer, 1991).

Similarly, justice and equity suggest the importance of the ethical principle of social solidarity in any number of forms, such as the Communitarian form (Bellah, et al., 1985; Minkler, 1994; Minkler & Robertson, 1991; The Responsive Communitarian Platform, 1991/1992). Social insurance by definition means that there is wisdom in assigning responsibility for payment by those who are young and working to support the health care of children and older people no longer completely independent. A public health orientation suggests that social solidarity forward and backward in time, across generations, is ethically persuasive. Those in the most productive stages of the life cycle today were once dependent children, and they are likely, one day, to be dependent older persons. Institutions such as Social Security and Medicare play a moral role in a democracy. They were established to attain common aims and are fair in that they follow agreed-upon rules (Bellah, et al., 1991). The alternatives to social solidarity between the young and the elderly are simply unacceptable. As members of a society made up of overlapping communities, our lives are intricately linked together. No man or woman is an island; not even the most wealthy or most "independent" can exist alone. The social pact that binds us to live in peace together requires cooperation of such a fundamental nature that we could not travel by car (assuming respect for traffic signals) to the grocery store to purchase food (or assume it safe for consumption) without appealing to social solidarity. These lessons apply to health care as well.

With the publication of the report of the 1994–1996 Advisory Council on Social Security on January 6, 1997, the nation has before it three approaches designed to protect the long-range solvency of the Social Security System (1994–1996 Advisory Council on Social Security, 1997). The report contains three different proposals. One proposal, based on the premise that as much of the program's benefits as possible should be maintained, labeled the "maintain benefits plan," keeps the Social Security benefits structure essentially intact by proposing small increases in the payroll tax and minor benefit cuts.

The second, the "individual account plan," seeks financial solvency through reductions in benefits and imposes mandatory employee contributions to individual savings accounts. The third, the "personal savings account plan," provides for a major redesign of the system, replacing a major portion of the Social Security retirement benefit with individ-

ual private savings accounts (Kollmann, 1997). While these may seem to be merely differing financial strategies to maintain the solvency of the Social Security system, they actually pose serious questions of ethics and equity. The second and third proposals represent departures from the basic Social Security system. In addition, they undermine the social solidarity built into the original law, adopted in 1935. Both compromise the risk protection of the Social Security system and jeopardize retirement benefits because they put the average citizen at the mercy of the vagaries of the market.

The passage of the Personal Responsibility and Work Opportunities Act of 1996 poses grave threats to our concepts of beneficence and justice. The new law abolishes the federal entitlement of Aid to Families with Dependent Children (AFDC) and replaces it with block grants to the states for temporary assistance for needy families (TANF). In severing the link between Medicaid and welfare assistance—a measure designed to preserve Medicaid—the law makes enrollment of eligible women and children in Medicaid more difficult. In tightening the rules for receipt of Supplemental Security Income (SSI), many disabled children will lose their support. The restriction of Medicaid benefits to legal immigrants for emergency care, immunizations, and testing and treatment for communicable diseases so flies in the face of ethics and fairness that Congress would do well to amend this portion of the legislation.

In 1983, the President's Commission for the Study of Ethical Problems in Medicine and Biomedical and Behavioral Research made as its first and principal recommendation on ethics in medicine that society has an obligation to assure equitable access to health care for all its citizens (President's Commission for the Study of Ethical Problems in Medicine and Biomedical and Behavioral Research, 1983). Equitable access, the commission said, requires that all citizens be able to secure an adequate level of care without excessive burdens. Implementation of this principle as an ethical imperative is even more urgent twelve years later as increasing numbers of people, of whom one-fourth are children, become uninsured. Fortunately, state and federal proposals are being considered for providing health insurance to all children in families under 150% or 200% of poverty—a strategy for remedying one of the most egregious injustices of the United States health care system.

ETHICAL ISSUES IN ORGANIZATION OF SERVICES

The principal ethical imperative in organization of health services is that services be organized and distributed in accordance with health needs. This ethical principle is illustrated by the issues of geographic and cultural access.

A system of health care, to be fair and just, must minimize geographic inequities in the distribution of care. Rural areas are underserved, as are inner cities. Any number of solutions have been proposed and tried to bring better access in health services to underserved areas, be they rural areas or inner cities. These include mandating a period of service for medical graduates as a condition of licensure, loan forgiveness and expansion of the National Health Service Corps, rural preceptorships, providing economic incentives for establishing practice in rural areas, and employment of physician assistants and nurse practitioners (Lewis, et al., 1976). Telemedicine may provide the best available medical consultants to rural areas in the near future (Smothers, 1942; Wheeler, 1994), but the technology involves initial start-up costs that are not trivial.

Similarly, the principles of autonomy and beneficence require health services to be culturally relevant to the populations they are designed to serve

(Marin & Marin, 1991; Orlandi, 1992). This means that medical care professionals need to be able to communicate in the language of those they serve and to understand the cultural preferences of those for whom they seek to provide care (Maher, 1993; Rafuse, 1993). The probability of success is enhanced if needed health professionals are from the same cultural background as those they serve. This suggests that schools of medicine, nursing, dentistry, and public health should intensify their efforts to reach out and extend educational and training opportunities to qualified and interested members of such populations. To carry out such programs, however, these schools must have the economic resources required to provide fellowships and teaching assistant positions.

The development of various forms of managed care—health maintenance organizations, prepaid group practices, preferred provider organizations, and independent practice associations—raises a different set of ethical questions. As experienced in the United States in recent years, managed care is designed more to minimize costs than to assure that health care is efficient and effective. If managed care ends up constraining costs by depriving individuals of needed medical attention (reducing medically appropriate access to specialists, for example), then it violates the ethical principle of beneficence because such management interferes with doing good for the patient. For example, if managed care is employed as a cost-containment scheme for Medicaid and Medicare without regard to quality of care, it risks increasing inequity. It could even contribute to a two-tiered health care system in which those who can avoid various forms of managed care by paying privately for their personal health services will obtain a higher quality of care.

The advantages of managed care are clear: team practice, emphasis on primary care, generous use of diagnostic and therapeutic outpatient services, and prudent use of hospitalization, all contributing to cost containment. At the same time, managed care systems have the disadvantage of restricted choice of provider, run the risk of underservicing, and may achieve cost containment through cost shifting (Luft, 1981).

The ethical issues in managed care are illustrated most sharply by the question of who decides what is medically necessary—the physician or others, such as the health plan, the insurer, the employer, the state legislature, or Congress (Mariner, 1994). This question is not unique to managed care; it has also arisen with respect to insurance companies and Medicaid (*Bush v. Barham,* 1980; *Pinneke v. Preisser,* 1980). On one hand, the physician has a legal and ethical duty to provide the standard of care that a reasonable physician in the same or similar circumstances would provide. On the other hand, insurers have traditionally specified what is covered or not covered as medically necessary in insurance contracts. The courts have reached different results in such cases, depending on the facts of the case, the character of the treatment sought (whether generally accepted or experimental), and the interpretation of medical necessity (Mariner, 1994).

As more and more integrated health care delivery systems are formed, as more mergers of managed care organizations occur, as pressures for cost containment persist, ethical issues concerning conflicts of interest, quality of care choices, restraints on expenditures, and patients' rights will attain increasing importance. The principles of autonomy, beneficence, and justice will be severely tested in the resolution of the ethical problems facing a complex, corporate health care system.

In response to these problems, the Advisory Commission on Consumer Protection and Quality in the Health Care Industry, headed by Secretary of Health and Human Services Donna E. Shalala and Secretary of Labor Alexis M. Herman, began deliberations in May 1997 to develop a much-needed patient's bill of rights. State legislatures are also considering bills to establish detailed standards for health plans (Peer, 1997).

If medicine is "for-profit," as seems to be the case today and for the near future in the United States, then the ethical dilemma between patients' interests and profits will be a continuing problem. Sometimes both can be served, but it is unlikely to be the case in all instances. That both consumers and employers are concerned about quality of care is clear from Paul Ellwood's statement expressing disappointment in the evolution of HMOs because "they tend to place too much emphasis on saving money and not enough on improving quality— and we now have the technical skill to do that" (Bayles, 1989; Callahan, 1988; Cederblom & Dougherty, 1990; Iannone, 1989; Noble, 1995).

ETHICAL ISSUES IN MANAGEMENT OF HEALTH SERVICES

Management involves *planning, administration, regulation,* and *legislation.* The style of management depends on the values and norms of the population. Planning involves determining the population health needs (with surveys and research, for example) and then assuring that programs are in place to provide the appropriate services. A public health perspective suggests that planning is appropriate to the extent that it provides efficient, appropriate health care (beneficence) to all who seek it (equity and justice). Planning may avoid waste and contribute to the rational use of health services. But it is also important that planning not be so invasive as to be coercive and deny the individual any say in his/her health care unless such intervention is necessary to protect public health interests. The ethical principle of autonomy preserves the right of the individual to refuse care and to determine his or her own destiny, especially when the welfare of others is not involved. A balance between individual autonomy and public health intervention that will provide benefit to the society is not easy to achieve. In some cases, however, the resolution of such dilemmas is clear, for example, the case for mandatory immunization programs. Equity and beneficence demand that the social burdens and benefits of living in a disease-free environment be shared. Therefore, immunization requirements should cover all those potentially affected.

Health administration has ethical consequences that may be overlooked because they appear ethically neutral: organization, staffing, budgeting, supervision, consultation, procurement, logistics, records and reporting, coordination, and evaluation (Roemer, 1991). All these activities involve ethical choices. The importance of privacy in record keeping, for example, once again raises the necessity of balancing the ethical principles of autonomy and individual rights with social justice and the protection of society, as, for example, in *Whalen v. Roe* (1977), upholding the constitutionality of a state law requiring that patients receiving legitimate prescriptions for drugs with an abuse potential have their names, addresses, ages, and other information reported to the state department of health.

The distribution of scarce health resources is another subject of debate. The principle of "first come, first served," may, at first, seem equitable. But it also incorporates the "rule of rescue" whereby a few lives are saved at great cost, and this policy results in the "invisible" loss of many more lives. The cost-benefit or cost-effectiveness analysis of health economics attempts to apply hard data to administrative decisions. This approach, however, does not escape ethical dilemmas because the act of assigning numbers to years of life, for example, is itself value-laden. If administrative allocation is determined on the basis of the number of years of

life saved, then the younger are favored over the older, which may or may not be equitable. If one factors into such an analysis the idea of "quality" years of life, other normative assumptions must be made regarding the importance of quality and what constitutes quality. Some efforts have been made to assign a dollar value to a year of life as a tool for administering health resources. But here, too, we encounter worrisome normative problems. Does not ability to pay deform such calculations (Hillman, et al., 1991)?

Crucial to management of health services are legal tools—legislation, regulations, and sometimes litigation—necessary for fair administration of programs. Legislation and regulations are essential for authorizing health programs; they also serve to remedy inequities and to introduce innovations in a health service system. Effective legislation depends on a sound scientific base, and ethical questions are especially troubling when the scientific evidence is uncertain.

For example, in a landmark decision in 1976, the Court of Appeals for the District of Columbia upheld a regulation of the Environmental Protection Agency restricting the amount of lead additives in gasoline based largely on epidemiological evidence (*Ethyl Corp. v. Environmental Protection Agency*, 1976). An analysis of this case and of the scope of judicial review of the regulatory action of an agency charged by Congress with regulating substances harmful to health underlines the dilemma the court faced: the need of judges trained in the law, not in science, to evaluate the scientific and epidemiological evidence on which the regulatory agency based its ruling (Silver, 1980). The majority of the court based its upholding of the agency's decision on its own review of the evidence. By contrast, Judge David Bazelon urged an alternative approach:

[I]n cases of great technological complexity, the best way for courts to guard against unreasonable or erroneous administrative decisions is not for the judges themselves to scrutinize the technical merits of each decision. Rather, it is to establish a decision making process that assures a reasoned decision that can be held up to the scrutiny of the scientific community and the public (*International Harvester Co. v. Ruckelshaus,* 1973).

Coping with conflicting scientific evidence is a persistent ethical dilemma, as reflected by a 1993 decision of the United States Supreme Court involving the question of how widely accepted a scientific process or theory must be before it qualifies as admissible evidence in a lawsuit. The case involved the issue of whether a drug prescribed for nausea during pregnancy, Bendectin, causes birth defects. Rejecting the test of "general acceptance" of scientific evidence as the absolute prerequisite for admissibility, as applied in the past, the Court ruled that trial judges serve as gate-keepers to ensure that pertinent scientific evidence is not only relevant but reliable. The Court also suggested various factors that might bear on such determinations (*Daubert v. Merrell Dow Pharmaceuticals,* 1993).

Epidemiological evidence, which is the core of public health, is increasingly recognized as helpful in legal suits—a significant advance for determination of ethical issues in cases where the scientific evidence is uncertain (Ginzburg, 1986). Of course, it should be noted that a court's or an agency's refusal to act because of uncertain scientific evidence is in itself a decision with ethical implications.

Enactment of legislation and issuance of regulations are important for management of a just health care system, but these strategies are useless if they are not enforced. For example, state legislation has long banned the sale of cigarettes to minors, but only recently have efforts been made to enforce these statutes rigorously through publicity, "stings"

(arranged purchases by minors), penalties on sellers, threats of license revocation, and banning cigarette sales from vending machines (Centers for Disease Control, 1989; Roemer, 1993).

A novel case of enforcement involves a Baltimore ordinance prohibiting billboards promoting cigarettes in areas where children live, recreate, and go to school, enacted in order to enforce the minors' access law banning tobacco sales to minors. Despite efforts by a billboard company to enjoin enforcement of the ordinance on First Amendment and federal preemption grounds, the ordinance was upheld in federal district court and in the United States Court of Appeals for the Fourth Circuit, and the United States Supreme Court has refused to review the case (Garner, 1996; *Penn Advertising of Baltimore, Inc. v. Mayor of Baltimore,* 1995). This ordinance is a model for other cities seeking to enforce the federal and state bans on sales of cigarettes to minors.

Thus, management of health services involves issues of allocating scarce resources, evaluating scientific evidence, measuring quality of life, and imposing mandates by legislation and regulations. Although a seemingly neutral function, management of health services must rely on principles of autonomy, beneficence, and justice in its decision-making process.

ETHICAL ISSUES IN DELIVERY OF CARE

Delivery of health services, the actual provision of health care services, is the end point of all the other dimensions discussed earlier. The ethical considerations of only a few of the many issues pertinent to delivery of care are discussed here.

Resource allocation in a time of cost containment inevitably involves rationing. While at first blush rationing by ability to pay may appear natural, neutral, and inevitable, the ethical dimensions for delivery of care may be overlooked. If ability to pay is recognized as a form of rationing, the question of its justice is immediately apparent. The Oregon Medicaid program is an example. It is equitable by design and is grounded in good part in the efficacy of the medical procedure in question, thus respecting the principle of ethical beneficence. It is structured to extend benefits to a wider population of poor people than is entitled to care under Medicaid. The plan does not qualify as equitable and fair, however, because it does not apply to the whole population of Oregon, but only to the poor. In addition, it reduces the level of services to some persons who used to be on Medicaid in order to widen the pool of beneficiaries. This also presents significant ethical problems (Annas, 1993; Rosenbaum, 1992).

Rationing medical care is not always ethically dubious but rather may conform to a public health ethic. In some cases, too much medical care is counterproductive and may produce more harm than good. For example, Canada "rations" health care, pays one-third less per population than the United States, and offers universal coverage; yet health status indicators do not suggest that Canadians suffer. In fact, on several performance indicators, Canada surpasses the United States (U.S. General Accounting Office, 1991). Because there is so little information about medical outcomes and the efficacy of many medical procedures, rationing would actually benefit patients if it discouraged unneeded and inappropriate treatment.

The rationing of organ transplants, similarly, is a matter of significant ethical debate. The number of organs available for transplant is less than the need. Rationing, therefore, must be used to determine who will be given a transplant. Employing tissue match makes medical sense and also seems ethically acceptable. But to the extent that ability to pay is a criterion, ethical conflict is inevitable. It may, in fact, go against scientific opinion and public health ethics if someone who can pay receives a transplant even though the tissue match is not as good as it would be for a patient who is also in need of a transplant but unable to pay the cost. Rationing on this basis seems ethically unfair and medically ill-advised. Although the sale of organs is unethical as well as scientifically unsound as a means of rationing, it exists and persists (Fox & Swazey, 1992; U.S. General Accounting Office, 1993).

One solution would be to make more organs available through mandatory donation from fatal automobile accidents without explicit consent of individuals and families. A number of societies have adopted this policy because the public health interest of society and the seriousness of the consequences are so great for those in need of a transplant that it is possible to justify ignoring the individual autonomy (preferences) of the accident victim's friends and relatives. This has not been the case in the United States to date (Associated Press, 1993; Roels, et al., 1991).

Delivery of services raises conflict-of-interest questions for providers that are of substantial public health importance. Hospitals pressed by competitive forces strain to survive and in some cases do so only by less-than-honest cost shifting, and even direct fraud. A recent General Accounting Office survey of hospital bills finds that more than 99% included "mistakes" that favored the hospital (Kerr, 1992; Rosenthal, 1993; U.S. General Accounting Office, 1993). Physicians have been found to refer patients to laboratories and medical testing facilities that they co-own to a far greater extent than can be medically justified (Hillman, et al., 1992; Hilts, 1994; Kolata, 1994; Mitchell & Scott, 1992; U.S. General Accounting Office, 1994; Winslow, 1994). The public health ethic of beneficence is called into question by such unnecessary tests.

The practice of medical and public health screening presents serious ethical dilemmas. Screening for diseases for which there is no treatment except where such information can be used to postpone onset or prevent widespread population infection is difficult to justify unless the information is explicitly desired by the patient for personal reasons (life planning and reproduction). In a similar case, screening without provision to treat those discovered to be in need of treatment is unethical. Public health providers need to be sure in advance that they can offer the health services required to provide care for those found to be affected. This is the ethical principle of beneficence and social justice (Heitman & Rosenau, 1993).

The tragic epidemic of HIV/AIDS has raised serious ethical questions concerning testing, reporting, and partner notification. The great weight of authority favors voluntary and confidential testing, so as to encourage persons to come forward for testing, counseling, and behavior change (Field, 1990; Fluss & Zeegers, 1989; World Health Organization, 1993). The majority of states require reporting of AIDS cases; only a few states require reporting of HIV positivity, and those have strong confidentiality protections in place (Bayer, 1991). Partner notification was at first generally disapproved on grounds of nonfeasibility and protection of privacy, but some states have enacted legislation permitting a physician to notify a partner of a patient's HIV+ status if the physician believes that the patient will not inform the partner (Bayer, 1992; California Health and Safety Code, 1990).

With the finding that administration of AZT during pregnancy to an HIV+ woman may protect the fetus, the question arises as to what extent pregnant women should be tested for HIV. Certainly, the option of voluntary, confidential testing should be offered. Should anyone else be tested involuntarily? Some guidance for resolving ethical questions in this difficult sphere is presented by Dr.

Stephen Joseph, former Commissioner of Health for New York City, who states that the AIDS epidemic is a public health emergency that carries within it extraordinary civil liberties issues, not a civil liberties emergency that carries within it extraordinary public health issues (Joseph, 1992).

The field of reproductive health is a major public health concern affecting women in their reproductive years. Here the principles of autonomy, beneficence, and justice apply to the provision of contraceptive services (including long-acting means of contraception), abortion (including medical abortion made possible by the approval of mifipristone and the promotion of emergency contraception after unprotected sex), and use of noncoital technologies for reproduction. The debate on these issues has been wide, abrasive, and divisive. Twenty-two years after abortion was legalized by the United States Supreme Court's decision in *Roe v. Wade* (1973), protests against abortion clinics escalated. Violence against clinics and murders of abortion providers threaten access to abortion services. In recognition of the necessity to promote a civil society and of the constitutional protection afforded to personal decisions relating to marriage, procreation, and contraception—matters involving "the most intimate and personal choices a person may make in a lifetime, choices central to personal dignity and autonomy," the United States Supreme Court in *Planned Parenthood of Southeastern Pennsylvania v. Casey* (1992) reaffirmed the right to choose abortion, stating that *Roe v. Wade* has acquired a "rare precedential force" and could be overturned under fire only at the cost of both profound and unnecessary damage to the Court's legitimacy, and to the nation's commitment to the rule of law.

Our position strongly favors the prochoice point of view in order to assure the autonomy of women, beneficence for women and their families faced with unwanted pregnancy, and justice in society. In the highly charged debate on teenage pregnancy, we believe that social realities, the well-being of young women and their children, and the welfare of society mandate access to contraception and abortion and respect for the autonomy of young people. The ethics of parental consent and notification laws, which often stand as a barrier to abortions needed and wanted by adolescents, is highly questionable (*Abortion Denied: Shattering Young Women's Lives,* 1990).

Of the many important ethical issues in the delivery of health care not discussed here because of space limitations, three examples may be mentioned briefly.

(1) The death debate is generally considered a matter of medical ethics involving the patient, his or her family, and the physician. But this issue is also a matter of public health ethics because services at the end of life entail administrative and financial dimensions that are part of public health and management of health services (Annas & Miller, 1994; Scitovsky, 1988; Temkin-Greener, et al., 1992).

(2) The conflict in the mental health field between the health needs and legal rights of patients, on one hand, and the need for protection of society, on the other, illustrates sharply the ethical problems facing providers of mental health services. This conflict has been addressed most prominently by reform of state mental hospital admission laws to make involuntary admission to a mental hospital initially a medical matter, with immediate and periodic judicial review as to the propriety of hospitalization—review in which a patient advocate participates (New York Mental Hygiene Law, 1988/1995; Special Committee to Study Commitment Procedures of the Association of the Bar of the City of New York in Cooperation with Cornell Law School, 1962). The *Tarasoff* case presents another problem in the provision of mental health services: the duty of a psychiatrist or psychologist to warn an identified person of a patient's intent to kill the person, despite the rule of confidentiality governing medical and psychiatric practice (*Tarasoff v. Regents of the University of California,* 1976). In both instances, a public health perspective favors protection of society against the legal rights of individuals.

(3) Records and statistics are basic to public health strategies and effective delivery of preventive and curative services. The moral and legal imperative of privacy to protect an individual's medical record gives way to public health statutes requiring reporting of gunshot wounds, communicable diseases, sexually transmitted diseases, child abuse, and AIDS (Grad, 1990). More generally, the right of persons to keep their medical records confidential conflicts with the need of society for epidemiological information to monitor the incidence and prevalence of diseases in the community and to determine responses to this information. A common resolution of this problem is to make statistics available without identifying information.

Ethical problems in the delivery of services will surely increase in number and kind in a period of great change in the health service system as private, fee-for-service, solo practice is being replaced by new ways of financing and providing health care. The most prominent problem will be the question of who decides the appropriateness of services—the payer or the provider, the managed care plan or the physician—and what role the consumer will have in the new system that is evolving.

ETHICAL ISSUES IN ASSURING QUALITY OF CARE

If a public health ethic requires fair and equitable distribution of medical care, then it is essential that waste and inefficiency be eliminated. Spending scarce resources on useless medical acts is a violation of a public health ethic. To reach this public health goal, knowledge about what is useful and medically efficacious is essential.

As strategies for evaluating the quality of health care have become increasingly important, the ethical dimensions of peer review, practice guidelines, and malpractice suits—all methods of quality assurance—have come to the fore. Established in 1972 to monitor hospital services under Medicare to assure that they were "medically necessary" and delivered in the most efficient manner, professional standards review organizations came under attack as overregulatory and too restrictive (Luce, 1986; Price, 1980). Congress ignored the criticism and in 1982 passed the Peer Review Improvement Act, which did not abolish outside review but consolidated the local peer review agencies, replaced them with statewide bodies, and increased their responsibility (Peer Review Improvement Act, 1982). In 1986, Congress passed the Health Care Quality Improvement Act, which established national standards for peer review at the state and hospital levels for all practitioners regardless of source of payment (Health Care Quality Improvement Act, 1986). The act also established a national data bank on the qualifications of physicians and provided immunity from suit for reviewing physicians acting in good faith.

The functions of peer review organizations (PROs) in reviewing the adequacy and quality of care necessarily involve some invasion of the patient's privacy and the physician's confidential relationship with his/her patient. Yet beneficence and justice in an ethical system of medical care mandate a process of control of the cost and quality of care. The work of PROs has been furthered by finding an accommodation between protection of privacy and confidentiality, on one hand, and necessary but limited disclosure, on the other. Physicians whose work is being reviewed are afforded the right to a hearing at which the patient is not present, and patients are afforded the protection of outside review in accord with national standards.

Practice guidelines developed by professional associations, health maintenance organizations and other organized providers, third-party payers, and governmental agencies are designed to evaluate the appropriateness of procedures. Three states—Maine, Minnesota, and Vermont—have passed legislation permitting practice guidelines to be used as a defense in malpractice actions under certain circumstances (U.S. Congress, Office of Technology Assessment, 1993). Such a simplistic solution, however, avoids the question of fairness: whose guidelines should prevail in the face of multiple sets of guidelines issued by different bodies, and how should accommodation be made to evolving and changing standards of practice (Capron, 1995; Halpern, 1995; Kane, 1995; Parker, 1995; Pauly, 1995)?

Malpractice suits constitute one method of regulating the quality of care, although an erratic and expensive system. This subject is discussed fully elsewhere (Andersen, et al., 1996). Here we raise only the ethical issue of the right of the injured patient to compensation for the injury and the need of society for a system of compensation that is more equitable and more efficient than the current system.

The various mechanisms for assuring quality of care all pose ethical issues. Peer review requires some invasion of privacy and confidentiality to provide surveillance of quality, although safeguards have been devised. Practice guidelines involve some interference with physician autonomy but in return provide protection for both the patient and the provider. Malpractice suits raise questions of equity, since many injured patients are not compensated. In the process of developing and improving strategies for quality control, the public health perspective justifies social intervention to protect the population.

MECHANISMS FOR RESOLVING ETHICAL ISSUES IN HEALTH CARE

Even in the absence of agreement on ethical assumptions and in the face of diversity and complexity that prohibit easy compromise, mechanisms for resolving ethical dilemmas in public health do exist. Among these are ombudsmen, institutional review boards, ethics committees, standards set by professional associations, practice guidelines, financing mechanisms, and courts of law. Some of these mechanisms are voluntary. Others are legal. None is perfect. Some, such as financing mechanisms, are particularly worrisome.

While ethics deals with values and morals, the law has been very much intertwined with ethical issues. In fact, the more that statutes, regulations, and court cases decide ethical issues, the narrower is the scope of ethical decision making by providers of health care (Grad, 1978). For example, because the *Cruzan* case defines the conditions for terminating life support for persons in a persistent vegetative state (clear and cogent evidence of a prior statement by the patient when competent of his or her desire not to be kept alive by artificial means in a persistent vegetative state), the scope of decision making by physicians and families is constrained (*Cruzan v. Missouri Department of Health,* 1990). Courts of law, therefore, are important mechanisms for resolving ethical issues.

The law deals with many substantive issues in numerous fields, including that of health care. It has also made important procedural contributions to resolving disputes by authorizing, establishing, and monitoring mechanisms or processes for handling claims and disputes. Such mechanisms are particularly useful for resolving ethical issues in health care because they are generally informal and flexible and often involve the participation of all the parties. Administrative mechanisms are much less expensive than litigation and in this respect potentially more equitable.

Ombudsmen in health care institutions are a means of providing patient representation and advocacy. They may serve as channels for expression of ethical concerns of patients and their families.

Ethics committees in hospitals and managed care organizations operate to resolve ethical issues involving specific cases in the institution. They may be composed solely of the institution's staff, or they may include an ethicist specialized in handling such problems. Institutional review boards, discussed earlier, are required to evaluate research proposals for their scientific and ethical integrity.

Practice guidelines, also discussed earlier, provide standards for ethical conduct and encourage professional behavior that conforms to procedural norms generally recognized by experts in the field.

Finally, financing mechanisms that provide incentives for certain procedures and practices have the economic power to encourage ethical conduct. At the same time, they may function to encourage the opposite behavior (Annas, 1993).

As the health care system continues to deal with budget cuts, greater numbers of uninsured persons, and restructuring into managed care and integrated delivery systems, ethical questions loom large. Perhaps their impact can be softened by imaginative and rational strategies to finance, organize, and deliver health care in accordance with the ethical principles of autonomy, beneficence, and justice.

Ethical issues in public health and health services management are likely to become increasingly complex in the future. New technology and advances in medical knowledge will challenge us and raise ethical dilemmas. These will need to be evaluated and applied in a public health context and submitted to a public health ethical analysis. Few of these developments are likely to be entirely new and without precedent, however. Already current discussions, such as that presented here, may inform these new developments.

REFERENCES

Abortion denied: Shattering young women's lives. (1990). Video produced by The Feminist Majority Foundation, 8105 W. 3rd Street, Los Angeles, CA 90048.

Andersen, R. M., Rice, T. H., & Kominski, G. F. (Eds.). (1996). *Changing the health care system: Key issues in health services, U.S. policy and management* (pp. 382–412). San Francisco: Jossey-Bass.

Annas, G. J. (1989, July–August). Who's afraid of the human genome? *Hastings Center Report, 19–21.*

Annas, G. J. (1991, May–June). Ethics committees: From ethical comfort to ethical cover. *Hastings Center Report, 18–21.*

Annas, G. J. (1993). *The standard of care: The law of American bioethics* (pp. 211–213). New York: Oxford University Press.

Annas, G. J., & Miller, F. H. (1994). The empire of death: How culture and economics affect informed consent in the U.S., the U.K., and Japan. *American Journal of Law & Medicine, XX, 4,* 359–394.

Associated Press. (1993, March 22–29). Bill would allow automatic donation. *American Medical News,* 10.

Ayanian, J., Hauptman, P. J., Guadagnoli, E., Antman, E., Pashos, C., & McNeil, B. (1994, October 27). Knowledge and practices of generalist and specialist physicians regarding drug therapy for acute myocardial infarction. *New England Journal of Medicine,* 1136.

Bayer, R. (1991, May 23). Public health policy and the AIDS epidemic: An end to AIDS exceptionalism. *New England Journal of Medicine, 324*(21), 1500–1504.

Bayer, R. (1992, August). HIV prevention and the two faces of partner notification. *American Journal of Public Health, 82*(8), 1156–1164.

Bayles, M. D. (1989). *Professional ethics* (2nd ed.). Belmont, CA: Wadsworth.

Beauchamp, T. L., & Childress, J. F. (1989). *Principles of biomedical ethics* (chaps. 3, 4, 5). New York: Oxford University Press.

Beauchamp, T. L., & Walters, L. (Eds.). (1994). *Contemporary issues in bioethics* (4th ed.). Belmont, CA: Wadsworth.

Bellah, R., Madsen, R., Sullivan, W., Swindler, A., & Tipton, S. (1985). *Habits of the heart.* New York: Harper & Row.

Bellah, R., Madsen, R., Sullivan, W., Swindler, A., & Tipton, S. (1991). *The good society.* New York: Knopf.

Braden, J. (1994). *Health status and access to care of rural and urban populations.* Rockville, MD: U.S. Department of Health and Human Services.

Braveman, P. A., Schaaf, M., Egerter, S., Bennett, T., & Schecter, W. (1994, August 18). Insurance-related differences in the risk of ruptured appendix. *New England Journal of Medicine,* 444.

Burns, J., Reardon, F., & Truog, R. (1994, December 15). Using newly deceased patients to teach resuscitation procedures. *New England Journal of Medicine, 331,* 1653.

Bush v. Barham, 625 F.2d 1150 (5th Cir. 1980).

California Health and Safety Code § 199.25 (1990).

Callahan, J. C. (1988). *Ethical issues in professional life.* New York: Oxford University Press.

Capron, A. M. (1995, Spring). Practice guidelines: How good are medicine's new recipes? *Journal of Law, Medicine & Ethics, 23*(1), 47–56.

Cederblom, J., & Dougherty, C. J. (1990). *Ethics at work.* Belmont, CA: Wadsworth.

Centers for Disease Control. (1989). *Reducing the health consequences of smoking: 25 years of progress. A report of the surgeon general* (DHHS Pub. No. CDC 89-8411, pp. 597–608). Rockville, MD: U.S. Department of Health and Human Services.

Comroe, Jr., J. H., & Dripps, R. D. (1976). Scientific basis for the support of biomedical science. *Science, 192,* 105–111.

Cooper, R. A. (1994, September 7). Seeking a balanced physician workforce for the 21st century. *Journal of the American Medical Association, 272,* 680–687.

Coster, J. M. (1992). Recombinant erythropoietin, orphan product with a silver spoon. *International*

Journal of Technology Assessment in Health Care, 8(635), 644–646.

Council on Ethical and Judicial Affairs, American Medical Association. (1991). Gender disparities in clinical decision making. *Journal of the American Medical Association, 266,* 559–562.

Cruzan v. Missouri Department of Health, 497 U.S. 261 (1990).

Daubert v. Merrell Dow Pharmaceuticals, Inc., 509 U.S. 579, 113 S. Ct. 2786, 125 L. Ed. 2d 469 (1993).

Eddy, D. (1994). Rationing resources while improving quality. *Journal of the American Medical Association, 272,* 818–820.

Ethyl Corp. v. Environmental Protection Agency, 541 F.2d 1 (1976).

Field, M. A. (1990). Testing for AIDS: Uses and abuses. *American Journal of Law and Medicine, 16*(1 & 2), 33–106.

Fluss, S. S., & Zeegers, D. (1989). AIDS, HIV, and health care workers: Some international perspectives (pp. 84–87). *Maryland Law Review, 48*(1), 77–92.

Foege, W. H. (1987). Public health: Moving from debt to legacy. 1986 presidential address. *American Journal of Public Health, 77,* 1276–1277.

Fogel, L. A., & MacQuarrie, C. (1994, November). Benefits and operational concerns of rural health clinics. *Healthcare Financial Management,* 40–46.

Fox v. Health Net of California, No. 219692 (Cal. Super. Ct. Dec. 23 and 28, 1993).

Fox, R., & Swazey, J. (1992). *Spare parts, organ replacement in American society.* New York: Oxford University Press.

Garner, D. W. (1996, April 24). Banning tobacco billboards: The case for municipal action. *Journal of the American Medical Association, 275*(16), 1263–1269.

Ginzburg, H. M. (1986). Use and misuse of epidemiologic data in the courtroom: Defining the limits of inferential and particularistic evidence in mass tort litigation. *American Journal of Law & Medicine, XII*(3 & 4), 423–439.

Grad, F. P. (1978, May). Medical ethics and the law. *Annals of the American Academy of Political and Social Science, 437,* 19–36.

Grad, F. P. (1990). *The public health law manual* (2nd ed.) (pp. 67–69). Washington, DC: American Public Health Association.

Haas, J., Udvarhelyi, S., & Epstein, A. (1993). The effect of health coverage for uninsured pregnant women on maternal health and the use of cesarean section. *Journal of the American Medical Association, 270*(1), 61–64.

Hafner-Eaton, C. (1994). When the phoenix rises, where will she go? The women's health agenda. In Pauline Vaillancourt Rosenau (Ed.), *Health care reform in the nineties.* Thousand Oaks, CA: Sage.

Halpern, J. (1995, Spring). Can the development of practice guidelines safeguard patient values? *Journal of Law, Medicine and Ethics, 23*(1), 75–81.

Health Care Quality Improvement Act, 42 U.S.C. § 11101 *et seq.* (1986).

Heitman, E., & Rosenau, P. V. (1993, October). *The new gene technology: Old material in fresh guise or tracking unexplored terrain?* Presented as a paper at the American Public Health Association's Annual Meeting, San Francisco, CA.

Helms, D. (1991). *Delivering essential health care services in rural areas.* Rockville, MD: U.S. Department of Health and Human Services.

Hillman, A. (1994, August 9). Center for health policy at the University of Pennsylvania. *New York Times,* p. A11.

Hillman, A. L., Eisenberg, J. M., Pauly, M. V., et al. (1991). Avoiding bias in the conduct and reporting of cost-effectiveness research sponsored by pharmaceutical companies. *New England Journal of Medicine, 324,* 1362–1365.

Hillman, B., Olson, G., Griffith, P., Sunshine, J., Joseph, C., Kennedy, S., Nelson, W., & Bernhardt, L. (1992, October 21). Physicians' utilization and charges for outpatient diagnostic imaging in a Medicare population. *Journal of the American Medical Association, 268,* 2050–2054.

Hilts, P. J. (1994, September 24). FDA seeks disclosures by scientists: Financial interests in drugs are at issue. *New York Times,* p. 7.

Hilts, P. J. (1995, January 15). Conference is unable to agree on ethical limits of research: Psychiatric experiment helped fuel debate. *New York Times,* p. A12.

Iannone, A. P. (Ed.). (1989). *Contemporary moral controversies in business.* New York: Oxford University Press.

International Harvester Co. v. Ruckelshaus, 478 F.2d 615, 652 (D.C. Cir. 1973), quoting from Silver, L. (1980). An agency dilemma: Regulating to protect the public health in light of scientific uncertainty. In R. Roemer & G. McKray (Eds.), *Legal aspects of health policy: Issues and trends* (p. 81). Westport, CT: Greenwood Press.

Joseph, S. C. (1992). *Dragon within the gates: The once and future AIDS epidemic* (pp. 53–54). New York: Carroll & Graf.

Kane, R. L. (1995, Spring). Creating practice guidelines: The dangers of over-reliance on expert judgment, *Journal of Law, Medicine and Ethics, 23*(1), 62–64.

Kerr, P. (1992, April 5). Glossing over health care fraud. *New York Times,* p. F17.

Kolata, G. (1994, July 29). Pharmacists help drug promotions; pharmacists paid by companies to recommend their drugs. *New York Times,* pp. A1, D2.

Kollmann, G. (1997). *Social security: Recommendations of the 1994–1996 advisory council on social security* (97-81 EPW, updated January 10). Washington, DC: Congressional Research Service, The Library of Congress.

Ladimer, I., & Newman, R. W. (Eds.). (1963). *Clinical investigation in medicine: Legal, ethical and moral aspects, an anthology and bibliography.* Boston: Law-Medicine Research Institute, Boston University.

Lewis, C. E., Fein, R., & Mechanic, D. (1976). *The right to health: The problem of access to primary medical care* (pp. 141–245). New York: Wiley.

Luce, G. M. (1986). The use of peer review organizations to control medicare costs. *ALI-ABA Course Materials Journal, 10,* 111–120.

Luft, H. S. (1981). *Health maintenance organizations: Dimensions of performance.* New York: Wiley.

Maher, J. (1993). Medical education in a multilingual and multicultural world. *Medical Education, 27,* 3–5.

Marin, G., & Marin, B. V. (1991). *Research with Hispanic populations* (chap. 3). Newbury Park: Sage.

Mariner, W. K. (1994, September). Patients' rights after health care reform: Who decides what is medically necessary? *American Journal of Public Health, 84*(9), 1515–1519.

Minkler, M. (1994, November). *Intergenerational equity: Divergent perspectives.* Paper presented at the Annual Meeting of the American Public Health Association, Washington, DC.

Minkler, M., & Robertson, A. (1991, August). Generational equity and public health policy: A critique of "age/race war" thinking. *Journal of Public Health Policy, 12*(3), 324–344.

Mitchell, J., & Scott, E. (1992, October 21). Physician ownership of physical therapy services: Effects on charges, utilization, profits, and service characteristics. *Journal of the American Medical Association, 268,* 2055–2059.

New York Mental Hygiene Law art. 9, §§ 9.01–9.59 (1988 and Supp. 1995).

1994–1996 Advisory Council on Social Security. (1997). *Report of the 1994–1996 Advisory Council on Social Security:* Vol. I: *Findings and recommendations.* Washington, DC: Author.

Noble, H. B. (1995, July 3). Quality is focus for health plans. *New York Times,* pp. A1–7.

Orlandi, M. (Ed.). (1992). *Cultural competence for evaluators.* Rockville, MD: U.S. Department of Health and Human Services.

Orlowski, J. P., Kanoti, G. A., & Mehlman, J. J. (1988). The ethics of using newly dead patients for teaching and practicing intubation techniques. *New England Journal of Medicine, 319,* 439–441.

Paehlke, R., & Vaillancourt Rosenau, P. (1993). Environment/equality: Tensions in North American politics. *Policy Studies Journal, 21*(4), 672–686.

Parker, C. W. (1995, Spring). Practice guidelines and private insurers. *Journal of Law, Medicine and Ethics, 23*(1), 57–61.

Pathman, D., Konrad, T., & Ricketts, T. (1994, November 2). The National Health Service Corps experience for rural physicians in the late 1980s. *Journal of the American Medical Association, 272,* 1341.

Patriarca, P. A. (1994, December 7). A randomized controlled trial of influenza vaccine in the elderly: Scientific scrutiny and ethical responsibility. *Journal of the American Medical Association, 272,* 1701.

Pauly, M. V. (1995, Spring). Practice guidelines: Can they save money? Should they? *Journal of Law, Medicine and Ethics, 23*(1), 65–74.

Peer, R. (1997, May 14). Health care panel considers need for patient bill of rights. *New York Times,* p. A12.

Peer Review Improvement Act, 42 U.S.C. § 1320c *et seq.* (1982).

Penn Advertising of Baltimore, Inc. v. Mayor of Baltimore, 63 F. 2d 1318 (4th Cir. 1995), *aff'g* 862 F. Supp. 1402 (D. Md. 1994), *cert. denied,* 65 U.S.L.W. 3727 (Apr. 28, 1997).

Pinneke v. Preisser, 623 F.2d 546 (8th Cir. 1980).

Planned Parenthood of Southeastern Pennsylvania v. Casey, 505 U.S. 833, 112 S. Ct. 2791 (1992).

President's Commission for the Study of Ethical Problems in Medicine and Biomedical and Behavioral Research, Alexander M. Capron, Executive Director. (1983). *Securing access to health care: The ethical implications of differences in the availability of health services* (Vol. 3, Appendices). Washington, DC: Author.

Price, S. J. (1980). Health systems agencies and peer review organizations: Experiments in regulating the delivery of health care. In R. Roemer & G. McKray (Eds.), *Legal aspects of health policy* (pp. 359–385; see pp. 380ff). Westport, CT: Greenwood.

Rafuse, J. (1993). Multicultural medicine. *Canadian Medical Association Journal, 148,* 282–284.

The Responsive Communitarian Platform. (1991/1992, Winter). Rights and responsibilities: A platform. *The Responsive Community, 4*–20.

Roe v. Wade, 410 U.S. 113 (1973).

Roels, L., Vanrenterghem, Y., Waer, M., et al. (1991). Three years of experience with a "presumed consent" legislation in Belgium: Its impact on multiorgan donation in comparison with other European countries. *Transplantation Procedures, 23,* 903–904.

Roemer, M. I. (1977). Primary care and physician extenders in affluent countries. *International Journal of Health Services, 7*(4), 545–555.

Roemer, M. I. (1991). *National health systems of the world, volume one—The countries* (pp. 33–80). New York: Oxford University Press.

Roemer, R. (1993). *Legislative action to combat the world tobacco epidemic* (2nd ed.) (pp. 117–126). Geneva: World Health Organization.

Rosenbaum, S. (1992). Mothers and children last: The Oregon Medicaid experiment. *American Journal of Law and Medicine, XVIII*(1 & 2), 97–126.

Rosenthal, E. (1993, January 27). Confusion and error are rife in hospital billing practices. *New York Times,* p. C16.

Sack, K. (1995, August 20). Public hospitals around country cut basic service. *New York Times,* p. A1.

Scitovsky, A. A. (1988). Medical care in the last twelve months of life: The relation between age, functional status, and medical care expenditures. *The Milbank Quarterly, 66*(4), 640–660.

Sekscenski, E., Sansom, S., Bazell, C., Salmon, M., & Mullan, F. (1994, November 10). State practice environments and the supply of physician assistants, nurse practitioners, and certified nurse-midwives. *New England Journal of Medicine,* 1266.

Silver, L. (1980). An agency dilemma: Regulating to protect the public health in light of scientific uncertainty. In R. Roemer & G. McKray (Eds.), *Legal aspects of health policy: Issues and trends* (pp. 60–93). Westport, CT: Greenwood Press.

Smothers, R. (1942, September 16). 150 miles away, the doctor is examining your tonsils. *New York Times,* p. C14.

Special Committee to Study Commitment Procedures of the Association of the Bar of the City of New York in cooperation with Cornell Law School. (1962). *Mental illness and due process, report and recommendations on admission to mental hospitals under New York law.* Ithaca, NY: Cornell University Press.

Tarasoff v. Regents of the University of California, 17 Cal. 3d 425, 551 P.2d 334, 131 Cal. Rptr. 14 (1976).

Temkin-Greener, H., Meiners, M. S., Petty, E. A., & Szydlowski, J. S. (1992). The use and cost of health services prior to death: A comparison of the Medicare-only and the Medicare-Medicaid elderly populations. *The Milbank Quarterly, 70*(4), 679–701.

U.S. Congress, Office of Technology Assessment. (1993, October). *Impact of legal reform on medical malpractice costs* (OTA-BP-H-19). Washington, DC: U.S. Government Printing Office.

U.S. General Accounting Office. (1991, June). *Canadian health insurance* (BAP/HRD-91-90, p. 16). Washington DC: Author. Also available on the Internet (info@www.gao.gov).

U.S. General Accounting Office. (1993, March 8). *Health insurance: Remedies Needed to reduce losses from fraud and abuse—Testimony* (GAO/T-HRD-9308). Washington, DC: Author.

U.S. General Accounting Office. (1993, April). *Organ transplants: Increased effort needed to boost supply and ensure equitable distribution of organs* (GAO/HRD-93-56). Washington, DC: Author. Also available on the Internet (info@www.gao.gov).

U.S. General Accounting Office. (1994, December). *Health care: School-based health centers can expand access for children* (GAO/HEHS-95-35). Washington, DC: Author. Also available on the Internet (info@www.gao.gov).

U.S. General Accounting Office. (1994, October). *Medicare: Referrals to physician-owned imaging facilities warrant HCFA's scrutiny* (GAO/HEHS-95-2). Washington, DC: Author.

U.S. Public Health Service, Women's Health. (1985). *Report of the Public Health Service Task Force on Women's Health Issues.* Washington, DC: U.S. Department of Health and Human Services.

U.S.C.A., vol. 42, §§ 289, 289a-1-6 (1995), C.F.R., vol. 21, pt. 56 (1995).

Wagner, J. (Ed). (1992). *International Journal of Technology Assessment in Health Care on Orphan Technologies, 8*(4) (special issue, entire issue).

Weissman, J. S., & Epstein, A. M. (1994). *Falling through the safety net: Insurance status and access to health care.* Baltimore: Johns Hopkins University Press.

Whalen v. Roe, 429 U.S. 589 (1977).

Wheeler, S. V. (1994, Fall). TeleMedicine. *BioPhotonics,* 34–40.

Winslow, R. (1994, October 28). Accreditation group to publish reports on performance of health providers. *Wall Street Journal,* p. B7A.

Winslow, R. (1994, September 8). Drug company's PR firm made offer to pay for editorial, professor says. *Wall Street Journal,* p. B12.

Wolfe, L. (1991, November 27). From the congressional office of technology assessment: The national service corps: Improving on past experience. *Journal of the American Medical Association,* 2808.

World Health Organization (1993). *WHO consultation on testing and counseling for HIV infection* (WHO/GPA/NF/93.2). Geneva: Global Programme on AIDS, World Health Organization.

INDEX

A

Abbott Laboratories, 388

Abbreviated New Drug Application, 395

Abortion:
   services, 502–503
   trends, U.S., 65–66t

Academic detailing, 480

Academic medical centers (AMCs), 278–279

Access to health care, 88, 475
   behavioral model of health services use, 88–91
   examples of key measures, 95–97t, 97–98
   future indicators and needed research, 107–108
   policy purposes of, 93f, 93–95
   trends in, 99t, 99–107
   types of, 91f, 91–93

Access to Personal Health Care Services, Committee on Monitoring, 94, 106–107

Accreditation Manual for Hospitals, 292

Acquired immune deficiency syndrome (AIDS), 9, 47–48, 502
   mortality rates, 78, 81t

Act for the Relief of Sick and Disabled Seamen, 448

Action for Mental Health Report, 357

Active medical staff, 290

Activities of daily living (ADL), 300, 316

Act Relative to Quarantine, 449

Acute inpatient care, 307

Aday, L.A., 92

Adult day care, 326–328

Adverse selection, 120

Advisory Commission on Consumer Protection and Quality in the Health Care Industry, 498

Advisory Council on Social Security, 496

Affective disorder, 364

African Americans:
   psychiatric disorder rates of diagnosis, 351, 354
   uninsured, 105, 147

Aged, 303–304f

Agency for Health Care Policy and Research, 104, 342

Aid to Families with Dependent Children (AFDC), 128, 496

Alaska, 251

Alcohol abuse, 82–83, 361

Alford, R.R., 447

Allied professionals, 371–372

Almshouses, 260–261, 450

Alternative therapy, 52–53

Alzheimer's disease, 301–302

Ambulatory health care, 228, 307–308
   government programs, 249–250
   history of, 228–230
   institutional services
      emergency services, 249
      outpatient clinics, 247–248
      surgery centers, 248–249
   levels of services, 230–231
   and managed care, 253–254
   for mental disorders, 364–366
   noninstitutional and public health services, 251
   organization of systems, 251–253
   practice settings, 237
      group, 239–247
      solo, 238–239
   use of office setting services, 234–238t
   use of services, 231–233t, 231–234

American Hospital Association, 120, 266

American Medical Association (AMA), 61, 120–121, 145, 175, 211, 241, 265, 450, 452
   Directory of Practice Parameters, 477

American Psychiatric Association, 352, 356, 368

American Psychological Association, 369

American Public Health Association, 219

Americans with Disabilities Act, 343, 359

Angina, 45

Annas, G.J., 494

Antibiotics, 8, 12, 263

Antisepsis, 262–263

Antisocial disorder, 365

Anxiety disorders, 364

APA Task Force Interagency Council, 361

Area Health Education Centers, 414–415

Asians, access to care, 106

Assessment, 214

Assisted living, 328

Associate medical staff, 290

Assurance, 214

Atherosclerosis, 45–46

Autonomy, 492

B

Balanced Budget Act, 339, 462–463

Base/major medical plans, 192

Basic insurance plans, 121–122

Baylor Hospital (Dallas), 173

Beecham Laboratories, 388

Behaviorism, 353–354

Bellevue Hospital, 4, 11

Benchmarking, 471–472

Biopsychosocial model, 354

Biotechnology, 389

Bipolar disorders, 364

Blind and visually impaired, 305

Block grants, 216, 454–455, 496

Blue Cross/Blue Shield, 16, 21, 120–121, 173, 176, 178–180, 266

Brizius, J.A., 443

Brokers, 153

Brook, Robert H., 104

Bureau of Labor Statistics, 192–193, 197

Bush, George, 145–146, 358